# Handbook of Children and Screens

Dimitri A. Christakis • Lauren Hale
Editors

# Handbook of Children and Screens

## Digital Media, Development, and Well-Being from Birth Through Adolescence

Springer

*Editors*
Dimitri A. Christakis
Seattle Children's Research Institute
University of Washington
Seattle, WA, USA

Lauren Hale
School of Medicine
Stony Brook University
Stony Brook, NY, USA

ISBN 978-3-031-69361-8    ISBN 978-3-031-69362-5 (eBook)
https://doi.org/10.1007/978-3-031-69362-5



This Springer imprint is published by the registered company Springer Nature Switzerland AG
The registered company address is: Gewerbestrasse 11, 6330 Cham, Switzerland

*To helping children lead healthy lives in a digital world*

# Foreword

As the Executive Director of Children and Screens: Institute of Digital Media and Child Development, it is with both pride and enthusiasm that I introduce this groundbreaking publication. Representing the expertise of nearly 400 leading scholars and practitioners, the handbook provides a unique synthesis of the intricate interplay between screen use and the health, development, and well-being of children and adolescents.

## Why a "Handbook?"

In 2017, Children and Screens produced a supplement to the journal *Pediatrics* on "Children, Adolescents, and Screens," which included 22 papers and 130 authors. Since that time, the domain of children and media has transformed—including the arrival of game-changing platforms as ubiquitous as TikTok, the introduction of novel media formats such as virtual reality, and groundbreaking technologies that have captured everyone's attention like generative artificial intelligence. With each advancement, we're faced with new and familiar opportunities and challenges. Each day, new reports document the potential risks posed by social media platforms and the complicity of their providers, which have fueled a global conversation about the urgent need to ensure that digital landscapes are being designed with children's basic rights and needs in mind. Parents and youth alike are joining these conversations, demanding better systems and support as they grapple with the challenge of enjoying the digital world's benefits while dodging its harms.

These seismic shifts and public concerns have amplified the enduring commitment of Children and Screens to help children lead healthy lives in a digital world. The result is this handbook, a comprehensive reflection and integration of the field itself, that brings together the scientific and clinical communities to answer progressively more complicated questions and to include more diverse voices, perspectives, and disciplines. This approach reflects Children and Screens' commitment to foster interdisciplinary collaboration in all of our work, founded on a belief that a kaleidoscopic view is necessary to achieve a true understanding of the complexities of digital media's impact on our youngest generation. It is our sincere hope that the reach and impact of this handbook will be significantly enhanced by the spirit of interdisciplinarity in which it was created.

We must remain steadfast in our commitment to foster a balanced approach to digital media that maximizes the benefits and mitigates the risks for children. I am confident that this comprehensive, open-access handbook will serve as an invaluable resource for researchers, practitioners, policymakers, educators, and caregivers alike, empowering us all to promote the optimal well-being of our children in the digital age.

## Appreciations

We extend our thanks to the many contributors who helped bring the handbook to fruition:

- Editors Drs. Dimitri A. Christakis and Lauren Hale, for their leadership and direction.
- The many section leaders, authors, collaborators, and reviewers, whose expertise shaped this publication.
- The researchers whose work is summarized herein, and who devote their time and energy year after year to the ongoing work of advancing our knowledge with objective science.
- Kate Blocker, Camara Brown, and Melinda Karth, members of Children and Screens' research team who carefully shepherded this project through every phase.
- Children and Screens' National Scientific Advisory Board and Board of Directors for their stalwart leadership and support.
- Children and Screens' individual donors, whose contributions enabled the full funding of this handbook in Open Access, ensuring accessibility for all at no cost.
- Our founder and Board Chair, Dr. Pamela Hurst-Della Pietra, for her leadership in conceiving, planning, and organizing this publication, and for soliciting and securing its section leaders and many of its authors.

Lastly, we extend our gratitude to every scholar, clinician, teacher, parent, policymaker, governmental organization, and media industry executive who takes a moment to read this and share it with others. We hope that this deep dive into the evidence will spark new, strategic discussions and action on the topic of children and media on a national scale. Together, we can use this handbook to construct a shared analytical, diagnostic, and educational toolkit to tackle the effects of media on children. By fostering collaboration, judiciously allocating resources, and harnessing the knowledge and research presented in this handbook, we can translate these efforts into effective interventions, pragmatic guidelines, and policies and practices grounded in data.

Children and Screens: Institute of Digital Media and Child Development — Kris Perry

# Acknowledgements

This Open Access handbook was made possible by the generous individual donors of Children and Screens: Institute of Digital Media and Child Development. The information, content, and conclusions are those of the author(s) and should not be construed as the official position or policy of, nor should any endorsements be inferred by, Children and Screens or its donors.

## Contents

---

The original version of the book has been revised. A correction to this book can be found at https://doi.org/10.1007/978-3-031-69362-5_88

# Editors and Contributors

## About the Editors

**Dimitri A. Christakis, MD MPH** is the George Adkins Professor of Pediatrics at the University of Washington, the Chief Health Officer at Special Olympics International, Editor in Chief of *JAMA Pediatrics*, and Chief Science Officer at Children and Screens: Institute of Digital Media and Child Development. He has devoted his career to investigating how early experiences impact children and to helping parents improve their children's early learning environments. He and his colleagues in the Christakis Lab have made a number of landmark findings, including discovering that young children who watch TV are more likely to develop attention problems and other health and behavioral issues. He is the author of more than 250 original research articles, a textbook on pediatrics, and co-author of the book, *The Elephant in the Living Room: Make Television Work for Your Kids*. He has appeared on CNN, NPR, Today, CBS News, ABC News, and NBC News and was featured as a TEDx speaker.

Dr. Christakis began serving as an expert witness in social media litigation in September 2023.

**Lauren Hale, PhD** is a Professor of Family, Population, and Preventive Medicine in the Program in Public Health at Stony Brook University's Renaissance School of Medicine. She studies the social patterning of sleep health and how it contributes to inequalities in health and well-being with current or previous funding from NICHD, NIDDK, NHLBI, NIA, and the Della Pietra Family Foundation. Dr. Hale is interested in sleep health equity, policies related to sleep health (i.e., high school start time, daylight saving time), and behavioral modifications (i.e., reducing evening screen use, increasing physical activity) for improving sleep health at the individual and population level. Dr. Hale has over 175 peer-reviewed journal articles. Dr. Hale recently served on the National Sleep Foundation's Board of Directors (including as Chair and Vice Chair) and is the founding Editor-in-Chief of the journal *Sleep Health*. She also serves on the Scientific Advisory Panes of the Pajama Program and Children and Screens: Institute of Digital Media and Child Development.

## Contributors

**Stephen J. Aguilar** Rossier School of Education, University of Southern California, Los Angeles, CA, USA

**Teki Akuetteh** Africa Digital Rights Hub, Accra, Ghana

**Fashina Aladé** Michigan State University, East Lansing, MI, USA

**Alyssa M. Alcorn** University of Edinburgh, Edinburgh, UK

**Jon-Patrick Allem** Rutgers School of Public Health, The State University of New Jersey, New Brunswick, NJ, USA

**Meryl Alper** Northeastern University, Boston, MA, USA

**Rachel Anderson** University of Kentucky, Lexington, KY, USA

**Nkemka Anyiwo** Columbia University, School of Social Work, New York, NY, USA

**Paola Araiza-Alba** Swinburne University of Technology, Melbourne, VIC, Australia

Liminal VR, Melbourne, VIC, Australia

**Merlin Ariefdjohan** Department of Psychiatry, University of Colorado Anschutz Medical Campus, Aurora, CO, USA

**Sumreen Asim** Indiana University Southeast, New Albany, IN, USA

**Randy P. Auerbach** Department of Psychiatry, Columbia University, New York, NY, USA

Division of Child and Adolescent Psychiatry, New York State Psychiatric Institute, New York, NY, USA

**Karla Badillo-Urquiola** University of Notre Dame, Notre Dame, IN, USA

**Isabel Baenas** Clinical Psychology Department, Bellvitge University Hospital-IDIBELL, Barcelona, Spain

Ciber Physiopathology of Obesity and Nutrition (CIBERObn), Instituto de Salud Carlos III, Madrid, Spain

Psychoneurobiology of Eating and Addictive Behaviors Group, Neuroscience Program, Bellvitge Biomedical Research Institute (IDIBELL), L'Hospitalet de Llobregat, Barcelona, Spain

**Jakki O. Bailey** University of Texas at Austin, Austin, TX, USA

**Rachel Barr** Department of Psychology, Georgetown University, Washington, DC, USA

**Ran Barzilay** Department of Psychiatry, University of Pennsylvania, Philadelphia, PA, USA

Department of Child and Adolescent Psychiatry and Behavioral Science, Children's Hospital of Philadelphia, Philadelphia, PA, USA

Lifespan Brain Institute of CHOP and Penn Medicine, Philadelphia, PA, USA

**Susanne E. Baumgartner** University of Amsterdam, Amsterdam, The Netherlands

**Daphné Bavelier** University of Geneva, Geneva, Switzerland

**Oliver W. J. Beer** The University of Plymouth, Plymouth, UK

**Mesfin A. Bekalu** Department of Social and Behavioral Sciences, Harvard T. H. Chan School of Public Health, Boston, MA, USA

**Ine Beyens** University of Amsterdam, Amsterdam, The Netherlands

**David S. Bickham** Boston Children's Hospital, Boston, MA, USA

**Stuart J. H. Biddle** Centre for Health Research, University of Southern Queensland, Springfield Central, QLD, Australia

Faculty of Sport & Health Sciences, University of Jyväskylä, Jyväskylä, Finland

**Candice Biernesser** University of Pittsburgh, Pittsburgh, PA, USA

**Joël Billieux** Institute of Psychology, University of Lausanne, Lausanne, Switzerland

Center for Excessive Gambling, Addiction Medicine, Lausanne University Hospitals (CHUV), Lausanne, Switzerland

**Ashley Blanchard** Department of Emergency Medicine, Columbia University Irving Medical Center, New York, NY, USA

**Elroy Boers** University of Montreal, Montreal, QC, Canada

**Bradley J. Bond** University of San Diego, San Diego, CA, USA

**Matthias Brand** General Psychology: Cognition and Center for Behavioral Addiction Research (CeBAR), University of Duisburg-Essen, Duisburg, Germany

Erwin L. Hahn Institute for Magnetic Resonance Imaging, Essen, Germany

**Joel Breakstone** Stanford University, Stanford, CA, USA

**Rosanna Breaux** Virginia Tech, Blacksburg, VA, USA

**André Brock** Georgia Tech, Atlanta, GA, USA

**Lionel Brossi** University of Chile, Millennium Nucleus for Improving the Mental Health of Adolescents and Youth, Santiago, Chile

**Dillon T. Browne** University of Waterloo, Waterloo, ON, Canada

**Matthew Bui** University of Michigan, Ann Arbor, MI, USA

**Julius Burkauskas** Lithuanian University of Health Sciences Neuroscience Institute, Kaunas, Lithuania

**Kaitlyn Burnell** The University of North Carolina at Chapel Hill, Chapel Hill, NC, USA

**Brad J. Bushman** School of Communication, The Ohio State University, Columbus, OH, USA

**Alyssa M. Button** Pennington Biomedical Research Center, Baton Rouge, LA, USA

**Angela Calvin** Department of Pediatrics, University of Wisconsin-Madison, Madison, WI, USA

**Natale Canale** Department of Developmental and Social Psychology, University of Padova, Padova, Italy

**Xavier Carbonell** Ramon Llull University, Department of Psychology, Barcelona, Spain

**Valerie Carson** Faculty of Kinesiology, Sport, and Recreation, University of Alberta, Edmonton, AB, Canada

**Justine Cassell** Carnegie Mellon University, Pittsburgh, PA, USA

PRAIRIE Paris Artificial Intelligence Research Institute and INRIA Paris, Paris, France

**Jesús Castro-Calvo** Department of Personality, Assessment, and Psychological Treatments, University of Valencia-Estudi General, Valencia, Spain

**Kenrick Cato** University of Pennsylvania School of Nursing, University of Pennsylvania, Philadelphia, PA, USA

Children's Hospital of Philadelphia, University of Pennsylvania, Philadelphia, PA, USA

**Bhaskar Chakravorti** The Fletcher School, Tufts University, Medford, MA, USA

**Linda Charmaraman** Wellesley Centers for Women, Wellesley College, Wellesley, MA, USA

**Jeffrey Chester** Center for Digital Democracy, American University, Washington, DC, USA

**Mai J. M. Chinapaw** Public and Occupational Health, Amsterdam Centre UMC, Vrije Universiteit, Amsterdam Public Health, Amsterdam, The Netherlands

**Koeun Choi** Virginia Polytechnic Institute and State University, Blacksburg, VA, USA

**Sophia Choukas-Bradley** Department of Psychology, University of Pittsburgh, Pittsburgh, PA, USA

**Dimitri A. Christakis** Seattle Children's Research Institute, Seattle, WA, USA

University of Washington, Seattle, WA, USA

Special Olympics, Washington, DC, USA

Children and Screens: Institute of Digital Media and Child Development, Jericho, NY, USA

**Drew P. Cingel** University of California Davis, Davis, CA, USA

**Elizabeth M. Clancy** School of Psychology, Deakin University, Geelong, VIC, Australia

**Lynn Schofield Clark** University of Denver, Denver, CO, USA

**Cristóbal Cobo** World Bank, Washington, DC, USA

**Courtney D. Cogburn** Columbia University, New York, NY, USA

**Anne Collier** The Net Safety Collaborative, Salt Lake City, UT, USA

**Ornella Corazza** Department of Psychology and Cognitive Science, University of Trento, Trento, Italy

University of Hertfordshire, Hatfield, UK

**Shelia R. Cotten** Clemson University, Clemson, SC, USA

**Dorothy Cowie** Durham University, Durham, UK

**Claire Coyne** Ann & Robert H. Lurie Children's Hospital of Chicago, Chicago, IL, USA

**Sarah M. Coyne** School of Family Life, Brigham Young University, Provo, UT, USA

**Wendy Craig** Queen's University, Kingston, ON, Canada

**Charles A. Czeisler** Departments of Medicine and Neurology, Division of Sleep and Circadian Disorders, Brigham and Women's Hospital, Boston, MA, USA

Division of Sleep Medicine, Harvard Medical School, Boston, MA, USA

**Judith H. Danovitch** Department of Psychological and Brain Sciences, University of Louisville, Louisville, KY, USA

**Jennifer Suzzane Darling-Aduana** Georgia State University, Atlanta, GA, USA

**Katie Davis** Information School, University of Washington, Seattle, WA, USA

**Emma Day** Tech Legality, Lisbon, Portugal

**Paul H. Delfabbro** School of Psychology, The University of Adelaide, Adelaide, SA, Australia

**Zsolt Demetrovics** Institute of Psychology, ELTE Eötvös Loránd University, Budapest, Hungary

Centre of Excellence in Responsible Gaming, University of Gibraltar, Europa Point, Gibraltar

College of Education, Psychology and Social Work, Flinders University, Adelaide, SA, Australia

**Jeffrey Derevensky** International Centre for Youth Gambling Problems and High Risk Behaviors, McGill University, Montreal, QC, Canada

**Jayson L. Dibble** Hope College, Holland, MI, USA

**Karen E. Dill-Shackleford** Fielding Graduate University, Santa Barbara, CA, USA

**Matías Dodel** Universidad Católica del Uruguay, Montevideo, Uruguay

**Sarah E. Domoff** Department of Psychology, University at Albany, State University of New York, Albany, NY, USA

**Rebecca A. Dore** The Ohio State University, Columbus, OH, USA

**Nicola Döring** Technische Universität Ilmenau, Thuringia, Germany

**Jennifer L. Doty** University of Oregon, Eugene, OR, USA

**Sarah Dryden-Peterson** Harvard University, Cambridge, MA, USA

**Adam K. Dubé** McGill University, Montreal, QC, Canada

**Bernadka Dubicka** Health Sciences, Hull & York Medical School, University of York, York, UK

Greater Manchester Mental Health Trust, Manchester, UK

Manchester Academic Health Science Centre (MAHSC), University of Manchester, Manchester, UK

**Dorothea Dumuid** Alliance for Research in Exercise, Nutrition and Activity, University of South Australia, Adelaide, SA, Australia

**Meenakshi Gigi Durham** School of Journalism and Mass Communication and Department of Gender, Women's and Sexuality Studies, University of Iowa, Iowa City, IA, USA

**Bobbie Eisenstock** California State University Northridge, Los Angeles, CA, USA

**Jon D. Elhai** Department of Psychology, University of Toledo, Toledo, OH, USA

Department of Psychiatry, University of Toledo, Toledo, OH, USA

**Nicole Ellison** University of Michigan, Ann Arbor, MI, USA

**Jennifer A. Emond** Geisel School of Medicine, Dartmouth College, Hanover, NH, USA

**Elizabeth Englander** Bridgewater State University, Bridgewater, MA, USA

**Devin English** Rutgers University, Newark, NJ, USA

**Rob Eschmann** Columbia University, School of Social Work, New York, NY, USA

**César Escobar-Viera** Department of Psychiatry, University of Pittsburgh School of Medicine, Pittsburgh, PA, USA

**Dorothy L. Espelage** The University of North Carolina at Chapel Hill, Chapel Hill, NC, USA

**Hannah Espeleta** Medical University of South Carolina, Charleston, SC, USA

**Rys Farthing** Centre for the Digital Child, Deakin University, Geelong, VIC, Australia

**Fernando Fernández-Aranda** Clinical Psychology Unit, University Hospital of Bellvitge-IDIBELL, Hospitalet del Llobregat, Barcelona, Spain

CIBER Fisiopatologia Obesidad y Nutrición, (CIBERobn), Hospitalet del Llobregat, Barcelona, Spain

Ciber Physiopathology of Obesity and Nutrition (CIBERObn), Instituto de Salud Carlos III, Madrid, Spain

Department of Clinical Sciences, School of Medicine, University of Barcelona, Hospitalet del Llobregat, Barcelona, Spain

Psychoneurobiology of Eating and Addictive Behaviors Group, Neuroscience Program, Bellvitge Biomedical Research Institute (IDIBELL), L'Hospitalet de Llobregat, Barcelona, Spain

**Prema Fillipone** New York University, New York, NY, USA

**Naomi A. Fineberg** School of Life and Medical Sciences, University of Hertfordshire, Hatfield, UK

**Maèva Flayelle** Institute of Psychology, University of Lausanne, Lausanne, Switzerland

**Frances Fleming-Milici** Rudd Center for Food Policy & Health, University of Connecticut, Storrs, CT, USA

**Arturo Franco** World Bank, Washington, DC, USA

**Sandra Fritsch** Department of Psychiatry, University of Colorado Anschutz Medical Campus, Aurora, CO, USA

Pediatric Mental Health Institute, Children's Hospital Colorado, Aurora, CO, USA

**Carter J. Funkhouser** Department of Psychiatry, Columbia University, New York, NY, USA

Division of Child and Adolescent Psychiatry, New York State Psychiatric Institute, New York, NY, USA

**Alessandro Gabbiadini** Mind and Behavior Technological Center, Department of Psychology, University of Milano-Bicocca, Milan, Italy

**Joy Gabrielli** University of Florida, Gainesville, FL, USA

**Sally M. Gainsbury** The University of Sydney, School of Psychology, Brain & Mind Centre, Gambling Treatment & Research Clinic, Sydney, NSW, Australia

**Christina R. Galanis** College of Education, Psychology & Social Work, Flinders University, Adelaide, SA, Australia

**Manuel Gámez-Guadix** Autonomous University of Madrid, Madrid, Spain

**Meredith Gansner** Department of Psychiatry, Boston Children's Hospital, Boston, MA, USA

**Antero Garcia** Stanford University, Stanford, CA, USA

**Michelle M. Garrison** Department of Public Health, Purdue University, West Lafayette, IN, USA

**Ashley N. Gearhardt** Department of Psychology, University of Michigan, Ann Arbor, MI, USA

**Susan A. Gelman** University of Michigan, Ann Arbor, MI, USA

**Douglas A. Gentile** Iowa State University, Ames, IA, USA

**Madeleine J. George** RTI International, Durham, NC, USA

**Gary W. Giumetti** Quinnipiac University, Hamden, CT, USA

**Biljana Gjoneska** Macedonian Academy of Sciences and Arts, Skopje, North Macedonia

**Tracy R. Gleason** Wellesley College, Wellesley, MA, USA

**Gary S. Goldfield** Healthy Active Living and Obesity Research Group, Children's Hospital of Eastern Ontario Research Institute, Ottawa, ON, Canada

**Thalia R. Goldstein** George Mason University, Fairfax, VA, USA

**Josh Golin** Fairplay, Boston, MA, USA

**Roberta Michnick Golinkoff** University of Delaware, Newark, DE, USA

**Jacob D. Gordon** Institute for Sexual and Gender Minority Health and Wellbeing, Northwestern University, Chicago, IL, USA

**Richard Graham** Good Thinking: The London Digital Mental Wellbeing Service, London, UK

**Michael A. Grandner** Department of Psychiatry, University of Arizona, Tucson, AZ, USA

**Don Grant** Center for Research and Innovation, Newport Healthcare, Sherman Oaks, CA, USA

Center for Research and Innovation, Newport Healthcare, Newport, RI, USA

Center for Research and Innovation, Newport Healthcare, Nashville, TN, USA

**Kishonna L. Gray** University of Kentucky, Lexington, KY, USA

**David Greenfield** The Center for Internet and Technology Addiction, West Hartford, CT, USA

**Christine Greenhow** Michigan State University, East Lansing, MI, USA

**Tobias Greitemeyer** Department of Psychology, University of Innsbruck, Innsbruck, Austria

**Sonya Grier** Kogod School of Business, American University, Washington, DC, USA

**Mark D. Griffiths** International Gaming Research Unit, Psychology Department, Nottingham Trent University, Nottingham, UK

**Lisa Guernsey** New America, Washington, DC, USA

**Michelle Schira Hagerman** University of Ottawa, Ottawa, ON, Canada

**Lauren Hale** Program in Public Health, Department of Family, Population, and Preventive Medicine, Renaissance School of Medicine, Stony Brook University, Stony Brook, NY, USA

**Jessica L. Hamilton** Rutgers University, New Brunswick, NJ, USA

**Rochelle F. Hanson** Medical University of South Carolina, Charleston, SC, USA

**Jennifer L. Harris** Rudd Center for Food Policy & Health, University of Connecticut, Storrs, CT, USA

**Kristen Harrison** University of North Carolina at Chapel Hill, Chapel Hill, NC, USA

**Heidi Hartikainen** University of Oulu, Oulu, Finland

**Lauren E. Hartstein** Department of Integrative Physiology, University of Colorado Boulder, Boulder, CO, USA

**Brenna Hassinger-Das** Pace University, New York, NY, USA

**Marie K. Heath** Loyola University Maryland, Baltimore, MD, USA

**Paul Heider** Medical University of South Carolina, Charleston, SC, USA

**Carolyn Heinrich** Vanderbilt University, Nashville, TN, USA

**Debby Herbenick** Department of Applied Health Science, Indiana University, Bloomington, IN, USA

**J. Maya Hernandez** Social Ecology, University of California, Irvine, Irvine, CA, USA

**Troy Hicks** Central Michigan University, Mount Pleasant, MI, USA

**Velislava Hillman** London School of Economics and Political Science, London, UK

**Kathy Hirsh-Pasek** Temple University, Philadelphia, PA, USA

**Jun Sung Hong** Wayne State University, Detroit, MI, USA
Ewha Womans University, Seoul, South Korea

**Wendy Yajun Huang** Department of Sport, Physical Education and Health, Hong Kong Baptist University, Kowloon Tong, Hong Kong, China

**Nicholas C. Jacobson** Center for Technology and Behavioral Health, Dartmouth College, Lebanon, NH, USA

**Carrie James** Harvard Graduate School of Education, Cambridge, MA, USA

**Hannah Javidi** Department of Applied Health Science, Indiana University School of Public Health-Bloomington, Bloomington, IN, USA

**Nancy Jennings** University of Cincinnati, Cincinnati, OH, USA

**Michaeline Jensen** University of North Carolina-Greensboro, Greensboro, NC, USA

**Susana Jiménez-Murcia** Clinical Psychology Unit, University Hospital of Bellvitge-IDIBELL, Hospitalet del Llobregat, Barcelona, Spain

CIBER Fisiopatologia Obesidad y Nutrición, (CIBERobn), Hospitalet del Llobregat, Barcelona, Spain

Ciber Physiopathology of Obesity and Nutrition (CIBERObn), Instituto de Salud Carlos III, Madrid, Spain

Department of Clinical Sciences, School of Medicine, University of Barcelona, Hospitalet del Llobregat, Barcelona, Spain

Psychoneurobiology of Eating and Addictive Behaviors Group, Neuroscience Program, Bellvitge Biomedical Research Institute (IDIBELL), L'Hospitalet de Llobregat, Barcelona, Spain

**Mengguo Jing** Boston College, Boston, MA, USA

**Samantha-Kaye Johnston** University of Oxford and Berkman Klein Centre for Internet and Society, Cambridge, MA, USA

**Tessa Jolls** Center for Media Literacy, Santa Monica, CA, USA

**Anya Kamenetz** Aspen Institute, Aspen, CO, USA

**Takayuki Kanda** Kyoto University, Kyoto, Japan

**Peter T. Katzmarzyk** Pennington Biomedical Research Center, Baton Rouge, LA, USA

**Jordy Kaufman** Swinburne University of Technology, Melbourne, VIC, Australia

**Therese Keane** La Trobe University, Melbourne, VIC, Australia

**Eunjoo Kim** Yonsei University College of Medicine, Seoul, South Korea

**Royce Kimmons** Brigham Young University, Provo, UT, USA

**Daniel L. King** Flinders University, College of Education, Psychology, & Social Work, Adelaide, SA, Australia

College of Education, Psychology & Social Work, Flinders University, Adelaide, SA, Australia

**Orsolya Király** Institute of Psychology, ELTE Eötvös Loránd University, Budapest, Hungary

ELTE Eötvös Loránd University, Budapest, Hungary

Institute of Psychology, ELTE Eötvös Loránd University, Budapest, Hungary

**Heather Kirkorian** University of Wisconsin-Madison, Madison, WI, USA

**Bianca Klettke** School of Psychology, Deakin University, Geelong, VIC, Australia

**Neta Kligler-Vilenchik** Hebrew University of Jerusalem, Jerusalem, Israel

**Eric Klopfer** Massachusetts Institute of Technology, Cambridge, MA, USA

**Ina Koning** Faculty of Behavioural and Movement Sciences, Clinical Child and Family Studies, Vrije Universiteit Amsterdam, Amsterdam, Netherlands

**Sara Konrath** Indiana University, Bloomington, IN, USA

University of Michigan, Ann Arbor, MI, USA

**Mariah Kornbluh** University of Oregon, Eugene, OR, USA

**Robin M. Kowalski** Clemson University, Clemson, SC, USA

**Colleen Kraft** Children's Hospital of Los Angeles, Los Angeles, CA, USA

**Barbara Krahé** Department of Psychology, University of Potsdam, Potsdam, Germany

**Shane W. Kraus** School of Psychology, Brain and Mind Centre, Science Faculty, University of Sydney, Sydney, NSW, Australia

**Daniel G. Krutka** University of North Texas, Denton, TX, USA

**Kaylee P. Kruzan** Northwestern University, Evanston, IL, USA

Northwestern University, Chicago, IL, USA

**Natalia Kucirkova** University of Stavanger, Stavanger, Norway

**Randy Kulman** LearningWorks for Kids, Wakefield, RI, USA

**Priya C. Kumar** Pennsylvania State University, State College, PA, USA

**Nicholas Kuzik** Children's Hospital of Eastern Ontario Research Institute, Ottawa, ON, Canada

**Rina Lai** University of Cambridge, Cambridge, UK

**Aviv Y. Landau** School of Social Policy & Practice, University of Pennsylvania, Philadelphia, PA, USA

**Elizabeth Langran** Marymount University, Arlington, VA, USA

**Monique K. LeBourgeois** Department of Integrative Physiology, University of Colorado Boulder, Boulder, CO, USA

**Ashley Lee** Harvard University, Cambridge, MA, USA

**Young-eun Lee** Massachusetts Institute of Technology, Cambridge, MA, USA

**Reg Leichty** Foresight Law + Policy, Washington, DC, USA

**Leslie Lenert** Medical University of South Carolina, Charleston, SC, USA

**Koen Leurs** Department of Media and Culture Studies, Utrecht University, Utrecht, Netherlands

**Eva Lievens** Ghent University, Ghent, Belgium

**Chung-Ying Lin** Institute of Allied Health Sciences, College of Medicine, National Cheng Kung University, Tainan, Taiwan

**Lisa Linder** Department of Child and Family Development, San Diego State University, San Diego, CA, USA

**Sonia Livingstone** The London School of Economics, London, UK

**Jiang Long** Shanghai Mental Health Center, Shanghai Jiao Tong University School of Medicine, Shanghai, China

**Olatz Lopez-Fernandez** Faculty of Psychology, Campus de Somosaguas, Universidad Complutense de Madrid, Madrid, Spain

Universidad Francisco de Vitoria, Psychology, Madrid, Spain

Centro de Estudios Universitarios Cardenal Cisneros, University College, Department of Psychology, Madrid, Spain

Hospital Universitario Fundación Jiménez Díaz, Servicio de Psiquiatría, Madrid, Spain

**Silvia Lovato** Public Broadcasting Service, Arlington, VA, USA

**Katerina Lukavska** Charles University, Prague, Czechia

**Megan K. Maas** Department of Human Development & Family Studies, Michigan State University, East Lansing, MI, USA

**Kathryn Macapagal** Northwestern University, Evanston, IL, USA

Institute for Sexual and Gender Minority Health and Wellbeing, Northwestern University, Chicago, IL, USA

Department of Medical Social Sciences, Feinberg School of Medicine, Northwestern University, Chicago, IL, USA

**Sheri Madigan** University of Calgary, Calgary, AB, Canada

Alberta Children's Hospital Research Institute, Calgary, AB, Canada

**Lucía Magis-Weinberg** Department of Psychology, University of Washington, Seattle, WA, USA

**Anne J. Maheux** Department of Psychology and Neuroscience, University of North Carolina at Chapel Hill, Chapel Hill, NC, USA

**Adriana Manago** Department of Psychology, University of California, Santa Cruz, CA, USA

**Jennifer A. Manganello** University at Albany, State University of New York, Albany, NY, USA

Department of Health Policy, Management, and Behavior, University at Albany School of Public Health, Rensselaer, NY, USA

**Jamie Manolev** Centre for Research in Educational and Social Inclusion, University of South Australia, Adelaide, SA, Australia

**Laura Marciano** Harvard T.H. Chan School of Public Health, Lee Kum Sheung Center for Health and Happiness, Dana-Farber Cancer Institute, Boston, MA, USA

**Lisa A. Marsch** Center for Technology and Behavioral Health, Dartmouth College, Lebanon, NH, USA

**Florence Martin** North Carolina State University, Raleigh, NC, USA

**Siva Mathiyazhagan** School of Social Policy & Practice, University of Pennsylvania, Philadelphia, PA, USA

**Ashley Maxie-Moreman** Children's National Hospital, Washington, DC, USA

**Angela Mazzone** University of Surrey, Stag Hill Campus, Guildford, UK

**Meghan McCoy** Bridgewater State University, Bridgewater, MA, USA

**Brandon T. McDaniel** Health Services and Informatics Research, Parkview Mirro Center for Research and Innovation, Fort Wayne, IN, USA

**Sarah McGrew** University of Maryland, College Park, MD, USA

**Lauren B. McInroy** The Ohio State University, Columbus, OH, USA

**Lara B. McKenzie** Abigail Wexner Research Institute at Nationwide Children's Hospital, Center for Injury Research and Policy, Columbus, OH, USA

**Tara McPherson** University of Southern California, Los Angeles, CA, USA

**Gemma Mestre-Bach** Instituto de Investigación, Transferencia e Innovación, Universidad Internacional de La Rioja, La Rioja, Spain

**Ellen Middaugh** San José State University, San Jose, CA, USA

**Tijana Milosevic** University College Dublin, Dublin, Ireland

**Elizabeth Milovidov** The LEGO Group, Digitalem S.A.S, Paris, France

**Christian Montag** Department of Molecular Psychology, Institute of Psychology and Education, Ulm University, Ulm, Germany

**Kathryn Montgomery** Center for Digital Democracy, American University, Washington, DC, USA

**Rosalba Morese** Faculty of Biomedical Sciences, Faculty of Communication, Culture and Society, Università della Svizzera italiana, Lugano, Switzerland

**Jorge Mota** Research Center on Physical Activity, Health and Leisure (CIAFEL), Faculty of Sport, University of Porto, Porto, Portugal

**Benjamin Mullin** Department of Psychiatry, University of Colorado Anschutz Medical Campus, Aurora, CO, USA

Pediatric Mental Health Institute, Children's Hospital Colorado, Aurora, CO, USA

**Tiffany Grace-Chung Munzer** University of Michigan, Ann Arbor, MI, USA

**Faisal Mushtaq** University of Leeds, Leeds, UK

**Lauren Myers** Lafayette College, Easton, PA, USA

**Shaylene E. Nancekivell** University of Manitoba, Winnipeg, MB, Canada

**Amy I. Nathanson** The Ohio State University, Columbus, OH, USA

**Kimberly M. Nelson** Department of Community Health Sciences, Boston University School of Public Health, Boston, MA, USA

Department of Psychiatry, Boston University Chobanian & Avedisian School of Medicine, Boston, MA, USA

**Jacqueline Nesi** Department of Psychiatry & Human Behavior, Alpert Medical School of Brown University, Providence, RI, USA

Bradley-Hasbro Research Center, Rhode Island Hospital, Providence, RI, USA

**Thomas Niederkrotenthaler** Medical University of Vienna, Vienna, Austria

**Safiya U. Noble** University of California, Los Angeles, CA, USA

**Jonathan Noel** Johnson & Wales University, Charlotte, NC, USA

**W. Ian O'Byrne** College of Charleston, Charleston, SC, USA

**Brian O'Neill** Technological University Dublin, Dublin, Ireland

**Cansu Oranç** Ronin Institute, Montclair, NJ, USA

**Stephanie M. Ortiz** University of Massachusetts Lowell, Sociology Department, Lowell, MA, USA

**Oyewole Oyekoya** City University of New York, New York, NY, USA

**Kathleen A. Paciga** Columbia College Chicago, Chicago, IL, USA

**David Pagliaccio** Department of Psychiatry, Columbia University, New York, NY, USA

Division of Child and Adolescent Psychiatry, New York State Psychiatric Institute, New York, NY, USA

**Luci Pangrazio** Deakin University, Melbourne, VIC, Australia

**Jinkyung Park** Vanderbilt University, Nashville, TN, USA

**Douglas A. Parry** Stellenbosch University, Stellenbosch, Western Cape, South Africa

**Katalin Parti** Virginia Tech, Blacksburg, VA, USA

**Justin Patchin** University of Wisconsin-Eau Claire, Eau Claire, WI, USA

**Russell R. Pate** Department of Exercise Science, Arnold School of Public Health, University of South Carolina, Columbia, SC, USA

**Manisha Pathak-Shelat** MICA, Ahmedabad, India

**Martin Paulus** University of California San Diego, La Jolla, CA, USA

**Dale Peeples** Augusta University, Augusta, GA, USA

Medical College of Georgia, Augusta, GA, USA

**Matthew Pesko** Department of Psychiatry, University of Colorado Anschutz Medical Campus, Aurora, CO, USA

Denver Health Medical Center, Denver, CO, USA

**Jochen Peter** University of Amsterdam, Amsterdam, Netherlands

**Morgan Scott Polikoff** Rossier School of Education, University of Southern California, Los Angeles, CA, USA

**Halley M. Pontes** University of London, Department of Organizational Psychology, Birkbeck, London, UK

**Marc N. Potenza** Department of Psychiatry, Yale University School of Medicine, New Haven, CT, USA

Departments of Psychiatry and Neuroscience, Child Study Center, Yale University School of Medicine, New Haven, CT, USA

Connecticut Mental Health Center, New Haven, CT, USA

Connecticut Council on Problem Gambling, Wethersfield, CT, USA

Department of Neuroscience, Yale University, New Haven, CT, USA

Wu Tsai Institute, Yale University, New Haven, CT, USA

Department of Psychology, University of Nevada, Las Vegas, NV, USA

**Kruakae Pothong** The London School of Economics, London, UK

**Yenda Prado** Digital Promise, Washington, DC, USA

**Detra Price-Dennis** The Ohio State University, Columbus, OH, USA

**Brian Primack** College of Public Health and Human Sciences, Oregon State University, Corvallis, OR, USA

**Srividya Ramasubramanian** Syracuse University, Syracuse, NY, USA

**Florian Rehbein** Department of Social Work, Münster University of Applied Sciences, Münster, Germany

**Justin Reich** Massachusetts Institute of Technology, Cambridge, MA, USA

**Stephanie M. Reich** University of California, Irvine, CA, USA

**Jazmin Reyes-Portillo** Montclair University, Montclair, NJ, USA

**Rebekah A. Richert** University of California, Riverside, Riverside, CA, USA

**Rebecca Robbins** Departments of Medicine and Neurology, Division of Sleep and Circadian Disorders, Brigham and Women's Hospital, Boston, MA, USA

Division of Sleep Medicine, Harvard Medical School, Boston, MA, USA

**Sarah T. Roberts** University of California, Los Angeles, CA, USA

**Thomas N. Robinson** Stanford Solutions Science Lab and Division of General Pediatrics, Department of Pediatrics, Stanford Prevention Research Center, Department of Medicine, and Department of Epidemiology and Population Health, Stanford University, Stanford, CA, USA

**Rachel R. Romeo** University of Maryland, College Park, MD, USA

**Maria Romo-Palafox** Nutrition and Dietetics, Saint Louis University, St. Louis, MO, USA

**Sarah Rosaen** University of Michigan-Flint, Flint, MI, USA

**Chad A. Rose** University of Missouri, Columbia, MO, USA

**Emily F. Rothman** Department of Occupational Therapy, Boston University, Boston, MA, USA

**Hans-Jürgen Rumpf** Department of Psychiatry and Psychotherapy, University of Lübeck, Lübeck, Germany

**Gillian Russell** Simon Fraser University, Burnaby, BC, Canada

**Colleen Russo Johnson** Toronto Metropolitan University, Toronto, ON, Canada

**Preeti G. Samudra** SUNY Plattsburgh, Plattsburgh, NY, USA

**Cheryl E. Sanders** Metropolitan State University of Denver, Denver, CO, USA

**James D. Sargent** The Koop Institute at Dartmouth College, Hanover, NH, USA

**Travis J. Saunders** Department of Applied Human Sciences, University of Prince Edward Island, Charlottetown, PE, Canada

**Brian Scassellati** Yale University, New Haven, CT, USA

**Erica Scharrer** University of Massachusetts Amherst, Amherst, MA, USA

**Florian Schaub** University of Michigan, Ann Arbor, MI, USA

**Stephen M. Schueller** Psychological Sciences and Informatics, University of California, Irvine, Irvine, CA, USA

**Anja Schultze-Krumbholz** Technische Universität Berlin, Berlin, Germany

**Tracy M. Scull** Innovation Research & Training, Durham, NC, USA

**Rachel L. Severson** University of Montana, Missoula, MT, USA

**Reem M. A. Shafi** Department of Psychiatry, Cairns and Hinterland Hospital and Health Services, Cairns, QLD, Australia

Mayo Clinic, Rochester, MN, USA

**Susan M. Sibert** Indiana University of Pennsylvania, Indiana, PA, USA

**Mark Smith** Stanford University, Stanford, CA, USA

**Tim J. Smith** Creative Computing Institute, University of the Arts London, London, UK

**Olivia Snow** University of California, Los Angeles, CA, USA

**Marcantonio M. Spada** School of Applied Sciences, London South Bank University, London, UK

**Amanda E. Staiano** Pennington Biomedical Research Center, Baton Rouge, LA, USA

**Elisabeth Staksrud** University of Oslo, Oslo, Norway

**Vladan Starcevic** FRANZCP, Discipline of Psychiatry, Sydney Medical School, Nepean Clinical School, Faculty of Medicine and Health, University of Sydney, Sydney, NSW, Australia

**Despina Stavrinos** Department of Psychology, University of Alabama at Birmingham, Birmingham, AL, USA

**Vasileios Stavropoulos** RMIT University, School of Health and Biomedical Sciences, Melbourne, VIC, Australia

**Stacey Steinberg** University of Florida, Gainesville, FL, USA

**Jennifer Stevens Aubrey** Department of Communication, University of Arizona, Tucson, AZ, USA

**Ashley Stewart** Georgia State University, Atlanta, GA, USA

**Mariya Stoilova** The London School of Economics, London, UK

**Leon Straker** School of Allied Health, Curtin University, Perth, WA, Australia

**Kaveri Subrahmanyam** University of North Florida, Jacksonville, FL, USA

Department of Psychology, University of Northern Florida, Jacksonville, FL, USA

**Annette S. Sundqvist** Linköping University, Linköping, Sweden

**Clifford Sussman** George Washington University School of Medicine, Washington, DC, USA

**Thomas B. Swanton** The University of Sydney, School of Psychology, Brain & Mind Centre, Gambling Treatment & Research Clinic, Sydney, NSW, Australia

**Attila Szabo** Faculty of Education and Psychology, ELTE Eötvös Loránd University, Budapest, Hungary

**Jessica Szczuka** University of Duisburg-Essen, Duisburg and Essen, Germany

**Hannah Szlyk** Washington University in St Louis, St Louis, MO, USA

**Lori Takeuchi** National Science Foundation, Alexandria, VA, USA

**Sisi Tao** University of Hong Kong, Hong Kong, SAR, China

**Mimi Tatlow-Golden** School of Education, Childhood, Youth and Sport, The Open University, Milton Keynes, UK

**Gemma Taylor** University of Salford, Salford, UK

**Valerie Jones Taylor** Rutgers University, New Brunswick, NJ, USA

**Jeff R. Temple** School of Behavioral Health Sciences, UTHealth Houston, Houston, TX, USA

**Moriah E. Thomason** New York University Langone Medical Center, New York, NY, USA

**Melina Throuvala** International Gaming Research Unit, NTU Psychology, Nottingham Trent University, Nottingham, UK

West Midlands Gambling Harms Clinic, Inclusion, Midlands Partnership NHS Trust, Stafford, UK

Paediatric Psychology, Child and Adolescent Mental health Services, Leicestershire Partnership NHS Trust, Leicester, UK

**Maxim Topaz** Columbia University School of Nursing, Columbia University, New York, NY, USA

Columbia University Data Science Institute, Columbia University, New York, NY, USA

**Noor Toraif** University of Pennsylvania, School of Social Policy and Practice, Philadelphia, PA, USA

**John Torous** Harvard University, Cambridge, MA, USA

**Jolien Trekels** The University of North Carolina at Chapel Hill, Chapel Hill, NC, USA

**Mark S. Tremblay** Children's Hospital of Eastern Ontario Research Institute, Ottawa, ON, Canada

Department of Pediatrics, University of Ottawa, Ottawa, ON, Canada

Department of Health Sciences, Carleton University, Ottawa, ON, Canada

**Torrey Trust** University of Massachusetts Amherst, Amherst, MA, USA

**Michael Tsappis** Boston Children's Hospital, Boston, MA, USA
Harvard Medical School, Boston, MA, USA

**Rebecca Tukachinsky Forster** Chapman University, Orange, CA, USA

**Kristen Hawley Turner** Drew University, Madison, NJ, USA

**Jean M. Twenge** San Diego State University, San Diego, CA, USA

**Lawrence Tychsen** Washington University School of Medicine, St. Louis, MO, USA
St. Louis Children's Hospital, St. Louis, MO, USA

**Brendesha M. Tynes** University of Southern California, Los Angeles, CA, USA

**Yalda T. Uhls** University of California Los Angeles, Center for Scholars & Storytellers, Los Angeles, CA, USA

**Melina Uncapher** University of California, San Francisco, CA, USA

**Desmond Upton Patton** University of Pennsylvania, School of Social Policy and Practice, Annenberg School for Communication, Philadelphia, PA, USA
Department of Child and Adolescent Psychiatry and Behavioral Sciences, University of Pennsylvania, Philadelphia, PA, USA

**Chikezie E. Uzuegbunam** Rhodes University, Makhanda, Eastern Cape, South Africa

**Patti M. Valkenburg** Amsterdam School of Communication Research, University of Amsterdam, Amsterdam, Netherlands

**Regina van den Eijnden** Department of Interdisciplinary Social Science, Utrecht University, Utrecht, Netherlands

**Amber van der Wal** University of Amsterdam, Amsterdam, Netherlands

**Johanna M. F. van Oosten** University of Amsterdam, Amsterdam School of Communication Research, Amsterdam, The Netherlands

**Joris Van Ouytsel** Hugh Downs School of Human Communication, Arizona State University, Tempe, AZ, USA

**Mariek M. P. Vanden Abeele** imec-mict, Department of Communication Sciences, Ghent University, Ghent, Belgium

**Tanner Vea** University of Washington, Seattle, WA, USA

**Alison K. Ventura** Department of Kinesiology and Public Health, Center for Health Research, California Polytechnic State University, San Luis Obispo, CA, USA

**Samantha Viano** George Mason University, Fairfax, VA, USA

**Carol Vidal** Johns Hopkins University, Baltimore, MD, USA

**Kasisomayajula Viswanath** Harvard T.H. Chan School of Public Health, Lee Kum Sheung Center for Health and Happiness, Dana-Farber Cancer Institute, Boston, MA, USA

**Gergana Vladova** University of Potsdam and Weizenbaum Institute, Berlin, Germany

**Sebastian Wachs** University of Münster, Münster, Germany

**Anthony D. Wagner** Stanford University, Stanford, CA, USA

**Eric R. Walsh-Buhi** Department of Applied Health Science, Indiana University School of Public Health-Bloomington, Bloomington, IN, USA

**L. Monique Ward** Department of Psychology, University of Michigan, Ann Arbor, MI, USA

**Ronald Warren** University of Arkansas, Fayetteville, AR, USA

**Ellen Wartella** Northwestern University, Evanston, IL, USA

**René Weber** Department of Communication, University of California, Santa Barbara, CA, USA

Department of Psychological & Brain Sciences, University of California, Santa Barbara, CA, USA

Department of Communication and Media, Ewha Womans University, Seoul, South Korea

**Paul Weigle** Department of Psychiatry, University of Connecticut School of Medicine, Farmington, CT, USA

**Aviv M. Weinstein** Ariel University, Ariel, Israel

**Emily Weinstein** Harvard Graduate School of Education, Cambridge, MA, USA

**Laura M. Widman** Department of Psychology, North Carolina State University, Raleigh, NC, USA

**Kofoworola D. A. Williams** Department of Community Health and Prevention, Drexel University Dornsife School of Public Health, Philadelphia, PA, USA

**Henry A. Willis** University of Pennsylvania, Philadelphia, PA, USA

**Sam Wineburg** Stanford University, Stanford, CA, USA

**Wisnu Wiradhany** University of Groningen, Groningen, The Netherlands

**Pamela Wisniewski** Vanderbilt University, Nashville, TN, USA

**Val Wongsomboon** Department of Psychology, Yale University, New Haven, CT, USA

**Xeturah Woodley** Doña Ana Community College, Las Cruces, NM, USA

**Susan J. Woolford** School of Public Health, University of Michigan, Ann Arbor, MI, USA

**Michelle F. Wright** Indiana State University, Terre Haute, IN, USA

**Paul J. Wright** Communication Science, The Media School, Indiana University, Bloomington, IN, USA

**Ying Xu** University of Michigan, Ann Arbor, MI, USA

**Chia-chen Yang** School of Education Foundations, Leadership and Aviation, Oklahoma State University, Stillwater, OK, USA

**Svetlana Yarosh** University of Minnesota, Minneapolis, MN, USA

**Elana Zeide** University of Nebraska, Lincoln, NE, USA

**Jamie Zelazny** University of Pittsburgh, Pittsburgh, PA, USA

**Jennifer M. Zosh** The Pennsylvania State University Brandywine, Media, PA, USA

# Introduction

Dimitri A. Christakis and Lauren Hale

## 1 Trends in Children's Media Research

The field of research related to children and media is likely to sustain its trajectory of rapid growth alongside an evolution in the available technologies and how, where, and when they are used. The past 15 years has seen a significant rise in scientific research into the effects of technology and media on child development, accompanied by a recent surge in government funding. This acceleration in research is mirrored by the significant increase in the number of publications stored within databases pertaining to children and media over the past 15 years (see Fig. 1).

In this period, children's media researchers have appropriately shifted their focus to a more nuanced exploration of the evolving landscape of digital media. For example, researchers are no longer concentrating solely on the amount of screen time but also on its quality, especially with respect to adolescents and their interaction with social media. TikTok has notably surfaced as the primary social media platform among teenagers. In 2022, it was reported that 67% of US teens were using TikTok [1]. Meanwhile, revelations regarding Instagram's adverse effects on the mental health of teenage girls have prompted significant action, including congressional hearings [2, 3].

A deeper understanding of media effects on child development and well-being will need a greater level of granularity, possibly in cooperation with industry. Passive sensing and usage tracking by scientists will require that phone manufacturers allow it, and this will likely require government intervention. Family and social context is also important, and collecting such data remains a challenge.

D. A. Christakis (✉)
Seattle Children's Research Institute,
Seattle, WA, USA

University of Washington, Seattle, WA, USA

Special Olympics, Washington, DC, USA

Children and Screens: Institute of Digital Media and Child Development, Jericho, NY, USA
e-mail: Dimitri.christakis@seattlechildrens.org

L. Hale
Program in Public Health, Department of Family, Population, and Preventive Medicine, Renaissance School of Medicine, Stony Brook University,
Stony Brook, NY, USA

## 2 About This Supplement

Representing the complexity of this expanding field, this handbook summarizes the insights of nearly 400 leading experts across the fields of pediatrics, psychiatry, psychology, epidemiology, communication, neuroscience, sociology, history, legal studies, social work, human development and family studies, gender studies, African American studies, education, information technology and design, and more.


D. A. Christakis, L. Hale (eds.), *Handbook of Children and Screens*,
https://doi.org/10.1007/978-3-031-69362-5_1

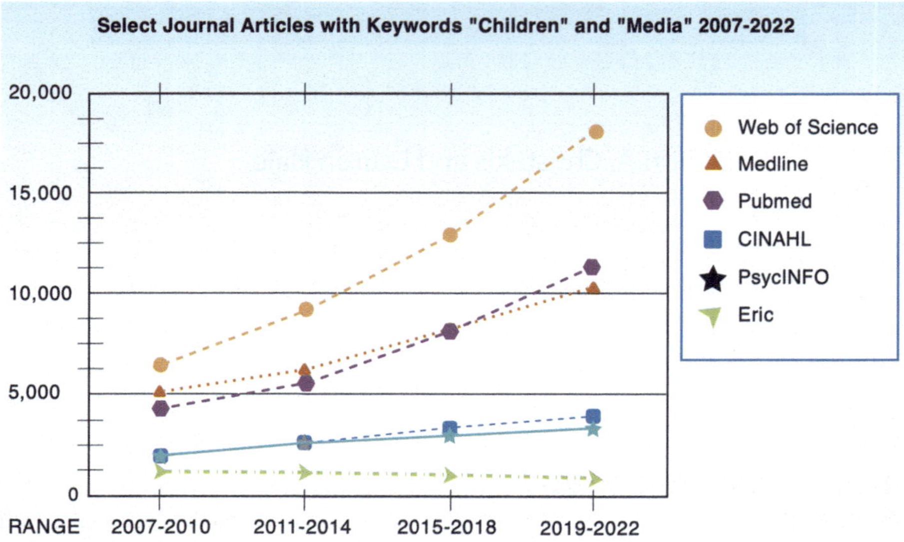


**Fig. 1** Select journal articles with the keywords "children" and "media": 2007–2022

This handbook is intended to serve as both a reference and a guide for current and future scientists as well as for parents and professionals alike who are interested in developing a stronger understanding of how to support healthy child development in an increasingly digital world. As such, it provides brief summaries of the current state of scientific evidence related to key domains and, equally important, an overview of salient research questions and recommendations for key stakeholders, including parents and caregivers, educators, clinicians, and policymakers. With a collection of 87 chapters, this handbook has been thoughtfully structured into 3 parts, each containing between 3 and 5 sections.

Part I of this compendium, titled "Research Concerning Cognitive, Physical, Mental, and Psychosocial Impacts on Children," brings together five distinct sections. These sections outline the intricate relationship between digital media and the cognitive, physical, and mental health of children and adolescents and address the potential risks associated with problematic Internet use. Importantly, this part emphasizes the multifaceted influence that digital media have on various aspects of child and adolescent development, providing insights into how media exposure can shape and inform their experiences and health outcomes.

The array of research encapsulated in Part II, "Research on How Media Influence Relationships, Family, Culture, and Society," navigates the intricate and complex terrain of digital media's influence on interpersonal relationships, family dynamics, societal norms, and cultural fabric. The five sections of Part II explore a range of digital media aspects, including an examination of how digital media represent and influence: 1.) race and racism, 2.) gender and sexuality, 3.) parenting, 4.) cyberbullying and digital incivility, and 5.) media policy.

The third and last part—"Digital Domains"—contains three sections that highlight research investigating specific digital domains such as education technology, video gaming, and emerging technologies and their influence on children's development. Part III fosters an in-depth exploration of the distinct realms of digital engagement, each of which presents unique challenges and opportunities.

Each section, and each chapter within each section, is designed to stand alone, representing the consensus of interdisciplinary authorship groups and additional input from the reviews of external experts. Accordingly, readers may find that sections have some overlap in the material covered or even diverse perspectives on complex issues. However, when read together, this handbook provides a robust collection of collaborative and peer-reviewed works and strengthens an already growing field by helping synthesize key findings, recommendations, and research opportunities for the future. We hope that this open-access handbook will serve the field as digital media research continues to evolve.

**Acknowledgments** We are grateful to all the section leaders and authors who contributed their expertise to this handbook and to the researchers whose work they cite. In addition to the nearly 400 authors, we also want to recognize those who supported this publication as expert reviewers of the chapters within:

**Vivien Wen Li Anthony, PhD, MSW**
Rutgers University
**Tracy Asamoah, MD, ACC**
Independent coaching practice
**Fiona Baker, PhD**
SRI International
**Kaitlyn Burnell, PhD**
University of North Carolina, Chapel Hill
**Jasmina Byrne, MA**
UNICEF
**Hilarie Cash, PhD, LMCH**
reSTART Center for Digital Technology Sustainability
**Meredith Clark, PhD**
Northeastern University
**Samuel Ehrenreich, PhD**
University of Nevada, Reno
**Kara Fox, MA**
University of North Carolina, Chapel Hill
**John Hutton, MD, MSc**
Cincinnati Children's Hospital
**Laura Jana, MD**
Pennsylvania State University
**Erica Kenney, ScD, MPH**
Harvard University
**Orsolya Kiss, PhD**
SRI International
**Daria Kuss, PhD**
Nottingham Trent University
**Benjamin Li, PhD**
Nanyang Technological University
**Lin Lin Lipsmeyer, EdD**
Southern Methodist University
**Camillia Matuk, EdD**
New York University
**Sherrel McArthur, PhD**
University of Georgia
**Kaitlynn Mendes, PhD**
Western University
**Dan Romer, PhD**
University of Pennsylvania
**Ellen Selkie, MD, MPH**
University of Wisconsin-Madison
**Tim Smith, PhD**
University of the Arts London
**Nicol Turner Lee, PhD**
Brookings
**Janis Whitlock, PhD**
Cornell University
**Nancy Willard, JD, MS**
Embrace Civility

We also gratefully acknowledge the support of Children and Screens: Institute of Digital Media and Child Development, for their sponsorship of this publication. Without their funding and dedicated staff support, this open-access resource would not be possible. We extend specific thanks to the following individuals for their indispensable facilitation: Pam Hurst-Della Pietra, DO, Founder, Kate Blocker, PhD, Director of Research and Programs, Camara Brown, MPhil, Project Coordinator, and Melinda Karth, PhD, Research and Programs Assistant.

**Conflict of Interest and Funding Disclosures** Dr. Christakis began serving as an expert witness in social media litigation in September 2023.

## References

1. Atske S. Teens, social media and technology 2022. Pew Research Center: Internet, Science & Tech. Published August 10, 2022. https://www.pewresearch.org/internet/2022/08/10/teens-social-media-and-technology-2022/. Accessed 29 May 2023.
2. Wells G, Horwitz J, Seetharaman D. Facebook knows Instagram is toxic for teen girls, company documents show. Wall Street J. Published September 14, 2021. https://www.wsj.com/articles/facebook-knows-instagram-is-toxic-for-teen-girls-company-documents-show-11631620739. Accessed 29 May 2023.
3. Time change: protecting our children online. Published online February 14, 2023. https://www.judiciary.senate.gov/committee-activity/hearings/protecting-our-children-online. Accessed 29 May 2023.

# Part I

# Research Concerning Cognitive, Physical, Mental, and Psychosocial Impacts on Children

# Introduction to the Section on Digital Media, Cognition, and Brain Development

Heather Kirkorian

Children's access to and use of screen media has increased markedly in the last decade, with children spending more time at younger ages with a wider range of media platforms than ever before [1, 2]. These changes have been met with both widespread concern about the potential impact of screen time on cognition and brain development and optimism for the educational potential of media access [3]. Proposed mechanisms for media impact on cognition and brain development include both direct effects, such as disrupted sleep or knowledge and skills gained from educational media, and indirect effects, such as displacement of time that could be spent doing activities believed to be more valuable for cognition, such as academic tasks (e.g., reading, homework), in-person social interactions, and the experience of boredom that might be a catalyst for creativity.

A careful examination of media effects on cognition and brain development requires a developmental lens. The brain develops rapidly in early childhood and continues to mature through adolescence and early adulthood, characterized by reductions in gray matter and increases in white matter that are shaped in part by experience [4, 5]. Notably, some regions of the brain mature faster than others [4]. As such, children are likely to be differentially susceptible to both positive and negative media effects at different points in development [6], with effects depending on the timing and nature of exposure. Studies examining associations between digital media use and the structure and function of the brain are just beginning to emerge, and they are cited throughout this section where available. However, most of what is known about digital media and brain development is inferred from behavioral research.

The chapters in this section tackle different aspects of cognition and brain development through critical reviews of the literature on digital media effects. Each chapter is written by a multidisciplinary team of experts in fields as far-ranging as behavioral pediatrics, psychology, psychiatry, neuroscience, family science, and communication studies. Each chapter concludes with calls for future research to fill the existing gaps and recommendations based on what is currently known. In this brief introduction, I provide an overview of each chapter and identify convergent themes across them.

## 1 Overview of Chapters in This Section

The first two chapters summarize the current state of research on media use, cognition, and brain development. Kirkorian et al. (see chapter "Digital Media, Cognition, and Brain Development in Infancy and Childhood") summarize research covering infancy through

H. Kirkorian (✉)
University of Wisconsin-Madison,
Madison, WI, USA
e-mail: kirkorian@wisc.edu


D. A. Christakis, L. Hale (eds.), *Handbook of Children and Screens*,
https://doi.org/10.1007/978-3-031-69362-5_2

childhood, while Marciano et al. (see chapter "Digital Media, Cognition, and Brain Development in Adolescence") summarize research covering adolescence. Both chapters situate the research in the context of brain development throughout these periods, underscoring that the potential for environmental impacts on brain structure and function depends on, among other things, the timing of exposure. The chapters review a small set of studies examining associations between media use and brain structure and function as well as a comparatively large body of literature on associations between media use and cognitive outcomes such as inhibitory control, attention, language, and academic achievement. Although these chapters cover different studies in the literature focusing on different periods, the general conclusions are notably similar. In general, meta-analytic studies report nonsignificant or small negative associations between overall screen time and cognitive outcomes. However, effects vary substantially between studies and individuals, with effects driven by the timing, content, context, and type of media used. Both chapters emphasize that research to date is primarily cross-sectional and based on parent- or self-reported media use, providing a relatively weak basis for causal inference but a useful foundation on which to build more rigorous research.

Other chapters focus on specific topics within the media effects literature. Baumgartner et al. (see chapter "The Short- and Long-Term Effects of Digital Media Use on Attention") summarize research on media multitasking and digital distractions, distinguishing between momentary, short-term effects of media use on task performance (e.g., homework) and cumulative, long-term effects of regular media distractions and multitasking over time. They find relatively strong evidence for momentary, short-term effects on concurrent task performance that vary based on motivational factors (e.g., relative importance placed on media versus the primary task), the degree to which the two tasks draw on the same sensory modalities (e.g., both require reading), and whether attention is forcefully interrupted by media (e.g., push notification). Baumgartner et al. find less support for longer-term, cumulative effects on attention skills, echoing themes in the chapters by Kirkorian et al. and Marciano et al. Baumgartner et al. note limitations in the current research that may explain the modest effects observed in the literature. They also suggest key areas for future research to better understand the potential links between media multitasking and cognitive abilities over time.

Dore et al. (see chapter "Digital Media Use and Language Development in Early Childhood") focus on the subset of studies examining media use and language development. Their conclusions are similar to those of Kirkorian et al. and Marciano et al., reporting that the average effects of media use on language development are small to negligible but with marked individual differences in media effects that seem to be driven by the content and context of media use. Dore et al. also consider whether media effects differ based on the type of media used, with interactive media that respond to children (e.g., digital games or apps) presenting different opportunities for word learning than noninteractive media (e.g., television programs). They call for more research on this topic. Richert et al. (see chapter "Imagination, Creativity, and Play") review a complementary but unique body of literature on media as it relates to children's imagination, creativity, and play. They describe how children understand media characters and build imagined relationships with them. Richert et al. also review studies examining the potential impacts of media use on creativity and play. The findings echo themes that emerged in other chapters, namely, that concurrent media use (e.g., background television) can interrupt children's play, but some types of media (e.g., storytelling with artificial intelligence (AI)-enhanced technology) may inspire pretend play and creativity.

Finally, Alper et al. (see chapter "Digital Media and Neurodevelopmental Differences") consider how children diagnosed with autism and/or attention-deficit/hyperactivity disorder use and experience media. They characterize media use in these populations as both high-risk and high-reward, emphasizing that media effects differ across individuals due to, among other things, the degree to which media use facilitates social connection (e.g., through shared interests and conversation topics) versus isolation or negative social experiences (e.g., cyberbullying victimization). Their chapter notes both similarities and differences in media use patterns compared to neurotypical youth. They also call for research that examines other aspects of human diversity (e.g., race, ethnicity, class, gender, geography) that are largely overlooked in media effects research.

## 2 Convergent Themes Across Chapters

Although the chapters in this section focus on different populations, outcomes, and ways of interacting with media, several consistent findings emerge. First, the degree and direction of media effects remain elusive. It seems clear that media use can have immediate, short-term effects. This includes positive effects, such as knowledge gained from media designed to teach specific concepts (Dore et al., Kirkorian et al.), as well as negative effects, such as disruption of concurrent activities (e.g., play, parent-child interactions; Kirkorian et al., Richert et al.) and reductions in task performance (e.g., homework), particularly when there is competition for processing capacity (Baumgartner et al.). However, causal evidence for cumulative, long-term effects of media use over time is lacking, necessitating rigorous research designs that go beyond cross-sectional analyses and self-report measures that collapse screen time into unidimensional quantity estimates (Baumgartner et al., Dore et al., Kirkorian et al., Marciano et al.).

The nature of media effects is likely more complex than most current research allows. First, all chapters in this section emphasize that media effects depend on the ways in which media are used. Content effects are common: Associations between media use and cognitive outcomes are generally neutral or positive for child-centered media content that is designed to teach and for joint parent-child media engagement, especially when compared to solitary media use and use of noneducational entertainment or adult-directed content (Dore et al., Kirkorian et al., Richert et al.). Less is known about the impact of media types, such as watching videos versus playing video games, but several authors consider differences that may emerge depending on the way media are designed and the type of skill measured (Dore et al., Kirkorian et al., Richert et al.). The impact of different content and design affordances is likely to be ever more important as the digital media and technology landscape continues to evolve.

Related, the context of media use matters. Effects are likely to differ depending on the degree to which media use facilitates positive interactions versus disrupts those interactions or creates opportunities for negative interactions such as cyberbullying (Alper et al., Dore et al., Kirkorian et al.). Several authors note that other contextual and structural factors (e.g., gender, race, ethnicity, socioeconomic status) may moderate media effects (Alper et al., Marciano et al.). For example, daily media use decreases with greater household income and parent education, is higher for boys than girls, and is higher for Black children and Hispanic/Latino children than for White children [1, 2]. However, while some studies of digital media and cognitive development consider these factors as control variables, few have sought to understand how these factors may moderate media effects. Sufficiently large and diverse samples would also allow for examination of differences both among and within subgroups, revealing a great deal about how different families use media to meet their different needs [7].

Moreover, small-to-negligible population effects likely mask individual differences in media effects. Several chapters in this section note that sensitivity to media effects is likely to change with age (Dore et al., Kirkorian et al., Marciano et al.). However, relatively few studies directly examine age-related correlates of media use that can explain age differences in media effects. Potential age-related correlates emerging from the chapters in this section include brain maturation (Kirkorian et al., Marciano et al.), experience and familiarity with media (Dore et al.), comprehension of media (Kirkorian et al.), and fantasy-reality boundaries (Richert et al.). Other individual differences raised in this section include gender (Marciano et al.), neurodiversity (Alper et al.), and motivational factors (Baumgartner et al., Marciano et al.). Children and youth who exhibit problematic media use behaviors (e.g., preoccupation with media, difficulty stopping media use) may be particularly susceptible to media effects (Kirkorian et al.). Some authors also call for research examining largely overlooked differences that may moderate or explain associations between media use and cognitive development, such as mental health conditions (Alper et al., Marciano et al.).

Finally, media effects are likely to be bidirectional. That is, just as media use may cause cognitive effects, so too might media use result from cognitive differences, as when parents turn to media to calm children with lower self-regulation (Kirkorian et al.), imaginative children seek out open-ended media that allow them to express their creativity (Richert et al.), and youth with poor inhibitory control become more easily distracted by media (Baumgartner et al.). Moreover, media effects are likely to be nonlinear. For example, some authors report optimal outcomes for moderate amounts of media use (Dore et al.). Future research should leverage longitudinal designs and more sophisticated quantitative approaches that allow for such complexity in media effects.

## 3 What Comes Next

Just as the chapters in this section reveal convergent findings about what is known, so do they reveal gaps in the literature and recurring themes about what is needed from future research. First, brain-behavior relations must be established to identify the potential mechanisms of influence and to explain whether and how associations between media use and brain structure and function are meaningful. Second, rigorous research methods are needed to advance the field and support causal inference. Most of our current knowledge is based on cross-sectional studies, self-report measures, and unidimensional global estimates of time spent with media. To advance our understanding of cognition and brain development in the digital age, we must invest in longitudinal studies that can help establish the temporal order of effects, allowing for bidirectionality while controlling for baseline measures and other potential confounds (e.g., parenting style, parent and child mental health). Similarly, randomized controlled trials are needed, where feasible, to test causality. Third, it will be critical to unpack individual differences in media effects. The research reviewed in this section points to some promising mechanisms, particularly as they relate to age differences in media effects. Finally, the field would benefit from shared, comprehensive measures that combine objective quantity estimates (e.g., continuous passive mobile sensing), subjective experiences (e.g., self-reported motivations for media use), and detailed reports that capture the complexity of media use "in the wild" (e.g., ecological momentary assessment or daily diaries). Studies such as these are currently underway and will build on a foundation of existing research to shed new light on cognition and brain development amid an ever-changing digital media landscape.

**Conflict of Interest and Funding Disclosures** None.

## References

1. Rideout V, Peebles A, Mann S, Robb MB. Common sense census: media use by tweens and teens, 2021. Common Sense Media; 2022. Retrieved from www.commonsensemedia.org.
2. Rideout V, Robb MB. Common sense census: media use by kids age zero to eight. Common Sense Media; 2020. Retrieved from www.commonsensemedia.org.
3. Lauricella AR, Blackwell CK, Wartella E. The "new" technology environment: the role of content and context on learning and development from mobile media. In: Media exposure during infancy and early childhood: the effects of content and context on learning and development. Springer International Publishing AG; 2017. p. 1–23. https://doi.org/10.1007/978-3-319-45102-2_1.
4. Gilmore JH, Knickmeyer RC, Gao W. Imaging structural and functional brain development in early childhood. Nat Rev Neurosci. 2018;19(3):123–37. https://doi.org/10.1038/nrn.2018.1.

5. Giedd JN, Blumenthal J, Jeffries NO, et al. Brain development during childhood and adolescence: a longitudinal MRI study. Nat Neurosci. 1999;2(10):861–3. https://doi.org/10.1038/13158.
6. Valkenburg P, Peter J. The differential susceptibility to media effects model. J Commun. 2013;63(2):221–43. https://doi.org/10.1111/jcom.12024.
7. Rideout V, Katz V. Opportunity for all? Technology and learning in lower-income families. The Joan Ganz Cooney Center at Sesame Workshop; 2016.

# Digital Media, Cognition, and Brain Development in Infancy and Childhood

Heather Kirkorian, Rachel Barr, Sarah M. Coyne, Tiffany Grace-Chung Munzer, Martin Paulus, and Moriah E. Thomason

## 1 Background

US children are using screen media more often and at younger ages than ever before. Daily reports of children's digital media use (i.e., "screen time") averaged roughly 49 minutes for children aged 0–2 years, 2.5 hours for those aged 2–4 years, just over 3 hours for those aged 5–8 years, and about 5.5 hours for those aged 8–12 years [1, 2]. The same studies showed that screen time at every age consists of watching TV and video content, particularly on streaming video platforms such as YouTube; however, preferences and behaviors change throughout childhood as gaming becomes more common and some children acquire their own devices. For more than half a century, the evolving media landscape has led to both widespread concern over the potential harms of media for cognition and brain development and optimism for the potential of media to teach and close achievement gaps [3].

An important consideration in the study of media effects is how early experience interacts with specific maturational processes; timing of exposure matters. Early childhood is a period of rapid brain development characterized by high sensitivity to early experience. The brain develops rapidly during the prenatal period such that the overall architecture of the brain is present at birth [4]. However, maturation is, by definition, a continuous process, and the brain is an organ in perpetual pursuit of environmental input. The early years are marked by the processes of synaptogenesis and pruning that are dynamic and nonlinear in nature, giving rise to systems known to be foundational to human cognition and lifelong brain health [5]. The brain continues to mature throughout childhood and into early adulthood, with girls generally attaining milestones earlier than boys [6]. Cortical thinning and synaptic pruning contribute to a reduction in gray matter volume, whereas white matter growth enhances neural communication and integration [5]. Both processes are shaped by environmental input in addition to genetic programs, creating opportuni-

H. Kirkorian (✉)
University of Wisconsin-Madison, Madison, WI, USA
e-mail: kirkorian@wisc.edu

R. Barr
Georgetown University, Washington, DC, USA

S. M. Coyne
Brigham Young University, Provo, UT, USA

T. G.-C. Munzer
University of Michigan, Ann Arbor, MI, USA

M. Paulus
University of California San Diego, La Jolla, CA, USA

M. E. Thomason
New York University Langone Medical Center, New York, NY, USA


D. A. Christakis, L. Hale (eds.), *Handbook of Children and Screens*,
https://doi.org/10.1007/978-3-031-69362-5_3

ties for early experience to affect brain development. Notably, regions associated with sensorimotor functions mature sooner than do those associated with higher-order cognitive functions [5]. As such, the impact of early experience on brain development depends on the timing and nature of exposure.

Potential mechanisms for media effects on cognition and brain development include both direct effects, as when sleep is disrupted by late-night media use or knowledge is gained by watching informational content, and indirect effects, as when media use displaces versus facilitates in-person interactions. Research on screen media, cognition, and brain development during the early lifespan falls into two broad categories. The first category considers how children process media in real time and the immediate effects of such use, including the degree to which early brain development and cognitive constraints shape whether and how children understand and learn from media. The second category considers the potential cumulative effects of repeated media use over time, including whether and how early media use relates to later cognitive abilities and the structure and function of the brain. In this chapter, we briefly summarize research in these areas, set a future research agenda, and propose recommendations for different stakeholder groups.

## 2 Current State

### 2.1 Children's Processing of Media

Cognitive constraints, such as emergent attention skills and working memory capacity, limit infants' comprehension of media [7]. Additionally, infants are primed for learning in the context of social interactions [8]. As such, infants exhibit a "transfer deficit," learning less from on-screen demonstrations than from equivalent real-life demonstrations [9]. This transfer deficit typically peaks at around 2 years of age, but it has also been observed in older children [10]. Nonetheless, even infants can learn from simple on-screen demonstrations, especially when those demonstrations are repeated [11]. Research is mixed regarding whether interactive media features (e.g., via video chat or touchscreen) help or hinder early learning from screens, likely depending on whether these features support versus distract from the lesson [12].

During their preschool years, children come to understand the relation between on-screen and real-life events [11] and they can learn from child-directed digital media that are designed to teach [13, 14]. However, they still have limited comprehension of more sophisticated TV content [15, 16] and touchscreen mechanics [17]. Through early adolescence, children gain a more advanced understanding of media conventions [18], and they show knowledge gains in wide-ranging domains after using carefully designed media [19–21].

Neural responses may help explain the differences in infants' learning from video versus real-life demonstrations. For example, electroencephalogram (EEG) studies show faster object recognition [22] and the presence of mu rhythm [23] (critical for social learning) when infants view objects and actions in person rather than on screen. Among preschool-aged children, neural responses also vary across media formats. For example, functional connectivity between and within neural networks (e.g., those associated with language versus visual processing) differ when young children listen to stories that vary in the degree of visual support (e.g., audio plus illustration or animation) [24, 25]. In older children, there may be other differences in neural network activation while using interactive media (e.g., digital games) versus viewing video [26], but this has not been tested directly. Together, current research suggests that the young brain processes information differently when presented in person versus on screen and that there may be other differences based on the type of media activity.

### 2.2 Associations Between Children's Media Use and Brain Structure and Function

Research on the associations between children's media use and their brain structure and function is beginning to emerge. Parent-reported adoption of less healthy media practices for their child (e.g., exceeding screen time recommendations, not co-using media with children) has been associated with lower white matter integrity in their 3- to 5-year-old children [27]. Additionally, higher screen use has been associated with lower cortical thickness in some regions of the brain in children aged 3–5 years [28] and 9–10 years [29]. It is unclear how to interpret findings in the cortical thickness studies because the nature of associations (i.e., higher versus lower cortical thickness) varies across brain regions and because cortical thinning is a natural part of the maturation process [5].

Most of these studies are cross-sectional and rely on parent reports of global screen time that overlook important moderators (e.g., media content and context). As such, much remains unknown regarding brain-behavior links and whether or how media use might play a causal role. For example, it is not clear whether early media experience alters brain circuitry, whether some early difference in brain circuitry leads to different media use patterns, or whether these associations are the result of some third factor that has not been considered. Nonetheless, this emergent literature provides a solid foundation on which to build future research.

## 2.3 Associations Between Children's Media Use and Cognitive Skills

There is a comparatively large body of research examining associations between early media use and cognitive skills. Findings across individual studies are mixed; meta-analytic reviews that average effects across studies typically report small negative associations or nonsignificant associations between children's overall screen time and cognitive skills, including attention, language, and academic achievement [30–33]. However, a careful examination of the literature reveals potential for both positive and negative effects of media use that vary across studies and individuals, driven in part by the content and context of media use. We consider each of these points below.

First, media content is an important moderator of media effects. By about 2 years of age, associations between screen time and cognitive skills are generally neutral or positive for child-directed educational media (i.e., media designed for children with an intent to incorporate informational content), especially when compared to noneducational entertainment (i.e., child-directed media without substantive informational content) or adult-directed content [13, 31]. Most research has focused on professionally produced media. User-generated content such as that found on YouTube may expose children to more consumerist, age-inappropriate, and violent content [34], but associations with young children's development have yet to be established.

In addition to media content, media design features influence children's learning and development. For example, studies have examined the impact of "hot spots" in touchscreen applications and digital books. In general, such features are more likely to support children's learning when they focus on, rather than distract from, the lesson [12, 35]. Other design features that are intended to prolong engagement (e.g., autoplay, behavioral reinforcement with frequent rewards) may be more likely to displace important developmental opportunities for young children and may have associations with greater child behavioral difficulties [36]. As such, these engagement-prolonging features merit further study.

The effects of media use on children also depend on both proximal (e.g., parenting style) and distal context factors (e.g., household income) [37]. For example, the impact of media use depends in part on its immediate social context. On the one hand, using media together can increase children's learning from media; on the other, solitary media use (by the parent or child) can disrupt ongoing parent-child interactions and children's play [11]. Moreover, parenting stress can predict how often children use media [38], and parents' specific use of media to calm young children may be particularly disruptive to children's development of self-regulatory abilities [39]. Together, this research underscores the importance of considering children's media use within the family system and the larger ecological context, both of which can influence the outcome of media use.

While studies to date have found that content and context moderate average media effects, it is clear that media effects also vary across individuals [40]. For instance, potentially problematic media use (e.g., preoccupation with media, sneaking media, meltdowns when media are removed) can emerge in some children as young as 4 years of age, and such behaviors were correlated with worse cognitive indicators such as hyperactivity and inattention [41]. In fact, negative associations with cognitive indicators were more consistent for parent reports of children's problematic media use behaviors than for parent reports of children's overall screen time [32]. Such findings indicate a need to better understand individual differences that might influence the degree of susceptibility to media effects and predict different developmental trajectories starting in early childhood [42].

One well-studied individual difference is age, which is a common proxy for developmental factors that may influence the degree of susceptibility to media effects [40]. As described earlier, the first few years after birth are characterized by rapid brain development, a strong orientation toward in-person interactions, and cognitive constraints that limit the degree to which infants learn from screen media. Thus, infants may be more susceptible to displacement effects (e.g., disruption of parent-child interaction) and less likely than older children to benefit from informational media content without joint media engagement [11]. This may explain why some studies find negative associations between media use and later cognitive skills when media use occurs in infancy but not when it occurs later in childhood [13]. Other periods of developmental susceptibility exist later in childhood, leading to different media effects in infants than in older children and adolescents [30]. For instance, television viewing may be particularly likely to displace leisure reading in the early school years, when reading is relatively difficult [43]. Together, this research illustrates the importance of a developmental lens, considering different windows of susceptibility to both positive and negative media effects across development.

Finally, the degree and direction of causality remain unclear since most research on children's media use and cognitive skills is based on cross-sectional research designs. Nonetheless, a growing set of longitudinal studies reveal complexity in associations. For example, some longitudinal studies suggest bidirectional effects such that media use could both contribute to and result from differences in cognition [44, 45]. Moreover, it is not clear whether longitudinal associations between early media use and later cognitive skills persist after controlling for potential confounding variables (e.g., demographic characteristics) [46–49]. Thus, while some meta-analytic studies report a small negative association between children's screen time and cognitive outcomes, the degree and direction of causality remain unclear.

## 3 Future Research

Research to date has revealed age-related changes in how children process media and the complex associations between children's media use and cognitive development. Moreover, studies are beginning to emerge regarding media use and brain structure and function. Collectively, research suggests that there is potential for both positive and negative effects of media use during early childhood, depending on its timing, content, and context. However, studies that lead to causal inference are still needed. It is critical for future research to leverage rigorous research designs that can isolate risk and protective factors to support positive development. Key questions for future research include:

- *How do different media experiences (e.g., variations in content and context) accumulate over time to produce divergent developmental trajectories?* Future research should use rigorous research designs to examine the potential mechanisms of media effects. For example, a small number of randomized controlled trials have compared the impact of different types of media content on developmental outcomes [50, 51]. Similarly, longitudinal studies should examine developmental trajectories over time while controlling for baseline skills (e.g., using cross-lagged analysis) and accounting for potential confounding or moderating variables.

- *Are there direct and/or indirect effects of early media use on brain structure and function, particularly as they relate to networks associated with higher-order skills (e.g., language)?* Future research should assess the degree and direction of causality, controlling for baseline measures and other confounds.
- *How do media design features for newer media affect cognitive development?* Future research should include careful examination of how children respond to persuasive design features (i.e., those designed to capture attention and prolong engagement) and new features designed to support learning from informational media (e.g., adaptive characters that respond to speech). Such research should apply a developmental lens, considering the role of cognitive, language, and motor constraints that change across development.
- *What is the interplay between direct and indirect effects of media use within the family system?* Future research should examine media use in context (e.g., in real time, in naturalistic settings) and seek to understand parents' motivations for their child's media use (e.g., whether and when benefits for one family member offset costs for another).
- *What modifiable factors can be targeted by personalized interventions designed to minimize problematic media use and promote positive media practices in the home?* Such research should include sufficiently large and diverse samples to enable subgroup analyses that identify differential susceptibilities (e.g., temperament, structural factors) to both negative and positive effects.

## 4 Recommendations

### 4.1 For Researchers

- Leverage cross-lagged longitudinal designs to examine temporal directionality and randomized controlled trials to test causality.
- Use rigorous, multi-method measures that can supplement self-report (e.g., continuous passive mobile sensing, direct observation) and that can capture the complexity of media use (e.g., time use diaries for media content and context).
- Adopt shared definitions and measurement of problematic versus supportive media use patterns, and measure systematically to enable comparison across studies.

### 4.2 For Parents and Other Caregivers

- Be mindful of digital distractions to ensure that each day has enough time for screen-free sleep, focused solitary activities, and high-quality family interactions (e.g., play, meals, reading).
- Be realistic about what young children can learn from digital media. Babies learn best from real people. For older children, try to use media together or ask questions about your child's media use to help your child connect what they see on the screen to their own life.
- When your child uses media, look for high-quality educational content and get freely available media tips and resources from non-profit organizations such as Common Sense Media, Zero to Three, PBS Kids, ChildTrends, and Children and Screens.

### 4.3 For Media Technology Providers

- Seek to incorporate child-centered design to maximize learning outcomes and healthy media habits while minimizing persuasive design practices that capture attention and keep kids engaged for extended periods of time.
- Share data with independent researchers seeking to minimize risks and maximize benefits of early media use.

### 4.4 For Policymakers

- Continue to invest in research on media in the lives of infants, children, and families, particularly for research that employs rigorous methods and measures, disentangles confounding factors, and seeks to establish temporal relations.
- Seek guidance from researchers to inform regulations aimed at reducing engagement-prolonging strategies that may be particularly detrimental to children.

### 4.5 For Clinicians

- Ask open-ended questions to understand how and why families use digital media.
- Encourage healthy media practices by focusing on quality (e.g., content and context).
- Watch for signs of potentially problematic media use (e.g., preoccupation with media, sneaking media, tantrums when media use ends), and help families identify strategies for managing challenging behaviors without digital media.

**Conflict of Interest and Funding Disclosures** HK, RB, and SMC are funded by the Eunice Kennedy Shriver National Institute of Child Health and Human Development (P01 HD109907). TG-CM is funded by the Eunice Kennedy Shriver National Institute of Child Health and Human Development (K23 HD105988-01). MET is funded by the National Institute on Drug Abuse (U01 DA055338), the National Institute of Mental Health (R01 MH122447; R01 MH126468; R01 MH125870), and the National Institute of Environmental Health Sciences (R01 ES032294).

## References

1. Rideout V, Peebles A, Mann S, Robb MB. Common sense census: media use by tweens and teens, 2021. Common Sense Media; 2022. Retrieved from www.commonsensemedia.org.
2. Rideout V, Robb MB. Common sense census: media use by kids age zero to eight. Common Sense Media; 2020. Retrieved from www.commonsensemedia.org.
3. Lauricella AR, Blackwell CK, Wartella E. The "new" technology environment: the role of content and context on learning and development from mobile media. In: Media exposure during infancy and early childhood: the effects of content and context on learning and development. Springer International Publishing AG; 2017. p. 1–23. https://doi.org/10.1007/978-3-319-45102-2_1.
4. van den Heuvel MI, Thomason ME. Functional connectivity of the human brain in utero. Trends Cogn Sci. 2016;20(12):931–9. https://doi.org/10.1016/j.tics.2016.10.001.
5. Gilmore JH, Knickmeyer RC, Gao W. Imaging structural and functional brain development in early childhood. Nat Rev Neurosci. 2018;19(3):123–37. https://doi.org/10.1038/nrn.2018.1.
6. Giedd JN, Blumenthal J, Jeffries NO, et al. Brain development during childhood and adolescence: a longitudinal MRI study. Nat Neurosci. 1999;2(10):861–3. https://doi.org/10.1038/13158.
7. Barr R, Kirkorian H. Reexamining models of early learning in the digital age: applications for learning in the wild. J Appl Res Mem Cogn. 2023;12(4):457–72. https://doi.org/10.1037/mac0000132.
8. Kuhl PK. Is speech learning 'gated' by the social brain? Dev Sci. 2007;10(1):110–20. https://doi.org/10.1111/j.1467-7687.2007.00572.x.
9. Strouse GA, Samson JE. Learning from video: a meta-analysis of the video deficit in children ages 0 to 6 years. Child Dev. 2021;92(1):e20–38. https://doi.org/10.1111/cdev.13429.
10. Kirkorian H, Simmering V. Searching in the sand: protracted video deficit in U.S. preschoolers' spatial recall using a continuous search space. Dev Sci:e13376. https://doi.org/10.1111/desc.13376.
11. Barr R. Growing up in the digital age: early learning and family media ecology. Curr Dir Psychol Sci. 2019;28(4):341–6. https://doi.org/10.1177/0963721419838245.
12. Kirkorian HL. When and how do interactive digital media help children connect what they see on and off the screen? Child Dev Perspect. 2018;12(3):210–4. https://doi.org/10.1111/cdep.12290.
13. Kostyrka-Allchorne K, Cooper NR, Simpson A. The relationship between television exposure and chil-

dren's cognition and behaviour: a systematic review. Dev Rev. 2017;44:19–58. https://doi.org/10.1016/j.dr.2016.12.002.
14. Griffith SF, Hagan MB, Heymann P, Heflin BH, Bagner DM. Apps as learning tools: a systematic review. Pediatrics. 2020;145(1):e20191579. https://doi.org/10.1542/peds.2019-1579.
15. Mares ML, Acosta EE. Be kind to three-legged dogs: Children's literal interpretations of TV's moral lessons. Media Psychol. 2008;11(3):377–99. https://doi.org/10.1080/15213260802204355.
16. Smith R, Anderson DR, Fischer C. Young children's comprehension of montage. Child Dev. 1985;56(4):962–71. https://doi.org/10.2307/1130108.
17. Cristia A, Seidl A. Parental reports on touch screen use in early childhood. PLoS One. 2015;10(6):e0128338. https://doi.org/10.1371/journal.pone.0128338.
18. Calvert SL, Scott MC. Television production feature effects on children's comprehension of time. J Appl Dev Psychol. 1988;9:263–73.
19. Clark DB, Tanner-Smith EE, Killingsworth SS. Digital games, design, and learning: a systematic review and meta-analysis. Rev Educ Res. 2016;86(1):79–122. https://doi.org/10.3102/0034654315582065.
20. Fisch SM. Bridging theory and practice: applying cognitive and educational theory to the design of educational media. In: Blumberg FC, Brooks PJ, editors. Cognitive development in digital contexts. Academic Press; 2017. p. 217–34. https://doi.org/10.1016/B978-0-12-809481-5.00011-0.
21. Fisch SM. Children's learning from educational television: sesame street and beyond. Routledge; 2004. https://www.routledge.com/Childrens-Learning-From-Educational-Television-Sesame-Street-and-Beyond/Fisch/p/book/9780805839364. Accessed 11 July 2021.
22. Carver LJ, Meltzoff AN, Dawson G. Event-related potential (ERP) indices of infants' recognition of familiar and unfamiliar objects in two and three dimensions. Dev Sci. 2006;9(1):51–62. https://doi.org/10.1111/j.1467-7687.2005.00463.x.
23. Ruysschaert L, Warreyn P, Wiersema JR, Metin B, Roeyers H. Neural mirroring during the observation of live and video actions in infants. Clin Neurophysiol. 2013;124(9):1765–70. https://doi.org/10.1016/j.clinph.2013.04.007.
24. Hutton JS, Dudley J, Horowitz-Kraus T, DeWitt T, Holland SK. Functional connectivity of attention, visual, and language networks during audio, illustrated, and animated stories in preschool-age children. Brain Connect. 2019;9(7):580–92. https://doi.org/10.1089/brain.2019.0679.
25. Hutton JS, Dudley J, Horowitz-Kraus T, DeWitt T, Holland SK. Differences in functional brain network connectivity during stories presented in audio, illustrated, and animated format in preschool-age children. Brain Imaging Behav. 2020;14(1):130–41. https://doi.org/10.1007/s11682-018-9985-y.
26. Anderson DR, Davidson MC. Receptive versus interactive video screens: a role for the brain's default mode network in learning from media. Comput Hum Behav. 2019;99:168–80. https://doi.org/10.1016/j.chb.2019.05.008.
27. Hutton JS, Huang G, Sahay RD, DeWitt T, Ittenbach RF. A novel, composite measure of screen-based media use in young children (ScreenQ) and associations with parenting practices and cognitive abilities. Pediatr Res. 2020;87(7):1211–8. https://doi.org/10.1038/s41390-020-0765-1.
28. Hutton JS, Dudley J, DeWitt T, Horowitz-Kraus T. Associations between digital media use and brain surface structural measures in preschool-aged children. Sci Rep. 2022;12(1):19095. https://doi.org/10.1038/s41598-022-20922-0.
29. Paulus MP, Squeglia LM, Bagot K, et al. Screen media activity and brain structure in youth: evidence for diverse structural correlation networks from the ABCD study. NeuroImage. 2019;185:140–53. https://doi.org/10.1016/j.neuroimage.2018.10.040.
30. Adelantado-Renau M, Moliner-Urdiales D, Cavero-Redondo I, Beltran-Valls MR, Martínez-Vizcaíno V, Álvarez-Bueno C. Association between screen media use and academic performance among children and adolescents. JAMA Pediatr. 2019;173(11):1058–67. https://doi.org/10.1001/jamapediatrics.2019.3176.
31. Madigan S, McArthur BA, Anhorn C, Eirich R, Christakis DA. Associations between screen use and child language skills: a systematic review and meta-analysis. JAMA Pediatr. 2020;174(7):665–75. https://doi.org/10.1001/jamapediatrics.2020.0327.
32. Mallawaarachchi SR, Anglim J, Hooley M, Horwood S. Associations of smartphone and tablet use in early childhood with psychosocial, cognitive and sleep factors: a systematic review and meta-analysis. Early Child Res Q. 2022;60:13–33. https://doi.org/10.1016/j.ecresq.2021.12.008.
33. Nikkelen SWC, Valkenburg PM, Huizinga M, Bushman BJ. Media use and ADHD-related behaviors in children and adolescents: a meta-analysis. Dev Psychol. 2014;50:2228–41. https://doi.org/10.1037/a0037318.
34. Radesky JS, Schaller A, Yeo SL, Weeks HM, Robb MB. *Young kids and YouTube: how ads, toys, and games dominate viewing*. Common Sense Media; 2020. https://www.commonsensemedia.org/research/young-kids-and-youtube-how-ads-toys-and-games-dominate-viewing.
35. Furenes MI, Kucirkova N, Bus AG. A comparison of children's reading on paper versus screen: a meta-analysis. Rev Educ Res. 2021;91(4):483–517. https://doi.org/10.3102/0034654321998074.
36. Munzer T, Torres C, Domoff SE, et al. Child media use during COVID-19: associations with contextual and social-emotional factors. J Dev Behav Pediatr. 2022;43(9):e573. https://doi.org/10.1097/DBP.0000000000001125.

37. Linebarger DL, Barr R, Lapierre MA, Piotrowski JT. Associations between parenting, media use, cumulative risk, and children's executive functioning. J Dev Behav Pediatr. 2014;35(6):367–77. https://doi.org/10.1097/DBP.0000000000000069.
38. Shin E, Choi K, Resor J, Smith CL. Why do parents use screen media with toddlers? The role of child temperament and parenting stress in early screen use. Infant Behav Dev. 2021;64:101595. https://doi.org/10.1016/j.infbeh.2021.101595.
39. Coyne SM, Shawcroft J, Gale M, et al. Tantrums, toddlers and technology: temperament, media emotion regulation, and problematic media use in early childhood. Comput Hum Behav. 2021;120:106762. https://doi.org/10.1016/j.chb.2021.106762.
40. Valkenburg P, Peter J. The differential susceptibility to media effects model. J Commun. 2013;63(2):221–43. https://doi.org/10.1111/jcom.12024.
41. Domoff SE, Harrison K, Gearhardt AN, Gentile DA, Lumeng JC, Miller AL. Development and validation of the problematic media use measure: a parent report measure of screen media "addiction" in children. Psychol Pop Media Cult. 2019;8:2–11. https://doi.org/10.1037/ppm0000163.
42. Barr R, Kirkorian H, Coyne S, Radesky J. Early childhood and digital media. Cambridge University Press; 2024. https://www.cambridge.org/core/elements/early-childhood-and-digital-media/226523438D797D8785837568EFCAB89B. Accessed 16 Apr 2024.
43. Ennemoser M, Schneider W. Relations of television viewing and reading: findings from a 4-year longitudinal study. J Educ Psychol. 2007;99:349–68. https://doi.org/10.1037/0022-0663.99.2.349.
44. Cliff DP, Howard SJ, Radesky JS, McNeill J, Vella SA. Early childhood media exposure and self-regulation: bidirectional longitudinal associations. Acad Pediatr. 2018;18(7):813–9. https://doi.org/10.1016/j.acap.2018.04.012.
45. Gentile DA, Swing EL, Lim CG, Khoo A. Video game playing, attention problems, and impulsiveness: evidence of bidirectional causality. Psychol Pop Media Cult. 2012;1:62–70. https://doi.org/10.1037/a0026969.
46. McBee MT, Brand RJ, Dixon WE. Challenging the link between early childhood television exposure and later attention problems: a multiverse approach. Psychol Sci. 2021;32(4):496–518. https://doi.org/10.1177/0956797620971650.
47. Portugal AM, Bedford R, Cheung CHM, Gliga T, Smith TJ. Saliency-driven visual search performance in toddlers with low– vs high–touch screen use. JAMA Pediatr. 2021;175(1):96–7. https://doi.org/10.1001/jamapediatrics.2020.2344.
48. Portugal AM, Bedford R, Cheung CHM, Mason L, Smith TJ. Longitudinal touchscreen use across early development is associated with faster exogenous and reduced endogenous attention control. Sci Rep. 2021;11(1):2205. https://doi.org/10.1038/s41598-021-81775-7.
49. Portugal AM, Hendry A, Smith TJ, Bedford R. Do pre-schoolers with high touchscreen use show executive function differences? Comput Hum Behav. 2023;139:107553. https://doi.org/10.1016/j.chb.2022.107553.
50. Christakis DA, Garrison MM, Herrenkohl T, et al. Modifying media content for preschool children: a randomized controlled trial. Pediatrics. 2013;131(3):431–8. https://doi.org/10.1542/peds.2012-1493.
51. Griffith SF, Hanson KG, Rolon-Arroyo B, Arnold DH. Promoting early achievement in low-income preschoolers in the United States with educational apps. J Child Media. Published online July 3, 2019. https://www.tandfonline.com/doi/full/10.1080/17482798.2019.1613246. Accessed 16 Apr 2024.

# Digital Media, Cognition, and Brain Development in Adolescence

Laura Marciano, Bernadka Dubicka, Lucía Magis-Weinberg, Rosalba Morese, Kasisomayajula Viswanath, and René Weber

## 1 Background

Today, digital media use is a ubiquitous aspect of adolescent life. In 2022, almost half of US adolescents reported being constantly online, with favorite activities including engaging in social media activities, playing games, and consuming short videos (95% YouTube, 67% TikTok, 62% Instagram, 59% Snapchat), primarily accessed through smartphones [1]. Among other devices, the smartphone is perceived as highly attractive since it provides quick, emotionally rewarding experiences, with potential mechanisms involving reward circuits in the brain. Due to its pervasiveness, there is concern about habitual engagement with smartphones and other digital devices, affirmed by prevalence data indicating that almost one out of four adolescents [2] report symptoms of problematic ("addictive") digital media use, including cognitive salience (e.g., constantly thinking about smartphone/social media activities), mood modification (e.g., experiencing negative mood when unable to use smartphone/social media), tolerance and withdrawal symptoms, conflict with other people due to excessive smartphone/social media use, loss of control over the use, and interference with functioning. However, the term "problematic media use" is preferred by experts, given the imprecision of the term "addictive." Rate estimates of problematic use are highly variable, depending

We thank Kylie Woodman, University of California Santa Barbara, Media Neuroscience Lab, Department of Communication, for her insightful contribution to this chapter.

L. Marciano (✉) · K. Viswanath
Lee Kum Sheung Center for Health and Happiness, Harvard T.H. Chan School of Public Health, Boston, MA, USA
e-mail: lmarciano@hsph.harvard.edu

B. Dubicka
Health Sciences, Hull & York Medical School, University of York, York, UK

Greater Manchester Mental Health Trust, Manchester, UK

Manchester Academic Health Science Centre (MAHSC), University of Manchester, Manchester, UK

L. Magis-Weinberg
Department of Psychology, University of Washington, Seattle, WA, USA

R. Morese
Faculty of Biomedical Sciences, Faculty of Communication, Culture and Society, Università della Svizzera italiana, Lugano, Switzerland

R. Weber
Department of Communication, University of California, Santa Barbara, CA, USA

Department of Psychological & Brain Sciences, University of California, Santa Barbara, CA, USA

Department of Communication and Media, Ewha Womans University, Seoul, South Korea
e-mail: renew@ucsb.edu


D. A. Christakis, L. Hale (eds.), *Handbook of Children and Screens*,
https://doi.org/10.1007/978-3-031-69362-5_4

on factors including population characteristics, measures used, contexts, and the presence of mental health problems [3].

In this chapter, we summarize selected recent studies focusing on how digital media use is related to measures of adolescent cognition and brain structure and function. Research in this field is still at an early stage and mainly based on cross-sectional studies, often measuring general self-reported screen time (including different types of media activities), which is now considered outdated [4] unless specific hypotheses (e.g., time displacement) are tested.

### 1.1 Cognitive and Brain Development in Adolescence

To understand how digital media use is related to adolescent brain development and cognition, we should first consider the underlying neural developmental processes. Adolescence is a period in which brain networks go through significant changes influenced by biological and environmental factors [5]. During adolescence, socio-emotional incentive and reward processing networks mature before brain regions necessary for cognitive control which undergo protracted development [6]. Maturation imbalance theories posit that this asynchrony predisposes adolescents to be overly influenced by the social environment and rewards, through the activity of the affective-motivational system [7]. Cognitive control is the ability to regulate behavior in line with goals and plans [8]. The prolonged development of the brain areas dedicated to cognitive control skills arises from the need to assemble "simpler" components, such as working memory, inhibition, and monitoring, into more complex processes such as reasoning, sustaining control across extended periods of time, abstract thinking, and decision and judgment making [9]. The increase in adolescent cognitive control drives advancements in learning and successful adaptations to varied social contexts and cultural influences [9]. The structural and functional development of the prefrontal cortex (PFC), in interaction with the more posterior parietal brain regions, underlies the maturation of higher cognitive abilities [10]. Different subregions participate in the maturational process of the PFC [8]: the dorsolateral prefrontal cortex (DLPFC), which guides the development of cognitive skills such as working memory, planning abilities, and self-control, and the orbitofrontal/ventromedial prefrontal cortex (OFC/VMPFC), which is related to the regulation of emotional responses.

Due to the still-maturing cognitive control system, adolescents' behavior is more strongly influenced by the affective or social context than is observed in adults. Adolescents are highly sensitive to the anticipation and receipt of rewards in affective tasks, when emotions are involved or peers are present [11]. As a result, socio-affective information is more salient and exerts a disproportionately strong modulation of decisions, actions, and regulation in adolescence [12]. The affective-motivational system includes subcortical regions like the amygdala, hippocampus, and striatum, including the nucleus accumbens, caudate, putamen, and globus pallidus [9]. During adolescence, increased dopaminergic activity increases reactivity to rewards and impulsivity [10] and the augmented functional connectivity between subcortical regions with the PFC enhances the regulation of motivation, emotions, and goal-oriented behaviors. However, the PFC does not reach complete maturation until 25 years of age [13]. When it comes to digital media use, large datasets have shown that the windows of developmental sensitivity vary between males (14–15 years) and females (11–13 years) depending on maturational processes, notably puberty. Yet, a common susceptibility window has been found in late adolescents at 19 years for both sexes, probably due to life-changing events like leaving home and social adjustments [14].

## 2 Current State

### 2.1 Digital Media Use and the Adolescent Brain

Although research on the neural correlates of digital media use in adolescents is still in its infancy, a scoping review [15] summarized the results of 16 neuroimaging studies of screen time and problematic digital media use. Mostly cross-sectional, the results showed that frequent and longer screen time (measured as hours per day) and problematic media usage behaviors (including Internet, social media, and smartphone problematic use)—defined as compulsive use with characteristics typical of behavioral addictions [16]—were related to diminished functional and structural connectivity of top-down cognitive control structures for that age. In particular, reduced connectivity was found in the brain areas involved in attentional and control networks (e.g., the default mode network, DMN; the central executive network, CEN). Additionally, digital media use was positively correlated with activations in the reward regions (including the striatum and the ventral tegmental area (VTA)). These findings align with the adolescent preference for motivational states valuing instant rewards. For example, one study showed that receiving "likes" on Instagram activates the gratification system to the same extent as receiving money [17]. In other words, we can draw an analogy for access to digital media content via smartphones by comparing it to "little sweets in adolescents' pockets" that are always available and with innovative and attractive new features like different "flavors." A narrative review found similar brain correlates of cognitive control in adolescents experiencing Internet gaming disorder (IGD) and problematic Internet use symptoms [3]. For example, adolescents with IGD and problematic Internet use also had structural changes in the anterior and posterior cingulate cortex, DLPFC, and OFC. Included studies suggested that inefficient regulation of the prefrontal cortical regions could augment the risk of developing compulsive habits, including overuse of the Internet. Moreover, alterations in the insula, which integrates interoceptive signals (i.e., information about the autonomic nervous system activities, including changes in respiration, blood pressure, gut functioning, and salivation) [18] to motivate future behaviors, would foster perseverance to reach the same rewarding goals.

Further results come from large-scale studies. In particular, structural imaging data were collected from 4277 youths taking part in the Adolescent Brain Cognitive Development (ABCD) study [19], the largest long-term study of brain development in the United States, including 21 research sites and started in 2015, with the aim of tracking biological and behavioral developmental outcomes from 9 to 10 years of age into young adulthood. This multicenter study assessed different health outcomes (including neurocognition, physical and mental health, social and emotional functions, and culture and environment) and brain development (using structural and functional brain imaging data and bioassays). However, although the ABCD study aims to follow participants throughout adolescence, current published data refer mostly to the earlier waves of data collection, which includes participants in late childhood (aged 9–10 years). Information on different screen media activities, including watching television, playing games, and using social media, were collected and analyzed in relation to brain correlates. Children who were frequently exposed to screens showed greater structural maturation of the brain areas related to the visual system and sensory processing [19]. In addition, the complex link between screen media activities and brain structure was examined by looking at psychopathological correlates, and the results showed correlations with the overall externalizing symptomatology, including rule breaking and aggressive behaviors assessed with the Child Behavior Checklist (CBCL).

## 2.2 Social Media and Socioemotional Development

A narrative review by Crone and Konijn [20] reported diverse mechanisms through which social media can impact adolescents' socioemotional cognitive development. Although some of the mechanisms are not drawn from studies looking directly at social media activities, they are an optimal starting point to comprehend the effects of the social dynamics that can happen online. For example, after an experience of social exclusion (using the Cyberball paradigm), brain imaging data (functional MRI (fMRI)) showed stronger activations in the regions implicated in arousal and negative affect, like the OFC, insula, and anterior cingulate cortex (ACC), indicating high sensitivity of the adolescent brain to social rejection. Considering that adolescents report higher expectations of being rejected by peers online (i.e., receiving negative feedback) when compared to adults, it seems reasonable to speculate that they might easily experience high arousal and negative emotions to others' feedback on social media when it involves exclusion, dislike, and cyberbullying. Frequent exposure to possible negative social experiences online at any time can foster negative mood over time in a way that is more pervasive with respect to real-time situations (which are limited in time and space). As a consequence, since the affective cognitive control system is still undeveloped and adolescents lack skills to manage strong negative emotions, this can predispose them to be more negatively affected by negative social experiences, especially if they have a mental health disorder [21]. However, few have examined the impact of mental health conditions, which can in themselves be the underlying driver of cognitive changes and digital media use. Hence, screen time can be just "one unfortunate correlate" of a broader underlying disorder. Adolescents are also generally highly sensitive to peer influence and adjust their behaviors to peer and group norms. In particular, adolescents tend to respond with increased emotional intensity and larger recruitment of socio-affective brain circuitry while processing social information [11]. This also occurs in social media, where youths might follow trends dictated by other peers. Increased peer orientation and sensitivity to peer approval make digital platforms such as social media and multi-player video games significantly more rewarding for teens. Adolescent sensitivity to social cues can be related to the type of social media use. In a recent study, social media checking behaviors (i.e., frequency) in early adolescence have been found to predict changes in neural sensitivity to rewards after completing a social incentive delay task in a 3-year longitudinal study [22]. Adolescents who habitually checked social media recruited different neural networks and showed increased sensitivity to social cues like anticipation of social rewards and punishments when compared to those engaging in fewer checking activities.

## 2.3 Digital Media Use and Adolescent Cognition

In addition to socioemotional impacts, there are increasing concerns about effects in terms of attention and academic disruption. Research investigating the role of smartphone (over-)use in academic achievement has consistently highlighted a negative relationship between the time spent using social media and academic performance [23]. A potential mechanism at play could be the balance between reward and cognitive effort. Attention allocated to media activities depends on a cognitive "priority map" [24, p. 19], which integrates top-down, bottom-up, and (learned) motivational signals into a common representational space that categorizes each media activity depending on how (i) rewarding it is and (ii) the amount of cognitive effort required. Rewarding tasks are preferred in the first place, and higher rewards for one task decrease the available attentional resource for another task. Considering that the adolescent brain is sensitive to rewarding content, and still developing cognitive capacities, it is likely that these effects are magnified during adolescence.

The cross-sectional ABCD data of children aged 9–10 years [25] showed that meeting recommendations for screen time (set at less than 2 hours per day), sleeping 9-11 hours per night, and doing at least 1 hour of physical activity per day, was positively related to higher global cognition. Similar results were found in a study looking at school grades at the end of the year [26], which were higher in adolescents meeting the recommendations for screen time, sleep, and physical activity assessed in spring during the school year. When students reported multitasking with different media during their leisure time, grades decreased with a negative gradient for each additional media multitasking activity [26]. One study with data from more than 12,000 adolescents performing psychometric tests of intelligence, spatial perception, information processing, and numeracy showed negligible-to-small correlations with overall social media usage time (including active, passive, and problematic use) [27]. When looking at the daily dynamics, a study using in situ assessments reported that digital media use and frequency of messaging activities were both associated with augmented symptoms of inattention on the same day [28], controlling for baseline reported symptoms. However, the results might have been related to other confounding factors that were not considered, like differences in socioeconomic status, or other ongoing daily activities.

## 3 Future Research

There is emerging evidence that adolescents' use of digital media for prolonged periods, very frequently, or in a problematic way is associated with differences in the brain regions related to cognitive control and reward systems, small associations with psychometric tests, and decreased school performance when teens frequently multitask. However, the majority of the MRI studies have been mainly cross-sectional using small, nonrepresentative samples, thus impeding the inference of cause-effect mechanisms, with the exception of the ABCD study. Several gaps should be addressed in future research.

### 3.1 Research Design and Assessment

Longitudinal studies with larger samples should assess causality and directionality and consider neural changes happening in early, middle, and late adolescence, possibly using accelerated longitudinal designs, which allow following different age cohorts simultaneously, or randomized controlled trials (of the effects of disconnection) and experiments (e.g., by exploring media effects on the brain and cognition during different tasks) to show causality. Experimental approaches [29] or computational modeling approaches [30, 31] hold promise to investigate mechanisms. Limited validity of self-report data of media use due to estimation, recall, and social desirability biases can be overcome by integrating trace data and in situ assessments of specific screen media use. Cognitive outcomes should be assessed through validated cognitive assessment measures and tests (e.g., borrowed from neuropsychology and adapted to the actual context), and mental health symptoms and well-being measures should be combined with biomarkers [32]. Considering that effects have been consistently reported as bidirectional, varying from adolescent to adolescent though overall small in the general population [33–35], we suggest assessing them in longitudinal studies looking at the direction of the effect. Importantly, considering that large-scale datasets showed that the links between social media use and constructs such as life satisfaction have been described as tiny, inconsistent, gender-dependent, and with great variability due to how data are analyzed [36], we can expect the same for cognitive development and brain correlates..

Moreover, there is still little research on the brain areas engaged in emotion regulation processes during adolescence, like the VMPFC, which crucially links the cortical and subcortical structures responsible for modulating negative emotions like the ones related to suicidal ideation [37]. More attention should be given to the investigation of brain correlates and cognitive processes related to the adverse consequences of digital media use such as gambling, bullying, grooming, self-harm, and exposure to eating disorder websites [38]. Importantly, digital media use may explain only an extremely small percentage of variance in adolescent well-being in the nonclinical population [36] and negligible-to-small effects have also been found regarding adolescent cognition and brain development [27]. However, considering that the majority of the studies are based on the general population, more specific studies are required in at-risk populations and specific minorities (e.g., LGBTQIA+ population, minoritized communities in the Global North, and teens living in the Global South), for which we still do not know the size and direction of the effect. Focusing on adolescents from different socioeconomic backgrounds, contexts (e.g., urban versus rural), genders, and ethnicities would allow us to delineate which groups are at risk of disproportionately negative effects of digital media use on cognitive and brain development, thus reducing the problem of "data absenteeism" [39]. Data on the potential correlates and impact of digital media use on the brain and cognition of adolescents with mental health conditions are also limited.

## 3.2 A Theory-Driven Approach

Additionally, studies should include more detailed and theory-driven assessments of digital media content, motivations, and meanings, thus moving beyond time and frequency. For example, theory-driven assessments can be guided by conceptual frameworks like social media elements, which comprise profiles, networks, messages, and streams (including relevant processes, challenges, and affordances) [40]. Similarly, research should define the concept of a digital "extended mind" [41] in adolescence, describing how human cognition may be coupled with the digital environment. Finally, more adolescent data are needed to explore the effects of short-term and simultaneous engagements with digital media (e.g., media multitasking) related to what is called "divided attention." Generalized recommendations for limits on digital media use should be considered only if screen time starts to displace activities needed for healthy living, such as sleep, diet, fresh air, exercise, and face-to-face social activities, or if there is a concern about potentially harmful types of online content or interactions, for example, gambling, bullying, or online grooming. Eventually, cognitive processes and brain correlates of digital media use can be mediated by third variables, including quantity and quality of sleep [42] and physical fitness [43].

## 3.3 Potential Positive Evidence of Media in Adolescence

More studies should also assess the positive effects of digital media use on cognition, especially with regard to learning at different ages of cognitive development. For example, adolescents from low- and-middle-income countries (LMICs) are usually the first to adopt new technologies compared to adults and caregivers, who might lack digital literacy skills to guide the safe use of social media and smartphones [44]. In LMICs, schools might be the first space where early adolescents learn digital skills, including digital resilience, and healthy habits. Empowering young people through education and developing digital resilience from an early age is an important strategy for the development of healthy digital use. Yet, at the same time, it is important to consider what adolescents access and are exposed to, especially when it comes to violent and harassing content. We should consider how different adolescents can be particularly vulnerable to the effects of digital media, leading to the presence of a "digital divide," which can be alleviated by parental digital literacy, active mediation, and discussion of online activity.

# 4 Recommendations

## 4.1 For Clinicians and Providers

- Clinicians and providers should consider the potential effects of digital media use on adolescents' cognition and brain development as well as mental health disorders.
- Generic recommendations regarding limiting screen time in adolescence is problematic when the underlying cause and effect mechanisms remain unclear. We suggest a personalized approach to digital resilience, including to better educate providers about what digital resilience is.
- In developing recommendations, both positive and negative impacts of digital media should be considered as well as individual vulnerabilities.

### 4.2 For Policymakers

- Policymakers need to compel tech companies to share their digital media use data and support independent, scholarly research within an appropriate ethical framework.
- Policymakers should also regulate access to inappropriate content, limit the possibility of engaging in cyberbullying and cyber stalking behaviors, establish common labeling standards to ensure consistency and facilitate content sharing, and moderate platform content in a rigorous and controlled way.

### 4.3 For Educators

- Educators should promote digital media literacy and help adolescents navigate the digital media environment safely, by creating new opportunities to learn through digital media and develop digital resilience.
- Educators should be able to promote healthy digital use by using screens in the classrooms and virtual learning when needed, minimizing multitasking, and vet content advertised as educational.
- Educators should also be aware of adolescents who can be more at risk of developing problematic use of digital technologies and redirect students to proper resources.

**Conflict of Interest and Funding Disclosures** LM is funded by the Swiss National Science Foundation (Grant No. P500PS_202974).

## References

1. Atske S. Teens, social media and technology 2022. Pew Research Center: Internet, Science & Tech. Published August 10, 2022. https://www.pewresearch.org/internet/2022/08/10/teens-social-media-and-technology-2022/. Accessed 7 Dec 2022.
2. Sohn S, Rees P, Wildridge B, Kalk NJ, Carter B. Prevalence of problematic smartphone usage and associated mental health outcomes amongst children and young people: a systematic review, meta-analysis and GRADE of the evidence. BMC Psychiatry. 2019;19(1):356. https://doi.org/10.1186/s12888-019-2350-x.
3. Cerniglia L, Zoratto F, Cimino S, Laviola G, Ammaniti M, Adriani W. Internet addiction in adolescence: neurobiological, psychosocial and clinical issues. Neurosci Biobehav Rev. 2017;76(Pt A):174–84. https://doi.org/10.1016/j.neubiorev.2016.12.024.
4. Valkenburg PM, Beyens I, Meier A, Vanden Abeele MMP. Advancing our understanding of the associations between social media use and well-being. Curr Opin Psychol. 2022;47:101357. https://doi.org/10.1016/j.copsyc.2022.101357.
5. Casey BJ, Getz S, Galvan A. The adolescent brain. Dev Rev. 2008;28(1):62–77. https://doi.org/10.1016/j.dr.2007.08.003.
6. Mills KL, Goddings AL, Clasen LS, Giedd JN, Blakemore SJ. The developmental mismatch in structural brain maturation during adolescence. Dev Neurosci. 2014;36(3–4):147–60. https://doi.org/10.1159/000362328.
7. van Duijvenvoorde ACK, Peters S, Braams BR, Crone EA. What motivates adolescents? Neural responses to rewards and their influence on adolescents' risk taking, learning, and cognitive control. Neurosci Biobehav Rev. 2016;70:135–47. https://doi.org/10.1016/j.neubiorev.2016.06.037.
8. Caballero A, Granberg R, Tseng KY. Mechanisms contributing to prefrontal cortex maturation during adolescence. Neurosci Biobehav Rev. 2016;70:4–12. https://doi.org/10.1016/j.neubiorev.2016.05.013.
9. Crone EA, Dahl RE. Understanding adolescence as a period of social–affective engagement and goal flexibility. Nat Rev Neurosci. 2012;13(9):636–50. https://doi.org/10.1038/nrn3313.
10. Larsen B, Luna B. Adolescence as a neurobiological critical period for the development of higher-order cognition. Neurosci Biobehav Rev. 2018;94:179–95. https://doi.org/10.1016/j.neubiorev.2018.09.005.
11. Somerville LH. The teenage brain: sensitivity to social evaluation. Curr Dir Psychol Sci. 2013;22(2):121–7. https://doi.org/10.1177/0963721413476512.
12. Casey BJ, Duhoux S, Cohen MM. Adolescence: what do transmission, transition, and translation have to do with it? Neuron. 2010;67(5):749–60. https://doi.org/10.1016/j.neuron.2010.08.033.
13. Arain M, Haque M, Johal L, et al. Maturation of the adolescent brain. Neuropsychiatr Dis Treat. 2013;9:449–61. https://doi.org/10.2147/NDT.S39776.
14. Orben A, Przybylski AK, Blakemore SJ, Kievit RA. Windows of developmental sensitivity to social media. Nat Commun. 2022;13(1):1649. https://doi.org/10.1038/s41467-022-29296-3.
15. Marciano L, Camerini AL, Morese R. The developing brain in the digital era: a scoping review of structural and functional correlates of screen time in adolescence. Front Psychol. 2021;12:671817. https://doi.org/10.3389/fpsyg.2021.671817.
16. Jo YS, Bhang SY, Choi JS, Lee HK, Lee SY, Kweon YS. Clinical characteristics of diagnosis for internet

gaming disorder: comparison of DSM-5 IGD and ICD-11 GD diagnosis. J Clin Med. 2019;8(7):945. https://doi.org/10.3390/jcm8070945.
17. Sherman LE, Payton AA, Hernandez LM, Greenfield PM, Dapretto M. The power of the like in adolescence: effects of peer influence on neural and behavioral responses to social Media. Psychol Sci. 2016;27(7):1027–35. https://doi.org/10.1177/0956797616645673.
18. Gasquoine PG. Contributions of the insula to cognition and emotion. Neuropsychol Rev. 2014;24(2):77–87. https://doi.org/10.1007/s11065-014-9246-9.
19. Paulus MP, Squeglia LM, Bagot K, et al. Screen media activity and brain structure in youth: evidence for diverse structural correlation networks from the ABCD study. Neuroimage. 2019;185:140–53. https://doi.org/10.1016/j.neuroimage.2018.10.040.
20. Crone EA, Konijn EA. Media use and brain development during adolescence. Nat Commun. 2018;9(1):588. https://doi.org/10.1038/s41467-018-03126-x.
21. Royal College of Psychiatrists. Technology use and the mental health of children and young people; 2020. https://www.rcpsych.ac.uk/docs/default-source/improving-care/better-mh-policy/college-reports/college-report-cr225.pdf.
22. Maza MT, Fox KA, Kwon SJ, et al. Association of habitual checking behaviors on social media with longitudinal functional brain development. JAMA Pediatr. 2023;177(2):160–7. https://doi.org/10.1001/jamapediatrics.2022.4924.
23. Cao X, Masood A, Luqman A, Ali A. Excessive use of mobile social networking sites and poor academic performance: antecedents and consequences from stressor-strain-outcome perspective. Comput Hum Behav. 2018;85:163–74. https://doi.org/10.1016/j.chb.2018.03.023.
24. Fisher JT, Hopp FR, Weber R. Mapping attention across multiple media tasks. Media Psychol. 2023;26(5):505–29. https://doi.org/10.1080/15213269.2022.2161576.
25. Walsh JJ, Barnes JD, Cameron JD, et al. Associations between 24 hour movement behaviours and global cognition in US children: a cross-sectional observational study. Lancet Child Adolesc Health. 2018;2(11):783–91. https://doi.org/10.1016/S2352-4642(18)30278-5.
26. Marciano L, Camerini AL. Recommendations on screen time, sleep and physical activity: associations with academic achievement in Swiss adolescents. Public Health. 2021;198:211–7. https://doi.org/10.1016/j.puhe.2021.07.027.
27. Stieger S, Wunderl S. Associations between social media use and cognitive abilities: results from a large-scale study of adolescents. Comput Hum Behav. 2022;135:107358. https://doi.org/10.1016/j.chb.2022.107358.
28. George MJ, Russell MA, Piontak JR, Odgers CL. Concurrent and subsequent associations between daily digital technology use and high-risk adolescents' mental health symptoms. Child Dev. 2018;89(1):78–88. https://doi.org/10.1111/cdev.12819.
29. Wikman P, Moisala M, Ylinen A, et al. Brain responses to peer feedback in social media are modulated by valence in late adolescence. Front Behav Neurosci. 2022;16:790478. https://doi.org/10.3389/fnbeh.2022.790478.
30. Lindström B, Bellander M, Schultner DT, Chang A, Tobler PN, Amodio DM. A computational reward learning account of social media engagement. Nat Commun. 2021;12(1):1311. https://doi.org/10.1038/s41467-020-19607-x.
31. Ferguson AM, Turner G, Orben A. Social uncertainty in the digital world. Trends Cogn Sci. 2024;28(4):286–9. https://doi.org/10.1016/j.tics.2024.02.005.
32. Carvalho AF, Solmi M, Sanches M, et al. Evidence-based umbrella review of 162 peripheral biomarkers for major mental disorders. Transl Psychiatry. 2020;10(1):1–13. https://doi.org/10.1038/s41398-020-0835-5.
33. Beyens I, Pouwels JL, van Driel II, Keijsers L, Valkenburg PM. Social media use and adolescents' well-being: developing a typology of person-specific effect patterns. Commun Res. Published online December 13, 2021:00936502211038196. https://doi.org/10.1177/00936502211038196.
34. Beyens I, Pouwels JL, van Driel II, Keijsers L, Valkenburg PM. The effect of social media on well-being differs from adolescent to adolescent. Sci Rep. 2020;10(1):10763. https://doi.org/10.1038/s41598-020-67727-7.
35. Marciano L, Driver CC, Schulz PJ, Camerini AL. Dynamics of adolescents' smartphone use and well-being are positive but ephemeral. Sci Rep. 2022;12(1):1316. https://doi.org/10.1038/s41598-022-05291-y.
36. Orben A, Przybylski AK. The association between adolescent well-being and digital technology use. Nat Hum Behav. 2019;3(2):173–82. https://doi.org/10.1038/s41562-018-0506-1.
37. Morese R, Longobardi C. Suicidal ideation in adolescence: a perspective view on the role of the ventromedial prefrontal cortex. Front Psychol. 2020;11:713. https://doi.org/10.3389/fpsyg.2020.00713.
38. Idelji-Tehrani S, Dubicka B, Graham R. The clinical implications of digital technology. Clin Child Psychol Psychiatry. 2023;28(1):338–53. https://doi.org/10.1177/13591045221145400.
39. Lee EWJ, Viswanath K. Big data in context: addressing the twin perils of data absenteeism and chauvinism in the context of health disparities research. J Med Internet Res. 2020;22(1):e16377. https://doi.org/10.2196/16377.
40. Bayer JB, Triệu P, Ellison NB. Social media elements, ecologies, and effects. Annu Rev Psychol. 2020;71:471–97. https://doi.org/10.1146/annurev-psych-010419-050944.
41. Barr N, Pennycook G, Stolz JA, Fugelsang JA. The brain in your pocket: evidence that smartphones

are used to supplant thinking. Comput Hum Behav. 2015;48:473–80. https://doi.org/10.1016/j.chb.2015.02.029.
42. Tarokh L, Saletin JM, Carskadon MA. Sleep in adolescence: physiology, cognition and mental health. Neurosci Biobehav Rev. 2016;70:182–8. https://doi.org/10.1016/j.neubiorev.2016.08.008.
43. Esteban-Cornejo I, Tejero-Gonzalez CM, Sallis JF, Veiga OL. Physical activity and cognition in adolescents: a systematic review. J Sci Med Sport. 2015;18(5):534–9. https://doi.org/10.1016/j.jsams.2014.07.007.
44. Magis-Weinberg L, Ballonoff Suleiman A, Dahl RE. Context, development, and digital media: implications for very young adolescents in LMICs. Front Psychol. 2021;12:632713. https://doi.org/10.3389/fpsyg.2021.632713.

# The Short- and Long-Term Effects of Digital Media Use on Attention

Susanne E. Baumgartner, Douglas A. Parry, Ine Beyens, Wisnu Wiradhany, Melina Uncapher, Anthony D. Wagner, and Daphné Bavelier

## 1 Background

Digital media, such as smartphones, tablets, and gaming consoles, are omnipresent in the lives of children and adolescents. With their highly gratifying nature, their promise of constant entertainment, and connection to friends, digital media exert a strong cognitive and emotional pull. It has become increasingly difficult for children to resist these omnipresent media temptations, and it is thus not surprising that most US teenagers report that they are "almost always online" [1]. Even though youth Internet access varies globally, most teenagers in the Global South also use digital technologies, with Asian countries showing the highest rates of child Internet use [2]. Digital media use is highly interwoven into youths' daily activities, and media multitasking—using media while engaging in other media or non-media-related tasks—has become a highly prevalent form of media use [3].

Due to the ubiquitous nature of digital media in youths' lives, concerns have been raised that digital media might negatively affect attention. For children and adolescents, these concerns mainly revolve around two questions. First, what are the momentary, short-term effects of digital media on attention and processing (e.g., while studying or doing homework)? Second, what are the sustained, long-term effects of frequent media distractions and media multitasking on youths' ability to focus and sustain attention? In this chapter, we provide an overview of the current state of the literature on these two issues and highlight the most important research gaps and directions for future research.

## 2 Current State

### 2.1 Momentary Effects of Digital Distractions

In the past decade, dozens of studies have investigated digital distractions. Most have focused on the immediate distractions posed by smartphones and social media during academic activities like attending classes and lectures or during

S. E. Baumgartner (✉) · I. Beyens
University of Amsterdam,
Amsterdam, The Netherlands
e-mail: s.e.baumgartner@uva.nl

D. A. Parry
Stellenbosch University,
Stellenbosch, Western Cape, South Africa

W. Wiradhany
Atma Jaya Catholic University of Indonesia,
Jakarta, Indonesia

M. Uncapher
University of California, San Francisco, CA, USA

A. D. Wagner
Stanford University, Stanford, CA, USA

D. Bavelier
University of Geneva, Geneva, Switzerland


D. A. Christakis, L. Hale (eds.), *Handbook of Children and Screens*,
https://doi.org/10.1007/978-3-031-69362-5_5

homework sessions. As smartphones are frequently kept on one's person and can be easily taken into the school or classroom, students are routinely distracted by their phones during academic activities. Illustrating this, a tracking study among Korean college students found that students were distracted by their smartphones every 3–4 minutes on average during class and used their phones for approximately 25% of their class time [4]. More recently, an experience sampling study conducted among Dutch secondary school students showed that adolescents reported that they were more distracted during times when they had used social media [5]. This study also showed that not all students experienced social media-related distractions—yet the majority did.

As highlighted by recent systematic reviews and meta-analyses, most cross-sectional and experimental studies have shown that digital distractions during class or while doing homework can impair academic performance and learning outcomes [6, 7]. For example, Waite et al. [8] found that answering text messages during class negatively impacted factual learning and the quality of note taking. In other studies, although task performance did not necessarily decrease when multitasking, students took longer to finish their tasks [9]. For example, Bowman et al. [9] found that students who received text messages during academic reading tasks had the same level of reading comprehension, but it took them longer to finish the reading than it did for students who read without media distractions.

Interestingly, some studies have found that the mere presence of a smartphone can negatively affect working memory performance [10]. In this body of work, participants do not actively interact with their phones during cognitive assessments. Rather, their devices are placed either on their person or within visible proximity to them. This "mere-presence" effect has been explained with the idea that performance suffers because people allocate attentional resources away from the primary task toward the highly salient smartphone within their line of sight [10]. Importantly, however, meta-analytical evidence suggests that the negative effects for task performance due to the mere presence of smartphones are less robust than initially reported [11].

Whether, and to what extent, media use is detrimental to task performance seems to depend on at least three boundary conditions. First, it depends on the extent to which the user is committed to the primary task, i.e., they view it as important. Szumowska and Kruglanski [12] found that students were more likely to use their phones during classes, which they perceived to be less important and thus they were less committed. In addition, the likelihood of media multitasking during task engagement increased when students perceived the goal related to the media distraction as more important (e.g., wanting to connect with peers). These findings indicate that students are more likely to be distracted either when they perceive the academic task as less relevant, and perhaps less motivating, or when they perceive the goal related to the media distraction as important or rewarding.

The second boundary condition related to whether media multitasking is detrimental to task performance depends on the extent to which users can adapt to the interference that is introduced by the digital distraction. Some media multitasking combinations are more cognitively demanding and thus more detrimental to task performance than are others, especially those combinations that require processing from the same sensory modality (e.g., auditory vs. visual) and those combinations that do not allow for task interruptions (e.g., continuous information flow) [13, 14]. For example, listening to music while doing homework is less detrimental than watching a television series while writing an essay, since the former has a minimal overlap of both sensory modalities. Most people appear to be aware of this interference and tend to select task combinations that produce lower levels of interference [15]. In addition, it has been shown that individuals at least partly tend to multitask strategically, by switching to a media distraction during "natural breaking points" when task interference is limited [16].

The third boundary condition relates to empirical evidence indicating that performance decrements depend on whether digital distractions are internally or externally initiated [17]. If an academic task is "forcefully" interrupted due to external cues, such as an incoming notification, then performance is more strongly impaired than during situations in which individuals can freely decide whether they use media. This is in line with the exploration-exploitation model of media multitasking [18], which postulates that attending to media distractions might occur as a natural process during the waxing and waning of task engagement. When primary task engagement (exploitation) begins to wane, alternative tasks become more attractive (exploration). When switches occur due to an internal cue (e.g., boredom, lack of concentration), the interruption might help recover cognitive resources and motivation [19]. However, in everyday life, media distractions might occur frequently due to external triggers (e.g., "push" notifications, phone vibrations) that then oftentimes impair task performance.

In sum, experimental studies point toward cognitive and academic performance decrements when using digital media. These performance decrements might be particularly strong when one perceives digital media to be more important than the primary task, when the digital distraction draws on the same sensory modalities than the primary task, and when one is forcefully interrupted by media (i.e., incoming messages).

## 2.2 Long-Term Effects of Digital Distractions

The second area of concern regarding digital media distraction pertains to potential *long-term* effects. That is, what happens if youth are continuously and repeatedly distracted by media? Does this have a sustained and generic impact on their cognitive processing abilities? The neuroplasticity of the brain—the potential of the brain to be malleable and adaptable—does suggest that continuous digital distractions can potentially change the structure and functioning of the brain over time [20].

In recent years, a plethora of studies have been conducted to begin to answer these questions. Most existing studies are cross-sectional and examine the differences in cognitive processes, such as working memory, task switching, and sustained attention between participants classified as heavy and light media multitaskers, which thus far have been based on a self-reported media multitasking index. Several reviews and meta-analyses of this cross-sectional research have found the relationship between media multitasking frequency and longer-term cognitive processing (e.g., working memory capacity, executive functioning, cognitive control) to be weakly negative [7, 21–24]. Overall, these studies indicate that individuals who multitask more with media have more problems sustaining attention, lower working memory capabilities, and lower inhibitory control. However, the reported effects tend to be small and heterogeneous across studies and samples. One reason for this heterogeneity in findings is likely due to the varying measures used for assessing media multitasking and cognitive functioning across studies. However, a recent study has shown that even if measures are kept constant across samples, the strength of the relationship between media multitasking and sustained attention varies across samples [25]. This finding strongly points toward the importance of examining individual differences in the relationship between media multitasking and cognitive control [25]. It seems likely that adolescents with specific cognitive profiles (e.g., attention problems) are more sensitive to highly stimulating digital distraction and, in turn, are at a higher risk of negative effects.

As with media multitasking, the use of screen media in general seems to be weakly related to longer-term attention problems experienced in everyday life, both among school-aged children and adolescents [26, 27]. For example, a study among Dutch 11- to 15-year-olds found that adolescents reported more attention problems when they had reported more problematic social media use (i.e., addiction-like social media use) 1 year before [28]. In addition, it has been shown that specific video content—particularly cognitively demanding videos and fast-paced content—depletes children's executive functions immediately after watching such content [29–31]. For example, Lillard et al. (2015) found that after only 10–20 minutes of watching fast-paced video content, children's executive functions were negatively affected [30]. These effects were not visible when children were exposed to slow-paced video content or when reading a story. However, the found effects were immediate effects after watching the videos and it remains unclear whether any long-term effects on executive functions persist when children frequently watch these shows.

If digital media affect children's attention and cognitive processing, a larger concern is whether this, in turn, hinders children's academic performance. While very few studies have investigated the potential long-term effects using longitudinal methods, one study showed that adolescents who used media more frequently during academic tasks found it increasingly difficult to focus their attention during academic activities [32]. However, using media during academic activities did not affect their subsequent school grades [32], which seems to indicate that children are able to at least partly compensate for these deficiencies. This is in line with a recent review of the literature that has revealed that among children and adolescents, there was no relationship between the frequency of social media use and academic achievement [33].

In sum, there is evidence that fast-paced video content depletes children's executive functioning immediately after watching. In addition, there is some evidence that the use of digital media in general, and media multitasking specifically, is weakly negatively related to cognitive control and attention problems. However, there is only limited evidence that digital media use increases attention problems in a sustained and generic manner over time [34]. In addition, there is, to date, no compelling evidence that the use of social media or engaging in media multitasking substantially affects adolescents' academic performance.

## 3 Future Research

Extant cross-sectional work has provided initial foundational knowledge about the short- and long-term effects of digital media on attention. However, the vast majority of existing studies are cross-sectional and therefore the causal direction of the relationships cited remains unknown. Moreover, without randomized manipulation, this body of research cannot rule out confounding nor reverse causality. If we are to truly progress the state of knowledge in this regard, then it is vital to move beyond small, cross-sectional studies and pursue causal inference. Future research should adopt state-of-the-art research designs and methodologies, such as (intensive) longitudinal designs and controlled field trials, and should address the following pressing research questions:

- What is the direction of the relationship between digital media distraction and cognitive profiles? Are some people more drawn to digital distractions or does the frequency/nature of digital distractions lead to different cognitive profiles over time?
- Are there reinforcing effects of specific individual susceptibilities making some children/adolescents more prone to digital distraction, which, in turn, reinforces preexisting vulnerabilities? Which individual differences make young people more vulnerable to the momentary and long-term effects of digital distractions?
- What is the neurobiological basis for the effects as well as predispositions toward digital distractions? Neurophysiological measures are needed (e.g., brain imaging) to understand this in more depth.
- Which situational cognitive, motivational, and emotional factors influence individuals' ability to ignore digital distractions and make them less/more vulnerable to the effects of digital distractions?
- To what extent do individuals adapt and habituate to digital distractions? As digital media have become a crucial part of our everyday lives, do individuals cognitively habituate to digital distractions, and do they adapt on the behavioral (e.g., notification management) and societal level (e.g., norm adjustment), which may make distractions less detrimental over time? Will individuals learn to cope with digital distractions and become more resilient over time?

- On which principles should interventions be designed? Should interventions target specific individual vulnerabilities (e.g., attention problems, low self-control), or should they target design factors of digital media that can potentially help individuals gain back control (e.g., grayscaling, notification management, etc.), or both?

## 4 Recommendations

While in some areas, empirical evidence is more robust, in other areas, particularly concerning long-term effects, critical caveats exist. These pertain particularly to the causal direction of the relationships as well as to potentially confounding factors. While the evidence is limited and extensive research is needed, given the potential vulnerability of children and adolescents and a rapidly shifting technological landscape, caution seems warranted, and we thus offer the following recommendations:

- *Media technology providers* should be mindful of the distracting and habit-creating nature of their technologies and should follow ethical guidelines when designing technologies, particularly when developing for younger audiences (e.g., minimizing notification alerts and infinite scrolling that trigger unintended app use).
- *Policymakers* need to provide legal frameworks and policies that are based on empirical evidence and that acknowledge the distracting nature of the persuasive design techniques used by digital technologies (e.g., European Union (EU)s rules to address digital addiction) [35].
- *Educators and parents* should acknowledge the appealing character of digital media for youth as well as their distracting potential. Instead of solely warning about the potential negative effects of using digital media during school or homework, they could do the following:
  - Educate youth about switching costs (i.e., switching back-and-forth between homework and digital technologies will require much more time to finish their task) but also about potential facilitating effects of taking digital breaks (i.e., sometimes it can help to take a break).
  - Educators should discuss with students an adaptive way to use technology in the classroom that allows for technology-enhanced/supported learning as opposed to uncontrolled distraction.
  - Facilitate digital-free spaces (e.g., during school, family dinners): With many adolescents wanting to use their phones less rather than more [1], parents and educators may want to encourage time off phones.
- *Researchers*: As the direct, concurrent effects of digital distractions during task performance are relatively well understood, there is particular value in researchers focusing on understanding the longer-term effects of digital media on attention, cognition, and performance. This will require interdisciplinary collaborations, long-term longitudinal projects, and employing a combination of objective (e.g., tracking screen time) and subjective measurements (e.g., self-reports of app usage, attention problems in everyday life) for both digital media use and cognitive functioning.

**Conflict of Interest and Funding Disclosures** None.

## References

1. Vogels EA, Gelles-Watnick R, Massarat N. Teens, social media and technology 2022. Pew Research Center: Internet, Science & Tech. Pew Research Center; 2022. Available at: https://www.pewresearch.org/internet/2022/08/10/teens-social-media-and-technology-2022/. Accessed 30 Mar 2023.
2. Ghai S, Magis-Weinberg L, Stoilova M, Livingstone S, Orben A. Social media and adolescent well-being in the Global South. Curr Opin Psychol. 2022;46:101318. https://doi.org/10.1016/j.copsyc.2022.101318.
3. Ettinger K, Cohen A. Patterns of multitasking behaviours of adolescents in digital environments. Educ Inf Technol. 2020;25(1):623–45. https://doi.org/10.1007/s10639-019-09982-4.
4. Kim I, Kim R, Kim H, et al. Understanding smartphone usage in college classrooms: a long-term measurement study. Comput Educ. 2019;141:103611. https://doi.org/10.1016/j.compedu.2019.103611.

5. Siebers T, Beyens I, Pouwels JL, Valkenburg PM. Social media and distraction: an experience sampling study among adolescents. Media Psychol. 2021;25(3):343–66. https://doi.org/10.1080/15213269.2021.1959350.
6. May KE, Elder AD. Efficient, helpful, or distracting? A literature review of media multitasking in relation to academic performance. Int J Educ Technol High Educ. 2018;15(1):1–17. https://doi.org/10.1186/s41239-018-0096-z.
7. van der Schuur WA, Baumgartner SE, Sumter SR, Valkenburg PM. The consequences of media multitasking for youth: a review. Comput Hum Behav. 2015;53:204–15. https://doi.org/10.1016/j.chb.2015.06.035.
8. Waite BM, Lindberg R, Ernst B, Bowman LL, Levine LE. Off-task multitasking, note-taking and lower- and higher-order classroom learning. Comput Educ. 2018;120:98–111. https://doi.org/10.1016/j.compedu.2018.01.007.
9. Bowman LL, Levine LE, Waite BM, Gendron M. Can students really multitask? An experimental study of instant messaging while reading. Comput Educ. 2010;54(4):927–31. https://doi.org/10.1016/j.compedu.2009.09.024.
10. Ward AF, Duke K, Gneezy A, Bos MW. Brain drain: the mere presence of one's own smartphone reduces available cognitive capacity. J Assoc Consum Res. 2017;2(2):140–54. https://doi.org/10.1086/691462.
11. Parry DA. Does the mere presence of a smartphone impact cognitive performance? A meta-analysis of the "brain drain effect". Media Psychol. 2022. https://doi.org/10.31234/osf.io/tnyda.
12. Szumowska E, Kruglanski AW. The psychology of getting busy: multitasking as a consequence of goal activation. J Exp Psychol Gen. 2022;151(1):137–60. https://doi.org/10.1037/xge0001077.
13. Salvucci DD, Taatgen NA. Threaded cognition: an integrated theory of concurrent multitasking. Psychol Rev. 2008;115(1):101–30. https://doi.org/10.1037/0033-295X.115.1.101.
14. Wang Z, Irwin M, Cooper C, Srivastava J. Multidimensions of media multitasking and adaptive media selection: cognitive dimensions of media multitasking. Hum Commun Res. 2015;41(1):102–27. https://doi.org/10.1111/hcre.12042.
15. Nijboer M, Taatgen NA, Brands A, Borst JP, van Rijn H. Decision making in concurrent multitasking: do people adapt to task interference? PLoS One. 2013;8(11):e79583. https://doi.org/10.1371/journal.pone.0079583.
16. Ralph BCW, Seli P, Wilson KE, Smilek D. Volitional media multitasking: awareness of performance costs and modulation of media multitasking as a function of task demand. Psychol Res. 2020;84(2):404–23. https://doi.org/10.1007/s00426-018-1056-x.
17. Puranik H, Koopman J, Vough HC. Pardon the interruption: an integrative review and future research agenda for research on work interruptions. J Manage. 2020;46(6):806–42. https://doi.org/10.1177/0149206319887428.
18. Wiradhany W, Baumgartner SE, de Bruin A. Exploitation–exploration model of media multitasking. J Media Psychol. 2021;33(4):169–80. https://doi.org/10.1027/1864-1105/a000303.
19. Ralph BCW, Smith AC, Seli P, Smilek D. The relation between task-unrelated media multitasking and task-related motivation. Psychol Res. 2021;85(1):408–22. https://doi.org/10.1007/s00426-019-01246-7.
20. Chiu M, Chein JM. Digital media and the developing brain. In: Nesi J, Telzer EH, Prinstein MJ, editors. Handbook of adolescent digital media use and mental health. Cambridge University Press; 2022. p. 104–34.
21. Parry DA, Le Roux DB. "Cognitive control in media multitaskers" ten years on: a meta-analysis. Cyberpsychology (Brno). 2021;15(2). https://doi.org/10.5817/cp2021-2-7.
22. Uncapher MR, Wagner AD. Minds and brains of media multitaskers: current findings and future directions. Proc Natl Acad Sci USA. 2018;115(40):9889–96. https://doi.org/10.1073/pnas.1611612115.
23. Uncapher MR, Lin L, Rosen LD, et al. Media multitasking and cognitive, psychological, neural, and learning differences. Pediatrics. 2017;140(Suppl 2):S62–6. https://doi.org/10.1542/peds.2016-1758D.
24. Wiradhany W, Nieuwenstein MR. Cognitive control in media multitaskers: two replication studies and a meta-analysis. Atten Percept Psychophys. 2017;79(8):2620–41. https://doi.org/10.3758/s13414-017-1408-4.
25. Rioja K, Cekic S, Bavelier D, Baumgartner SE. Unravelling the link between media multitasking and attention across three samples. Technol Mind Behav. 2023;4:tmb0000106.
26. Beyens I, Valkenburg PM. Children's media use and its relation to attention, hyperactivity, and impulsivity. In: The Routledge international handbook of children, adolescents, and media. Routledge; 2022. p. 202–10.
27. Beyens I, Valkenburg PM, Piotrowski JT. Screen media use and ADHD-related behaviors: four decades of research. Proc Natl Acad Sci USA. 2018;115(40):9875–81. https://doi.org/10.1073/pnas.1611611114.
28. Boer M, Stevens G, Finkenauer C, van den Eijnden R. Attention deficit hyperactivity disorder-symptoms, social media use intensity, and social media use problems in adolescents: investigating directionality. Child Dev. 2020;91(4):e853–65. https://doi.org/10.1111/cdev.13334.
29. Lillard AS, Peterson J. The immediate impact of different types of television on young children's executive function. Pediatrics. 2011;128(4):644–9. https://doi.org/10.1542/peds.2010-1919.
30. Lillard AS, Drell MB, Richey EM, Boguszewski K, Smith ED. Further examination of the immediate impact of television on children's executive function. Dev Psychol. 2015;51(6):792–805. https://doi.org/10.1037/a0039097.

31. Kostyrka-Allchorne K, Cooper NR, Simpson A. The relationship between television exposure and children's cognition and behaviour: a systematic review. Dev Rev. 2017;44:19–58. https://doi.org/10.1016/j.dr.2016.12.002.
32. van der Schuur WA, Baumgartner SE, Sumter SR, Valkenburg PM. Exploring the long-term relationship between academic-media multitasking and adolescents' academic achievement. New Media Soc. 2020;22(1):140–58. https://doi.org/10.1177/1461444819861956.
33. Appel M, Marker C, Gnambs T. Are social media ruining our lives? A review of meta-analytic evidence. Rev Gen Psychol. 2020;24(1):60–74. https://doi.org/10.1177/1089268019880891.
34. Baumgartner SE, van der Schuur WA, Lemmens JS, te Poel F. The relationship between media multitasking and attention problems in adolescents: results of two longitudinal studies: media multitasking and attention problems. Hum Commun Res. Published online 2017. https://doi.org/10.1111/hcre.12111.
35. New EU rules needed to address digital addiction. News: European parliament. (12-12-2023). Available at: https://www.europarl.europa.eu/news/en/press-room/20231208IPR15767/new-eu-rules-needed-to-address-digital-addiction. Accessed 08 Apr 2024.

# Digital Media Use and Language Development in Early Childhood

Rebecca A. Dore, Mengguo Jing, Gemma Taylor, Sheri Madigan, Preeti G. Samudra, Annette S. Sundqvist, and Ying Xu

## 1 Background

Language skills are vital for young children's academic, social, and occupational success [1]. Given the pervasiveness of digital media [2], there is a pressing need to understand their role in language development. The aim of the current review is to summarize current evidence related to the effects of digital media use during early childhood, defined as birth to 6 years of age, given the rapid development of language during these years. We include a diverse range of activities under "digital media," including watching television/videos, using apps/games, video chatting, looking at, listening to, or being read e-books, and interacting with conversational agents, such as Apple's Siri or Amazon's Alexa. Notably, the diversity of these activities contributes to challenges in determining the impacts of digital media as a whole on language development. This topic is crucial as understanding such links can inform digital media use guidelines distributed by organizations such as the American Academy of Pediatrics and the World Health Organization.

## 2 Current State

Historically, research involving digital media has focused on the *duration* of use (i.e., the amount of time that children spend using media, primarily television). It has been proposed that the duration of media use may have a negative impact on language development to the extent that it replaces other more traditional developmentally beneficial activities (known as the "displacement hypothesis;" e.g., Mutz et al. [3]). Indeed, some evidence suggests that children's television viewing is inversely associated with the time spent with their parents or siblings, doing homework, engaging in creative play [3], and reading [4]. Furthermore, a recent meta-analysis of more than 18,000 participants from 42 studies has demonstrated that the association between media use duration and early language skills is negative, albeit with a small-to-medium effect size [5].

R. A. Dore (✉)
The Ohio State University, Columbus, OH, USA
e-mail: dore.13@osu.edu

M. Jing
Boston College, Boston, MA, USA

G. Taylor
University of Salford, Salford, UK

S. Madigan
University of Calgary, Calgary, AB, Canada

P. G. Samudra
SUNY Plattsburgh, Plattsburgh, NY, USA

A. S. Sundqvist
Linköping University, Linköping, Sweden

Y. Xu
University of Michigan, Ann Arbor, MI, USA


D. A. Christakis, L. Hale (eds.), *Handbook of Children and Screens*,
https://doi.org/10.1007/978-3-031-69362-5_6

In recent years, however, there has been an increased focus on *content* (i.e., what kinds of media children are using), *context* (i.e., who they are using digital media with), and *interactivity* (i.e., whether they are watching videos or using media like apps or games that can respond contingently) of media use as well as technoference (i.e., adult technology use around children). Two of these factors, content and context, have been exemplified by recent meta-analyses demonstrating that both content intended to be educational and media that is co-used with an adult are positively associated with language skills [5, 6]. Some researchers have also argued that more technologically advanced forms of media that can be interactive, or respond contingently to children, may also be more supportive of language development (e.g., Barr [7]), although more research is needed to investigate this possibility. In this chapter, we focus on these components of digital media use in early childhood, as they have been a primary source of exploration in research studies over the last decade.

## 2.1 Content

It is vital to consider the content of media when examining links to language development, as media can have different goals, with some primarily aiming to entertain, whereas others intend to inform or impart knowledge to children (i.e., educational content). Research on the impacts of educational content can vary, depending on the age of the child. Notably, for the youngest children, infants, and toddlers under 2.5 or 3 years of age, research has demonstrated a *transfer deficit*, in which children have trouble transferring learning between two-dimensional (2D) formats (i.e., media or storybooks) and real-world situations, even when the content is intended to be educational (e.g., DeLoache et al. [8]). A recent meta-analysis has shown that this deficit was smaller for language tasks than for other types of tasks (e.g., imitation, object retrieval) but was still a significant deficit [9]. Although live interactions may most consistently lead to robust word learning, individual studies show that older toddlers can learn words from media sources under certain circumstances. For example, one study found that toddlers can learn words from video chat interactions similarly to live interactions (e.g., Roseberry et al. [10]). Interestingly, newer studies report smaller deficits than do older ones [9], although notably even recent studies have demonstrated small but significant deficits (see Kirkorian and Choi [11] for a similar effect).

In contrast, in the preschool years, studies have found that educational content may be positive for language development [5]. Specifically, studies show that children learn new words from well-designed, developmentally appropriate media, including both videos and apps (e.g., Mares and Pan [12] and Dore et al. [13]). It has also been hypothesized that preschoolers may be developmentally ready to learn from educational media due to an increased understanding of the symbolic nature of media and improved memory flexibility [7]. Indeed, research has shown that although e-book features unrelated to the narrative can distract from comprehension [14], a meta-analysis [15] found that well-designed e-books with features like intentionally integrated animations and sound effects were supportive of children's word learning.

## 2.2 Context

Adults' co-use of media with children, or *joint media engagement*, may promote language because media does not completely replace contingent caregiver–child interactions and instead provides a new context for conversation. Thus, to the extent that caregivers use media with children and engage in conversation around media, any potential negative effects of digital media on language may be at least partially offset. Indeed, in laboratory studies, young children appear to comprehend and learn more from media when adults use it with them and engage in conversation around the content (e.g., Strouse and Troseth [16]). However, while this is an ideal scenario, it is important to note that research suggests that parents do not necessarily engage in language-supportive conversations during co-use of media, with language quality typically decreasing during media use, in tandem with an increase in more functional language about the media format [17]. Furthermore, an individual study showed that the link between television and preschoolers' language growth is fully explained by fewer adult–child conversations [18], suggesting that adult language input is a critical mechanism and a potential lever for interventions.

Higher-quality forms of engagement, such as asking questions to enhance understanding of words and content of media, are more likely to support language development than other forms of co-use [19]. Well-designed media have the potential to support these higher-quality forms of interaction. For example, one study found that an interactive e-book that includes prompts giving parents ideas on how to engage with their children can promote richer language and interactions, which may foster children's language skills [20]. Furthermore, media may support adults in finding new topics to discuss with children after its use (such as talking about astronauts after viewing a show about outer space), potentially promoting language skills (e.g., Lavigne et al. [21]).

## 2.3 Interactivity

Although the devices and platforms that children use to access media have changed drastically in the last decade, young children's media use is still predominated by video viewing [2] rather than using more interactive forms of media, like apps or video chat, which might be supportive of language skills [7]. Furthermore, there have been mixed findings regarding the role of interactivity in children's learning across domains, showing inconsistencies in whether children learn better from noninteractive or interactive media (e.g., Kirkorian et al. [22]) and little research specifically comparing interactive and noninteractive media has examined word learning (c.f., Russo-Johnson et al. [23]). Newer technologies like conversational agents (e.g., Amazon's Alexa or Apple's Siri) have also been explored in recent studies in relation to their potential for supporting children's interactions with books and media. For example, studies have explored incorporating conversational agents into children's educational television programs so that they can interact with the shows' characters. These studies have found that such interactions promote children's engagement and learning of educational content, like science, from the shows. Similarly, conversational agents have been used to support preschoolers' comprehension of storybooks by posing comprehension questions and providing immediate feedback [24]. Although these interactions have been shown to improve comprehension to a degree comparable to interactions with a human partner, the key qualities of children's verbal engagement differed depending on whether they were interacting with a conversational agent or an adult language partner [25].

## 2.4 Technoference

Beyond children's direct use of media, both background television and adults' use of mobile devices while interacting with children, or technoference, can interrupt interactions between parents and children [26]. Research shows that parents are commonly distracted by digital devices while around their children and that this behavior is linked to lower sensitivity and fewer verbal interactions [26], thus potentially impacting language development. In one experimental study, children failed to learn new words taught by their parents if the learning event was disrupted by a short phone call [27]. The mechanisms by which technoference may disrupt language development include disruptions to gaze following parental responsiveness and joint attention [28].

# 3 Future Research

There are several pressing research questions and critical avenues for future research:

- First, to what extent is there a link between media use, and characteristics of media use, and children's language development over time (e.g., longitudinal designs) [5] and in naturalistic settings (i.e., in real-world environments rather than lab-based studies) [29]?

Many researchers have called for increasing methodological rigor in study designs, via longitudinal research with repeated measurements over time to examine the bidirectional links in which media and development both predict each other over time (e.g., Madigan et al. [5]) as well as scaled-up interventions or quasi-experiments implemented in naturalistic settings (e.g., McArthur et al. [29]).

- Second, to what extent does the effect of media on language development depend on individual child-level factors, such as gender, temperament, and cognitive skills, in line with the Differential Susceptibility to Media Effects Model [30] (e.g., McArthur et al. [31])? This model proposes that individual differences may act as moderators of media effects, such that children with different qualities will be more or less likely to be negatively (or positively) impacted by media use, but this has not been commonly applied to language development.
- Third, to what extent does the link between media and language development differ for different groups, such as those from non-Western cultures, underresourced backgrounds, or multilingual homes? Cultural differences in family dynamics and how media is used in the home may influence the way that links between media use and language development manifest across groups.
- Fourth, are there nonlinear (e.g., quadratic) relations between media use and language development, in line with some recent research (e.g., McArthur et al. [29], Taylor et al. [32], and Dore et al. [33]), such that effects are apparent at high but not moderate levels of media use?
- Lastly, how do educational media compare to other methods for language learning (e.g., storybooks, games, direct instruction) and how can they best be used in tandem with other methods?

## 4 Recommendations

### 4.1 For Clinicians and Advocacy Groups

- Focus on the content and context of young children's media use, in addition to time-based recommendations for preschoolers and older children.
- Better define and communicate about what makes media educational and create rigorous, evidence-based guidelines for helping families and practitioners distinguish between high-quality educational content and low-quality content or media meant primarily for entertainment.
- Emphasize the "why" behind guidelines and the importance of adult–child interactions regardless of whether or not the child is using media.

### 4.2 For Policymakers

- Encourage and fund research on media use and language development in naturalistic contexts, especially in light of the 2022 passing of the Children and Media Research Advancement (CAMRA) Act directing the National Institutes of Health to pursue a research program on technology and media's effects in childhood.
- Continue to provide funding for high-quality educational media focused on promoting language development, in addition to the recent emphasis on STEM content, as children's language skills are foundational for subsequent learning.
- Provide better guidelines and regulations for categorizing only high-quality and developmentally appropriate media content as educational.

## 4.3 For Educators, Parents, and Other Caregivers

- Encourage children to use high-quality educational media, including media that are developed with educational consultants and introduce sophisticated but age-appropriate language and concepts in accessible ways, connect educational information to children's real-world experiences, and give children the opportunity to answer questions and solve problems. Use sources such as CommonSenseMedia.org to find age-based recommendations.
- Use media with children (co-use), helping them understand and contextualize the content and relating it to their own lives.
- Face-to-face interactions and conversational turns are the best way to support children's language development; find some times of the day/week to have device-free family time.
- Be aware of disruptions from adult mobile device use and background television.
- Visit childrenandscreens.com/tips-for-parents to see additional recommendations for how to manage family screen time, from early childhood to teenage years.

## 4.4 For Media Technology Providers

- Focus on evidence-based language-promoting content in video as well as apps and newer technologies, as video still makes up most of children's media use.
- Create media that support adult–child interactions and provide examples of positive ways for adults to interact with children around media.
- Use high-quality language in children's media and embed opportunities for language learning even within content primarily focused on other domains, such as science, math, or social and emotional skills.

## 4.5 For Researchers

- Consider using novel (e.g., neuroimaging, video observation, passive device sensing) and mixed method approaches (e.g., combining surveys and direct child assessments with case studies) to develop a deeper understanding of the role of media in children's language development.
- Use more optimal study designs (e.g., randomized controlled trials, quasi-experiments), conduct longitudinal research with repeated measurements of digital media use and language, and consider including more relevant covariates in studies to better isolate the unique relation between media use and language development.
- Measure media use in more robust ways, including measures of content and context, and work collaboratively to converge on universal measures to facilitate comparison across studies and labs.
- Consider conducting research to inform the accuracy and utility of specific time-based limits on children's media use to elucidate the nature of any links between media use quantity and language development and inform guidelines provided to families.

**Conflict of Interest and Funding Disclosures** None.

## References

1. Lee VE, Burkham DT. Inequality at the starting gate: social background differences in achievement as children begin school. Washington, DC: Economic Policy Institute; 2002.
2. Rideout V, Robb M. The Common Sense census: Media use by kids age zero to eight, 2020. San Francisco: Common Sense Media; 2020.
3. Mutz DC, Roberts DF, Vuuren DV. Reconsidering the displacement hypothesis: Television's influence on children's time use. Commun Res. 1993;20(1):51–75.
4. Khan KS, et al. Association between television viewing and parent-child reading in the early home environment. J Dev Behav Pediatr. 2017;38(7):521–7.

5. Madigan S, McArthur BA, Anhorn C, Eirich R, Christakis D. Associations between screen use and child language skills: a systematic review and meta-analysis. JAMA Pediatr. Published online 2020:1–11. https://doi.org/10.1001/jamapediatrics.2020.0327.
6. Jing M, Ye T, Kirkorian H, Mares L. Screen media exposure and young children's vocabulary learning and development: a meta-analysis. Child Dev. 2023;94:1398–418.
7. Barr RF. Growing up in the digital age: early learning and family media ecology. Curr Dir Psychol Sci. Published online 2019:096372141983824. https://doi.org/10.1177/0963721419838245.
8. DeLoache JS, Chiong C, Sherman K, et al. Do babies learn from baby media? Psychol Sci. 2010; 21(11):1570–4. https://doi.org/10.1177/0956797610384145.
9. Strouse GA, Samson JE. Learning from video: a meta-analysis of the video deficit in children ages 0 to 6 years. Child Dev. 2021;92(1):e20–38. https://doi.org/10.1111/cdev.13429.
10. Roseberry S, Hirsh-Pasek K, Golinkoff RM. Skype me! Socially contingent interactions help toddlers learn language. Child Dev. 2014;85(3):956–70. https://doi.org/10.1111/cdev.12166.
11. Kirkorian HL, Choi K. Associations between toddlers' naturalistic media experience and observed learning from screens. Infancy. 2016;2007:1–7. https://doi.org/10.1111/infa.12171.
12. Mares M-L, Pan Z. Effects of Sesame Street: a meta-analysis of children's learning in 15 countries. J Appl Dev Psychol. Published online March 2013. https://doi.org/10.1016/j.appdev.2013.01.001.
13. Dore RA, et al. Education in the app store: using a mobile game to support US preschoolers' vocabulary learning. J Child Media. 2019;13(4):452–71.
14. Parish-Morris J, et al. Once upon a time: parent–child dialogue and storybook reading in the electronic era. Mind Brain Educ. 2013;7(3):200–11.
15. Takacs ZK, Swart EK, Bus AG. Benefits and pitfalls of multimedia and interactive features in technology-enhanced storybooks: a meta-analysis. Rev Educ Res. Published online 2015:1–42. https://doi.org/10.3102/0034654314566989.
16. Strouse GA, Troseth GL. Supporting toddlers' transfer of word learning from video. Cogn Dev. 2014;30(1):47–64. https://doi.org/10.1016/j.cogdev.2014.01.002.
17. Ewin CA, Reupert AE, McLean LA, Ewin CJ. The impact of joint media engagement on parent–child interactions: a systematic review. Hum Behav Emerg Technol. 2021;3(2):230–54. https://doi.org/10.1002/hbe2.203.
18. Zimmerman FJ, et al. Teaching by listening: the importance of adult-child conversations to language development. Pediatrics. 2009;124(1):342–9.
19. Strouse GA, O'Doherty K, Troseth GL. Effective coviewing: preschoolers' learning from video after a dialogic questioning intervention. Dev Psychol. 2013;49(12):2368–82. https://doi.org/10.1037/a0032463.
20. Troseth GL, Strouse GA, Flores I, Stuckelman ZD, Johnson CR. An enhanced eBook facilitates parent–child talk during shared reading by families of low socioeconomic status. Early Child Res Q. 2020:1–14. https://doi.org/10.1016/j.ecresq.2019.02.009.
21. Lavigne HJ, Hanson KG, Anderson DR. The influence of television coviewing on parent language directed at toddlers. J Appl Dev Psychol. 2015;36:1–10. https://doi.org/10.1016/j.appdev.2014.11.004.
22. Kirkorian HL, Choi K, Pempek TA. Toddlers' word learning from contingent and non-contingent video on touchscreens. Child Dev. 2016;29(1):91–102. https://doi.org/10.3233/SW-140134.
23. Russo-Johnson C, Troseth GL, Duncan C, Mesghina A. All tapped out: touchscreen interactivity and young children's word learning. Front Psychol. 2017;8(April):578. https://doi.org/10.3389/fpsyg.2017.00578.
24. Xu Y, Aubele J, Vigil V, Bustamante AS, Kim YS, Warschauer M. Dialogue with a conversational agent promotes children's story comprehension via enhancing engagement. Child Dev. 2022;93(2):e149–67. https://doi.org/10.1111/cdev.13708.
25. Xu Y, Wang D, Collins P, Lee H, Warschauer M. Same benefits, different communication patterns: comparing Children's reading with a conversational agent vs. a human partner. Comput Educ. 2021;2021(161):104059. https://doi.org/10.1007/bf02527095.
26. McDaniel BT, Radesky JS. Parent distraction with phones, reasons for use, and impacts on parenting and child outcomes: a review of the emerging research. Hum Behav Emerg Technol. 2019;(February):72–80. https://doi.org/10.1002/hbe2.139.
27. Reed J, Hirsh-pasek K, Golinkoff RM. Learning on hold: cell phones sidetrack parent-child interactions. Dev Psychol. 2017;53:1428–36.
28. Morris AJ, Filippetti ML, Rigato S. The impact of parents' smartphone use on language development in young children. Child Dev Perspect. 2022;16(2):103–9.
29. McArthur BA, Browne D, Tough S, Madigan S. Trajectories of screen use during early childhood: predictors and associated behavior and learning outcomes. Comput Hum Behav. Published online 2020:106501. https://doi.org/10.1016/j.chb.2020.106501.
30. Valkenburg PM, Peter J. The differential susceptibility to media effects model. J Commun. 2013;63(2):221–43. https://doi.org/10.1111/jcom.12024.

31. McArthur BA, Hentges R, Christakis DA, McDonald S, Tough S, Madigan S. Cumulative social risk and child screen use: the role of child temperament. J Pediatr Psychol. 2022;47(2):171–9. https://doi.org/10.1093/jpepsy/jsab087.
32. Taylor G, Monaghan P, Westermann G. Investigating the association between children's screen media exposure and vocabulary size in the UK. J Child Media. 2018;12(1):51–65. https://doi.org/10.1080/17482798.2017.1365737.
33. Dore RA, Logan J, Lin TJ, Purtell KM, Justice LM. Characteristics of children's media use and gains in language and literacy skills. Front Psychol. 2020;11:2224. https://doi.org/10.3389/fpsyg.2020.02224.

# Imagination, Creativity, and Play

Rebekah A. Richert, Koeun Choi, Tracy R. Gleason,
Thalia R. Goldstein, and Susan M. Sibert

## 1 Background

Imagination, or the process of mentally representing people, objects, and ideas, is critical to healthy cognitive development, as well as to the ways in which children engage with and learn from the people, objects, and events that populate their worlds [1, 2]. Throughout development, but especially from early childhood through adolescence, using imagination to engage in creative thought and expression leads to scientific and artistic innovations [2] and helps children process and understand their everyday experiences [1]. The prevalence of digital media and technology in children's lives has engendered concerns regarding the harmful effects of exposure on children's creativity and play [3]. These effects may be either direct, as when children center imaginative play around themes and storylines encountered in media, or indirect, as when engagement in media undermines the time spent on alternative, real-world activities such as reading or playing outside [4]. For example, access to and use of digital technologies may restrict children's experience of boredom, which is often characterized as a cognitive space in which creativity can thrive (e.g., Bronson and Merryman [5]). The use of digital devices might also interfere with creativity because screens are presumed to provide simulation that is "impoverished" when compared to the cognitive stimulation children receive through interactions in the real world [6]. Furthermore, children who use devices for more than 1 hour per day are likely to be negatively impacted in five developmental domains: physical health and well-being, social competence, emotional maturity, language and cognitive development, and communication skills [7]. As such, understanding the ways in which media use relates to the development of imagination, creativity, and play is critical for creating developmental contexts as well as digital media that support healthy development.

R. A. Richert (✉)
University of California, Riverside,
Riverside, CA, USA
e-mail: rebekahr@ucr.edu

K. Choi
Virginia Polytechnic Institute and State University,
Blacksburg, VA, USA

T. R. Gleason
Wellesley College, Wellesley, MA, USA

T. R. Goldstein
George Mason University, Fairfax, VA, USA

S. M. Sibert
Indiana University of Pennsylvania,
Indiana, PA, USA

## 2 Current State

Early research into the relations between media exposure and imaginative play found that children who were heavy television viewers demon-


D. A. Christakis, L. Hale (eds.), *Handbook of Children and Screens*,
https://doi.org/10.1007/978-3-031-69362-5_7

strated less engagement in pretend play [2]. Similarly, longitudinal studies have found a negative relation between creativity and foreground media (i.e., media with which children are currently engaging), particularly for receptive media such as television and videos [8]. Greater overall time spent with digital media has also been linked to reduced mental imagery among children in early and middle childhood over the course of 10 months, after controlling for other potential influences such as working memory and vocabulary [9]. Likewise, experimental studies involving infants and young children have documented that the quality and quantity of children's solitary and parent–child (dyadic) play decrease when technological distractions are present, such as background television [10, 11] and when parents use mobile media ("technoference") [12]. A proposed mechanism through which indirect exposure to screen media interferes with creativity and play is that this exposure may interfere with the concentrated mental effort required for imagination and creativity [13]; however, this specific relation has not yet been directly tested with children.

While the overall frequency and duration of exposure to media have been found to negatively influence creativity and imagination, other studies emphasize the importance of the content of programs and games. For example, children who tend to be highly imaginative (e.g., those who gravitate toward fantasy toys and play or create imaginary companions) also tend to watch educational programs, such as those on public television, which are intended to foster imagination and creativity [2]. While correlational, such findings raise the question of how closely, and in what ways, media content is linked to children's creativity and imagination, particularly in play. Media and media characters often appear in children's play since children's play is often (although not always) closely tied to their experiences [1]. A more thorough exploration of the relations between media use and imagination and play, particularly the role of content and child temperament, is needed.

## 2.1 Creativity and Fantasy Play

Educational television programs designed intentionally to model imaginative behaviors (e.g., scenes of children engaging in pretend play) have been found to stimulate preschool-aged children's imaginative and pretend play immediately after viewing [14]. These have also been linked to greater divergent thinking and higher participation in creative activities in adolescence. In contrast, exposure to violent media content in the preschool age range has been found to be negatively related to subsequent creative abilities in adolescence [15].

Because fantasy play in early childhood is often based upon mundane scenarios with which children are highly familiar, such as playing house [1], media would be expected to be a source of ideas for play for children who spend a lot of time engaged with it. On one end of the spectrum, children's fantasy or make-believe scenarios might be faithful enactments of media stories, whereas, in the middle of the spectrum, they might co-opt elements of media, such as characters or storylines but not both, and, at the other end of the spectrum, they might bear no relation to any mediated content at all. However, a comprehensive, cross-cultural study of the intersection between media and fantasy found that a significant proportion of children (37%) did not use any obviously media-related content either explicitly or implicitly in their observed fantasy play [16]. Similarly, although some imaginary companions might draw a name or appearance from the characters encountered in media, an imaginary companion fully based on a media character, including the character's personality, characteristics, and behaviors, is rare [17]. On the whole, these studies suggest that while media elements do sometimes provide inspiration for fantasy play, most media themes, storylines, and characters might not be readily adopted into play.

In middle childhood, as cognitive capacities increase, interactive games providing high levels of control, feedback, and opportunities for creativity support metacognitive skills (i.e., children's reflection on their own cognitive strategies during game play) [18]. In addition, the interactive nature of newer technologies provides opportunities for children to create and shape media content themselves. Emerging interactive technologies, such as social robots and voice assistant systems powered by artificial intelligence (AI), may expand children's range of imaginative and creative activities by enabling them to ask and answer questions, provide and receive feedback, and generate and perform stories [19, 20]. Social robots resembling humans and animals have been introduced to co-create musical theater with children, thus allowing them to express their creativity through acting, dancing, music, and drawing [19]. These activities go beyond guiding children through scripted actions by purposefully encouraging open-ended activities to stimulate imaginative thinking and original expression across diverse artistic mediums (e.g., designing unique robot motions and expressions, creating original music and sound, crafting costumes and performance scenes based on imagination). A recent study has revealed an increase in 6- to 10-year-old children's verbal and figurative creativity as they engaged in storytelling experiences in collaboration with AI that transforms children's speech into drawings and generates sketches semantically similar to the story content [20].

## 2.2 Understanding Media Characters

One of the primary ways in which children's imagination and creativity is activated while engaging with media is in their processing of and interactions with media characters, thus highlighting the social nature of their media interactions [21]. Contrary to popular belief, extensive research in cognitive and emotional development shows that during their preschool years, children come to an understanding of the line between what is real and what is pretend, although fantasy content that is highly emotional is more difficult for children to differentiate from reality [22, 23]. Children's beliefs about whether media content is real or fantastical are important because this is related to children's abstract transfer of learning from media content to real-world problems as well as to their divergent and creative problem-solving skills [24, 25]. For example, although children seem to be more likely to learn from realistic than fantastical characters, they are also more likely to engage in abstract, analogical transfer of learning when presented with fantastical characters that can violate real-world, physical laws than with fantastical characters who can otherwise do nothing particularly special [25]. Children in early childhood who playfully interact with a character while viewing subsequently display more creative problem-solving skills when presented with a challenge immediately after viewing [24].

The effects of media characters on children's lives are certainly not uniformly positive, and viewing of violent and aggressive media is related to children's beliefs that violence and aggression are permissible and to children's use of aggressive behavior subsequent to viewing violence and aggression [26]. However, as related to promoting children's imagination and creativity, findings in this area suggest that children's cognition can benefit from engagement with fantastical media when the storylines involve moderate levels of fantasy that grab children's attention and bring them into the fantastical world but not so much fantasy that it overwhelms their ability to process what they are viewing [27].

## 2.3 Media and Social Cognition

One newer line of research relates to children's social cognitive understanding and processing of the nature of acting itself [28, 29]. While children's television shows and films contain a mix of genres and elements, including hand-drawn and computer-generated animation, puppets, muppets, and real people, the *agents* that children see on screens are typically represented in some way by human beings (whether being the puppeteer or actually portraying the characters) or anthropomorphized creatures [29, 30]. Regardless of the genre, children must determine not just whether the events on TV are real [31] but also that in acting there is a real person behind each character. While adults (mostly) have a common sense view of how acting and actors work [32], developmental science knows little about how children develop social cognitive understanding to process actors and performers. This topic is particularly important because sometimes children's television shows and films involve obvious cues to their pretense [33, 34], but, at other times, performers act as realistically as possible within their worlds, occasionally confusing even adults as to their emotions and personalities [35].

Children's understanding of acting develops significantly in early childhood. For instance, 3- and 4-year-olds think that both realistic and nonrealistic actors experience the emotions and physical states they portray, whereas 5-year-olds can make finer distinctions [28]. These older children believe that realistic, but not unrealistic, actors experience the emotions they portray and occasionally the physical characteristics as well (e.g., a stomachache or a hurt leg) [28]. At this age, children do not show a preference between unrealistic and realistic acting. However, they do choose unrealistically acted performances as "harder to do" when given a direct comparison with realism [36]. Beyond the performance itself, other work has shown that age (from 3 to 8 years), but not viewing experience, predicts children's beliefs that the people they see in instructional YouTube videos are "real" [37]. Children's reality status judgments are not, however, affected by the content of the videos—scientific or other educational information on YouTube is not more likely to be seen as being provided by "real" people [37]. This finding has implications for both children's developing social understanding of the people they see on screen and whether and how they learn from such people. If children believe that the people they see on screens are not real, then researchers and parents may want to think about how children understand and frame any information those actors provide and the kinds of modeling children may be socialized to as a result of judging the actors as real or not.

## 2.4 Imagined Relationships with Characters

One area of research receiving heightened attention in recent years has been the nature of the relationships that children form with on-screen characters. Many children have favorite media characters and develop parasocial relationships with them—one-sided, emotional ties to media personae [38]. Even so, when children pretend with media characters (e.g., with a stuffed animal or a puppet based on the character), the play often manifests themes and behaviors of pretend play with real others, such as nurturing the character by feeding or bathing it [39]. As with imaginary companions [40], media characters that provide parasocial relationships appear to be appreciated for their human-like qualities and the social relationships and behaviors that they afford [41], more so than for the details of their mediated scripts and storylines. While most children develop parasocial relationships with slightly older characters with positive characteristics that they admire [42], children might also create parasocial relationships with characters that engage in rude or immoral behaviors if they are interested in exploring negative relationship affordances.

Because media characters do not typically age, children often "break up" with their favorite characters in favor of new ones as they grow [42]. Abandoned favorites sometimes become identified as too young or babyish. Just as the criteria that children explain as the basis for real friendship shift with development, so too do the characteristics that children appreciate in media characters, becoming more mature and often more gendered with age [42]. These findings suggest that the relationships imagined with media characters might fulfill a developmentally specific niche in children's social networks. However, much of the research in this area is based on parent report rather than direct interviews with children, meaning that the reasons children choose particular characters for parasocial attention, and the affordances of these relationships, are filtered through parents' perspectives.

## 3 Future Research

In summary, the current findings suggest several key takeaways regarding the impact of digital media use on creativity, imagination, and play. First, a higher frequency of digital media exposure has been linked to lower levels of creativity. Furthermore, background and foreground television has been linked to decreases in creative play. However, media content that engages children's imagination can promote creativity and imagination, especially when children are engaged with their beloved on-screen characters. The current state of research on the relation between media use and imagination, creativity, and play leaves several critical questions for future research:

- How might frequent media use reduce the frequency of boredom in the lives of children?
- Related, does ubiquitous media access interfere with the focus and effort required for imagination and creativity [13]?
- How do media, especially newer media such as AI and social robots, engage and scaffold children's imagination and creativity?
- What are the individual differences in children whose imagination and creativity are benefitted or harmed by interactions with digital media?
- When and to what extent is media content incorporated into children's fantasy play?
- How and when do young children understand acting, and what are the implications of this understanding? How is children's understanding of actors incorporated into their imagination and role play?

## 4 Recommendations

- *Parents and educators* should limit children's exposure to violent, aggressive, or otherwise negative media content and be particularly mindful of background media. Engaging with media might be best considered an activity, much the same as playing with toys, reading, or playing outside, rather than a backdrop to or constant interruption of other activities. As such, parents and educators should be intentional about when children are engaged with media and when to remove media from children's contexts. Parents also should engage children in conversations around what they are seeing, such as the behaviors of characters and the extent to which children may actually face in the real world the situations that the characters find themselves in. Media are likely to influence children's fantasy play, just as stories from books and adult behaviors do. Observers or participants in children's play might suggest expansions or alterations to a storyline that seems rigidly adherent to a media source. However, adults should remember that children likely choose themes and narratives from media that resonate.
- *Policymakers and media creators should* understand the links between media content and children's behavior—with respect to both creativity-enhancing media and violent or prosocial media. These connections suggest that media can be both a powerful tool for fostering imaginative thinking and behavior and a source of anxiety and a model of aggressive behavior. Regulation of media content for children would help leverage its influence in an appropriate and positive way.
- *Researchers* should consider that understanding the content of media experiences is more critical than broad measures of exposure (such as frequency and duration) for delineating the mechanisms through which digital media engagement influences imagination, creativity, and play.

**Conflict of Interest and Funding Disclosures** None.

## References

1. Harris PL. Early constraints on the imagination: the realism of young children. Child Dev. 2021;92(2):466–83. https://doi.org/10.1111/cdev.13487.
2. Calvert SL, Wilson BJ. The handbook of children, media, and development. Wiley eBooks; 2008. https://doi.org/10.1002/9781444302752.

3. Levin DE, Rosenquest B. The increasing role of electronic toys in the lives of infants and toddlers: should we be concerned? Contemp Issues Early Child. 2001;2(2):242–7. https://doi.org/10.2304/ciec.2001.2.2.9.
4. Oswald TK, Rumbold A, Kedzior SGE, Moore V. Psychological impacts of "screen time" and "green time" for children and adolescents: a systematic scoping review. PLoS One. 2020;15(9):e0237725. https://doi.org/10.1371/journal.pone.0237725.
5. Bronson P, Merryman A. The creativity crisis. Newsweek. August 2010. https://www.immagic.com/eLibrary/ARCHIVES/GENERAL/GENPRESS/N100710B.pdf.
6. Ruder DB. Screen time and the brain: digital devices can interfere with everything from sleep to creativity. Harvard Medical School News and Research. 2019. https://hms.harvard.edu/news/screen-time-brain.
7. Kerai S, Almas AN, Guhn M, Forer B, Oberle E. Screen time and developmental health: results from an early childhood study in Canada. BMC Public Health. 2022;22(1):310. https://doi.org/10.1186/s12889-022-12701-3.
8. Calvert SL, Valkenburg PM. The influence of television, video, games, and the Internet on children's imagination and creativity. In: Taylor M, editor. Oxford handbook of the development of imagination. New York: Oxford University Press; 2013. p. 438–50.
9. Suggate S, Martzog P. Screen-time influences children's mental imagery performance. Dev Sci. 2020;23(6):e12978. https://doi.org/10.1111/desc.12978.
10. Kirkorian HL, Pempek TA, Murphy LA, Schmidt M, Anderson DR. The impact of background television on parent–child interaction. Child Dev. 2009;80(5):1350–9. https://doi.org/10.1111/j.1467-8624.2009.01337.x.
11. Schmidt M, Pempek TA, Kirkorian HL, Lund AF, Anderson DR. The effects of background television on the toy play behavior of very young children. Child Dev. 2008;79(4):1137–51. https://doi.org/10.1111/j.1467-8624.2008.01180.x.
12. Gaudreau C, Hirsh-Pasek K, Golinkoff RM. What's in a distraction? The effect of parental cell phone use on parents' and children's question-asking. Dev Psychol. 2022;58(1):55–68. https://doi.org/10.1037/dev0001268.
13. Sternberg RJ, Lubart T. An investment theory of creativity and its development. Hum Dev. 1991;34(1):1–31. https://doi.org/10.1159/000277029.
14. Friedrich-Cofer LK, Huston-Stein AC, Kipnis D, Susman EJ, Clewit A. Environmental enhancement of prosocial television content: effects on interpersonal behavior, imaginative play, and self-regulation in a natural setting. Dev Psychol. 1979;15(6):637–46. https://doi.org/10.1037/0012-1649.15.6.637.
15. Anderson DR, Huston AC, Schmitt K, Linebarger D, Wright JC. Early childhood television viewing and adolescent behavior. Monogr Soc Res Child Dev. 2001;68(1):1–143.
16. Götz M, Lemish D, Moon H, Aidman A. Media and the make-believe worlds of children: when Harry Potter meets Pokemon in Disneyland. 2005. https://ci.nii.ac.jp/ncid/BA73402359.
17. Ruben E, Ffrench JA, Lee HJ, Aguiar NA, Richert R, Gleason T. Let it go: media influences on imaginary companions in early childhood. Poster presented at the 2023 meeting of the Society for Research in Child Development, Salt Lake City, UT; 2023.
18. Ricker AA, Richert RA. Digital gaming and metacognition in middle childhood. Comput Hum Behav. 2021;115:106593. https://doi.org/10.1016/j.chb.2020.106593.
19. Dong J, Choi K, Yu S, et al. A child-robot musical theater afterschool program for promoting STEAM education: a case study and guidelines. Int J Hum Comput Interact. 2023:1–17. https://doi.org/10.1080/10447318.2023.2189814.
20. Zhang C, Yao C, Wu J, et al. StoryDrawer. In: CHI conference on human factors in computing systems; April 2022. https://doi.org/10.1145/3491102.3501914.
21. Richert RA, Robb MB, Smith EI. Media as social partners: the social nature of young children's learning from screen media. Child Dev. 2011;82(1):82–95. https://doi.org/10.1111/j.1467-8624.2010.01542.x.
22. Sobel D. Understanding pretense as causal inference. Dev Rev. 2023;68:101065. https://doi.org/10.1016/j.dr.2023.101065.
23. Wellman HM, Liu D. Scaling of theory-of-mind tasks. Child Dev. 2004;75(2):523–41. https://doi.org/10.1111/j.1467-8624.2004.00691.x.
24. Calvert SL, Strong BL, Jacobs EL, Conger EE. Interaction and participation for young Hispanic and Caucasian girls' and boys' learning of media content. Media Psychol. 2007;9(2):431–45. https://doi.org/10.1080/15213260701291379.
25. Richert RA, Schlesinger MA. Relations between fantasy and transfer of learning from storybooks. J Exp Child Psychol. 2022;222:105474. https://doi.org/10.1016/j.jecp.2022.105474.
26. Wiedeman AM, Black JA, Dolle AL, Finney EJ, Coker KL. Factors influencing the impact of aggressive and violent media on children and adolescents. Aggress Violent Behav. 2015;25:191–8. https://doi.org/10.1016/j.avb.2015.04.008.
27. Weisberg DS, Richert RA. How, when, and what do young children learn from fictional stories? J Exp Child Psychol. 2022;221:105445. https://doi.org/10.1016/j.jecp.2022.105445.
28. Goldstein TR, Bloom P. Characterizing characters: how children make sense of realistic acting. Cogn Dev. 2015;34:39–50. https://doi.org/10.1016/j.cogdev.2014.12.001.
29. Nguyentran G, Weisberg DS. Should the cat in the hat keep talking like that? Educational correlates of anthropomorphism in children's science media. Psychol Pop Media. 2023;13:274. https://doi.org/10.1037/ppm0000467.
30. Goldstein TR, Alperson K. Dancing bears and talking toasters: a content analysis of supernatu-

ral elements in children's media. Psychol Pop Media. 2020;9(2):214–23. https://doi.org/10.1037/ppm0000222.

31. Hui L, Boguszewski K, Lillard AS. Can that really happen? Children's knowledge about the reality status of fantastical events in television. J Exp Child Psychol. 2015;139:99–114. https://doi.org/10.1016/j.jecp.2015.05.007.
32. Goldstein TR, Filipe A. The interpreted mind: understanding acting. Rev Gen Psychol. 2018;22(2):220–9. https://doi.org/10.1037/gpr0000116.
33. Lillard AS, Nishida T, Massaro D, Vaish A, Ma L, McRoberts GW. Signs of pretense across age and scenario. Infancy. 2007;11(1):1–30. https://doi.org/10.1207/s15327078in1101_1.
34. Lillard AS, Witherington DC. Mothers' behavior modifications during pretense and their possible signal value for toddlers. Dev Psychol. 2004;40(1):95–113. https://doi.org/10.1037/0012-1649.40.1.95.
35. Gunn A. I have a character issue. New York Times. 23 August 2013. Retrieved from: https://www.nytimes.com/2013/08/24/opinion/i-have-a-character-issue.html.
36. Goldstein TR, Bloom P. Is it Oscar-worthy? Children's metarepresentational understanding of acting. PLoS One. 2015;10(3):e0119604. https://doi.org/10.1371/journal.pone.0119604.
37. Hassinger-Das B, Dore RA. "Sometimes people on YouTube are real, but sometimes not": Children's understanding of the reality status of YouTube. E-Learn Digit Media. 2022;20(6):618–30. https://doi.org/10.1177/20427530221140679.
38. Calvert S. Parasocial relationships with media characters: imaginary companions for young children's social and cognitive development. In: Blumberg FC, Brooks PJ, editors. Cognitive development in digital contexts. Academic Press; 2017. p. 93–118.
39. Gola AAH, Richards MN, Lauricella AR, Calvert SL. Building meaningful parasocial relationships between toddlers and media characters to teach early mathematical skills. Media Psychol. 2013;16(4):390–411. https://doi.org/10.1080/15213269.2013.783774.
40. Gleason TR. The psychological significance of play with imaginary companions in early childhood. Learn Behav. 2017;45(4):432–40. https://doi.org/10.3758/s13420-017-0284-z.
41. Aguiar NR, Richards MN, Bond BJ, Brunick KL, Calvert SL. Parents' perceptions of their children's parasocial relationships: the Recontact Study. Imagin Cogn Pers. 2018;38(3):221–49. https://doi.org/10.1177/0276236618771537.
42. Aguiar NR, Richards MN, Bond BJ, Putnam MM, Calvert SL. Children's parasocial breakups with media characters from the perspective of the parent. Imagin Cogn Pers. 2018;38(3):193–220. https://doi.org/10.1177/0276236618809902.

# Digital Media and Neurodevelopmental Differences

Meryl Alper, Alyssa M. Alcorn, Kristen Harrison, Jennifer A. Manganello, and Rachel R. Romeo

## 1 Background

From birth through late adolescence, young people today are encountering more digital media and of various types (e.g., smartphones, computers, video games, virtual reality) than ever before, all with increasing potential for interactivity and immersion. Accordingly, "screen media" guidance is not a one-size-fits-all, and this is especially true for young people whose development occurs outside the window of linear "typical" development. This population includes those with brain differences that emerge during pregnancy, infancy, and early childhood, which alter neural functioning. Developmental differences may be present at birth but can also manifest with age relative to events and critical stages [1]. There have been significant cultural and social shifts over the past three decades in the recognition and diagnosis of neurodevelopmental differences in children, though much progress is still to be made with respect to reducing global, racial, ethnic, socioeconomic, and gendered health disparities [2].

Given the wide range of developmental differences in children, our research review of the effects of digital media use primarily focuses on those diagnosed with autism and/or attention-deficit/hyperactivity disorder (ADHD)—conditions that differ (e.g., by the degree of communication and social interaction difficulties) but often co-occur and share many underlying cognitive and clinical characteristics (e.g., attention and impulsivity challenges) [3]. Children with a diagnosis of autism and/or ADHD (as well as those with conditions such as dyslexia and dyscalculia) can be described as "neurodivergent" [4], meaning that their developmental trajectories and neurocognitive functioning are in the minority compared to those in the majority population (i.e., neurotypical development). The neurodiversity paradigm acknowledges these variations as conferring some possible cognitive strengths (e.g., problem-solving, pattern recognition) while also recognizing that neurodivergent people may need more support than those with "typical" development and experience substantial impacts on their daily lives (e.g., challenges in executive functioning) [5].

M. Alper (✉)
Northeastern University, Boston, MA, USA
e-mail: m.alper@northeastern.edu

A. M. Alcorn
University of Edinburgh, Edinburgh, Scotland, UK

K. Harrison
University of North Carolina at Chapel Hill, Chapel Hill, NC, USA

J. A. Manganello
University at Albany, State University of New York, Albany, NY, USA

R. R. Romeo
University of Maryland, College Park, MD, USA


D. A. Christakis, L. Hale (eds.), *Handbook of Children and Screens*,
https://doi.org/10.1007/978-3-031-69362-5_8

Our chapter organizes the major findings into (1) the effects of digital media on several developmental domains and (2) ecological contents for media engagement among these populations. While the evidence base is highly uneven and incomplete, existing research reviews [6–11] indicate that digital media use by children and adolescents with an autism and/or ADHD diagnosis can be not only high-risk (for example, in terms of experiencing sensory overwhelm from media, being victimized online, and vulnerability to excessive or compulsive technology use) but also high-reward (with respect to pursuing interest-based learning online and seeking networked social connection, for instance). Seeing as most scholarship has largely focused on maladaptive effects, it is equally (if not more) important to investigate and recognize adaptive benefits that may lead to improved quality of life. We begin by reviewing the current state of research on children, autism, ADHD, and digital media use, followed by suggestions for future work and recommendations for key stakeholders.

## 2 Current State

Media effects research on children with an autism and/or ADHD diagnosis is incomplete in several ways. Thus far, it has predominantly included short-term studies with small samples that focus on single settings/use cases/technologies and collected data from White and socioeconomically privileged samples in highly industrialized countries. Children diagnosed with autism and/or ADHD who have an intellectual disability and/or who do not reliably use spoken language have often been excluded. Little work on digital media use among young people diagnosed with autism and/or ADHD is demographically representative or longitudinal in nature, which limits the validity, applicability, and replicability of findings. Research also tends to prioritize parental reports over child perspectives, which presents a partial view of media engagement.

Research to date has found that media use rates may be higher or comparable for children with an ADHD and/or autism diagnosis relative to neurotypical young people [12]. However, motivations, usage patterns, and sensory sensitivities to digital media in these child populations can differ greatly [13]. For example, autistic adolescents reportedly use social media more for entertainment than for social interaction [14]. It is also important to note that while age is a significant factor, it is not necessarily the most helpful differentiator for children with significant communication and intellectual challenges [15]. Developmental age and chronological age may not fully align with respect to independent technology use and media content preferences [16].

### 2.1 Developmental Domains

Young people with an ADHD and/or autism diagnosis engage in digital media use that may impact several different yet overlapping domains of their development. These populations can experience unique challenges in their daily lives regarding behavior (e.g., executive functioning), physical health (e.g., sleep), social well-being (e.g., play and interaction), emotional regulation (e.g., recognizing emotions), sensory processing (e.g., avoidance and seeking of sensory input), cognition and learning (e.g., attention and focus), and communication (e.g., expressive and receptive language) [17]. In some aspects, the effects of digital media on these domains might be similar to those related to neurotypical young people but can also diverge.

For autistic children with limited social connections, for instance, playing video games can be considered a leisure activity and a topic of conversation to share with their friends and family, and social media offer ways to engage with others who share similar interests with less pressure than what they experience during in-person interactions [18]. However, individual usage of digital media and mobile devices may exacerbate social isolation for some of these children, specifically for those with limited access to in-person community engagement and recreational opportunities [19]. Adolescents with a diagnosis of autism and/or ADHD have reportedly higher rates of cybervictimization than do their neurotypical peers [20]. Although autistic adolescents may be more vulnerable to being cyberbullied, research also indicates that they are more risk-averse online (e.g., not revealing personal information to strangers) than are the typically developing youth [20–22].

## 2.2 Ecological Contexts

In addition to developmental domains, it is important to consider the mainstream and assistive/adaptive digital media uses of autistic young people and/or those with ADHD within their varied and interconnected social contexts [23, 24]. Besides everyday universal uses (e.g., accessible information seeking and messaging), these contexts include family and the home environment (e.g., parental mediation of disabled children's technology use), education and schooling (e.g., adaptive games for learning; to complete lessons and homework), health care (e.g., telehealth screenings), usage in the broader community (e.g., mobile apps for building daily life skills and managing tasks), and general communication (e.g., augmentative and alternative communication [AAC] devices for non- and minimally speaking young people).

As an example, virtual learning can potentially be more effective than in-person options for neurodivergent children with mental health struggles (e.g., those with social anxiety), which was seen for some during the COVID-19 pandemic [25]. Yet, while online learning and therapy platforms may reduce certain access barriers, they have also been inadequate substitutes for in-person support for many neurodivergent young people, especially those already experiencing resource inequities prior to the pandemic (e.g., related to race/ethnicity, class, immigration status, and geography) [26].

In all of these social contexts, there are also economic incentives and pressures to incorporate media and technology (e.g., machine learning algorithms, artificial intelligence) as replacements for more expensive, though potentially more effective, human forms of assistance for autistic children and/or those with ADHD (e.g., teachers, therapists) [27]. Despite significant financial investment in the development of novel intervention technologies for neurodivergent children (e.g., social robots), there is scant research evidence and evaluation base [28] as well as limited quality control in terms of market entry [29].

# 3 Future Research

Given the many unknowns and lack of empirical grounding in terms of media effects for children with autism and/or ADHD diagnoses (e.g., directionality, causality), and a lack of clarity regarding how autism and ADHD traits are linked to differential susceptibility to positive and negative effects, we offer several understudied questions for researchers building a body of work on autism, ADHD, neurodivergence, and children's digital media use to pursue and suggest actively involving those with lived experiences of autism and/or ADHD to take part in developing and engaging in such research projects:

- What is the true global heterogeneity of young people in terms of neurodevelopmental differences, and how do these individual differences influence, or how are they influenced by media and technology use?
- Seeing as online gaming can be an essential type of social connection and participation for neurodivergent young people, how could risks to their well-being (e.g., safety, privacy) best be minimized on these interactive digital platforms?
- How do potentially co-occurring mental health conditions (e.g., anxiety, eating disorders) among youth with an autism and/or ADHD diagnosis interact with mass, social, and interactive media use?
- To what extent could screen-based telehealth options support appropriate health-care treatment for neurodivergent young people, and in what ways?
- Which social and environmental factors lead to a greater or lesser reliance on media and technology for neurodivergent youth and their families (e.g., parent stress, limited affordable activities, poor access to health services), and how do these relate to well-being?

# 4 Recommendations

It is now a given that neurodivergent children engage with digital media at least as much if not more than neurotypical children do. Conversations about their technological engagement should be driven less by popular opinion and more by evidence-based approaches. Digital media are unlikely to cause autism and/or ADHD, akin to environmental exposure, despite frequent speculation [30]. It may, though, be an important moderator of positive and/or negative effects at various ages, with the potential to either shift or alter clinical presentation and developmental trajectories. There is also a reasonable need for technology providers to provide meaningful evidence that their products are beneficial or are at least not harmful to children who may qualify for, or who receive, an autism and/or ADHD diagnosis. As such, we offer the following recommendations for researchers, clinicians and care providers, policymakers, educators, and technologists:

## 4.1 For Researchers

- Create a transferrable evidence base (e.g., a data clearinghouse) regarding screen media use among neurodivergent children, which can be utilized by the key stakeholders (e.g., parents, teachers).
- Conduct more representative, longitudinal, and global studies that prioritize the perspectives of neurodivergent children and adolescents.

## 4.2 For Clinicians and Care Providers

- Improve training and education for healthcare providers on the benefits and risks of media use for young people with an autism and/or ADHD diagnosis.
- Reconsider one-size-fits-all recommendations and instead focus on which media are preferable for which developmental tasks (e.g., "scheduling/reminder apps can support executive functioning for adolescents with ADHD").

## 4.3 For Policymakers

- Provide more government research funding to understand the associations between various measures of screen usage (e.g., time, content, context) and health outcomes (e.g., mental health, social support, physical activity) among neurodivergent young people.

## 4.4 For Educators

- Utilize assistive and adaptive screen-based technology to support the meaningful inclusion of neurodivergent children and adolescents in schools, classrooms, and communities.

## 4.5 For Technologists

- Prioritize universal accessibility, user safety, and flexible use in developing mainstream technologies, including tools to support responsible usage by neurodivergent children.

**Conflict of Interest and Funding Disclosures** MA is currently paid as an educational consultant for PBS KIDS. AMA is a creator of the Learning About Neurodiversity at School (LEANS) program, a free-to-use classroom resource for teaching children about neurodiversity, and receives occasional income from paid speaking and training engagements related to this program. The other authors have no potential conflicts of interest or financial relationships relevant to this chapter to disclose.

## References

1. Boettcher L, Dammeyer J. Development and learning of young children with disabilities a Vygotskian perspective. Cham: Springer International Publishing; 2016.
2. Wiggins LD, Durkin M, Esler A, et al. Disparities in documented diagnoses of autism spectrum disorder based on demographic, individual, and service factors. Autism Res. 2019;13(3):464–73.
3. Astle DE, Holmes J, Kievit R, Gathercole SE. Annual research review: the transdiagnostic revolution in neurodevelopmental disorders. J Child Psychol Psychiatry. 2022;63(4):397–417.

4. Milton D, Ridout S, Martin N, Mills R, Murray D, editors. The neurodiversity reader: exploring concepts, lived experience and implications for practice. Pavilion Publishing and Media Ltd; 2020.
5. Kapp SK, Gillespie-Lynch K, Sherman LE, Hutman T. Deficit, difference, or both? Autism and neurodiversity. Dev Psychol. 2013;49(1):59–71.
6. Beyens I, Valkenburg PM, Piotrowski JT. Screen media use and ADHD-related behaviors: four decades of research. Proc Natl Acad Sci. 2018;115(40):9875–81.
7. Lane R, Radesky J. Digital media and autism spectrum disorders. J Dev Behav Pediatr. 2019;40(5):364–8.
8. Slobodin O, Heffler KF, Davidovitch M. Screen media and autism spectrum disorder: a systematic literature review. J Dev Behav Pediatr. 2019;40(4):303–11.
9. Stiller A, Mößle T. Media use among children and adolescents with autism spectrum disorder: a systematic review. Rev J Autism Dev Disord. 2018;5(3):227–46.
10. Cibrian FL, Lakes KD, Schuck SE, Hayes GR. The potential for emerging technologies to support self-regulation in children with ADHD: a literature review. Int J Child Comput Interact. 2022;1(31):100421.
11. Lakes KD, Cibrian FL, Schuck SE, Nelson M, Hayes GR. Digital health interventions for youth with ADHD: a mapping review. Comput Hum Behav Rep. 2022;1(6):100174.
12. Montes G. Children with autism spectrum disorder and screen time: results from a large, nationally representative US study. Acad Pediatr. 2016;16(2):122–8.
13. Harrison K. Rude or shrewd? Reframing media devices as care structures and child use as accommodation. J Child Media. 2019;13(3):367–75.
14. Alhujaili N, Platt E, Khalid-Khan S, Groll D. Comparison of social media use among adolescents with autism spectrum disorder and non-ASD adolescents. Adolesc Health Med Ther. 2022;13:15–21.
15. Alper M. Digital youth with disabilities. MIT Press; 2014.
16. Martins N, King A, Beights R. Audiovisual media content preferences of children with autism spectrum disorders: insights from parental interviews. J Autism Dev Disord. 2020;50(9):3092–100.
17. White SW, Maddox BB, Mazefsky CA, editors. The Oxford handbook of autism and co-occurring psychiatric conditions. Oxford University Press; 2020.
18. Pavlopoulou G, Usher C, Pearson A. "I can actually do it without any help or someone watching over me all the time and giving me constant instruction": autistic adolescent boys' perspectives on engagement in online video gaming. Br J Dev Psychol. 2022;40(4):557–71.
19. Alper M. Kids across the spectrums: growing up autistic in the digital age. MIT Press; 2023.
20. Beckman L, Hellström L, von Kobyletzki L. Cyber bullying among children with neurodevelopmental disorders: a systematic review. Scand J Psychol. 2020;61(1):54–67.
21. Gillespie-Smith K, Hendry G, Anduuru N, Laird T, Ballantyne C. Using social media to be 'social': perceptions of social media benefits and risk by autistic young people, and parents. Res Dev Disabil. 2021;118:104081.
22. Rocheleau JN, Chiasson S. Privacy and safety on social networking sites: autistic and non-autistic teenagers' attitudes and behaviors. ACM Trans Comput Hum Interact. 2022;29(1):1139.
23. Bronfenbrenner U. The ecology of human development. Harvard University Press; 1979.
24. Takeuchi LM, Levine MH. Learning in a digital age: toward a new ecology of human development. In: Jordan AB, Romer D, editors. Media and the well-being of children and adolescents. Oxford University Press; 2014. p. 20–43.
25. Averett KH. Remote learning, COVID-19, and children with disabilities. AERA Open. 2020;7(1):1–12.
26. Bakaniene I, Dominiak-Świgoń M, Meneses da Silva Santos MA, et al. Challenges of online learning for children with special educational needs and disabilities during the COVID-19 pandemic: a scoping review. J Intellect Dev Disabil. Published online August 9, 2022:1–12.
27. Iannone A, Giansanti D. Breaking barriers: the intersection of AI and assistive technology in autism care: a narrative review. J Pers Med. 2023;14(1):41.
28. Spiel K, Frauenberger C, Keyes O, Fitzpatrick G. Agency of autistic children in technology research—a critical literature review. ACM Trans Comput Hum Interact. 2019;26(6):1–40.
29. Kim JW, Nguyen TQ, Gipson SYMT, Shin AL, Torous J. Smartphone apps for autism spectrum disorder—understanding the evidence. J Technol Behav Sci. 2018;3:1–4.
30. Pouretemad HR, Sadeghi S, Badv RS, Brand S. Differentiating post-digital nannying autism syndrome from autism spectrum disorders in young children: a comparative cross-sectional study. J Clin Med. 2022;11(22):6786.

# Introduction to the Section on Screens and Physical Health

Lauren Hale

While much of the scientific literature on the effects of digital screen media use on child well-being focuses on the wide-ranging psychological, cognitive, and social effects, in recent years, there has been growing evidence of the implications of digital screen media use in physical health as well. In this handbook, we include five chapters discussing the distinct effects on physical health outcomes (i.e., physical activity, nutrition, food marketing, marketing of other health risk behaviors, sleep health, and physical injuries). While some of these chapters address overlapping topics, they each delve into the mechanisms and strengthen the case that the pervasive role of screens in our children's lives have a complex relationship with potentially both positive and negative impacts on physical health.

The first two chapters address the role of digital screen media use in physical activity and nutrition. First, Tremblay et al. (see Chap. 10) use the 24-h movement behavior framework (physical activity, sedentary behavior, sleep) to discuss current knowledge and research challenges regarding how digital screen media use relates to child growth and development. Then, Staiano et al. (see Chap. 11) summarize the evidence of digital screen media use on nutrition through increased eating while viewing screens and exposure to food advertising, contributing to higher energy intake, lower nutritional quality, and more nighttime eating. Both chapters report that more passive screen time (e.g., television) has stronger effects than do other types of screen uses (e.g., video game playing or computer use) for physical activity and nutritional outcomes.

The next two chapters explore the role of digital marketing in children's diet and several high-risk products. Harris et al. (see Chap. 12) discuss how digital marketing has amplified the promotion of unhealthy foods and products, thus influencing the child's food preferences. These food advertisements have penetrated the evolving digital media landscape with promotions in traditional television commercials, sponsored ads on websites and social media platforms, promotions in gaming sites, branded games (advergames), company-sponsored apps, and paid online personalities (influencers) often featuring music, sports, cars, and celebrities that appeal to the youth. Relatedly, Emond et al. (see Chap. 13) write about how marketing tactics used in current digital media target adolescents for alcohol, tobacco, and firearms. Alcohol and e-cigarette companies routinely reach out to underage populations due to the latter's ability to misrepresent their birth dates on social media. In addition, the firearms imagery in current video games has become much more realistic and the weapons used are often commercially available. Given the

L. Hale (✉)
Family, Population, and Preventive Medicine, Renaissance School of Medicine, Stony Brook University, Stony Brook, NY, USA
e-mail: lauren.hale@stonybrook.edu


D. A. Christakis, L. Hale (eds.), *Handbook of Children and Screens*,
https://doi.org/10.1007/978-3-031-69362-5_9

massive user base of social media and violent video games and the extended amount of time spent using these devices, there may be implications for changing attitudes and behaviors about all of these categories of products.

Hale et al. (see Chap. 14) update the literature on the relatively consistent finding that digital screen media use, particularly at night, is associated with later bedtimes, shorter sleep duration, and lower sleep quality. In particular, they note that recent review articles have shown that interactive digital screen media use is likely worse for sleep health than more passive viewing of digital media, which interestingly contrasts with the finding for nutrition and physical activity described above.

In the final chapter, Manganello et al. (see Chap. 15) accurately delineate four distinct ways in which digital screen media use can cause injuries to young individuals, including risks of injury from impact with the device itself (e.g., a screen tipping over), distraction causing an injury (e.g., distracted driving), overuse of the device (e.g., a strained neck), and media effects on high-risk physical activities. In particular, since social media videos can be created by anyone, there are often videos of youth engaging in risky behavior (ranging from not wearing a seatbelt to a high-risk "fire challenge" viral video), with very little or even misleading educational content warning about safety risks.

Each of these brief chapters summarizes the scientific literature within their topic area, providing key references for future inquiry and identifying gaps in the literature. A consistent limitation across all the chapters is the concern about our limited ability to accurately measure digital screen-based media use and the challenges of incorporating the nuances of content. Another limitation is the ability to address a causal impact. After the summary of the current state of the literature, each team of authors identified their top research questions for future scholars to pursue. Finally, each chapter concludes with recommendations aimed at mitigating the effects of digital screen media use on the range of physical health outcomes addressed. Together, the chapters included in this section provide a compelling overview of the role of digital media use in the healthy physical development of children.

**Conflict of Interest and Funding Disclosures** LH is partially supported by grants from NICHD (R01 HD073352 and R21 HD097491) and the Della Pietra family. She has received consulting fees from Idorsia Pharmaceuticals and honoraria/travel support for lectures and consulting supported by Brown University, Harvard University, University of Miami, New York University, Columbia University/Princeton University, and the National Sleep Foundation. She ended her term as the editor-in-chief of *Sleep Health* in 2020.

# Digital Screen Media Use, Movement Behaviors, and Child Health

Mark S. Tremblay, Nicholas Kuzik, Stuart J. H. Biddle, Valerie Carson, Mai J. M. Chinapaw, Dorothea Dumuid, Wendy Yajun Huang, Travis J. Saunders, Amanda E. Staiano, and Russell R. Pate

## 1 Background

"Movement behaviors" is an umbrella term encompassing sleep, sedentary behaviors, and physical activity [1]. The adoption of this term coincides with recognition of the importance of the interaction of these three behaviors throughout a 24-h day, as opposed to traditional approaches that examined each separately [1, 2]. Digital screen media use (DSMU; defined for this chapter as the use of mediums of digitized information transmitted via screens), sometimes referred to as screen time, typically falls under the sedentary behavior category, since it is generally consumed while sedentary—though it would be erroneous to assume equivalence between the two concepts [1, 2]. According to several countries around the world, a healthy DSMU duration is considered ≤2 h per day of recreational screen time for children aged 5–17 years, ≤1 h for


M. S. Tremblay (✉)
Children's Hospital of Eastern Ontario Research Institute, Ottawa, ON, Canada

Department of Pediatrics, University of Ottawa, Ottawa, ON, Canada

Department of Health Sciences, Carleton University, Ottawa, ON, Canada
e-mail: mtremblay@cheo.on.ca

N. Kuzik
Children's Hospital of Eastern Ontario Research Institute, Ottawa, ON, Canada

S. J. H. Biddle
Centre for Health Research, University of Southern Queensland, Springfield Central, QLD, Australia

Faculty of Sport & Health Sciences, University of Jyväskylä, Jyväskylä, Finland

V. Carson
Faculty of Kinesiology, Sport, and Recreation, University of Alberta, Edmonton, AB, Canada

M. J. M. Chinapaw
Public and Occupational Health, Amsterdam Centre UMC, Vrije Universiteit, Amsterdam Public Health, Amsterdam, The Netherlands

D. Dumuid
Alliance for Research in Exercise, Nutrition and Activity, University of South Australia, Adelaide, SA, Australia

W. Y. Huang
Department of Sport, Physical Education and Health, Hong Kong Baptist University, Hong Kong, China

T. J. Saunders
Department of Applied Human Sciences, University of Prince Edward Island, Charlottetown, PE, Canada

A. E. Staiano
Pennington Biomedical Research Center, Baton Rouge, LA, USA

R. R. Pate
Department of Exercise Science, Arnold School of Public Health, University of South Carolina, Columbia, SC, USA



D. A. Christakis, L. Hale (eds.), *Handbook of Children and Screens*,
https://doi.org/10.1007/978-3-031-69362-5_10

children 2–4 years, and no screen time is recommended for children <2 years [1–3]. The consideration of DSMU in relation to all movement behaviors in a 24-h day has important implications for children's healthy growth and development (Fig. 1) [4]. Specifically, a day is a fixed amount of time, and engaging in one movement behavior necessarily displaces the amount of time remaining for other behaviors (e.g., an extra hour of sedentary behavior means an hour less for physical activity and/or sleep). Additionally, the benefits or risks of one behavior (e.g., excessive DSMU) can be mitigated, compounded, or increased depending on the individual's other daily movement behaviors. However, DSMU is a complex behavior to fully conceptualize within an integrated 24-h movement behavior framework because of the many ways that it can be categorized and subcategorized. For instance, the impact of DSMUs on all movement behaviors could vary by the types, content, format, and context of media that youth engage in, irrespective of whether the media promote active or passive engagement and whether the youth are simultaneously engaging in more than one DSMU (media multitasking). Furthermore, within existing public health guidelines for preschool- and school-aged children and adolescents, DSMU can be framed as either recreational [1, 2] or educational [5]. The purpose of this brief review is to examine the relationship between DSMUs and children's healthy growth and development, within a 24-h movement behavior framework, while providing recommendations for healthy DSMUs and directions for future research.

## 2 Current State

### 2.1 Displacement

The displacement hypothesis states that DSMU demonstrates adverse associations with children's health and development [4, 6, 7] because it reduces the available time for behaviors that are beneficial to health and development such as sleep, physical activity, and in-person socializing [8]. Displacement of healthy movement behaviors is one explanation for the simultaneous increases in DSMU and mental health concerns of the last ~20 years [8]. While the evidence for DSMU displacing physical activity is mixed, a

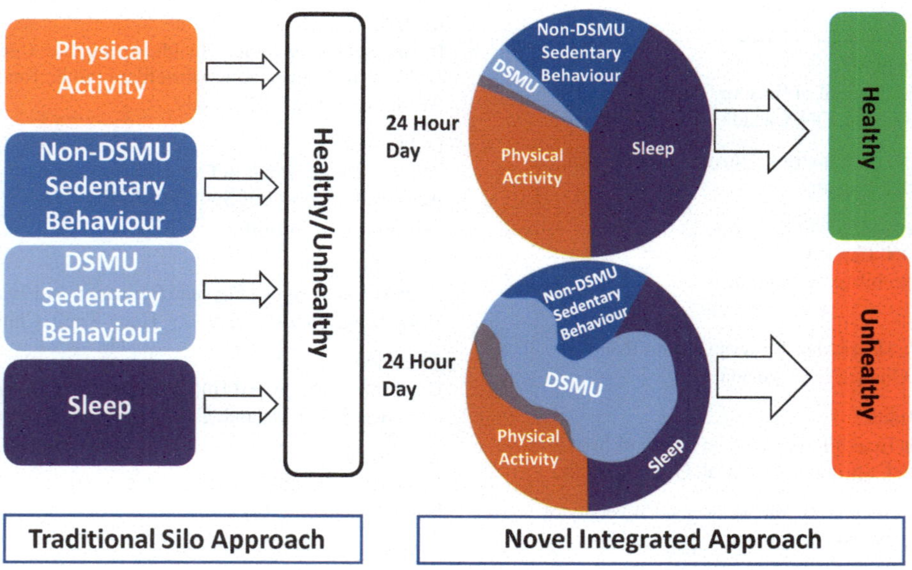


**Fig. 1** The traditional siloed approach to conceptualizing associations between movement behaviors and health, compared to the paradigm shift using an integrated approach. The two right illustrations of movement behavior compositions in a 24-h day depict how digital screen media use (DSMU) creep can lead to unhealthy outcomes

meta-analysis examining the association between screen time and physical activity demonstrated small negative associations for physical activity with total screen time, Internet time, and television, whereas null associations were found for computer time and video games [9]. Longer screen time in children aged 2–3 years was associated with more sedentary behavior and less physical activity in later childhood [10] and displacement of time spent playing with peers [11]. A recent clustered randomized controlled trial has demonstrated substantial increases in children's physical activity among families randomized to the recreational screen media reduction arm of the intervention [12]. Another study showed no evidence overall for the displacement hypothesis in a cohort of 755 adolescents followed prospectively for more than 3 years; though when examined by gender, there was partial displacement in boys [13]. The authors reported that girls engaged in more smartphone time, whereas boys engaged in more video games time, and, thus, the type of screen time may be an important consideration for displacement, especially when considering smartphones have a level of portability that may allow for simultaneous engagement in physical activity compared to computer- and television-based screen time [13].

Displacing time spent in physical activity toward more sedentary pursuits, such as DSMU, is unfavorable from a health perspective [4, 6, 7], but engaging in such pursuits for entertainment or stimulation can be inherently reinforcing and appealing behaviors for children, especially given that many DSMU apps or interfaces are engineered to catch and keep one's attention. The effort minimization and affective-reflective theories examine the motivations involved in transitioning from sedentary behavior to physical activity. The effort minimization theory is rooted in evolutionary biology and explains the drive for humans to avoid unnecessary physical exertion, whereas the affective-reflective theory articulates that if people learn to associate negative affect with physical activity, then it will require additional cognitive resources to overcome [14]. Thus, choosing to displace physical activity with DSMU is reinforced through our biology and could be the easiest and most rewarding choice. While limited research for these theories exists on practical ways to replace sedentary behavior with physical activity at the individual level, some suggestions include strengthening an individual's cognitive resources and self-control capacity, to overcome the tendency to minimize energy expenditure, and creating positive experiences around physical activity to develop positive affective valuations of physical activity [14]. Interventions to channel sedentary DSMU propensities toward healthy or otherwise beneficial sedentary options such as reading, board games, or playing a musical instrument deserve exploration. At the societal level, policies that make physical activity affordable and accessible are also likely to support those families looking to shift time from DSMUs to more active pursuits [15].

Screen time could also displace or disturb sleep through heightened physiological arousal, suppression of melatonin release, or simply being woken due to incoming messages or other notifications [16–20]. Decreased sleep quantity and quality could cause fatigue, resulting in less motivation for physical activity and more motivation for physically and mentally passive screen time [18]. See the chapter focusing on sleep and DSMU in this handbook for further details.

DSMUs may displace other modes of sedentary behavior, for example, displacement of traditional classroom activities with screen-based learning or displacement of traditional sedentary media (e.g., books, magazines, newspapers, television, movies) with digital media alternatives (e.g., Internet, texting, social media, gaming) [21]. Recent international school-related sedentary behavior recommendations for children and youth have suggested that child health and well-being may be promoted through limiting education-based DSMU (preferentially replacing it with non-screen-based learning activities), similar to constraining recreational use [5]. While the review informing the international school-related sedentary behavior recommendations for children and youth found no benefits for replacing traditional non-screen-based learning with DSMUs [22], it could be argued that an integration of DSMUs could compliment or enhance non-screen-based learning. To understand the implications for child health, these other sedentary displacements deserve further attention by the research community.

## 2.2 Combined Associations

Beyond behavior displacement, understanding how different movement behavior patterns integrate throughout a 24-h day is important for a fulsome understanding of the relationship with child health. Excessive DSMU alone has been shown to be harmful for numerous aspects of children's health and development [4, 6, 7], but, when combined with inadequate levels of physical activity and sleep, the risks may increase [1, 4]. For instance, one US study found that high levels of screen time were not associated with obesity for the most physically active children, but, in combination with lower physical activity levels, the risk of obesity increased, with the highest risk seen for the least active and most screen time [23]. In an international sample of ~600,000 children, the mitigating benefits of physical activity for children with excessive screen time for mental health were not seen, but the combination of higher levels of physical activity and lower levels of screen time were still the most beneficial in a dose-response manner [24]. Likewise, replacing screen time with physical activity or sleep has demonstrated benefits for adiposity, psychosocial health, and academic achievement cross-sectionally and depressive symptom changes over a year [25, 26]. Interestingly, replacing social media or television with team sports was beneficial for emotional distress, but similar associations were not seen when replacing video gaming or general computer use [27]. Thus, the types of behaviors being combined or replaced are important considerations and provide further support for understanding and managing movement behaviors, including DSMU, as a collective when promoting child health. Such efforts are further complicated by differing sociodemographic profiles of users across media platforms, making it difficult to disentangle and find causal associations of movement behaviors and health. Furthermore, the optimal distributions of movement behaviors and DSMUs may vary by the health outcome being examined (e.g., optimal combinations may vary when comparing obesity and mental health risks).

## 2.3 Content and Context

To understand what constitutes a healthy combination of movement behaviors for a particular age, one needs to consider the content and context of DSMU. A recent meta-analysis has found that passive viewing, gaming, socio-recreational, and total screen time were unfavorable for children's health while the limited number of studies prevented any firm conclusions for educational screen time [28]. Likewise, a recent systematic review has found limited and mixed research evidence on school-related screen time, but benefits were seen when school-related screen time was intentionally implemented to serve a specific pedagogical purpose [29]. Possible benefits of cognitively active DSMU require further research, especially in the context of 24-h movement behaviors. When considering video games, an important distinction may be passive vs. active (video games requiring physical activity) gaming, as the latter has demonstrated benefits for children's adiposity and cardiorespiratory fitness [30].

The distinctions between healthy and unhealthy digital media content and context require further research before firm conclusions can be drawn, and, currently, most research is lumping all types into a total DSMU or screen time variable [28]. However, total screen time is a heterogeneous collection of devices (e.g., televisions, smartphones, computers), contents (e.g., video streaming channels, online classes), and contexts (e.g., co-viewing television with parents, dancing with friends, watching a video, active video games). Furthermore, media multitasking is particularly problematic when conceptualizing the displacement of behaviors, since various types of DSMUs can be co-occurring, thus complicating accurate measurement [31].

### 2.4 Measurement and Analysis Issues

Common methodologies for measuring movement behaviors include self- or proxy-reports and device-based measures (e.g., accelerometers, inclinometers), each with their own strengths and limitations [32]. DSMU measures include an abundance of self- or proxy-report questionnaires that trade high levels of feasibility for low (and often unknown) levels of validity and reliability—with limited exploration of the key contents and contexts (e.g., educational vs. recreational, active vs. sedentary, shared vs. solitary, productive vs. consumptive) [33]. A small, but growing, number of studies have examined alternative measurements of DSMU with in-device tracking of screen use [34], or passive sensing, which could greatly enhance the validity and reliability of digital media measurement [33], assuming that only one individual accumulates their DSMU on one particular device. In reality, individuals use multiple devices (e.g., smartphones, televisions, tablets), and devices may also be shared (e.g., family television, library computer) or used concurrently. Even if techniques capable of accurately measuring DSMUs arise, including multitasking, consideration is also needed for how to treat the data in relation to other movement behaviors in a 24-h day. For instance, an earlier report estimated that 29% of digital media exposure occurs while multitasking [35], so should analyses expand beyond the 24-h window to accommodate the extra 29% of DSMU or contract the duration of DSMU by 29% to account for overlap? Contracting reintroduces the previous issue of losing the nuances of content and context, whereas expanding distorts real-world recommendations by creating a synthetic >24-h day. Advances in measurement technology and analyses methods are needed to integrate all movement behaviors while determining the optimal doses of combinations of various digital media types, formats, and platforms, to fully elucidate DSMU–movement behavior relationships with child health.

Methods of analysis are also central to understanding how various movement behaviors, including sedentary DSMU, interact to impact measures of child health. For example, some analyses show that the effect sizes of screen time alone lack clinical significance or are too small to be of any concern [36]. However, such analyses of one behavior miss the relevance of combinations of all movement behaviors across the whole day and the idea that small changes in individual behaviors may collectively result in bigger changes to overall movement behavior profiles and health indicators at a population level. Indeed, the principle of multifinality—any one component of a system may function differently depending on the organization of the system in which it operates—supports the importance of an integrated movement behavior and health approach. For example, DSMU may contribute to small unfavorable changes (e.g., increases in anxiety, depression, insufficient sleep) but collectively aggregate to meaningful improvements and variation for global health/functioning [33]. Future research examining global health/functioning and patterns of DSMUs and movement behaviors are warranted to explore the aggregation of effects for time use exposures and global health outcomes.

## 3 Future Research

With the novelty of the 24-h movement behavior paradigm and rapid evolution in digital media technology and consequent usage, there are many more research questions than answers. Research priorities and some of their subsets are presented below.

### 3.1 Healthy Behavior Displacement

- What movement behaviors are displaced when DSMU increases? Is the displacement similar in educational, recreational, and family settings? How do movement behavior displacement patterns differ by age, gender, socioeconomic status, cultural background, and/or their intersections? Furthermore, when

displacement patterns differ among diverse groups, research is needed that explores the underlying mechanisms driving these differences (e.g., neighborhood safety).
- Does DSMU displace outdoor time? Is increasing outdoor time a feasible intervention to displace excessive DSMU? If so, what are the health benefits? Can DSMU be used to increase outdoor time (e.g., augmented reality games)? If so, are health benefits the same as non-DSMU outdoor time?
- What are the health effects of displacing traditional sedentary behaviors with sedentary DSMU (e.g., paper-based vs. DSMU recreational reading), even if the total volume of sedentary behavior remains constant?

## 3.2 Combined Associations

- How does DSMU influence the composition of movement behaviors associated with optimal child health (i.e., what does the "best day" look like and does this vary by child characteristics)?
- Can healthy movement behavior compositions moderate the adverse influence of excessive DSMU? Does this vary among indicators of physical and mental health? Are there differences by age, gender, socioeconomic status, cultural background, and/or their intersections?
- Beyond the ideal distribution of movement behaviors, including DSMU, for health and wellness, what are the feasible distributions of movement behaviors for children to adopt? How can we make the optimal movement behavior patterns feasible?

## 3.3 Content and Context

- What are the ideal combinations or compositions of DSMU types (e.g., social DSMU, educational DSMU, co-viewing DSMU) with other movement behaviors in a 24-h day? How does this distribution differ by age, gender, socioeconomic status, cultural background, and/or their intersections?
- Can DSMU be used to improve healthy movement behaviors, and does it depend on the type, context, content, or intersections of age, gender, socioeconomic status, and cultural background?
- Develop a clear, common, and accepted terminology for DSMU that encapsulates the emerging and existing types, contexts, and contents.
- How can the above information be most effectively distributed to clinicians, parents, children, adolescents, and educators?

## 3.4 Measurement and Analysis

- How can we accurately measure 24-h movement behaviors incorporating the nuances of DSMU (e.g., multitasking, content, context) with adequate reliability, validity, feasibility, and generalizability across different countries, ages, genders, socioeconomic status, and cultural backgrounds?
- What are the shared correlates or determinants that would create parsimonious intervention targets for healthy movement behaviors and DSMU?
- How does timing (e.g., digital screen use before bed and during the night), pattern (e.g., long bouts vs. intermittent) and proportional distribution of DSMU as a component of sedentary time change the interactions of DSMU with movement behaviors?

## 3.5 Research Designs

- Better quality research designs (e.g., longitudinal, interventional, experimental) are required.
- More representative samples are needed (e.g., including marginalized groups, rural samples, low- and middle-income countries, early years).

## 4 Recommendations

While the evidence base remains incomplete, there is sufficient guidance from existing research to inform recommendations that conform to the principle *primum non nocere* (first, do no harm). Below is a list of recommendations, segmented to help guide parents and families, educators, clinicians and public health leaders, policymakers and governments, and researchers to promote habitual movement behaviors and responsible DSMU for healthy growth and development [37].

Increases in DSMU may adversely affect healthy child movement behaviors such as physical activity and sleep, having undesirable healthy outcomes. However, not all DSMUs may be adversely associated with health (e.g., active video games, digital physical activity accessories, motivating digital music), and some devices may be used for self-monitoring and goal setting (e.g., wearable movement monitors), technology-delivered support like just-in-time adaptive interventions, virtual coaches, prompts/nudges, and for setting limits for screen use (e.g., parental controls). Whether the lure of DSMU can be balanced with the need for a healthy combination of physical activities, sedentary behaviors, and sleep requires diligent monitoring and study to ensure adherence to the principle *primum non nocere*.

### 4.1 For Parents and Families

- Create positive physical activity experiences that could help children displace sedentary DSMU with physical activity in the future.
- Protect sleep time by encouraging sleep hygiene (e.g., no DSMU 1 h before bed, no screens in the bedroom).
- Promote healthy movement behaviors by encouraging, facilitating, role modeling, and monitoring healthy behaviors.
- Develop household rules and goal setting that limit excessive DSMU and create opportunities for healthy physical activity and sleep habits.
- Prevent personal and familial DSMU from displacing or disrupting important family activities (e.g., playing, socializing, bonding, mealtimes).

### 4.2 For Educators [4]

- When school-related DSMU is warranted:
  - Ensure that it is meaningful, mentally or physically active, and serves a specific pedagogical purpose that enhances learning.
  - Limit time on devices, especially for students <12 years of age.
  - Take a device break at least once every 30 min.
  - Discourage media multitasking in the classroom and while doing homework.
- Teach and promote the importance of a healthy balance of movement behaviors and the consequences of excessive sedentary DSMU.

### 4.3 For Clinicians and Public Health Leaders

- Talk with families about the importance of all movement behaviors, including the role that DSMU may be playing in displacing other healthy movement behaviors.
- Encourage families to create family plans to establish agreed-upon household DSMU rules (e.g., daily/weekly limits on recreational DSMU; screen-free mealtimes).
- Encourage parents to adopt healthy DSMU and movement behavior habits themselves, as parental modeling of behaviors will influence child DSMU habits.
- Understand that DSMU should be considered in relation to other movement behaviors.

### 4.4 For Policymakers and Governments

- Implement evidence-informed legislation around DSMU limits or restrictions on children (e.g., Utah Social Media Regulation

Amendments, Social Media NUDGE Act; China and South Australia have banned children from using mobile phones in school).
- Provide resources for enhancing infrastructure and access to inclusive physical activity opportunities (e.g., parks, playgrounds, recreation centers, bike lanes, sports fields) for all intersections of age, gender, socioeconomic status, and cultural background.
- Provide resources for developing, promoting, and implementing national 24-h movement behavior guidelines, including recommendations for healthy DSMU.

## 4.5 For Researchers

- When presenting total DSMU, include the various contents and contexts and their potential associations with health and other health behaviors.
- Develop better methods to measure and analyze DSMU quantity, quality, and context.
- Develop consensus on the best practice DSMU measurements and analyses that reflect the complexities of DSMU multitasking, incorporation into a 24-h day of movement behaviors, and feasibility when conducting national/international surveillance research.
- Compare and contrast associations between DSMU and any one health outcome in relation to overall well-being and all movement behaviors.
- Conceptualize strategies for research to keep pace with rapidly evolving DSMU.
- Examine whether and how DSMU could be an agent of positive change (e.g., wearables for goal setting, active video games, remote education).

**Conflict of Interest and Funding Disclosures** There was no specific funding support for this project. NK was supported by a Canadian Institutes of Health Research Postdoctoral Fellowship.

## References

1. Tremblay MS, Carson V, Chaput J-P, et al. Canadian 24-hour movement guidelines for children and youth: an integration of physical activity, sedentary behaviour, and sleep. Appl Physiol Nutr Metab. 2016;41(6):S311–27.
2. World Health Organization. Guidelines on physical activity, sedentary behaviour and sleep for children under 5 years of age. Geneva: World Health Organization; 2019.
3. Parrish AM, Tremblay MS, Carson S, Veldman SL, Cliff D, Vella S, Chong KH, Nacher M, del Pozo CB, Ellis Y, Aubert S. Comparing and assessing physical activity guidelines for children and adolescents: a systematic literature review and analysis. Int J Behav Nutr Phys Act. 2020;17:1–22.
4. Rollo S, Antsygina O, Tremblay MS. The whole day matters: understanding 24-hour movement guideline adherence and relationships with health indicators across the lifespan. J Sport Health Sci. 2020;9(6):493–510.
5. Saunders TJ, Rollo S, Kuzik N, et al. International school-related sedentary behaviour recommendations for children and youth. Int J Behav Nutr Phys Act. 2022;19(1):39.
6. Carson V, Hunter S, Kuzik N, et al. Systematic review of the relationships between sedentary behaviour and health indicators in school-aged children and youth: an update. Appl Physiol Nutr Metab. 2016;6(Suppl. 3):S240–65.
7. Stiglic N, Viner RM. Effects of screen time on the health and well-being of children and adolescents: a systematic review of reviews. BMJ Open. 2019;9:e023191.
8. Twenge JM. Increases in depression, self-harm, and suicide among U.S. adolescents after 2012 and links to technology use: possible mechanisms. Psychiatr Res Clin Pract. 2020;2(1):19–25.
9. Pearson N, Braithwaite R, Biddle SJ, van Sluijs EM, Atkin AJ. Associations between sedentary behaviour and physical activity in children and adolescents: a meta-analysis. Obes Rev. 2014;15(8):666–75.
10. Chen B, Bernard JY, Padmapriya N, et al. Associations between early-life screen viewing and 24 hour movement behaviours: findings from a longitudinal birth cohort study. Lancet Child Adolsec Health. 2020;4(3):201–9.
11. Putnick DL, Trinh M-H, Sundaram R. Displacement of peer play by screen time: associations with toddler development. Pediatr Res. 2023;93:1425–31. https://doi.org/10.1038/s41390-022-02261-y.
12. Pedersen J, Rasmussen MGB, Sørensen SO, et al. Effects of limiting recreational screen media use on physical activity and sleep in families with children: a cluster randomized clinical trial. JAMA Pediatr. 2022;176(8):741–9.

13. Lizandra J, Devís-Devís J, Valencia-Peris A, Tomás JM, Peiró-Velert C. Screen time and moderate-to-vigorous physical activity changes and displacement in adolescence: a prospective cohort study. Eur J Sport Sci. 2019;19(5):686–95.
14. Brand R, Cheval B. Theories to explain exercise motivation and physical inactivity: ways of expanding our current theoretical perspective. Front Psychol. 2019;10:1147.
15. Global action plan on physical activity 2018–2030: more active people for a healthier world. Geneva: World Health Organization; 2018. Licence: CC BY-NC-SA 3.0 IGO.
16. Cain N, Gradisar M. Electronic media use and sleep in school-aged children and adolescents: a review. Sleep Med. 2010;11(8):735–42.
17. Exelmans L, Van den Bulck J. Binge viewing, sleep, and the role of pre-sleep arousal. J Clin Sleep Med. 2017;13(8):1001–8.
18. Hale L, Guan S. Screen time and sleep among school-aged children and adolescents: a systematic literature review. Sleep Med Rev. 2015;21:50–8.
19. Saunders TJ, McIsaac T, Campbell J, et al. Timing of sedentary behaviour and access to sedentary activities in the bedroom and their association with sleep quality and duration in children and youth: a systematic review. Health Promot Chronic Dis Prev Can. 2022;42(4):139–49.
20. Wood B, Rea MS, Plitnick B, Figueiro MG. Light level and duration of exposure determine the impact of self-luminous tablets on melatonin suppression. Appl Ergon. 2013;44(2):237–40.
21. Twenge JM, Martin GN, Spitzberg BH. Trends in U.S. adolescents' media use, 1976–2016: the rise of digital media, the decline of TV, and the (near) demise of print. Psychol Pop Media Cult. 2019;8:329–45.
22. Kuzik N, da Costa BG, Hwang Y, Verswijveren SJ, Rollo S, Tremblay MS, Bélanger S, Carson V, Davis M, Hornby S, Huang WY. School-related sedentary behaviours and indicators of health and well-being among children and youth: a systematic review. Int J Behav Nutr Phys Act. 2022;19(1):40.
23. Sisson SB, Broyles ST, Baker BL, Katzmarzyk PT. Screen time, physical activity, and overweight in U.S. youth: national survey of children's health 2003. J Adolesc Health. 2010;47(3):309–11.
24. Khan A, Lee EY, Rosenbaum S, Khan SR, Tremblay MS. Dose-dependent and joint associations between screen time, physical activity, and mental wellbeing in adolescents: an international observational study. Lancet Child Adolesc Health. 2021;5(10):729–38.
25. Dumuid D, Olds T, Wake M, et al. Your best day: an interactive app to translate how time reallocations within a 24-hour day are associated with health measures. PLoS One. 2022;17(9):e0272343.
26. Sampasa-Kanyinga H, Colman I, Dumuid D, et al. Longitudinal association between movement behaviours and depressive symptoms among adolescents using compositional data analysis. PLoS One. 2021;16(9):e0256867.
27. Kandola A, del Pozo CB, Hayes JF, Owen N, Dunstan DW, Hallgren M. Impact on adolescent mental health of replacing screen-use with exercise: a prospective cohort study. J Affect Disord. 2022;301:240–7.
28. Zahedi S, Jaffer R, Iyer A. A systematic review of screen-time literature to inform educational policy and practice during COVID-19. Int J Educ Res Open. 2021;1(2):100094.
29. Kuzik N, da Costa BG, Hwang W, et al. School-related sedentary behaviours and indicators of health and well-being among children and youth: a systematic review. Int J Behav Nutr Phys Act. 2022;19(1):1–32.
30. Oliveira CB, Pinto RZ, Saraiva BTC, et al. Effects of active video games on children and adolescents: a systematic review with meta-analysis. Scand J Med Sci Sports. 2020;30(1):4–12.
31. Browne DT, May SS, Colucci L, et al. From screen time to the digital level of analysis: a scoping review of measures for digital media use in children and adolescents. BMJ Open. 2021;11(5):e046367.
32. Fairclough SJ, Noonan RJ. Introduction to physical activity measurement. In: Brusseau T, Fairclough S, Lubans D, editors. The Routledge handbook of youth physical activity. New York: Routledge; 2020. p. 251–60.
33. Browne D, Thompson DA, Madigan S. Digital media use in children: clinical vs scientific responsibilities. JAMA Pediatr. 2020;174(2):111–2.
34. Wade NE, Ortigara JM, Sullivan RM, Tomko RL, Breslin FJ, Baker FC, Fuemmeler BF, Delrahim Howlett K, Lisdahl KM, Marshall AT, Mason MJ, Neale MC, Squeglia LM, Wolff-Hughes DL, Tapert SF, Bagot KS, Novel Technologies ABCD, Workgroup. Passive sensing of preteens' smartphone use: an adolescent brain cognitive development (ABCD) cohort substudy. JMIR Ment Health. 2021;8(10):e29426. https://doi.org/10.2196/29426. PMID: 34661541; PMCID: PMC8561413
35. Rideout VJ, Foehr UG, Roberts DF. Generation M$^2$: media in the lives of 8-to 18-year-olds. Henry J. Kaiser Family Foundation; 2010.
36. Orben A, Przybylski AK. The association between adolescent well-being and digital technology use. Nat Hum Behav. 2019;3:173–82.
37. Rhodes RE, Guerrero MD, Vanderloo LM, et al. Development of a consensus statement on the role of the family in the physical activity, sedentary, and sleep behaviours of children and youth. Int J Behav Nutr Phys Act. 2020;17:74.

# Screen Media, Obesity, and Nutrition

Amanda E. Staiano, Alyssa M. Button, Gary S. Goldfield, Thomas N. Robinson, Jorge Mota, Susan J. Woolford, and Peter T. Katzmarzyk

## 1 Background

Globally, obesity (body mass index percentile ≥95th) affects 39 million children under the age of 5 and 340 million children and adolescents aged 5–19 years, and it leads to lifelong physical, mental, and psychological challenges [1]. Screen media use is a well-documented contributor to obesity and is the most prevalent activity in a day for most children aside from school or sleep [2]. A review of 130 surveillance studies indicated that children and adolescents report 3.6 h/day of total screen time, though some studies report as high as 7 h/day [3].

This chapter provides an update on a previous report on screen media exposure and obesity, which suggested that the primary mechanism linking screen media use to children's obesity is dietary intake, specifically excess eating while viewing screen media and repeated exposures to high-calorie and low-nutrient food and beverage marketing [2]. Since the initial publication, the media landscape has evolved significantly, warranting an updated perspective. Screen time continues to evolve with the advent of continuous and immersive video reels, voice-activated assistants, social media influencers, augmented and virtual reality, targeted advertising, immersive worlds where children can virtually shop for food and beverages, cook, or work in a fast-food outlet from a smartphone, a tablet, a computer, or an Internet-connected TV, and more. When in-person interactions were limited during the COVID-19 pandemic [4], schools, parents, and children increasingly relied on screen media as an educational tool, for entertainment, and for peer and family connections. Post-pandemic, children aged 6–10 years reported the largest increases in total and leisure screen time of any age group (approximately 1.4 h more per day) [5]. The associations between screen media use, obesity, and nutrition may be more complex than previously recognized, with multifactorial mech-

A. E. Staiano (✉) · A. M. Button · P. T. Katzmarzyk
Pennington Biomedical Research Center, Baton Rouge, LA, USA
e-mail: Amanda.Staiano@pbrc.edu

G. S. Goldfield
Healthy Active Living and Obesity Research Group, Children's Hospital of Eastern Ontario Research Institute, Ottawa, ON, Canada

T. N. Robinson
Stanford Solutions Science Lab and Division of General Pediatrics, Department of Pediatrics, Stanford Prevention Research Center, Department of Medicine, and Department of Epidemiology and Population Health, Stanford University, Stanford, CA, USA

J. Mota
Research Center on Physical Activity, Health and Leisure (CIAFEL), Faculty of Sport, University of Porto, Porto, Portugal

S. J. Woolford
School of Public Health, University of Michigan, Ann Arbor, MI, USA



D. A. Christakis, L. Hale (eds.), *Handbook of Children and Screens*,
https://doi.org/10.1007/978-3-031-69362-5_11

anisms and influences explaining the effects of prolonged, frequent, and pervasive use on children's nutrition and weight gain. A better understanding of the media landscape and how children's continuous interactions with media impact food availability, food choice, food preference, and amount consumed could point to novel intervention targets and more effective ways to mitigate the potentially harmful effects of screen media.

This chapter examines the current state of the science on the associations between and the purported mechanisms underlying screen media use, obesity, and nutrition, delineates effective strategies to reduce screen media use or to convert media time to promote healthier food intake, identifies limitations to the current state of evidence and future research directions, and provides recommendations for researchers, policymakers, clinicians, educators, and media technology providers.

## 2 Current State

Children's time spent viewing screens is related to their nutritional intake [6] and consequently their risk of obesity [6, 7]. A recent umbrella review of 13 reviews has found strong evidence of associations between screen time and greater obesity/adiposity and moderate evidence between screen time and higher energy intake [6]. However, most of the findings supporting the link to obesity were specific to television screen time, with mixed results for other forms of screen time or for overall screen time, and there was no strong evidence for a dose-response association or specific threshold of screen time related to the incidence or risk of obesity [6]. Similarly, television screen time was the predominant screen type linked to higher energy intake and poor dietary quality [6]. There is less or mixed evidence of associations for other types of media uses such as video game play, computer, or smartphone use. One study that did collapse total media use, including television, computer, and video game in an analysis of 659,288 adolescents, indicated that adolescents who reported using screen media for 6 or more h per day, compared to those who used screen media for less than 2 h/day, had a higher odds of nighttime eating, inadequate sleep, poor dietary intake, and increased risk of obesity [7].

The degree of sedentary vs. physically active engagement with screen media may change the relationship with nutrition and obesity. In a systematic review and a dose-response meta-analysis, screen time was defined based on the World Health Organization's definition as *passive* time spent watching screen-based entertainment, excluding active screen-based games that involve physical activity or movement. Adolescents under the highest category of *passive* screen time were 1.27 times more likely to develop overweight/obesity (44 studies including a total $N = 112{,}489$) [8]. Similarly, a meta-analysis of 54 studies including a total of 45,638 children and adolescents observed a higher body mass index among those in the highest vs. lowest *passive* screen users and daily screen time was 0.3 h higher in children and adolescents with obesity vs. without obesity [9]. In another recent study, youth who had reported using their smartphones for nonphysical active gaming for more than 2 h/day were two times more likely than were their peers who had done the same for less than 2 h/day to be overweight or obese [10]. Conversely, several studies showed inverse associations between time spent playing *physically active* video games and obesity [8], indicating that energy expenditure with screen media use may portend different effects on nutrition and obesity.

### 2.1 Purported Mechanisms

The most researched and consistent mechanism that links screen media use to nutrition and obesity is the advertising effects on dietary consumption [11–13]. Children are uniquely vulnerable to persuasive advertisements given their developing critical thinking skills, limited ability to distinguish persuasive from non-persuasive content or understand advertising intent, and poor impulse inhibition [14]; moreover, children respond more positively to unhealthy food advertisements versus healthy food or nonfood ads [11]. Social media present an opportunity for significant targeted advertisements. For example, an analysis of YouTube ads targeted toward children determined that food and beverage ads appeared most frequently, with over half of them promoting food with low nutritional value [12]. Children view unhealthy food advertising posts for longer periods of time than other types of ads, and children who are heavy media users (>3 h/day) are more willing to engage with food ads on Instagram (i.e., "liking") [13]. Food advertising targeting children, particularly Black and Hispanic children [15], intensified during the COVID-19 pandemic [11], thus further exacerbating the pervasive influence of food ads on children's dietary consumption and contributing to racial disparities in weight.

The non-advertising effects of media use on dietary consumption have also been recognized, including neurocognitive effects of non-advertising screen media content on children's executive functioning, which may prime young viewers with salient food cues that elicit hunger signals and make it difficult to inhibit the urges to eat long after the screen viewing is over [16]. Media use mechanisms may distract from or interrupt internal signals of satiety and satiation (i.e., interoceptive awareness); may divert attention away from viewers' habitual control of food intake; may condition the viewer with cues to eat, thus decreasing temporal windows of delayed gratification; may impair memory of how much food has been eaten; and may contribute to hedonic eating [16]. Each mechanism has preliminary associative evidence but warrants further confirmation (see Fig. 1). Experimental studies are needed to examine the complexities of these relationships. Furthermore, adolescents are frequently exposed to unattainable beauty standards, where digital tools, filters, and posing create images and messages of body shapes and sizes that are idealized and unnatural. This contributes to poor self-image and body dissatisfaction [17], which directly and indirectly cause emotional distress and related disordered eating [18]. Compared to peers with healthy weight, youth with obesity are at a greater risk of developing unhealthy dieting behaviors that trigger and maintain disordered eating symptoms and, in many cases, increase energy intake, as a result of emotional distress and body dissatisfaction [19].

## 2.2 Interventions to Reduce Screen Time and Effects on Improving Obesity and Nutrition

Given the evidence that screen media use exerts harmful effects on children's nutrition and puts them at risk for obesity [6, 7], there have been widespread efforts to reduce children's screen time [20, 21]. A systematic review concluded that interventions to reduce recreational screen time did successfully do so while also increasing physical activity, improving diet, and improving or maintaining weight status among children aged 13 and younger [20]. The interventions varied: coaching/counseling and monitoring screen media use for the child and family, building family and peer support, delivering classroom-based lessons, and issuing mass educational appeals [21]. Similarly, a meta-analysis of 23 studies evaluating interventions to reduce screen time and sedentary behavior indicated a small but significant reduction in television viewing from interventions designed to promote healthy screen use, along with a small reduction in sedentary behavior [21], with each mechanism associated with child adiposity and cardiometabolic health [6]. It is unclear which characteristics (e.g., intensity and duration) and components (e.g., family-based social support, electronic monitoring) are the most effective in reducing screen time, and it is also unclear how long the intervention effects are maintained after the active intervention ends [20, 21]. Effects of reducing mobile device use were rarely reported, so it remains unknown the extent to which reducing children's time spent with these devices is achievable and is associated with improvements in nutrition and reductions in the risk for obesity.

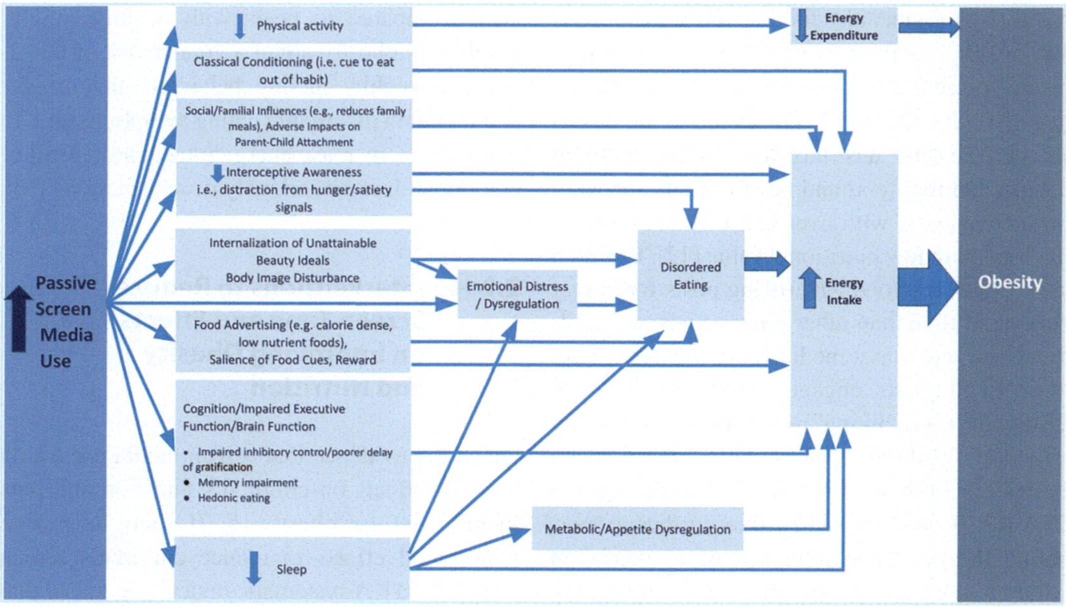


**Fig. 1** Proposed mechanisms for passive, noneducational screen media's influence on children's energy intake and obesity

## 2.3 Interventions Incorporating Screen Media to Improve Nutrition and Obesity Outcomes

Instead of reducing time spent on screens, many are turning to these devices to administer nutritional and obesity reduction interventions. Screen media are being integrated into treatment delivery for weight management and nutritional counseling, including health information technology in primary care that supports the healthcare provider [22] and technology-based interventions such as telehealth, exergames (i.e., video games that require physical activity to play), apps, wearables, and other platforms and devices to promote healthy nutrition and facilitate health behavior change. The 2023 American Academy of Pediatrics clinical practice guidelines on the treatment of children and adolescents with obesity identified technology-based interventions as an effective adjunctive tool for intensive health behavior and lifestyle interventions, citing evidence that exergames have helped children increase their physical activity and reduce weight [23].

However, systematic reviews also indicated mixed results on the effectiveness of these screen-based interventions, likely due to heterogeneity in age, parent involvement, intervention, the use of outdated technology, and limited rigor in the study design [24–27]. The evidence is limited on newer technologies like immersive gamification through augmented reality and virtual reality as ways to prevent or treat obesity. There are few studies utilizing technology to deliver adaptive or just-in-time interventions such as voice-activated assistants to provide immediate, personalized, timely support to children and families related to nutrition and obesity [25].

Children and adolescents are also using screen media for self-management and information seeking related to nutrition and obesity. A systematic review of 16 studies concluded that adolescents utilize smartphones (via apps, blogs/discussion boards, messaging services, social media) to easily access health and nutrition information, to partake in nutrition counseling, to communicate with clinicians and peers, and to engage with social influencers who advertise food brands and share video reels of themselves eating, cooking, or exercising and that these types of screen interactions can also facilitate behavior logging and self-assessment [28]. Screen-based interventions that capitalize on the platforms that adolescents are currently using for health information have demonstrated improvements in weight, sedentary behavior, dietary intake, physical activity, and peer support [28]. While these studies offer promising results for dietary interventions, limited measures of feasibility have been collected and a decline in participation is evident over time. A further concern is that youths are increasingly turning to social media for weight loss and nutrition information that may convey misinformation or harmful strategies, which may then contribute to unhealthy or overly restrictive eating attitudes and behaviors [11].

## 2.4 Limitations of Our Knowledge

Difficulties in measuring both habitual dietary intake in children and habitual media use due to inaccurate measurements complicate the examination of the associations, mechanisms, and interventions targeting screen media, obesity, and nutrition [3, 29, 30]. Television remains the most commonly used proxy for screen time, accounting for 64% of measures used in 130 population-based surveillance studies [3]. Despite the shift in children's media use toward portable devices, only <5% of reviewed studies measured mobile phone use and <1% measured active gaming [3]. Furthermore, the accuracy of self-report screen usage is limited, with documented discrepancies between objective measures vs. self-report media use [29]. A systematic review of 622 articles that used screen time measures in children aged 0–6 years identified that only 11% of studies reported psychometric properties to support the measures' validity and reliability and that these had generally weak or moderate validity [30]. The known poor accuracy of self-reports and/or parent reports of screen time may result in attenuated and/or biased associations and frequently do not attempt to measure the content of what users are seeing and doing on their digital screens.

Obtaining ecologically valid estimates of screen use often overlooks the type, content, and quality (i.e., opportunities for cognitive and physical development) of screen time [6]. These potentially important characteristics of screen use may differentially impact nutritional intake and obesity risk, such as the amount of passive vs. physically active engagement of the child, whether the screen media is co-viewed or discussed with a parent, whether the content is meaningful to the child and promotes or allows for social interaction, the context and setting, and the presence of foods or food advertisements. Moreover, few studies examine the potential longer-term influence of screen media use on children's consumption, dietary preferences, and attitudes toward food or household food availability throughout childhood and into adolescence.

# 3 Future Research

Despite the pervasive nature of screen media use in children's lives [3] and the associations demonstrated with both nutritional intake and obesity [7, 8], there remains a wide gulf to better contextualize children's real-world experiences with screen media as it relates to nutritional intake and obesity and the underlying mechanisms that can be targeted to either mitigate or disrupt harmful health effects. The following are proposed as timely research questions:

- What are the nutrition- and obesity-related exposures that children and adolescents experience with screen media (i.e., what is the content, where do they occur)? Which contextual factors, including the timing and environment of exposure, moderate these impacts?
- What are the effects of screen media use on children's acute and long-term nutritional intake, moving beyond a focus solely on the duration of screen time? Are there differential impacts of screen media on populations with the highest prevalence of obesity? What are the novel mechanisms linking media use to nutrition and obesity, such as neural vulnerabilities associated with media use that could impact nutrition and obesity outcomes, particularly

through effects on children's brain structure and neurocognitive function? Can these vulnerabilities be addressed through intervention?
- What are the effective, sustainable strategies to reduce sedentary screen media use in children and adolescents? What are the individual, family, and sociodemographic characteristics that moderate the impacts of interventions?
- What makes health-promoting media interventions effective in improving children's nutrition and lowering obesity risk? How well do newer technologies (such as smartphone apps, telehealth, wearables, augmented/virtual reality, and voice assistants) complement traditional in-person nutrition and obesity counseling?

## 4 Recommendations

The following recommendations are made for mitigating the harmful effects of screen media use on children's obesity and nutrition:

- *Clinicians and providers* should talk with parents and youth about the impact of screen media use on nutrition and weight and help families establish healthy limits and practices tailored to their needs.
- *Policymakers and advocates* should increase funding for research on screen media, obesity, and nutrition, including:
  - Develop and validate passive, accurate, reliable methods for capturing the content, context, functions, timing, and quantity of children's screen use across multiple devices throughout the day and night for use in real-world and research settings and also develop mechanisms for privacy-protected data sharing for the research community.
  - Update current public health surveillance systems (e.g., Youth Risk Behavior Surveillance System, National Health and Nutrition Examination Survey) to capture both screen use beyond television viewing and engagement with other types of screens as well as the content, quality, and interactivity of screen usage.
  - Develop and validate simple self-report measures that identify the risk of problematic children's media for use as screening and monitoring tools in clinical and school settings and connect families to appropriate resources and counseling.
  - Develop and test theory-driven strategies (individual, family, school, community, and policy) to mitigate the harmful effects of screen media use on children's nutrition and obesity and utilize screen media to promote healthful behaviors and nutritious diets.
- *Industry leaders* should expand parental control and user control features, including for food advertisements, food placement, and content, which promote disordered eating and/or weight control behaviors in children, especially on newer platforms and devices that are not currently regulated.
- *Policymakers* should develop regulations and legislation to reduce exposure of children and adolescents to unhealthy food marketing in screen media by eliminating targeted ads that track what users do online, digital advertising engagement activities, and manipulative design features specifically targeting children and adolescents.

**Conflict of Interest and Funding Disclosures** None.

## References

1. World Health Organization. Obesity and overweight. https://www.who.int/news-room/fact-sheets/detail/obesity-and-overweight. Accessed 27 Jan 2023.
2. Robinson TN, Banda JA, Hale L, et al. Screen media exposure and obesity in children and adolescents. Pediatrics. 2017;140(Supplement 2):S97–S101.

3. Thomas G, Bennie JA, De Cocker K, Castro O, Biddle SJ. A descriptive epidemiology of screen-based devices by children and adolescents: a scoping review of 130 surveillance studies since 2000. Child Indic Res. 2020;13:935–50.
4. Abouk R, Heydari B. The immediate effect of COVID-19 policies on social-distancing behavior in the United States. Public Health Rep. 2021;136(2):245–52. https://doi.org/10.1177/0033354920976575.
5. Trott M, Driscoll R, Iraldo E, Pardhan S. Changes and correlates of screen time in adults and children during the COVID-19 pandemic: a systematic review and meta-analysis. EClinicalMedicine. 2022;48:101452. https://doi.org/10.1016/j.eclinm.2022.101452.
6. Stiglic N, Viner RM. Effects of screentime on the health and well-being of children and adolescents: a systematic review of reviews. BMJ Open. 2019;9(1):e023191.
7. Cha EM, Hoelscher DM, Ranjit N, et al. Effect of media ese on adolescent body weight. Prev Chronic Dis. 2018;15:E141.
8. Haghjoo P, Siri G, Soleimani E, Farhangi MA, Alesaeidi S. Screen time increases overweight and obesity risk among adolescents: a systematic review and dose-response meta-analysis. BMC Prim Care. 2022;23(1):1–24.
9. Wu Y, Amirfakhraei A, Ebrahimzadeh F, Jahangiry L, Abbasalizad-Farhangi M. Screen time and body mass index among children and adolescents: a systematic review and meta-analysis. Front Pediatr. 2022;10:822108.
10. Brodersen K, Hammami N, Katapally TR. Is excessive smartphone use associated with weight status and self-rated health among youth? A smart platform study. BMC Public Health. 2023;23(1):234. https://doi.org/10.1186/s12889-023-15037-8.
11. Bozzola E, Spina G, Agostiniani R, et al. The use of social media in children and adolescents: scoping review on the potential risks. Int J Environ Res Public Health. 2022;19(16):9960.
12. Tan L, Ng SH, Omar A, Karupaiah T. What's on YouTube? A case study on food and beverage advertising in videos targeted at children on social media. Child Obes. 2018;14(5):280–90.
13. Lutfeali S, Ward T, Greene T, et al. Understanding the extent of adolescents' willingness to engage with food and beverage companies' Instagram accounts: experimental survey study. JMIR Public Health Surveill. 2020;6(4):e20336. https://doi.org/10.2196/20336.
14. Albuquerque P, Brucks M, Campbell MC, et al. Persuading children: a framework for understanding long-lasting influences on children's food choices. Cust Needs Solut. 2018;5(1):38–50. https://doi.org/10.1007/s40547-017-0083-x.
15. Harris JL. Targeted food marketing to Black and Hispanic consumers: the tobacco playbook. Am J Public Health. 2020;110(3):271.
16. Marsh S, Ni Mhurchu C, Maddison R. The non-advertising effects of screen-based sedentary activities on acute eating behaviours in children, adolescents, and young adults. A systematic review. Appetite. 2013;71:259–73. https://doi.org/10.1016/j.appet.2013.08.017.
17. Fioravanti G, Bocci Benucci S, Ceragioli G, Casale S. How the exposure to beauty ideals on social networking sites influences body image: a systematic review of experimental studies. Adolesc Res Rev. 2022;7(3):419–58. https://doi.org/10.1007/s40894-022-00179-4.
18. Cruz-Sáez S, Pascual A, Wlodarczyk A, Echeburúa E. The effect of body dissatisfaction on disordered eating: the mediating role of self-esteem and negative affect in male and female adolescents. J Health Psychol. 2020;25(8):1098–108. https://doi.org/10.1177/1359105317748734.
19. Jebeile H, Lister NB, Baur LA, Garnett SP, Paxton SJ. Eating disorder risk in adolescents with obesity. Obes Rev. 2021;22(5):e13173. https://doi.org/10.1111/obr.13173.
20. Buchanan LR, Rooks-Peck CR, Finnie RK, et al. Reducing recreational sedentary screen time: a community guide systematic review. Am J Prev Med. 2016;50(3):402–15.
21. Oh C, Carducci B, Vaivada T, Bhutta ZA. Interventions to promote physical activity and healthy digital media use in children and adolescents: a systematic review. Pediatrics. 2022;149(Supplement 6):e2021053852I.
22. Kepper M, Walsh-Bailey C, Staiano A, et al. Health information technology use among healthcare providers treating children and adolescents with obesity: a systematic review. Curr Epidemiol Rep. 2021;8:151–71.
23. Hampl SE, Hassink SG, Skinner AC, et al. Clinical practice guideline for the evaluation and treatment of children and adolescents with obesity. Pediatrics. 2023;151:e2022060640.
24. Hsu MS, Rouf A, Allman-Farinelli M. Effectiveness and behavioral mechanisms of social media interventions for positive nutrition behaviors in adolescents: a systematic review. J Adolesc Health. 2018;63(5):531–45.
25. Kouvari M, Karipidou M, Tsiampalis T, et al. Digital health interventions for weight management in children and adolescents: systematic review and meta-analysis. J Med Internet Res. 2022;24(2):e30675.
26. Hammersley ML, Jones RA, Okely AD. Parent-focused childhood and adolescent overweight and obesity eHealth interventions: a systematic review and meta-analysis. J Med Internet Res. 2016;18(7):e203. https://doi.org/10.2196/jmir.5893.
27. McMullan M, Millar R, Woodside JV. A systematic review to assess the effectiveness of technology-based interventions to address obesity in children. BMC Pediatr. 2020;20(1):1–14.

28. Chau MM, Burgermaster M, Mamykina L. The use of social media in nutrition interventions for adolescents and young adults—a systematic review. Int J Med Inform. 2018;120:77–91.
29. Parry DA, Davidson BI, Sewall CJR, Fisher JT, Mieczkowski H, Quintana DS. A systematic review and meta-analysis of discrepancies between logged and self-reported digital media use. Nat Hum Behav. 2021;5(11):1535–47. https://doi.org/10.1038/s41562-021-01117-5.
30. Byrne R, Terranova CO, Trost SG. Measurement of screen time among young children aged 0–6 years: a systematic review. Obes Rev. 2021;22(8):e13260.

# Digital Food Marketing and Children's Health and Well-being

Jennifer L. Harris, Frances Fleming-Milici, Ashley N. Gearhardt, Sonya Grier, Kathryn Montgomery, Maria Romo-Palafox, and Mimi Tatlow-Golden

## 1 Background

Food, beverage, and restaurant (henceforth "food") companies spend billions in marketing directed at children, including adolescents (henceforth "children"), predominantly promoting calorie-dense products that are high in sugar, fat, and sodium [1, 2]. A large body of research on marketing to children has concluded that exposure to food marketing is associated with significant increases in choice, preferences, and requests to parents for unhealthy foods and increased caloric intake, with lifelong negative health impacts [1–3]. The World Health Organization (WHO) calls for dramatic reductions in unhealthy food marketing to children to reverse the global epidemic of childhood obesity and poor diet [1, 4, 5]. Most countries have ceded responsibility of this critical public health issue to food industry self-regulatory initiatives, which typically apply industry-defined nutrition criteria to food products advertised in traditional media directed at younger children (under age 13, primarily children's TV) [1]. Yet, self-regulation has failed to produce meaningful reductions in children's exposure to unhealthy food marketing [1, 6].

Moreover, food marketing has been transformed in the past 20 years. The amount of time children spend watching traditional TV has declined, whereas time spent online has skyrocketed [6, 7]. Unhealthy food brands have innovated digital marketing techniques to engage young people on mobile devices [8], where they now spend the majority of their screen time [7]. Food companies now market unhealthy products directly to children on their smartphones virtually anytime anywhere, using their online behaviors to precisely target marketing messages [8]. Companies place this marketing on digital sites popular with children, including social media, influencer videos, and gaming platforms, using techniques that encourage viral dissemination through peers, thus deepening children's engagement with brands and amplifying their negative impact [6, 8].

J. L. Harris (✉) · F. Fleming-Milici
Rudd Center for Food Policy & Health, University of Connecticut, Storrs, CT, USA
e-mail: Jennifer.Harris@uconn.edu

A. N. Gearhardt
Department of Psychology, University of Michigan, Ann Arbor, MI, USA

S. Grier
Kogod School of Business, American University, Washington, DC, USA

K. Montgomery
Center for Digital Democracy, American University, Washington, DC, USA

M. Romo-Palafox
Nutrition and Dietetics, Saint Louis University, St. Louis, MO, USA

M. Tatlow-Golden
School of Education, Childhood, Youth and Sport, The Open University, Milton Keynes, UK


D. A. Christakis, L. Hale (eds.), *Handbook of Children and Screens*, https://doi.org/10.1007/978-3-031-69362-5_12

This chapter summarizes the current state of digital food marketing to children, including adolescents, why this raises substantial concerns about their health and well-being, and how to effectively reduce the significant negative consequences.

## 2 Current State

Digital marketing refers to any form of product promotion that occurs online, including on computers, mobile devices, and smart TVs. Since the 1990s, food brands have been at the forefront in adopting youth-targeted digital marketing techniques, including advertisements on websites, branded games (advergames), and company-sponsored apps (e.g., online ordering, loyalty programs) [6, 8]. Food brands have also led in marketing on social media platforms [6, 8], including YouTube, Instagram, TikTok, and Snapchat, the most popular online destinations for US children as young as 3 years [7, 9]. In addition to purchasing advertising on these sites, food brands maintain accounts where young people engage with company- and user-generated posts, which often prominently feature music, sports, and other youth-appealing celebrities [10]. Followers like and share these posts, spreading marketing messages virally through peer networks [10]. As with traditional advertising aimed at children, numerous content analyses have found that these forms of digital marketing primarily promote products that are detrimental to health, including fast food, sugary drinks, candy, and snacks [6, 10].

In recent years, youth-targeted online entertainment has expanded while food brands continuously pioneer new marketing techniques. Similar to branded product placements in streaming TV, music, and online games, paid online personalities (influencers) post videos endorsing branded products on YouTube and other social media platforms while engaging in entertaining activities, such as playing with toys or applying makeup [8]. Influencers with millions of young followers endorse or integrate food brands into their content [8]. Popular live-streaming gaming sites (Twitch, Facebook Gaming) enhance connectedness to influencers touting brands, whereas the metaverse provides a platform that rewards children's "avatar selves" for engaging with brands in a fantasy world [11]. Approximately three-quarters of children aged 9–12 years visit the most popular gaming platform Roblox [8].

Thus, digital food marketing is designed to achieve maximum reach and appeal to young people [6, 8, 12]. In one study, 70% of adolescents reported engaging with up to 48 food brands on social media [13]. More than 60% of social media posts viewed by adolescents in another study contained food promotions, the majority of which were embedded within influencer or other entertainment content [14]. On YouTube, children as young as 5 years of age regularly watch child influencer channels with millions of followers, where more than one-third of videos feature branded, primarily unhealthy, food products [15].

Reviews of the existing literature have found that exposure to social media marketing and advergames has similar effects as traditional TV advertising exposure does on young people's diets, including food choices, preferences, purchase requests, and intake of marketed and other available foods [10, 16, 17]. Digital marketing is highly effective at increasing positive attitudes about and consumption of unhealthy foods and beverages for all youth, including adolescents and young adults [10, 16].

### 2.1 How Digital Marketing Differs from Traditional Advertising

Although online food marketing to children promotes the same unhealthy products with similar negative effects as food advertising in traditional media such as TV, digital marketing raises unique concerns. In traditional advertising (e.g., TV commercials), brands communicate in one direction to a broadly defined target audience (e.g., children's TV viewers) through marketing content clearly separated from programming. Effectively counteracting traditional advertising messages requires conscious attention and recognition of the marketing attempt and the ability and motivation to counterargue the persuasive message, a difficult task even for adults [18]. Yet, much of food marketing (traditional and digital) is specifically designed to bypass conscious rational message processing [18].

Branded messages embedded within online content often come disguised as games, videos, and other entertainment or as social media posts from peers and celebrities and are thus more difficult to recognize than traditional advertising [19]. This stealth marketing also distracts users from conscious attention to its persuasive intent while the entertainment content activates positive emotions that transfer to the brand through a classical conditioning process [18]. Food marketing gets "under the skin" by activating the neural circuitry implicated in reward, motivation, and attention [20], and these neural systems can be activated outside of conscious awareness [21]. Adolescents who exhibit greater reward and motivation activation when viewing TV commercials for both healthy and unhealthy foods are more likely to order and consume unhealthy food options and may be more prone to gain weight over time [21].

Social media marketing disguised as messages from friends also taps into peer networks and makes children unwitting promoters of branded content as they engage with and share content online [16]. Adolescents attend to, like, and share social media posts for unhealthy foods more, compared to healthy food or nonfood posts, and they rate peers whose social media feeds contain unhealthy food advertising posts more positively [22]. Online marketing enables brands to cultivate direct relationships with children, including through parasocial relationships with beloved influencers and celebrities and via children's "avatar selves" in the metaverse [10, 12].

In addition, users' personal data and marketing are inextricably intertwined online, especially on mobile devices where every behavior can be tracked, measured, integrated, and used to target entertainment and advertising content in real time [6, 12]. The world's largest food companies together with the technology industry utilize big data and AdTech tools to tap into children's online cultural spaces [8]. Even the majority of children's education websites, including those used by schools, feature targeted advertising and/or unclear policies on behavioral and contextual advertising [23].

Moreover, digital marketing amplifies everything through repetitive exposure across multiple channels. Children's lives are now hybrid, and food marketing flows and interacts between their off- and online worlds [6, 8]. Yet, the entire digital enterprise is highly complex and remains inaccessible to outsiders, including academic researchers. Neither technology platforms nor food companies provide clear, publicly available data on their techniques, demographic targets, or the impacts of their efforts [8, 12]. Most digital marketing also takes place completely under the radar of parents, policymakers, and health professionals [6]. Due to the highly personalized and targeted nature of digital marketing, public health researchers face significant challenges to studying what children are exposed to online [12, 17].

## 2.2 Adolescents May Be Uniquely Vulnerable

Worldwide, existing policies to limit unhealthy food marketing, including government and industry self-regulatory initiatives, typically only address advertising to children up to 13 years of age [5, 24], based on decades of research demonstrating that young children do not have the cognitive ability to recognize and actively defend against persuasive attempts [18]. These policies assume that adolescents' ability to recognize marketing attempts and greater advertising skepticism than younger children protect them from potentially harmful marketing attempts. Although cognitive abilities develop throughout adolescence, they do not reduce adolescents' enjoyment of advertising, its positive impact on product attitudes [25], nor remove positive associations with brands firmly established through years of food marketing experiences from earliest childhood [26].

Moreover, some developmental gains during adolescence bring greater vulnerabilities, which many features of digital food marketing exploit. Due to the importance of peer relationships during this developmental stage, marketing messages shared virally through social media may be especially effective with adolescents and establish peer norms around preferred foods [16]. Adolescents are disproportionately sensitive to social affiliation and standing [27], thus increasing vulnerability to marketing that emphasizes peer acceptance or utilizes high-status influencers and celebrities. Adolescents may also be particularly vulnerable to the highly rewarding nature of food marketing due to their stage of brain development, characterized by heightened reward sensitivity compared to younger children and adults and their less developed impulse control capacities [27].

Adolescents also have the means and opportunity to make their own food purchases. US-based research demonstrates that adolescents begin establishing dietary habits that persist through adulthood. Thus, adolescent-targeted food marketing has direct and long-term effects on unhealthy consumption [19]. Worldwide, in jurisdictions where unhealthy foods cannot be advertised in media primarily viewed by younger children, sugary drinks, energy drinks, candy, snack foods, and fast food are highly advertised and directly targeted at adolescents with no restrictions [19, 24]. Moreover, restrictions on the collection and use of personal data (e.g., through the US Children's Online Privacy and Protection Act) [28] typically only apply to younger children [6, 8]. Therefore, adolescents' personal data and online behavior can be used by marketers to craft highly targeted messages designed specifically to appeal to their unique developmental vulnerabilities.

## 2.3 Marketing Targeted at Minoritized Children

Digital marketing aimed at US children of color also raises significant concerns [29, 30]. Likely accrued from greater exposure and engagement with digital media reinforced by socioenvironmental factors and circumstances, Black and Hispanic children face a higher risk of health-related impacts of marketing relative to non-Hispanic White children [29]. Yet, they have been largely overlooked in the research on food marketing.

The limited existing research primarily examines the marketing environment of Black and Hispanic adolescents, including the amount and frequency of exposure and targeting strategies. These children experience greater exposure to unhealthy food marketing due to the greater time spent with all screens compared to non-Hispanic White children [7] as well as targeted marketing in media and their communities. Hispanic children are also more likely to visit food company websites than are non-Hispanic children [31] and to visit websites for brands targeting Hispanic consumers [32]. Black adolescents and Hispanic adolescents in Spanish-speaking households are more likely to engage with junk food brands on social media [13]. Unhealthy food brands targeting Black adolescents have disproportionately higher percentages of Black followers on their social media accounts [32]. Moreover, online marketing for sugary drinks, snacks, candy, and fast-food brands often features Black and Hispanic music and sports celebrities to target children of color and portray a "cool" image to attract a wider youth audience [8].

Yet, this research rarely delves into the important questions of how digital food marketing affects minoritized children, leaving important unanswered research questions. For example, the use of Black celebrities in social media may heighten its impact on Black children's consumption via their shared racial identity [33]. Does it also evoke behavior consistent with these celebrities' behavior (i.e., consumption of unhealthy foods)? Black parents have expressed concerns about celebrity promotion of unhealthy products to their children and identify a potential role for celebrities to endorse counter-marketing efforts [34]. Systemic factors such as differences in family wealth and neighborhood resources, along with racism and discrimination, influence adolescent identity development, including self-esteem [29, 35]. Do these factors also affect their response to targeted marketing? Research is also needed to understand the synergistic effect of Black and Hispanic children's heightened exposure to diverse forms of food marketing as well as the meaning and functions of digital marketing in their lives.

### 2.4 Exploring Potential Solutions

Existing evidence strongly suggests that commonly proposed information-based solutions to protect young people from harmful food marketing online are unlikely to neutralize its effects. Advertising literacy and awareness of commercial data collection practices increase with age but do not mature fully until late adolescence [25]. Media literacy education teaches young people to identify and counterargue marketing messages but may not be effective in deactivating digital marketing messages disguised as entertainment or messages from peers [12, 18], which are designed specifically to appeal to young people's emotions and core motivations [6]. Similarly, disclosure requirements for influencers to reveal the funding of branded messages and ad identifiers on other types of digital marketing are unlikely to reduce the impact of marketing that appeals to emotions and core motivations [18]. Education cannot be expected to unravel well-established positive brand associations conditioned through years of marketing experiences from early childhood [18, 26]. Moreover, marketing of healthy foods does not appear to increase preferences for healthy foods and instead may activate associations with unhealthy brands or settings (e.g., fast-food restaurants) [21, 36] and/or increase consumption of unhealthy foods by priming a generalized desire to eat [17, 22, 37]. To date, research has not identified any promising solutions to inoculate children or adolescents from the negative influence of unhealthy digital food marketing.

## 3 Future Research

The preponderance of evidence on digital food marketing to children points to significant negative influences on food-related attitudes and behaviors. However, relatively few studies have examined how digital marketing may uniquely affect children, including adolescents. Research is needed to increase our understanding of how food companies reach young people online and how to effectively address digital marketing harms.

- What are the underlying processes and mechanisms through which digital food marketing affects young people's diets and health, and what are the synergistic effects of increasing exposure to diverse amounts, types, and content of food marketing on- and offline?
- How do social media and other forms of unhealthy digital food marketing uniquely impact adolescents, including through engagement with reward, motivation, and attentional networks and identity formation?
- How can we better understand the nature of marketing targeted at minoritized children in the digital marketplace? Are Black and Hispanic children impacted differently by digital food marketing? If so, to what extent and how?
- What strategies can adequately protect young people against the harmful effects of exposure to digital food marketing? Are dramatic reductions in the amount and types of marketing aimed at children the only effective options?
- What data sources and research methods can be used to stay abreast of the rapid changes in digital marketing to design up-to-date studies that address children's engagement with the complex, multi-platform techniques deployed by food companies and their impacts?

## 4 Recommendations

Key stakeholders must take action to address the harmful effects of digital marketing on children (Table 1):

- *Governments* should enact legislative and/or regulatory actions to restrict unhealthy food marketing aimed at children, including online [1, 6].
- *Governments* should also enact legislative and/or regulatory actions to restrict unfair data collection and use for targeting marketing online [8, 12]. The misuse of online data to target children with digital marketing is increasingly recognized as a threat to chil-

**Table 1** Current and potential actions to address harms from digital food marketing to children and adolescents

| Key factors | Initiatives | Examples of existing and proposed actions |
|---|---|---|
| Governments | Legislative and/or regulatory actions to restrict unhealthy food marketing aimed at children, including online [1, 6] | Implement the WHO Set of Recommendations on the Marketing of Foods and Non-alcoholic Beverages to Children [5]<br>Countries with existing government regulations of food marketing should expand them to restrict:<br>Digital marketing in all forms<br>Marketing to children up to the age of 18<br>Collection and use of data<br>Brand marketing (e.g., marketing that uses logos and brand names but does not promote a specific product)<br>All marketing with large child audiences<br>Cross-border marketing<br>The United Kingdom passed legislation in 2022 to remove marketing of unhealthy food products on TV before 9 pm and completely online, but implementation has been delayed until October 2025 |
| Governments | Legislative and/or regulatory actions to restrict unfair data collection and use, including targeted marketing online [8, 12] | The US Children's Online Privacy Protection Act (COPPA) requires parental permission to collect any personal information from children under age 13<br>COPPA was updated in 2013 to specifically address practices on social media, mobile, and other platforms<br>The proposed "COPPA 2.0" update would extend requirements to children under the age of 17<br>The 2016 European Union (EU) General Data Protection Regulation (GDPR) protects children's data and their right to privacy<br>**Policymaking under the UN Convention on the Rights of the Child (UNCRC)**<br>The UN General Comment no.25 (2021) on the rights of children (up to the age of 18 years) in relation to the digital environment provides guidance for states to fulfill their obligations under the UNCRC<br>Make the best interests of the child a primary consideration when regulating advertising and marketing addressed to and accessible to children<br>Prohibit by law the profiling or targeting of children of any age for commercial purposes on the basis of a digital record of their actual or inferred characteristics, including group or collective data, targeting by association, or affinity profiling<br>Practices that rely on neuromarketing, emotional analytics, immersive advertising, and advertising in virtual and augmented reality environments to promote products, applications, and services should also be prohibited from engagement directly or indirectly with children<br>The 2022 EU Digital Services Act, effective from 2024, recognizes the rights of the child under the UNCRC<br>It bans advertising targeted at children and restricts data harvesting for profiling<br>Large platforms must conduct risk assessments for impacts on rights, including those of children<br>The Fundamentals for a Child-Oriented Approach to Data Processing (2021) from Ireland's Data Protection Commission provides guidance for requirements for implementing the EU's GDPR, taking a child rights approach<br>Protects children in "mixed use" internet t environments where personal data are used to target advertising<br>Notes the additional need for advertising standards to address contextual advertising, including for food<br>**Other US policies**<br>The proposed American Data Privacy and Protection Act (ADPPA) would create a comprehensive privacy and civil rights framework for everyone; prohibition of targeted advertising for children under 17<br>The proposed Kids Online Safety Act (KOSA) would impose a "duty of care" for social media platforms, including a duty to prevent and mitigate "predatory, unfair, or deceptive marketing practices"<br>The California Age-Appropriate Design Code Act, modeled on the United Kingdom's Age-Appropriate Design Code, will be effective from 2024. Similar efforts are underway in other states<br>The proposed US Federal Trade Commission rulemaking on commercial surveillance (2021), including prohibition of data targeting with a strong focus on children and adolescents |

| | | |
|---|---|---|
| Technology companies | Eliminate unfair data collection and targeting practices aimed at children [8, 12] | Tech companies should follow the UK Age-Appropriate Design Code, issued in 2020, which sets expected default privacy protections in digital media for children under 18 years (although not legally binding)<br>Take the age of individual users into account<br>Not limited to child-directed sites; rather encompasses services that children access<br>Implement data protection assessments<br>Follow best practices for data privacy, including services accessed by children:<br>Set privacy settings to "high" and data profiling to "off" by default<br>Institute data minimization to replace consent models<br>Eliminate uses of data that are harmful to the well-being of young people, such as any use of data that are detrimental to children's physical or mental health<br>Ban collection of geolocation data from minors<br>Ban discriminatory ad and data practices<br>Stop use of manipulative and unfair marketing techniques, including tactics that trick users into taking unwanted actions, such as sharing their data<br>Curb "engagement" techniques that encourage children to share digital marketing messages with their peers online |
| Food, beverage, technology, and entertainment companies | Improve self-regulatory initiatives to restrict unhealthy food marketing to children [1, 2, 8] | Address the many limitations of current food industry self-regulation (such as the US Children's Food and Beverage Advertising Initiative), including:<br>Cover all forms of digital marketing with large child audiences (in addition to media primarily directed at children)<br>Restrict marketing to children under age 18<br>Utilize uniform science-based nutrition criteria to identify unhealthy foods and beverages that cannot be marketed to children<br>Google's policy is that it does not allow ads (including on YouTube) for unhealthy products to be served to children under age 18 in the United Kingdom and the EU<br>Establish similar policies in all countries and at other technology and entertainment companies with large child audiences |
| Parents, child educators, healthcare providers, and the public health community | Increase awareness of the scope and potentially harmful effects of digital food marketing aimed at children. Identify potential opportunities to empower individuals to protect children and adolescents [2, 23] | Establish policies to restrict digital food marketing in schools, including:<br>On school networks and school-issued devices<br>Digital instructional materials<br>On student-owned devices during school days<br>Increase understanding that marketing engages "hot" affective and reward circuitry and can motivate behavior outside of conscious awareness and that educational materials focused on advertising literacy and decision-making about the nutritional value of foods will not adequately address these responses to food marketing<br>Examine potential interventions designed to diminish the ability of digital food marketing to engage reward, motivation, and attention neural systems in adolescents and children, such as approach–avoidance training methods used in treating substance use disorders to strengthen implicit tendencies and reduce motivational approach tendencies to highly rewarding cues. However, recognize the limitations of individual solutions in an obesogenic environment<br>Design education initiatives to empower children to identify and advocate for their right to participate in digital media that are not exploitative<br>Implement counter-marketing campaigns to increase awareness of the harmful effects of digital food marketing to children and the need for protections<br>Engage in advocacy to enact government policies and other systemic changes to address harmful digital marketing practices |

dren's rights to privacy and freedom from exploitation, and some governments have begun to address these issues [8, 12].

- *Technology companies* should eliminate unfair data collection and targeting practices aimed at children [8, 12]. The threat of potential government regulation has led some technology companies to establish policies restricting children's exposure to harmful marketing on their platforms and the use of children's personal data [8, 12].
- *Food, beverage, technology, and entertainment companies* should improve self-regulatory initiatives to close the loopholes that allow them to continue to market unhealthy products to children [1, 2, 8].
- *Parents, educators, healthcare providers*, and others who care about children's health and well-being currently have few options to protect children from digital food marketing, but greater awareness and an understanding of children's online experiences and potential harms from exposure among these key actors would further pressure the food, beverage, and tech industries to take meaningful actions.
- *The public health community* can act to increase awareness of the scope and potentially harmful effects of digital food marketing aimed at children and to identify potential opportunities to empower individuals to protect children and adolescents [2, 23].

Digital marketing has deepened young people's relationships with food brands and has amplified negative effects on diets, long-term health outcomes, and basic human rights [6, 8, 12]. Government-sponsored restrictions on digital food marketing aimed at children are needed to address the power that food and technology corporations now hold in shaping desires, tastes, identities, and bodies through marketing of unhealthy foods.

**Conflict of Interest and Funding Disclosures** JH, FF-M, and KM received support from the Robert Wood Johnson Foundation. MT-G receives consultancy funding from UNICEF and from the Center for Digital Democracy.

## References

1. World Health Organization. Evaluating implementation of the set of recommendations on the marketing of foods and non-alcoholic beverages to children; 2018. http://www.euro.who.int/__data/assets/pdf_file/0003/384015/food-marketing-kids-eng.pdf.
2. Radesky J, Chassiakos YLR, Ameenuddin N, Navsaria D. Digital advertising to children. Pediatrics. 2020;146(1):e20201681. https://doi.org/10.1542/peds.2020-1681.
3. Boyland E, McGale L, Maden M, et al. Association of food and nonalcoholic beverage marketing with children and adolescents' eating behaviors and health. JAMA Pediatr. 2022;176(7):e221037. https://doi.org/10.1001/jamapediatrics.2022.1037.
4. World Health Organization. Ending childhood obesity; 2016. https://apps.who.int/iris/bitstream/handle/10665/204176/9789241510066_eng.pdf?sequence=1&isAllowed=y
5. World Health Organization. Policies to protect children from the harmful impact of food marketing: WHO guidelines; 2023. https://www.who.int/publications/i/item/9789240075412
6. World Health Organization. Tackling food marketing to children in a digital world: transdisciplinary perspective; 2016. https://www.euro.who.int/__data/assets/pdf_file/0017/322226/Tackling-food-marketing-children-digital-world-trans-disciplinary-perspectives-en.pdf
7. Rideout V, Peebles A, Mann S, Robb MB. Common sense census: media use by Tweens and Teens; 2022. https://www.commonsensemedia.org/sites/default/files/research/report/8-18-census-integrated-report-final-web_0.pdf
8. Chester J, Montgomery KC, Kopp K. Big Food, Big Tech, and the global childhood obesity epidemic; 2021. https://democraticmedia.org/assets/resources/full_report.pdf
9. Radesky JS, Weeks HM, Ball R, et al. Young children's use of smartphones and tablets. Pediatrics. 2020;146(1) https://doi.org/10.1542/peds.2019-3518.
10. Kucharczuk AJ, Oliver TL, Dowdell EB. Social media's influence on adolescents' food choices: a mixed studies systematic literature review. Appetite. 2022;168:105765. https://doi.org/10.1016/j.appet.2021.105765.
11. Pollack CC, Kim J, Emond JA, Brand J, Gilbert-Diamond D, Masterson TD. Prevalence and strategies of energy drink, soda, processed snack, candy and restaurant product marketing on the online streaming platform Twitch. Public Health Nutr. 2020;23(15):2793–803. https://doi.org/10.1017/S1368980020002128.
12. Tatlow-Golden M, Garde A. Digital food marketing to children: exploitation, surveillance and rights violations. Glob Food Sec. 2020;27:100423. https://doi.org/10.1016/j.gfs.2020.100423.

13. Fleming-Milici F, Harris JL. Adolescents' engagement with unhealthy food and beverage brands on social media. Appetite. 2020:146. https://doi.org/10.1016/j.appet.2019.104501.
14. van der Bend DLM, Jakstas T, van Kleef E, Shrewsbury VA, Bucher T. Adolescents' exposure to and evaluation of food promotions on social media: a multi-method approach. Int J Behav Nutr Phys Act. 2022;19(1):74. https://doi.org/10.1186/s12966-022-01310-3.
15. Fleming-Milici F, Phaneuf L, Harris J. Prevalence of food and beverage brands in "made-for-kids" child-influencer YouTube videos: 2019–2020. Pediatr Obes. 2023;18(4) https://doi.org/10.1111/ijpo.13008.
16. Buchanan L, Kelly B, Yeatman H, Kariippanon K. The effects of digital marketing of unhealthy commodities on young people: a systematic review. Nutrients. 2018;10(2):148. https://doi.org/10.3390/nu10020148.
17. McCarthy CM, Vries R, Mackenbach JD. The influence of unhealthy food and beverage marketing through social media and advergaming on diet-related outcomes in children—a systematic review. Obes Rev. 2022;23(6) https://doi.org/10.1111/obr.13441.
18. Harris JL, Brownell KD, Bargh JA. The food marketing defense model: integrating psychological research to protect youth and inform public policy. Soc Issues Policy Rev. 2009;3(1):211–71. https://doi.org/10.1111/j.1751-2409.2009.01015.x.
19. Harris JL, Yokum S, Fleming-Milici F. Hooked on junk: emerging evidence on how food marketing affects adolescents' diets and long-term health. Curr Addict Rep. 2021;8(1):19–27. https://doi.org/10.1007/s40429-020-00346-4.
20. Arrona-Cardoza P, Labonté K, Cisneros-Franco JM, Nielsen DE. The effects of food advertisements on food intake and neural activity: a systematic review and meta-analysis of recent experimental studies. Adv Nutr. 2023;14(2):339–51. https://doi.org/10.1016/j.advnut.2022.12.003.
21. Gearhardt AN, Yokum S, Harris JL, Epstein LH, Lumeng JC. Neural response to fast food commercials in adolescents predicts intake. Am J Clin Nutr. 2020;111(3):493–502. https://doi.org/10.1093/ajcn/nqz305.
22. Murphy G, Corcoran C, Tatlow-Golden M, Boyland E, Rooney B. See, like, share, remember: adolescents' responses to unhealthy-, healthy- and non-food advertising in social media. Int J Environ Res Public Health. 2020;17(7):2181. https://doi.org/10.3390/ijerph17072181.
23. Emond JA, Fleming-Milici F, McCarthy J, et al. Unhealthy food marketing on commercial educational websites: remote learning and gaps in regulation. Am J Prev Med. 2021;60(4):587–91. https://doi.org/10.1016/j.amepre.2020.10.008.
24. Taillie LS, Busey E, Stoltze FM, Dillman Carpentier FR. Governmental policies to reduce unhealthy food marketing to children. Nutr Rev. 2019;77(11):787–816. https://doi.org/10.1093/nutrit/nuz021.
25. Zarouali B, Verdoodt V, Walrave M, Poels K, Ponnet K, Lievens E. Adolescents' advertising literacy and privacy protection strategies in the context of targeted advertising on social networking sites: implications for regulation. Young Consum. 2020;21(3):351–67. https://doi.org/10.1108/YC-04-2020-1122.
26. Tatlow-Golden M, Hennessy E, Dean M, Hollywood L. Young children's food brand knowledge. Early development and associations with television viewing and parent's diet. Appetite. 2014;80:197–203. https://doi.org/10.1016/j.appet.2014.05.015.
27. Casey BJ, Getz S, Galvan A. The adolescent brain. Dev Rev. 2008;28(1):62–77. https://doi.org/10.1016/j.dr.2007.08.003.
28. BBB National Programs. Children's food and beverage advertising initiative; 2023. https://bbbprograms.org/programs/all-programs/cfbai
29. Barnhill A, Ramírez AS, Ashe M, et al. The racialized marketing of unhealthy foods and beverages: perspectives and potential remedies. J L Med & Ethics. 2022;50(1):52–9. https://doi.org/10.1017/jme.2022.8.
30. Grier SA. Targeted research for well-being: dissecting the effects of marketing on youth of color. J Public Policy Mark. 2023;42(4):348–50. https://doi.org/10.1177/07439156231183515.
31. Hyary M, Harris JL. Hispanic youth visits to food and beverage company websites. Health Equity. 2017;1(1):134–8. https://doi.org/10.1089/heq.2016.0026.
32. Rummo PE, Arshonsky JH, Sharkey AL, Cassidy OL, Bragg MA. Social media accounts of food and beverage brands have disproportionately more black and Hispanic followers than white followers. Health Equity. 2021;5(1):414–23. https://doi.org/10.1089/heq.2020.0068.
33. Grier SA. African American & Hispanic youth vulnerability to target marketing: implications for understanding the effects of digital marketing; 2009. https://dra.american.edu/islandora/object/auislandora%3A65669
34. Eaton TM, Kumanyika S, DiSantis KI, Yadeta K, Grier S. Black community conversations about opposing ethnically targeted marketing of unhealthy foods and beverages. J Racial Ethn Health Disparities. 2022;9(5):1946–56. https://doi.org/10.1007/s40615-021-01133-1.
35. Tao X, Fisher CB. Exposure to social media racial discrimination and mental health among adolescents of color. J Youth Adolesc. 2022;51(1):30–44. https://doi.org/10.1007/s10964-021-01514-z.
36. Gearhardt AN, Bueno NB, DiFeliceantonio AG, Roberto CA, Jiménez-Murcia S, Fernandez-Aranda F. Social, clinical, and policy implications of ultra-processed food addiction. BMJ. 2023:e075354. https://doi.org/10.1136/bmj-2023-075354.
37. Harris JL, Bargh JA, Brownell KD. Priming effects of television food advertising on eating behavior. Health Psychol. 2009;28(4):404–13. https://doi.org/10.1037/a0014399.

# Alcohol, Tobacco, and Firearm Promotion in Digital Media: Corporate Influences on Adolescent Health

Jennifer A. Emond, Jeffrey Chester, Jonathan Noel, Jon-Patrick Allem, Brad J. Bushman, Brian Primack, and James D. Sargent

## 1 Background

Alcohol and tobacco use are the primary causes of chronic diseases, disability, and mortality in the United States [1]. Adolescence is a critical time when the use of these products often begins, and this increases the risk of dependency and leads to serious consequences across the lifespan [2–5]. Additionally, firearm-related injuries are now the leading cause of death among children and adolescents [6]. Taken together, this cluster of products has a remarkable impact on health.

Adolescents are attractive targets for companies marketing these products because of the potential to shape brand alliances and lifelong use. A large and diverse body of research has documented that alcohol, tobacco, and firearm marketing in traditional media (e.g., TV, movies, billboards) glamorizes these products, thus positively impacting cognition and use among adolescents [7–9]. Social media platforms and online, multiplayer video games are now the most popular media sources among adolescents [10]. However, how the marketing of these products in digital spaces impacts adolescent attitudes and product use is unclear.

Adolescents confront a pervasive, sophisticated, and personalized marketing environment when online [11], with few privacy and marketing protections [11]. Digital marketing often uses artificial intelligence (AI)-driven models to leverage data about a user, including their online activity across multiple platforms, to create psychometric profiles of the user for targeted marketing [12]. Companies promote their brands through social media via explicit advertisements, thinly veiled promotional posts, paid promotions via influencers, and product placement. Online exposure to marketing is guided by sophisticated

J. A. Emond (✉) · J. D. Sargent
Geisel School of Medicine, Dartmouth College, Hanover, NH, USA

The Koop Institute at Dartmouth College, Hanover, NH, USA
e-mail: Jennifer.A.Emond@Dartmouth.edu

J. Chester
Center for Digital Democracy, American University, Washington, DC, USA

J. Noel
Johnson & Wales University, Charlotte, NC, USA

J.-P. Allem
Rutgers School of Public Health, The State University of New Jersey, New Brunswick, NJ, USA

B. J. Bushman
The Ohio State University, Columbus, OH, USA

B. Primack
Oregon State University, Corvallis, OR, USA


D. A. Christakis, L. Hale (eds.), *Handbook of Children and Screens*,
https://doi.org/10.1007/978-3-031-69362-5_13

algorithms that leverage user behaviors, geolocation, and other data sources [11, 13]. Extensive market research, often in collaboration with social media platforms themselves, results in "best practices" to maximize brand awareness, positive emotional encoding, and subsequent behavioral outcomes such as purchase and use [14]. Importantly, this type of marketing capitalizes on the participatory nature of social media and online gaming, blurring the line between traditional marketing and product use [13].

## 2 Current State

### 2.1 Marketing Alcohol, Tobacco, and Firearms in Digital Media

#### 2.1.1 Alcohol

Digital alcohol marketing is one of the most progressive, data-driven, and cutting-edge marketing [11] techniques to build brand awareness and create positive perceptions [13]. For example, Anheuser-Busch InBev (AB InBev) was named the "Creative Marketer of the Year" in 2022 and 2023 by Cannes Lions (a global organization that honors creativity in advertising and marketing) because of the company's marketing that resulted in record sales [15].

Digital alcohol marketing is highly interactive; users engage with company-generated content via liking, commenting on, and resharing digital content from companies or influencers [13]. Alcohol companies can reach adolescents by posting directly on social media using brand accounts and paying "influencers" to promote their products [16]. This content is then delivered to an adolescent audience whose preferences and online behaviors mirror the young adult target group. Additionally, users often participate in marketing campaigns by uploading their own images of product use [13]. Alcohol marketing campaigns also creatively reach adolescents in specific popular digital environments. For example, AB InBev created a "bot" that can be added to a Discord server. While the explicit purpose is to allow gamers to "play royalty-free music from emerging artists," its purpose in fact is to deliver prominent branding for Budweiser [17].

Alcohol companies also market in the "metaverse," a virtual social environment. For example, the 2022 "Absolut.Land" marketing campaign uses multiple techniques known to appeal to adolescents, including a tie-in with a popular music festival, games, and dressing an avatar in Absolut-branded gear. The campaign amassed more than $450,000 of increased sales during the two-weekend period when Absolut.Land was launched [18].

There are no federal regulations specific to limiting the reach of alcohol marketing to minors [19]. Instead, alcohol companies self-regulate marketing to minors (<21 years). Guidelines are based on audience composition data but allow companies to reach an audience with up to 25% underage persons [20, 21]. Many social media sites also have marketing codes that mirror industry codes. TikTok, which has an extremely high youth usership, has currently banned any alcohol promotion. Despite self-regulation, alcohol marketing routinely reaches adolescents via social media and online marketing [22]. Minors can also engage with alcohol company websites directly by entering a false date of birth when confronted with an age verification system.

#### 2.1.2 Tobacco

E-cigarettes are the most commonly used tobacco product among US youth, and their use during adolescence both curbs brain development and increases the risk of smoking combustible cigarettes in adulthood [23]. Child-targeted marketing of tobacco and tobacco-related products is largely absent because of the 1998 Master Settlement Agreement [24]. Other litigation has dampened child-directed marketing. For example, a 2022 settlement with the prominent e-cigarette brand Juul barred the company from using marketing material appealing to those <35 years of age [25]. Cigarette websites require verified proof of age for any online sale per federal law [26], and, in practice, this is commonly at the point of entry. Many social media companies—including X (formally Twitter) [27], Pinterest [28], Meta (Facebook and Instagram) [29]—have explicitly banned tobacco or vaping-related marketing. However, e-cigarette marketing reaches adolescents when companies post their own content and share/re-tweet e-cigarette-related content from other uses or when users share coupons or other promotional material [30]. E-cigarette marketing themes appeal to youth by focusing on safety and risk reduction; however, they also leverage commonly used cigarette marketing themes of freedom, friendship, and independence [31, 32]. Smaller e-cigarette companies maintain a more prominent social media presence than do larger e-cigarette companies, likely because larger corporations are more reluctant to face scrutiny or litigation around their marketing practices. About a quarter to a third of adolescents (21–36%) across national cohorts recall being exposed to digital e-cigarette marketing [33, 34].

### 2.1.3 Firearms

Firearm manufacturers have carefully crafted a false narrative about the power and importance of guns in the United States since their inception, and marketing has always driven this narrative [35]. Firearms are promoted as symbols of patriotism, power, independence, and military adventure [36]. Targeted marketing with those themes drove the surge in popularity of the semiautomatic AR-15, a weapon that accounted for only 1.2% of US-manufactured firearms in 1990 yet 23.4% in 2020 [37].

A likely part of the gun industry's marketing is product placements in movies, TV shows, music videos, and video games [37, 38]. In 2016, Fox News reported that the gunmaker Beretta paid $250,000 to place their product in *Lone Survivor*, a biographical war film [39]. Glock, a firearm manufacturer, won a "lifetime product placement achievement award" in 2010 from Brandchannel for placement of their products in action movies [38]. Firearm violence depictions in PG-13 movies tripled between 1985 and 2015 [40]. Gun violence in prime-time dramas doubled between 2000 and 2018 [41]. Violent video games can be another considerable source of firearm exposure for youth. Video game imagery, weapons used, and situations encountered have become increasingly realistic, and the guns used in these games often map directly onto commercially available products [42, 43]. For example, two firearms in *Call of Duty, Modern Warfare 2* bear striking resemblances to the Colt M4 rifle and the Glock G17 firearm [44, 45]. According to investigative reporting by the *Washington Post*, technicians from the developer of *Call of Duty* met with representatives of the two firearm manufacturers to record the sounds of firearms, including the AR-15 [37]. Collaborations between firearm manufacturers and video game makers claimed to have ceased after the Sandy Hook elementary school shooting in 2012 [37]. Whether exposure to violence in media, and in video games specifically, impacts behavior is debated [46, 47], and observable effects on behavior are modest [48, 49]. However, a small effect could translate into a large population-level impact [50].

Strikingly, there are no studies that have considered whether the marketing described above influences firearms purchase or whether adolescent exposure to firearms within media specifically impacts the attitudes and beliefs about those weapons. Such an effect is supported by communication research regarding persuasive messaging [51]. Robust media effects research studies show that tobacco and alcohol receptivity resulting from media and marketing exposures relates to subsequent product use among adolescents and young adults [7–9, 52–57] via an increasing level of identification with the brands as a reflection of the promotional themes used for those products [55]. It is imperative to extend this line of research to media exposures to firearms to understand whether such exposures have a measurable impact on shaping the acceptance and potential use of firearms for harm during adolescence and beyond. This research is warranted given the high prevalence of firearm injury and mortality among adolescents and young adults [6, 58, 59].

### 2.1.4 Summary

Adolescence is a critical life stage when alcohol and tobacco use can affect lifelong health; promoting firearm use at this stage can have deadly consequences. Adolescents are an attractive target for the marketing of these products because of the potential to build lifelong loyalties. The marketing of these products is cutting-edge and reaches adolescents in emerging digital spaces.

Research to understand causal relationships between marketing exposure and use of these products is critical for understanding the implications on adolescent health. Greater transparency and oversight are needed for digital marketing practices among companies that promote harmful products to ensure that their marketing does not target minors, and researchers need to understand these marketing practices and prepare for what is on the horizon while supporting advocacy efforts to shape policy to protect adolescent health.

## 3 Future Research

The following is proposed for future research. Addressing these items can further prepare researchers to monitor the marketing of emerging products. For example, cannabis is legal for adult recreational use in 24 US states and the District of Columbia as of November 2023 [60] Cannabis marketing in social media uses the same techniques used to market alcohol and tobacco, which are techniques that appeal to adolescents [61].

- *How to quantify adolescent exposure to digital marketing of harmful products?* Digital marketing is difficult to define because it is tailored to the user. Social media marketing can also be difficult for adolescents to identify and understand as promotional content. Methods to objectively capture digital marketing exposures are needed given the limitations of self-reported measures, particularly for marketing exposures that may be brief. Research could utilize intermittent screen captures, such as in an ecological momentary assessment framework [62, 63], or record sessions for coding [64]. Data and computer scientists are needed to facilitate the capture, transmission, and storage of data. Machine learning methods could be implemented to automate coding of brand appearances in captured content to avoid manual coding [65]. Ensuring the privacy and confidentiality of the data collected will be critical.
- *What characteristics of digital marketing make a message more salient?* Digital marketing occurs in many forms, and there is an urgent need to understand how the context of digital marketing affects receptivity to product use. How is marketing from online ads, paid social media posts, or from influencers differentially received? How does engagement with immersive environments, such as virtual reality or first-person shooter video games, affect the saliency of imagery exposed to? How is the context of marketing exposure more (or less) important than the quantity of exposure on adolescent perceptions, attitudes, and behaviors?
- *What is needed to conclude whether causal associations exist between exposure to digital marketing of harmful products and adolescent health?* Engagement with alcohol and tobacco social media marketing clearly relates to positive product cognitions and product use among adolescents, yet studies rigorously testing causality are lacking. There is an urgent need to better understand the likely bidirectional relationships between marketing exposure and product use. Research should investigate the predisposing factors that influence an adolescent's selection of content and also assess whether engagement with digital marketing contributes to an earlier initiation of product use.

## 4 Recommendations

Risks to adolescent health from the marketing of harmful products in the digital space demands change. The following recommendations can be made:

- Research examining the marketing of harmful products can be controversial. Philanthropies and independent research organizations have always played an important role in this type of research. Since 2019, the US Congress has earmarked funds for firearm research and more recently for research to study the effects of technology and media on the physical and socioemotional health of infants, children, and adolescents (the CAMRA (Children and

Media Research Advancement) Act). However, the National Institutes of Health (NIH) should dedicate resources specifically to youth-directed marketing in digital media because of the potential impact on adolescent health, well-being, and development. Any efforts by the NIH must be independent of corporations that produce these products, as companies have worked hard to capture government agencies, including the NIH, in the past. For example, between 2013 and 2020, there were extensive communications between the alcohol industry and personnel at the National Institute of Alcohol and Alcoholism (NIAAA), including heavy criticism of public health research and researchers by NIAAA personnel in correspondence with the industry [66].

- Importantly, there is a wealth of data on the data-driven marketing practices of companies used to target youth [11], including those used by alcohol and tobacco companies. Researchers and clinicians should examine these resources along with company market research to understand the extent of industry practices and further collaborate with advocacy groups to define future research and policy needs to eliminate targeted marketing that impacts adolescent health.
- In the absence of a unifying set of regulations, companies that sell harmful products including alcohol, tobacco including e-cigarettes, and firearms must have a standardized code to eliminate purposeful and inadvertent digital marketing to minors. Social media platforms must also support and enforce these codes. The information companies use to target marketing, including the age of a targeted user and the age distribution of an intended audience, should also be transparent and readily available to ensure that companies are acting as pledged. More resources should be extended to government agencies like the Federal Trade Commission (FTC) charged with enforcing these codes, and every effort should be made to prevent industry capture of the agency charged with oversight.
- Better government oversight of marketing within digital spaces is needed when it comes to minors' exposure to harmful products. Efforts to protect children and adolescents online have been slow. The Kids Internet Design and Safety (KIDS) Act (H.R.5439) [67], introduced to the US House of Representatives in 2021, was proposed to stop manipulative practices that threaten children and adolescents <16 years of age online, including the amplification of harmful content via algorithms and damaging design features. The Act prohibited online platforms from using data-driven algorithms to present influencer advertising, content with product placement, and advertising or material with alcohol, nicotine, or commercial tobacco content (Sect. 4.c of the Act). The Act was not voted on and has expired. In 2022, the Kids Online Safety Act (S.3663) was introduced to the Senate. This Act requires transparency in how data from minors are used for marketing purposes, disclosures for all marketing material, and online platforms to "prevent or mitigate" exposure to marketing for narcotics, tobacco, gambling, or alcohol [68]. The 2022 American Data Privacy and Protection Act would ban all digital targeted marketing to those <17 years of age [69]. Enacting any marketing regulations in the United States is complicated by the company's first amendment rights. However, regulations have a greater likelihood of passing when company behaviors are clearly connected to adolescent health outcomes via rigorous research. Furthermore, dissemination of that research could shift public perception and sway congressional actions.
- State and city attorneys general also play a role. When government agencies fail to appropriately regulate harmful products and companies successfully target minors, the judicial system could intervene. For example, after the publication of a scholarly editorial describing vape pen product placements in music videos [70], the Los Angeles City Attorney's Office reached out to the authors for assistance in their primary case against the vape company.

The research team's contributions helped the City Attorney's Office obtain an injunction against product placement, including a $1.2 million fine [71]. Litigation can change corporate behavior, and scientists should be encouraged to participate in such activities, with their institution's support, to enhance the public health impact of their research.

**Conflict of Interest and Funding Disclosures** JE was supported by a grant from the NIH (5K01DK117971). J-PA has received fees for consulting services in court cases pertaining to the content on social media platforms. He reports no other conflicts of interest. JP-A was supported by the California Tobacco Control Branch, Center for Healthy Communities of the California Department of Public Health through contract number 21-10032 Tobacco Industry Monitoring Evaluation (TIME), Grant #U54 CA 180905 from the National Cancer Institute and the Food and Drug Administration Center for Tobacco Products, and The Regents of the University of California, Research Grants Program Office, Tobacco-Related Diseases Research Program, Grant Number No. T30IR0891. The findings and conclusions in this chapter are those of the authors and do not necessarily represent the views or opinions of the California Department of Public Health, the NIH, or the California Health and Human Services Agency. The other authors have no conflicts of interest to disclose.

## References

1. Harris KM, Majmundar MK, Becker T. High and rising mortality rates among working-age adults. National Academies Press; 2021. https://doi.org/10.17226/25976.
2. Youth and tobacco use | Smoking and tobacco use | CDC. https://www.cdc.gov/tobacco/data_statistics/fact_sheets/youth_data/tobacco_use/index.htm. Accessed 28 Mar 2024.
3. Fast facts and fact sheets | Smoking and tobacco use | CDC. https://www.cdc.gov/tobacco/data_statistics/fact_sheets/fast_facts/index.htm. Accessed 28 Mar 2024.
4. Underage drinking | CDC. https://www.cdc.gov/alcohol/fact-sheets/underage-drinking.htm. Accessed 28 Mar 2024.
5. Nelson LF, Weitzman ER, Levy S. Prevention of substance use disorders. Med Clin North Am. 2022;106(1):153–68. https://doi.org/10.1016/J.MCNA.2021.08.005.
6. Goldstick JE, Cunningham RM, Carter PM. Current causes of death in children and adolescents in the United States. N Engl J Med. 2022;386(20):1955–6. https://doi.org/10.1056/nejmc2201761.
7. National Center for Chronic Disease Prevention and Health Promotion (US) Office on Smoking and Health. Centers for Disease Control and Prevention (US); 2012.
8. Prescott AT, Sargent JD, Hull JG. Metaanalysis of the relationship between violent video game play and physical aggression over time. Proc Natl Acad Sci USA. 2018;115(40):9882–8. https://doi.org/10.1073/pnas.1611617114.
9. Hanewinkel R, Sargent JD, Poelen EAP, et al. Alcohol consumption in movies and adolescent binge drinking in 6 European countries. Pediatrics. 2012;129(4):709–20. https://doi.org/10.1542/peds.2011-2809.
10. Common Sense Media. The common sense census: media use by tweens and teens, 2021 | common sense media. Published 2021. https://www.commonsensemedia.org/research/the-common-sense-census-media-use-by-tweens-and-teens-2021. Accessed 6 June 2022.
11. World Health Organization. Understanding the digital media ecosystem. How the evolution of the digital marketing ecosystem impacts tobacco, alcohol and unhealthy food marketing. Published 2022. https://www.who.int/europe/publications/i/item/9789289057950. Accessed 21 Mar 2023.
12. World Health Organization. Reducing the harm from alcohol by regulating cross-border alcohol marketing, advertising and promotion: a technical report. World Health Organization; 2022. https://www.who.int/publications/i/item/9789240046504. Accessed 26 Mar 2023
13. Carah N, Brodmerkel S. Alcohol marketing in the era of digital media platforms. J Stud Alcohol Drugs. 2021;82(1):18–27. https://doi.org/10.15288/jsad.2021.82.18.
14. What we know about social media effectiveness | WARC. https://www.warc.com/content/paywall/article/bestprac/what-we-know-about-social-media-effectiveness/en-GB/111562? Accessed 23 Mar 2023.
15. Cannes Lions. Cannes Lions honours AB InBev with the 2023 creative marketer of the year. Published 2023. https://www.canneslions.com/news/cannes-lions-honours-ab-inbev-with-the-2023-creative-marketer?utm_campaign=cmoty23&utm_medium=email&utm_source=mkt-email-gen&utm_content=2023.03.17-ecc-vet&utm_term=noterm&mkt_tok=ODk3LU1CQy0yMDcAAAGKjwXmM17Yaf2jJXg2Df3qkJszbb-o4IdzJsn6UfWMbBhS3DowOtL5a4IFQAKAlatY9aSchc2XcUVVosla086HaoKFYpUkJ3X48qcEKIXwQiUdHA. Accessed 23 Mar 2023.
16. Hendriks H, Wilmsen D, van Dalen W, Gebhardt WA. Picture me drinking: alcohol-related posts by Instagram influencers popular among adolescents and young adults. Front Psychol. 2020;10:497588. https://doi.org/10.3389/FPSYG.2019.02991/BIBTEX.
17. Budweiser: Royalty Free Bot • Ads of the World™ | Part of The Clio network. https://www.adsoftheworld.

com/campaigns/royalty-free-bot. Accessed 23 Mar 2023.
18. Absolut.Land – The shorty awards. https://shortyawards.com/15th/absolutland. Accessed 23 Mar 2023.
19. TTBGov – Alcohol beverage advertising. https://www.ttb.gov/advertising/alcohol-beverage-advertising. Accessed 28 Mar 2024.
20. Advertising & marketing code – Beer Institute. https://www.beerinstitute.org/policy-responsibility/responsibility/advertising-marketing-code/. Accessed 7 Mar 2023.
21. Code of responsible practices – Distilled Spirits Council of the United States. https://www.distilledspirits.org/code-of-responsible-practices/. Accessed 7 Mar 2023.
22. Lobstein T, Landon J, Thornton N, Jernigan D. The commercial use of digital media to market alcohol products: a narrative review. Addiction. 2017;112:21–7. https://doi.org/10.1111/add.13493.
23. McCabe SE, West BT, McCabe VV. Associations between early onset of e-cigarette use and cigarette smoking and other substance use among us adolescents: a national study. Nicotine Tob Res. 2018;20(8):923–30. https://doi.org/10.1093/ntr/ntx231.
24. The Tobacco Master Settlement Agreement (MSA) – NAAG. https://www.naag.org/our-work/naag-center-for-tobacco-and-public-health/the-master-settlement-agreement/. Accessed 28 Mar 2024.
25. Juul to pay about $439 million to settle e-cigarette marketing probe | Reuters. https://www.reuters.com/legal/litigation/juul-pay-about-439-mln-settle-e-cigarette-marketing-probe-2022-09-06/. Accessed 7 Mar 2023.
26. Prevent All Cigarette Trafficking (PACT) Act | Bureau of alcohol, tobacco, firearms and explosives. https://www.atf.gov/alcohol-tobacco/prevent-all-cigarette-trafficking-pact-act. Accessed 28 Mar 2024.
27. Tobacco and tobacco accessories. https://business.x.com/en/help/ads-policies/ads-content-policies/tobacco-and-tobacco-accessories.html. Accessed 28 Mar 2024.
28. Community guidelines | Pinterest Policy. https://policy.pinterest.com/en-gb/community-guidelines-2022. Accessed 28 Mar 2024.
29. Tobacco and related products | Transparency Center. https://transparency.fb.com/policies/ad-standards/dangerous-content/tobacco. Accessed 28 Mar 2024.
30. Collins L, Glasser AM, Abudayyeh H, Pearson JL, Villanti AC. E-cigarette marketing and communication: how E-cigarette companies market E-cigarettes and the public engages with E-cigarette information. Nicotine Tob Res. 2019;21(1):14–24. https://doi.org/10.1093/ntr/ntx284.
31. Farrelly MC, Duke JC, Crankshaw EC, et al. A randomized trial of the effect of E-cigarette TV advertisements on intentions to use E-cigarettes. Am J Prev Med. 2015;49(5):686–93. https://doi.org/10.1016/j.amepre.2015.05.010.
32. Vogel EA, Ramo DE, Rubinstein ML, et al. Effects of social media on adolescents' willingness and intention to use e-cigarettes: an experimental investigation. Nicotine Tob Res. 2021;23(4):694–701. https://doi.org/10.1093/ntr/ntaa003.
33. Wang Y, Duan Z, Weaver SR, et al. Association of e-cigarette advertising, parental influence, and peer influence with US adolescent e-cigarette use. JAMA Netw Open. 2022;5(9):E2233938. https://doi.org/10.1001/jamanetworkopen.2022.33938.
34. Singh T, Marynak K, Arrazola RA, Cox S, Rolle IV, King BA. Vital signs: exposure to electronic cigarette advertising among middle school and high school students—United States, 2014. MMWR Morb Mortal Wkly Rep. 2016;64(52):1403–8. https://doi.org/10.15585/mmwr.mm6452a3.
35. How did guns get so powerful? | The New Yorker. https://www.newyorker.com/tech/annals-of-technology/how-did-guns-get-so-powerful. Accessed 7 Mar 2023.
36. Analysis | Decades of marketing reinvented the AR-15 into a top-selling firearm – Washington Post. https://www.washingtonpost.com/business/interactive/2023/history-of-ar-15-marketing/. Accessed 23 Apr 2023.
37. How the AR-15 became a powerful political, cultural symbol in America – Washington Post. https://www.washingtonpost.com/nation/interactive/2023/ar-15-america-gun-culture-politics/. Accessed 27 Mar 2023.
38. Apple, Glock Grab Most Movie Placements. https://www.forbes.com/sites/briancaulfield/2011/02/22/apple-glock-top-movie-placement-list/?sh=2d86017414e3. Accessed 7 Mar 2023.
39. McKay H. How Hollywood helps gun makers sell their guns. Fox News. Published online 24 Mar 2015.
40. Bushman BJ, Jamieson PE, Weitz I, Romer D. Gun violence trends in movies. Pediatrics. 2013;132(6):1014–8. https://doi.org/10.1542/peds.2013-1600.
41. Jamieson PE, Romer D. The association between the rise of gun violence in popular US primetime television dramas and homicides attributable to firearms, 2000–2018. Brenner MH, ed. PLoS One. 2021;16(3):e0247780. https://doi.org/10.1371/journal.pone.0247780.
42. Games Atlas | Video game guides, databases & walkthroughs. https://www.gamesatlas.com/. Accessed 31 Mar 2024.
43. Internet Movie Firearms Database – Guns in movies, TV and Video Games. https://imfdb.org/wiki/Main_Page. Accessed 16 Apr 2023.
44. M4 | Blueprints list in Warzone and MW2. https://www.gamesatlas.com/cod-modern-warfare-2/weapons/m4. Accessed 28 May 2024.
45. X12 | Blueprints list in Warzone and MW2. https://www.gamesatlas.com/cod-modern-warfare-2/weapons/x12. Accessed 28 May 2024.
46. Drummond A, Sauer JD, Ferguson CJ. Do longitudinal studies support long-term relationships between aggressive game play and youth aggressive behav-

iour? A meta-analytic examination. R Soc Open Sci. 2020;7(7) https://doi.org/10.1098/RSOS.200373.
47. Bushman BJ, Huesmann LR. Twenty-five years of research on violence in digital games and aggression revisited: a reply to Elson and Ferguson (2013). Eur Psychol. 2014;19(1):47–55. https://doi.org/10.1027/1016-9040/a000164.
48. Bushman BJ. Violent media and hostile appraisals: a meta-analytic review. Aggress Behav. 2016;42(6):605–13. https://doi.org/10.1002/AB.21655.
49. Prescott AT, Sargent JD, Hull JG. Metaanalysis of the relationship between violent video game play and physical aggression over time. Proc Natl Acad Sci USA. 2018;115(40):9882–8. https://doi.org/10.1073/PNAS.1611617114/ASSET/D504A2A6-FEC7-4375-AFC7-09004C2E7C6D/ASSETS/GRAPHIC/PNAS.1611617114FIG01.JPEG.
50. Götz FM, Gosling SD, Rentfrow PJ. Small effects: the indispensable foundation for a cumulative psychological science. Perspect Psychol Sci. 2022;17(1):205–15. https://doi.org/10.1177/1745691620984483.
51. Rosenberg BD, Marshburn A, Siegel JT. Persuasive communication: source, message, Audience Oxford Research Encyclopedia of Psychology. Published online 15 Sept 2022. https://doi.org/10.1093/ACREFORE/9780190236557.013.285
52. Chang JH, Bushman BJ. Effect of exposure to gun violence in video games on children's dangerous behavior with real guns a randomized clinical trial. JAMA Netw Open. 2019;2(5) https://doi.org/10.1001/jamanetworkopen.2019.4319.
53. Anderson CA, Bushman BJ, Bartholow BD, et al. Screen violence and youth behavior. Pediatrics. 2017;140(Supplement_2):S142–7. https://doi.org/10.1542/peds.2016-1758T.
54. Dillon KP, Bushman BJ. Effects of exposure to gun violence in movies on children's interest in real guns. JAMA Pediatr. 2017;171(11):1057–62. https://doi.org/10.1001/jamapediatrics.2017.2229.
55. McClure AC, Stoolmiller M, Tanski SE, Engels RCME, Sargent JD. Alcohol marketing receptivity, marketing-specific cognitions, and underage binge drinking. Alcohol Clin Exp Res. 2013;37(Suppl. 1) https://doi.org/10.1111/j.1530-0277.2012.01932.x.
56. Gabrielli J, Brennan ZLB, Stoolmiller M, Jackson KM, Tanski SE, McClure AC. A new recall of alcohol marketing scale for youth: measurement properties and associations with youth drinking status. J Stud Alcohol Drugs. 2019;80(5):563–71. https://doi.org/10.15288/JSAD.2019.80.563.
57. Pierce JP, Choi WS, Gilpin EA, Farkas AJ, Berry CC. Tobacco industry promotion of cigarettes and adolescent smoking. JAMA. 1998;279(7):511–5. https://doi.org/10.1001/JAMA.279.7.511.
58. Lawrence WR, Freedman ND, McGee-Avila JK, et al. Trends in mortality from poisonings, firearms, and all other injuries by intent in the US, 1999–2020. JAMA Intern Med. 2023;183(8):849–56. https://doi.org/10.1001/JAMAINTERNMED.2023.2509.
59. Johns Hopkins Center for gun violence solutions T. US gun violence in 2021: an accounting of a public health crisis. Published online 2023.
60. State Medical Cannabis Laws. https://www.ncsl.org/health/state-medical-cannabis-laws. Accessed 28 Mar 2024.
61. Trangenstein PJ, Whitehill JM, Jenkins MC, Jernigan DH, Moreno MA. Active cannabis marketing and adolescent past-year cannabis use. Drug Alcohol Depend. 2019:204. https://doi.org/10.1016/j.drugalcdep.2019.107548.
62. Chiatti A, Cho MJ, Gagneja A, et al. Text extraction and retrieval from smartphone screenshots: building a repository for life in media. Published online 4 Jan 2018. http://arxiv.org/abs/1801.01316. Accessed 7 Mar 2023.
63. Reeves B, Ram N, Robinson TN, et al. Screenomics: a framework to capture and analyze personal life experiences and the ways that technology shapes them. Hum Comput Interact. 2021;36(2):150–201. https://doi.org/10.1080/07370024.2019.1578652.
64. Lara-Mejía V, Franco-Lares B, Lozada-Tequeanes AL, Villanueva-Vázquez C, Hernández-Cordero S. Methodologies for monitoring the digital marketing of foods and beverages aimed at infants, children, and adolescents (ICA): a scoping review. Int J Environ Res Public Health. 2022;19(15) https://doi.org/10.3390/ijerph19158951.
65. Ricard BJ, Hassanpour S. Deep learning for identification of alcohol-related content on social media (reddit and twitter): exploratory analysis of alcohol-related outcomes. J Med Internet Res. 2021;23(9) https://doi.org/10.2196/27314.
66. Mitchell G, McCambridge J. Interactions between the U.S. National Institute on alcohol abuse and alcoholism and the alcohol industry: evidence from email correspondence 2013–2020. J Stud Alcohol Drugs. 2023;84(1):11–26. https://doi.org/10.15288/jsad.22-00184.
67. Rep. Castor K [D F 14]. Text – H.R.5439 – 117th congress (2021–2022): KIDS Act Published online 2021.
68. Sen. Blumenthal R [D C. Text – S.3663 – 117th congress (2021–2022): Kids Online Safety Act. Published online 2022.
69. Rep. Pallone FJr [D N 6]. Text – H.R.8152 – 117th congress (2021–2022): American Data Privacy and Protection Act. Published online 2022.
70. Allem JP, Escobedo P, Cruz TB, Unger JB. Vape pen product placement in popular music videos. Addict Behav. 2019;93:263–4. https://doi.org/10.1016/j.addbeh.2017.10.027.
71. LA City Atty Gets $1.2M penalty, injunction against Vape Co. – Law360. https://www.law360.com/articles/1376690. Accessed 12 Mar 2023.

# What Do We Know About the Link Between Screens and Sleep Health?

Lauren Hale, Lauren E. Hartstein, Rebecca Robbins, Michael A. Grandner, Monique K. LeBourgeois, Michelle M. Garrison, and Charles A. Czeisler

## 1 Background

Screen-based digital media devices are ubiquitous in the daily lives of children and adolescents [1, 2]. Given that these digital technology and mobile devices are often used during the evening and nighttime hours, the impact of screen use on sleep health is a critical concern. In this updated review of a related summary article [3], we provide current evidence on the importance of sleep health among pediatric populations and what recent research has revealed about screen use and sleep. After discussing the limitations of screen use and sleep health research (including bidirectionality and measurement issues), we then elucidate pressing research questions. We conclude with recommendations for youth, families, and clinicians to help mitigate the possible negative effects of screen use on sleep.

### 1.1 Importance of Sleep Among Pediatric Populations

Sleep plays many physiological roles, including regulation and maintenance of cardiovascular, metabolic, immune, cognitive, behavioral, and mental health [4]. For these and other reasons, healthy sleep is an integral part of healthy development [5]. Current guidelines reiterate the need for sufficient restorative sleep in pediatric populations and that the recommended sleep duration is greater for children than for adults [6, 7]. Across childhood, the recommended sleep duration decreases with age; toddlers need between

In loving memory of Monique LeBourgeois, whose unique combination of heartfelt compassion and scientific curiosity advanced circadian and sleep research in childhood. We will miss you dearly.

L. Hale (✉)
Program in Public Health, Department of Family, Population, and Preventive Medicine, Renaissance School of Medicine, Stony Brook University, Stony Brook, NY, USA
e-mail: lauren.hale@stonybrook.edu

L. E. Hartstein · M. K. LeBourgeois
Department of Integrative Physiology, University of Colorado Boulder, Boulder, CO, USA

R. Robbins · C. A. Czeisler
Departments of Medicine and Neurology, Division of Sleep and Circadian Disorders, Brigham and Women's Hospital, Boston, MA, USA

Division of Sleep Medicine, Harvard Medical School, Boston, MA, USA

M. A. Grandner
Department of Psychiatry, University of Arizona, Tucson, AZ, USA

M. M. Garrison
Department of Public Health, Purdue University, West Lafayette, IN, USA


D. A. Christakis, L. Hale (eds.), *Handbook of Children and Screens*,
https://doi.org/10.1007/978-3-031-69362-5_14

11 and 14 h per night, preschoolers need between 10 and 13 h per night, school-aged children need between 9 and 11 h per night, and teens need between 8 and 10 h [6].

Sufficient habitual sleep duration among school-aged children has been positively associated with cognitive function (especially executive function and school performance), according to two recent meta-analyses of children aged 5–12 years [8, 9]. Beyond cognitive outcomes, insufficient sleep duration is associated with behavioral problems, including both internalizing and externalizing behavioral issues [8]. Similar research in younger age groups reports consistent findings. Both sleep quality and duration are associated with cognitive performance according to a systematic review of preschool-aged children [10]. Shorter sleep duration was also associated with poorer emotional regulation in both early childhood and among school-aged children [11, 12].

In addition to cognitive and emotional outcomes, research has explored the relationship between sleep and physical health outcomes. In the early years of life, longer sleep duration and a higher number of bouts of sleep are associated with better growth among infants [13]. Furthermore, there was a consistent, strong association between longer sleep and lower adiposity, as well as risk factors for obesity, across child development [11, 12]. Additionally, according to a review of 75 published studies among children and adolescents, there is a significant association between inadequate sleep and cardiovascular risk factors, including adiposity, decreased insulin sensitivity, and high blood pressure [14].

In summary, there is strong evidence that sufficient, restorative sleep is associated with cognitive, emotional, and physical outcomes linked to healthy development in young children from birth through adolescence.

## 2 Current State

Recent research on digital media use and sleep has been consistent with earlier systematic literature reviews demonstrating an association between digital media use and poor sleep health among pediatric populations ranging from preschool-aged children through adolescents. In the vast majority of relevant studies that research digital media use and sleep, more digital media use is associated with delayed bedtimes, longer sleep-onset latency, shorter total sleep time, and more daytime sleepiness among children and adolescents [15–22]. Several more recent themes that may inform screen use recommendations have emerged:

### 2.1 Types of Digital Media and How They Are Used May Affect Sleep Health Outcomes

Interactive types of digital media (e.g., gaming, social media, messaging) and smartphones that interrupt nighttime sleep are associated with a range of sleep outcomes, including later bedtimes, longer sleep-onset latency, shorter sleep duration, and poorer sleep quality [15, 18, 23]. Systematic reviews demonstrate that more passive types of media uses (e.g., streaming video content and watching television) show inconsistent results regarding associations with sleep health outcomes [15, 19].

### 2.2 Digital Media and Light Exposure Before Bed and During the Night May Have Strong Effects on Sleep

Timing of the exposure to both the media content and the light from devices before going to bed also relates to sleep health [22]. Bedtime and nighttime use of screens may have a particular impact on poor sleep outcomes due to both content and light effects [20, 24, 25]. A 2016 meta-analysis including 20 cross-sectional studies from >125,000 children showed that bedtime mobile phone use was associated with higher rates of insufficient sleep duration (odds ratio (OR) = 2.17, 95% confidence interval (95% CI) 1.42–3.32 poor sleep quality (OR = 1.46, 95% CI 1.14–1.88), and excessive daytime sleepiness (OR = 2.72, 95% CI, 1.32–5.61) [20]. Studies of screen use during the day or further from bedtime have shown more inconsistent effects [15, 22].

## 2.3 Effects of Interventions Are Small and Difficult to Achieve

Effective and sustainable interventions to reduce children's screen use and improve their sleep health outcomes remain limited. In a 2020 meta-analysis of 11 intervention studies, encompassing 4656 children aged 2–13 years, screen time was reduced by an average of 33 min/day and the mean sleep duration increased by 11 min/day [26]. More recent studies that involve parent–child interventions have seen both reductions in screen time and improvements in sleep [27, 28], though other studies aimed at reducing screen time have found limited or no effects of an intervention on sleep health [29, 30]. Some limitations to these findings include the presence of co-interventions, such as those aimed at parenting or weight-related behaviors, as well as the difficulty in subject recruitment, as adolescents are reluctant to make changes to their evening device use [31].

## 2.4 What Are the Mechanisms for This Association Between Screen Time and Sleep?

There are five plausible pathways through which scientists explain the widely observed association between screen use and sleep outcomes:

1. *Activity displacement*: The first pathway acknowledges that the time spent using screens can replace the time that could be spent preparing for sleep (e.g., reading a book, preparing for the next morning) or actually sleeping [16]. Similarly, screen use may also displace other health behaviors that may be beneficial for sleep, such as daytime exposure to outdoor light and engaging in physical activities.
2. *Decreased interoceptive awareness*: Screen time use has been experimentally linked to decreased awareness of internal sensations—including feelings of tiredness, muscle stiffness, and the passage of time [32]. As these are some of the very cues that might otherwise prompt discontinuation of media use for the night, they are likely responsible for some degree of the activity displacement described above.
3. *Psychological and emotional stimulation from content*: The third pathway involves content-related stimulation that increases the likelihood of youth becoming more alert and less able to fall asleep. This could include arousal from engaging in video game playing or emotional arousal from social media or messaging with peers [16]. Examples of this type of effect are social comparison and cybervictimization, both of which can lead to repetitive and obsessive thoughts, emotions, and memories [24, 33].
4. *Physiological effects of light on circadian timing and alertness*: The artificial light emitted by electronic devices can cause arousal and decreased sleepiness at bedtime. A 2015 experimental study of young adults demonstrated that reading on a light-emitting device before bedtime compared to reading a paper book suppressed the sleep-promoting hormone melatonin, delayed the circadian phase of the melatonin rhythm, increased sleep-onset latency, and decreased the duration of rapid eye movement sleep [25]. Children, who have a larger pupil size and increased light transmission rate of the crystalline lens, may be more sensitive to this light than mature adults [34–36].
5. *Noises, vibrations, and other middle of the night phone checks*: In 2019, Common Sense Media conducted a survey in which over one-third of teens reported checking their phones in the middle of the night [2]. While these awakenings may be triggered by noises or vibrations, they may also be routine checks in anticipation of messaging or social media content from other users (e.g., awaiting likes or replies), reducing both sleep efficiency and sleep duration [23]. While it is normal to experience brief

arousals from sleep during the night, engagement with screen media during these times can increase the duration of waking and may increase the frequency of further wakings that night.

### 2.5 What Are the Limitations of the Current Research?

Despite general agreement on the association between screen time and adverse sleep health outcomes using cross-sectional studies, many of these studies lack rigorous experimental design, making it difficult to identify causality when there are likely bidirectional relationships. For example, one study showed that experimentally reducing children's sleep led to increased television watching [37]. Beyond the issue of causality, the field struggles with concerns about measurement error for both the predictor (i.e., screen use variables) and the outcomes (i.e., sleep health variables), with a primary reliance on self- or parent-reported data for both sets of measures [19]. In addition, the screen use variables are often limited to assessments of screen time (duration/timing) or binary characterizations of content as violent/nonviolent, rather than those related to interactivity, level of engagement, or other aspects of content, all of which are factors that may affect the impact on the user's stimulation/alertness and sleep health outcomes.

Finally, additional work is needed to clarify the effects of digital media on sleep that may influence and/or amplify other aspects of child health and development, such as anxiety, depression, or other elements of daytime performance. Sleep health has not been fully incorporated into studies in which researchers investigate the effects of media on other outcomes. Finally, there is little information about whether and why there are moderating factors with differential effects of digital media use on sleep by age, sex, socioeconomic, neighborhood, and cultural factors, trauma history, neurodiversity, and/or personality characteristics.

## 3 Future Research

Below, we offer several key research questions we believe should be addressed in the forthcoming research on screen use and sleep:

- How can the prevalence, duration, and timing of digital media use be accurately measured and also capture components such as content and interactivity? This is complicated by the regular use of multiple devices simultaneously as well as by challenges researchers face when aiming to integrate data from different platforms (e.g., android, iOS).
- What are effective sustainable interventions to mitigate the effects of screen use on sleep health? What are the psychological and social barriers to changing behaviors around screen use in the evening?
- Do the effects of digital media on sleep influence and/or amplify other aspects of child health and development, such as anxiety, depression, or other elements of daytime performance? Understanding the potential range and magnitude of the downstream consequences of digital media use on sleep health may help bring attention to the concerns.
- Are there moderating factors (e.g., age, sex, socioeconomic factors, clinical conditions) that affect the association between screen use and sleep health?
- What are messages and distribution channels for effectively reaching and then nudging and navigating pediatric audiences and families toward healthier screen practices?

## 4 Recommendations

We offer the following public-facing recommendations to youth, families, teachers, coaches, clinicians, and policymakers. These are based on the most recent research as well as our prior recommendations [3] and those endorsed by the American Academy of Pediatrics [1]:

- Make sleep a priority: Talk about the importance of sleep and healthy sleep expectations in a range of environments (e.g., homes, classrooms, after-school activities, doctor visits).

- Facilitate a bedtime routine that includes calming activities and avoids disruptive electronic media use.
- Encourage families to remove all electronic media from their children or teenagers' bedrooms, including televisions, video games, computers, tablets, and smartphones—and to set a good example by doing so themselves.
- Promote tools that parents/caregivers can use to support healthier electronic media use at home (e.g., parental controls etc.)
- Talk with families about the negative consequences of bright light in the evening on sleep.
- If the child or adolescent in your care is exhibiting mood or behavioral problems, consider sleep disturbance as a contributing factor and screen for sleep disorders where appropriate.
- Support policies that benefit population sleep health, including later school start times and permanent standard time.

**Conflict of Interest and Funding Disclosures** LH is partially supported by grants from NICHD (R01 HD073352 and R21 HD097491) and the Della Pietra family. LEH receives research support from NICHD (F32 HD103390). MAG is partially supported by R01DA051321 and R01MD011600. LH has received consulting fees from Idorsia Pharmaceuticals and honoraria/travel support for lectures and consulting from Brown University, Harvard University, University of Miami, New York University, Columbia University/Princeton University, and the National Sleep Foundation. She ended her term as the editor-in-chief of *Sleep Health* in 2020. MKL reports receiving travel funds from the Australian Research Council and research support from the National Institutes of Health, beyond the submitted work. LEH has no conflicts to disclose. MAG has received grants from Jazz Pharmaceuticals, and CeraZ has received honoraria/travel support from New York University, University of Miami, and Yale University and has received consulting support from Fitbit, Natrol, Smartypants Vitamins, Simple Habit, Idorsia, Eisai, and Canyon Ranch. RR has received consulting fees from Sonesta Hotels International, byNacht GmbH, Savoir Beds Ltd., Castle Hot Springs, and Oura Ring Ltd. MG has received research grant funding from the National Institutes of Health and the Verizon Foundation. CAC serves as the incumbent of an endowed professorship provided to Harvard Medical School by Cephalon, Inc. and reports institutional support for a Quality Improvement Initiative from Delta Airlines and Puget Sound Pilots; education support to Harvard Medical School Division of Sleep Medicine and support to Brigham and Women's Hospital from Jazz Pharmaceuticals PLC, Inc., Philips Respironics, Inc., Optum, and ResMed, Inc.; research support to Brigham and Women's Hospital from Axome Therapeutics, Inc., Dayzz Ltd., Regeneron Pharmaceuticals, Sanofi SA, Casey Feldman Foundation, Summus, Inc., Takeda Pharmaceutical Co., LTD, Abbaszadeh Foundation, and CDC Foundation; educational funding to the Sleep and Health Education Program of the Harvard Medical School Division of Sleep Medicine from ResMed, Inc., Teva Pharmaceuticals Industries, Ltd., and Vanda Pharmaceuticals; royalty payments on sales of the Actiwatch-2 and Actiwatch-Spectrum devices from Philips Respironics, Inc; personal consulting fees from Bryte Foundation, With Deep, Inc., and Vanda Pharmaceuticals; honoraria for Thomas Roth Lecture of Excellence at SLEEP 2022 and from the Massachusetts Medical Society for a *New England Journal of Medicine* Perspective article, from the National Sleep Foundation for serving as chair of the Sleep Timing and Variability Consensus Panel, for lecture fees from Teva Pharma Australia PTY Ltd. and Emory University, and for serving as an advisory board member for the Institute of Digital Media and Child Development, the Klarman Family Foundation, and the UK Biotechnology and Biological Sciences Research Council. CAC has served as an expert witness on a number of civil matters, criminal matters, and arbitration cases, including those involving the following commercial and government entities: Amtrak; Bombardier, Inc.; C&J Energy Services; Dallas Police Association; Delta Airlines/Comair; Enterprise Rent-A-Car; FedEx; Greyhound Lines, Inc./Motor Coach Industries/FirstGroup America; PAR Electrical Contractors, Inc.; Puget Sound Pilots; and the San Francisco Sheriff's Department; Schlumberger Technology Corp.; Union Pacific Railroad; United Parcel Service; and Vanda Pharmaceuticals. CAC has received travel support from the Stanley Ho Medical Development Foundation for travel to Macao and Hong Kong; equity interest in Vanda Pharmaceuticals, With Deep, Inc, and Signos, Inc.; and institutional educational gifts to Brigham and Women's Hospital from Johnson & Johnson, Mary Ann and Stanley Snider via Combined Jewish Philanthropies, Alexandra Drane, DR Capital, Harmony Biosciences, LLC, San Francisco Bar Pilots, Whoop, Inc., Harmony Biosciences LLC, Eisai Co., LTD, Idorsia Pharmaceuticals LTD, Sleep Number Corp., Apnimed, Inc., Avadel Pharmaceuticals, Bryte Foundation, f.lux Software, LLC, and Stuart F. and Diana L. Quan Charitable Fund. In addition, CAC has a patent for "Actiwatch-2 and Actiwatch-Spectrum devices" with royalties paid to Philips Respironics Inc., a patent for "Assessment and Modification of a Subject's Endogenous Circadian Cycle," a patent for "Test for Evaluation of Visual Functioning in Visually Impaired Subjects," a patent for "Assessment and Modification of a Subject's Endogenous Circadian Cycle," a patent for "Assessment and Modification of Endogenous Circadian Phase and Amplitude," a patent for "Assessment and Modification of Circadian Phase and Amplitude," a patent for "Assessment and Modification of a Subject's Endogenous Circadian Cycle," a patent for "Assessment and Modification of a Human Subject's Circadian Cycle, " a patent for "Apparatus for Producing and Delivering High-Intensity Light to a Subject," a patent for "Intermittent Use of Bright Light to Modify the Circadian Phase," a patent for "Method of Facilitating the Physiological Adaption to an Activity/Rest Schedule and Apparatus for Prescribing a Substantially Optimum Stimulus Regimen of Pulses of Bright Light to Allow a Subject's Circadian Cycle to be Modified to a Desired State," a patent for "Method and Device for Modifying the Circadian Cycle in Humans," a patent for "Assessment and Modification of a Subject's Endogenous Circadian Cycle," a patent for "Modification of Endogenous Circadian Pacemaker," a patent for "Test for evaluation of visual functioning in visually impaired subjects," a patent for "Method for modifying or resetting the circadian cycle using short wavelength light," and a patent for "High sensitivity of the human circadian pacemaker to resetting by short wavelength light.". As none of these patents issued to the Brigham and Women's Hospital has been licensed, no royalties have been generated from them.

## References


1. Council on Communications and Media. Media use in school-aged children and adolescents. Pediatrics. 2016;138(5) https://doi.org/10.1542/peds.2016-2592.
2. Common Sense Census: Media Use by Tweens and Teens. 2019. https://www.commonsensemedia.org/research/the-commonsense-census-media-use-by-tweens-and-teens-2019.
3. LeBourgeois MK, Hale L, Chang AM, Akacem LD, Montgomery-Downs HE, Buxton OM. Digital media and sleep in childhood and adolescence. Pediatrics Nov 2017;140(Suppl 2):S92-S96. doi:https://doi.org/10.1542/peds.2016-1758J.
4. Grandner MA, Fernandez FX. The translational neuroscience of sleep: a contextual framework. Science. 2021;374(6567):568–73. https://doi.org/10.1126/science.abj8188.
5. Meltzer LJ, Williamson AA, Mindell JA. Pediatric sleep health: it matters, and so does how we define it. Sleep Med Rev. 2021;57:101425. https://doi.org/10.1016/j.smrv.2021.101425.
6. Hirshkowitz M, Whiton K, Albert SM, et al. National Sleep Foundation's updated sleep duration recommendations: final report. Sleep Health. 2015;1(4):233–43. https://doi.org/10.1016/j.sleh.2015.10.004.
7. Paruthi S, Brooks LJ, D'Ambrosio C, et al. Pediatric sleep duration consensus statement: a step forward. J Clin Sleep Med. 2016;12(12):1705–6. https://doi.org/10.5664/jcsm.6368.
8. Astill RG, Van der Heijden KB, Van Ijzendoorn MH, Van Someren EJ. Sleep, cognition, and behavioral problems in school-age children: a century of research meta-analyzed. Psychol Bull. 2012;138(6):1109–38. https://doi.org/10.1037/a0028204.
9. Short MA, Blunden S, Rigney G, et al. Cognition and objectively measured sleep duration in children: a systematic review and meta-analysis. Sleep Health. 2018;4(3):292–300. https://doi.org/10.1016/j.sleh.2018.02.004.
10. Reynaud E, Vecchierini MF, Heude B, Charles MA, Plancoulaine S. Sleep and its relation to cognition and behaviour in preschool-aged children of the general population: a systematic review. J Sleep Res. 2018;27(3):e12636. https://doi.org/10.1111/jsr.12636.
11. Chaput JP, Gray CE, Poitras VJ, et al. Systematic review of the relationships between sleep duration and health indicators in the early years (0–4 years). BMC Public Health. 2017;17(Suppl 5):855. https://doi.org/10.1186/s12889-017-4850-2.
12. Chaput JP, Gray CE, Poitras VJ, et al. Systematic review of the relationships between sleep duration and health indicators in school-aged children and youth. Appl Physiol Nutr Metab. 2016;41(6 Suppl 3):S266–82. https://doi.org/10.1139/apnm-2015-0627.
13. Lampl M, Johnson ML. Infant growth in length follows prolonged sleep and increased naps. Sleep. 2011;34(5):641–50. https://doi.org/10.1093/sleep/34.5.641.
14. Quist JS, Sjodin A, Chaput JP, Hjorth MF. Sleep and cardiometabolic risk in children and adolescents. Sleep Med Rev. 2016;29:76–100. https://doi.org/10.1016/j.smrv.2015.09.001.
15. Brautsch LA, Lund L, Andersen MM, Jennum PJ, Folker AP, Andersen S. Digital media use and sleep in late adolescence and young adulthood: a systematic review. Sleep Med Rev. 2022;68:101742. https://doi.org/10.1016/j.smrv.2022.101742.
16. Cain N, Gradisar M. Electronic media use and sleep in school-aged children and adolescents: a review. Sleep Med. 2010;11(8):735–42. https://doi.org/10.1016/j.sleep.2010.02.006.
17. Duch H, Fisher EM, Ensari I, Harrington A. Screen time use in children under 3 years old: a systematic review of correlates. Int J Behav Nutr Phys Act. 2013;10:102. https://doi.org/10.1186/1479-5868-10-102.
18. Alonzo R, Hussain J, Stranges S, Anderson KK. Interplay between social media use, sleep quality, and mental health in youth: a systematic review. Sleep Med Rev. 2021;56:101414. https://doi.org/10.1016/j.smrv.2020.101414.
19. Hale L, Guan S. Screen time and sleep among school-aged children and adolescents: a systematic literature review. Sleep Med Rev. 2015;21:50–8. https://doi.org/10.1016/j.smrv.2014.07.007.
20. Carter B, Rees P, Hale L, Bhattacharjee D, Paradkar MS. Association between portable screen-based media device access or use and sleep outcomes: a systematic review and meta-analysis. JAMA Pediatr. 2016;170(12):1202–8. https://doi.org/10.1001/jamapediatrics.2016.2341.
21. Lund L, Solvhoj IN, Danielsen D, Andersen S. Electronic media use and sleep in children and

adolescents in western countries: a systematic review. BMC Public Health. 2021;21(1):1598. https://doi.org/10.1186/s12889-021-11640-9.
22. Saunders TJ, McIsaac T, Campbell J, et al. Timing of sedentary behaviour and access to sedentary activities in the bedroom and their association with sleep quality and duration in children and youth: a systematic review. Health Promot Chronic Dis Prev Can. 2022;42(4):139–49. Revue systematique des liens entre, d'une part, l'horaire des comportements sedentaires et l'acces a des activites sedentaires dans la chambre et, d'autre part, la qualite et la duree du sommeil chez les enfants et les adolescents. https://doi.org/10.24095/hpcdp.42.4.03.
23. Rod NH, Dissing AS, Clark A, Gerds TA, Lund R. Overnight smartphone use: a new public health challenge? A novel study design based on high-resolution smartphone data. PLoS One. 2018;13(10):e0204811. https://doi.org/10.1371/journal.pone.0204811.
24. Scott H, Biello SM, Woods HC. Identifying drivers for bedtime social media use despite sleep costs: the adolescent perspective. Sleep Health. 2019;5(6):539–45. https://doi.org/10.1016/j.sleh.2019.07.006.
25. Chang AM, Aeschbach D, Duffy JF, Czeisler CA. Evening use of light-emitting eReaders negatively affects sleep, circadian timing, and next-morning alertness. Proc Natl Acad Sci U S A. 2015;112(4):1232–7. https://doi.org/10.1073/pnas.1418490112.
26. Martin KB, Bednarz JM, Aromataris EC. Interventions to control children's screen use and their effect on sleep: a systematic review and meta-analysis. J Sleep Res. 2021;30(3):e13130. https://doi.org/10.1111/jsr.13130.
27. Lin YM, Kuo SY, Chang YK, et al. Effects of parental education on screen time, sleep disturbances, and psychosocial adaptation among Asian preschoolers: a randomized controlled study. J Pediatr Nurs. 2021;56:e27–34. https://doi.org/10.1016/j.pedn.2020.07.003.
28. Flint Bretler O, Tzischinsky O, Asraf K, Shochat T. The effects of parental intervention on sleep patterns and electronic media exposure in young adolescents. Clocks Sleep. 2022;4(1):129–44. https://doi.org/10.3390/clockssleep4010013.
29. Pedersen J, Rasmussen MGB, Sorensen SO, et al. Effects of limiting recreational screen media use on physical activity and sleep in families with children: a cluster randomized clinical trial. JAMA Pediatr. 2022;176(8):741–9. https://doi.org/10.1001/jamapediatrics.2022.1519.
30. Mahalingham T, Howell J, Clarke PJF. Assessing the effects of acute reductions in mobile device social media use on anxiety and sleep. J Behav Ther Exp Psychiatry. 2023;78:101791. https://doi.org/10.1016/j.jbtep.2022.101791.
31. Bartel K, Scheeren R, Gradisar M. Altering adolescents' pre-bedtime phone use to achieve better sleep health. Health Commun. 2019;34(4):456–62. https://doi.org/10.1080/10410236.2017.1422099.
32. Khoshnoud S, Alvarez Igarzabal F, Wittmann M. Brain-heart interaction and the experience of flow while playing a video game. Front Hum Neurosci. 2022;16:819834. https://doi.org/10.3389/fnhum.2022.819834.
33. Jose PE, Vierling A. Cybervictimisation of adolescents predicts higher rumination, which in turn, predicts worse sleep over time. J Adolesc. 2018;68:127–35. https://doi.org/10.1016/j.adolescence.2018.07.011.
34. Eto T, Ohashi M, Nagata K, Shin N, Motomura Y, Higuchi S. Crystalline lens transmittance spectra and pupil sizes as factors affecting light-induced melatonin suppression in children and adults. Ophthalmic Physiol Opt. 2021;41(4):900–10. https://doi.org/10.1111/opo.12809.
35. Hartstein LE, Behn CD, Akacem LD, Stack N, Wright KP Jr, LeBourgeois MK. High sensitivity of melatonin suppression response to evening light in preschool-aged children. J Pineal Res. 2022;72(2):e12780. https://doi.org/10.1111/jpi.12780.
36. Hartstein LE, Diniz Behn C, Wright KP Jr, Akacem LD, Stowe SR, LeBourgeois MK. Evening light intensity and phase delay of the circadian clock in early childhood. J Biol Rhythm. 2023;38(1):77–86. https://doi.org/10.1177/07487304221134330.
37. Hart CN, Hawley N, Davey A, et al. Effect of experimental change in children's sleep duration on television viewing and physical activity. Pediatr Obes. 2017;12(6):462–7. https://doi.org/10.1111/ijpo.12166.

# Screen Use, Physical Injuries, and Orthopedic Health

Jennifer A. Manganello, Lara B. McKenzie, Despina Stavrinos, and Leon Straker

## 1 Background

Children and adolescents are using screen media more than ever before. The use of screen media, which include devices such as cell phones, tablets, computers, and televisions, can result in a range of health outcomes, many of which are related to physical health. Much research has examined the impact of screen use on obesity, physical activity, and sedentary behavior as well as sleep and eye strain. The use of screens can also lead to physical injuries, including orthopedic issues, for children and adolescents.

In this chapter, we review the impact of screens on orthopedic health through four distinct mechanisms. One focuses on the ways in which devices themselves can lead to injury (e.g., a television tipping over). One study found 230,325 incidents of television tip overs during a 30-year period [1]. Another explains how screen use can cause distractions, leading to physical injury, as youth often use phones when walking, biking, and driving, which can result in injury [2]. The third mechanism relates to overuse. Screen use has been linked to neck pain in young people across multiple studies [3]. Finally, the fourth mechanism considers the role of media effects. In other words, it involves thinking about how screen use can lead to exposure to content that can influence users to engage in behaviors that result in physical harm. As an example, 41% of scenes from movies rated G and PG from 2008 to 2012 showed unsafe behaviors [4].

Each of these four mechanisms has its own literature that examines the ways in which these mechanisms may explain links between screen use and physical injury or orthopedic health for children and adolescents. Below, we present a brief overview about each of these four areas of research. We also offer important research questions to address going forward and identify recommendations for key audiences.

## 2 Current State

### 2.1 Devices

One possible way for injuries to occur is from the devices themselves that are used during screen time. Most research in this area focuses on televi-

J. A. Manganello (✉)
Department of Health Policy, Management, and Behavior, University at Albany School of Public Health, Rensselaer, NY, USA
e-mail: jmanganello@albany.edu

L. B. McKenzie
Abigail Wexner Research Institute at Nationwide Children's Hospital, Center for Injury Research and Policy, Columbus, OH, USA

D. Stavrinos
Department of Psychology, University of Alabama at Birmingham, Birmingham, AL, USA

L. Straker
School of Allied Health, Curtin University, Perth, WA, Australia


D. A. Christakis, L. Hale (eds.), *Handbook of Children and Screens*,
https://doi.org/10.1007/978-3-031-69362-5_15

sion (TV) tip overs. TVs are used to entertain and educate, so many parents are surprised to learn that they pose a hazard, particularly to young children. Between 2000 and 2021, 167 child fatalities involved a television falling and another 170 involved both a television and the furniture it was on falling [5]. Despite the trends and changes in the design (shift from cathode ray tube to flat screen), size, and affordability of TVs, the number and types of injuries associated with TVs have remained constant. This is true even with declines in TV ownership over the last several decades (96% owned at least one television set in 2020, down from 98% in 2011) [6]. Flat screen televisions are top-heavy, have relatively narrow bases, and can tip over from a table or entertainment center. Due to the weight of some TVs relative to a child's small size and strength [7], combined with their inability to get out of the way quickly (when a TV or furniture on which the TV is placed is tipping), tip overs can lead to severe and sometimes fatal injuries.

Parents' attitudes, knowledge, and behaviors related to securing TVs demonstrate that the hazard of falling TVs and possible resulting injuries are not on most parents' minds. Three out of four parents have not heard of this type of hazard, and only one in four parents mount their flat screen TV on the wall. Reasons given for not mounting TVs are related to concern about damage to the wall; being unsure of whether mounting matters; and worry that the TV might fall off the wall [8]. TVs are most often placed on a dresser or TV stand and are not secured. Dressers and other furniture not designed to support TVs are commonly involved in TV tip overs as well.

Other device injuries include those from video games and cell phones. Video gaming has expanded in the last several decades, and this expansion of games, players, and experiences brings with it the risk of possible injury. A review of the literature has identified acute injuries from traumatic events such as falling while gaming as well as the risk of overuse injuries from performing repetitive motions for long periods of time.[2] Some studies have looked at injury from electronic gaming. Acute trauma injuries have been reported during active game use, ranging from bone fractures [9] occurring as a result of game use to injuries from unintended collisions with furniture or co-players [10]. Skin issues from gaming have also been reported, mainly with the palm and fingers, resulting from friction or allergies [11].

With respect to cell phones, one study found that children under age 13 were more likely to sustain a direct mechanical injury from cell phones than to be otherwise injured from cell phone use [12]. Examples of direct mechanical injuries include injuries sustained from a cell phone battery exploding or being hit in the face with a cell phone, estimated to be 36,091 over a 20-year period [12]. The types of cell phone-related injuries included lacerations, contusions or abrasions, internal organ injury, strains or sprains, concussions, foreign body, fractures, and others or not stated [12].

## 2.2 Distractions

Another way that screen use can lead to physical injuries is when people are distracted while using screen devices. This is particularly problematic when screen devices are used in road environments, leading to distracted walking, distracted cycling, or distracted driving [2]. Adolescents are more likely to sustain cell phone-related injuries while walking and driving compared to other age groups [13]. The general prevalence of distracted walking and cycling for youth is currently unknown. However, one observational study found that almost 19% of high school students were distracted while walking [14]. Most of what is currently known about distractions during cell phone use among children and adolescents concerns distracted driving.

Motor vehicle crashes (MVCs) have consistently been the leading cause of death for children and adolescents in the United States, only recently overtaken by firearm injuries [13]. Distracted driving, or the reallocation of resources necessary for driving to a competing activity or secondary task, has emerged as a significant contributor to MVCs, especially for new drivers who lack adequate experience with the cognitively complex task of driving [15]. In the United States, more than 310C people have been killed and about 424,000 have been injured in crashes involving a distracted driver [15]. Distracted driving is especially a problem for adolescents aged 15–20, who comprise the largest proportion of drivers who were distracted at the time of a fatal crash (9%) [15].

Many studies have documented the impairing effects of distracted driving among adolescents. Distractions can take various forms, such as peer passengers, eating and drinking, and reaching for objects. However, cell phone use remains one of the most prevalent and impairing behaviors behind the wheel. Tasks that involve interaction with an electronic device involve visual, manual, and cognitive distractions that significantly impair driving. On the other hand, tasks like conversing on a cell phone may have a lesser impact on safety compared to texting or visually intensive tasks, but still involve cognitive distraction, so they are not risk-free. Meta-analyses of the current work indicate that electronic device use significantly impairs adolescent driving, regardless of the developmental level (younger vs. older), type of task (cell phone conversation vs. interaction with an electronic device), and study methodology (driving simulation vs. naturalistic "on-road" studies) [2].

Despite efforts to mitigate distracted driving, it continues to be a pervasive issue. Graduated driver licensing laws restricting usage of electronic devices for beginner drivers indicate that cell phone restrictions may not result in long-term avoidance of cell phone use [16]. Distraction-specific legislation (e.g., hands-free laws) shows some promise [17] and supports the science suggesting that manual and visual distractions significantly increase crash risk. However, adolescents often perceive hands-free devices as risk-free [18] despite research suggesting that cognitive distraction increases crash risk [19], and, while cell phone blocking technology is effective at mitigating interaction with electronic devices for adolescent drivers [20], they may find alternate ways to "cheat" the system.

## 2.3 Overuse

Screen use can also lead to physical injury or orthopedic health issues through overuse. Musculoskeletal issues related to prolonged or repetitive postures and movements during screen use are a common concern for families and health professionals. However, research evidence is surprisingly weak. For example, although associations between various types of screen uses and musculoskeletal issues are commonly reported [21], a recent systematic review of epidemiological studies on adults has reported an inconsistent and weak increased risk of musculoskeletal symptoms with screen work based on self-reported exposure and no increased risk with objectively measured exposure [22].

Evidence showing that screen use among children and adolescents can lead to neck and back problems is limited. Prolonged neck flexion has been reported in a number of studies of children using small screens such as laptop and tablet computers, handheld electronic games, and smartphones. For example, a short-term observational study found that children aged 5–12 had a small (2 degree) increase in head tilt while using a smartphone [23]. There is reported to be a widespread belief among health professionals and in the wider community that habitual prolonged neck flexion increases the risk of chronic neck pain [24]. Whilst this belief is supported by increased discomfort with acute exposure to sustained neck flexion and some cross-sectional studies [25], longitudinal epidemiological studies have not provided supportive evidence. As an example, a longitudinal study of young adults found no increase in neck pain risk with increased habitual neck flexion posture [26]. Similarly, although there are concerns that prolonged screen use in flexed/slouched lumbar postures may increase the risk of chronic low back pain, there is little evidence to support this.

Although there is limited research with children and adolescents concerning hand issues from screen use, high exposure to repetitive movements of the hands in computer keyboard typing and mouse use has some evidence of being related to thumb, wrist, and elbow pain in adults [21]. There is also some weak evidence of mobile phone use and texting being related to thumb or hand pain in adults; a laboratory study found differences in thumb kinematics and muscle activity during phone use between young adults with and without musculoskeletal symptoms [26]. In children, rare cases of distal upper extremity overuse inflammation have been reported related to electronic game use as early as 1991 [10]. Similarly, cases of neck/shoulder pain have been reported following unaccustomed use of active electronic games involving wrist and arm movements.

Finally, some also believe that the use of screens may displace other activities that provide important physical demands to stimulate muscle and bone development, coordination, and energy expenditure. However, children and adolescents are likely to have sufficient time in their awake day to include required physical activities [27]. In fact, screen use may actually provide some benefit in terms of the development of fine motor control from touch screen device use [28] and gross motor control from active electronic games, although real-world activities are likely to provide better three-dimensional training [29].

## 2.4 Content

Another important area of study related to screens and physical injury comes from exposure to content through the use of devices. Messages included in a variety of screen media have the potential to influence the attitudes and behaviors of children and adolescents. A number of studies over the years have examined the influence of media content, and more recently social media, on health behaviors such as violence, nutrition, smoking, and more. Various health behavior theories, including social cognitive theory and the integrated behavioral model, suggest that exposure to media messages can influence attitudes and behaviors [30].

Injury prevention has been one of the least studied health topics with respect to media influences on health. However, some studies have examined media content with the goal of identifying potential influences on behaviors that can result in injury. For instance, one study of driving behaviors in television shows popular with adolescents found that only 17% of teen drivers were shown wearing a seat belt [31]. Viewers of such programs could observe a lack of seat belt use and come to the conclusion that wearing a seat belt is not important or typical for people their age.

With social media, content can be created by anyone. This has led to an increase in content depicting unsafe behaviors or injuries, including "challenge" videos that encourage people to engage in behaviors that can sometimes lead to injury [32]. A study of 50 YouTube videos showing a fire challenge (where someone sets themselves on fire and tries to put out the flames before injury occurs) found that over half of people in the videos were under the age of 20 [33]. Experts have suggested that such challenge videos encourage viewers to engage in risky behavior with the promise that their video can go viral [33]. People, including adolescents, are also more likely to engage in challenges when they see others doing them and perceive them to be a "common behavior." [30]

At the same time, media can also provide a platform to help educate children and adolescents and prevent physical injury, as messages can also educate and promote safe behaviors [34]. However, research has found there are few educational messages provided. For instance, a study of TikTok videos using the keywords "concussion" and "head injury" found that only 1 of the 92 concussion-related videos provided any type of educational message [35]. Another study of choking game videos on YouTube found that even when educational messages were provided, they were often "not accurate or representative." [36]

# 3 Future Research

There is much evidence to suggest that screen use can lead to a range of physical injuries through different mechanisms, but there is still more to learn. Questions to guide future work include the following:

- What are the best strategies for children and adolescents to avoid screen use or manage screens while doing other activities, including driving, especially as cell phones continue to dominate our lives?
- How can we encourage users to develop lifelong habits to vary their postures and avoid prolonged and awkward postures whilst using screens?
- Can we develop clear evidence of dose–response relationships between screen use, biomechanical and physiological parameters, and musculoskeletal disorders?
- What are the best ways to educate parents and caregivers about how to decrease physical injury resulting from screen use, such as installation of tip restraint devices for televisions?
- What injury-promoting or injury-preventing messages are screen users seeing in different types of media, and how do these messages influence attitudes, knowledge, and behavior that can result in or prevent physical injury?

# 4 Recommendations

While more research is needed, several actions have already been recommended to help address these issues.

## 4.1 For Clinicians and Providers

- Remind parents to be good role models by not engaging in distracted driving themselves.
- Encourage users to be aware of discomfort arising from postures and movements and use this as a trigger to move and suggest that parents help their children develop habits of varying their posture during screen use.
- Remind parents to secure TVs with restraint devices, attach furniture to walls, rearrange household items, and recycle old TVs.
- Help screen users, including parents, be aware of social media trends and challenges and the dangers of participating in such challenges [26].

## 4.2 For Policymakers

- Strengthen and enforce legislation related to screen use while driving.
- Encourage organizations to develop codes of practice (or guidelines) that encourage children and adolescents to move regularly.
- Continue the use of warning labels and strengthen and enforce stability requirements for furniture and TVs.
- Consider how regulations could be implemented to provide warnings on media content that could lead to injuries.

## 4.3 For Educators

- Help debunk the perception that hands-free driving is completely risk-free.
- Teach children and adolescents to vary their postures and move regularly when using screens.
- When screens are being used at school, consider providing screen breaks or supporting correct posture with reminders or ergonomic furniture.
- Make parents aware of the hazards of TV tip overs and the need for tip restraints through warnings on TVs.
- Provide media literacy education in schools to help students learn how to be informed and critical media consumers.

## 4.4 For Industry

- Make technological modifications to remind users to stay focused on the activity they are engaged in, such as driving.
- Provide frequent opportunities in electronic games for users to be able to save and stop playing.

- Ensure that warning labels remind parents of the dangers of devices and the need to secure TVs and other large devices.
- Determine whether media content produced or allowed to be created can result in the promotion of injury-causing behaviors, and consider restricting or editing such content or adding content warnings.

Continuing needed research related to injuries and orthopedic health can expand the evidence and allow for more refined recommendations. Additional funding for research and design changes is needed to continue to reduce injuries among children and adolescents. These complex problems will require innovative solutions to mitigate the risks of physical injury and orthopedic issues stemming from screen use. As screen use and devices continue to change and develop, researchers, practitioners, industry professionals, and parents must all remain observant of how the use of such devices can result in injury and orthopedic health issues.

**Conflict of Interest and Funding Disclosures** None.

## References

1. Lu C, Badeti J, Mehan TJ, Zhu M, Smith GA. Furniture and television tip-over injuries to children treated in United States emergency departments. Injury Epidemiol. 2021;8(1):53. https://doi.org/10.1186/s40621-021-00346-6.
2. Stavrinos D, Pope CN, Shen J, Schwebel DC. Distracted walking, bicycling, and driving: systematic review and meta-analysis of mobile technology and youth crash risk. Child Dev. 2018;89(1):118–28. https://doi.org/10.1111/cdev.12827.
3. David D, Giannini C, Chiarelli F, Mohn A. Text neck syndrome in children and adolescents. Int J Environ Res Public Health. 2021;18(4):1565. https://doi.org/10.3390/ijerph18041565.
4. Pelletier AR, Tongren JE, Gilchrist J. Injury prevention practices as depicted in G- and PG-rated movies, 2008–2012. J Commun Health. 2015;40(4):613–8. https://doi.org/10.1007/s10900-014-9974-z.
5. Suchy A. Product instability or tip-over injuries and fatalities associated with televisions, furniture, and appliances: 2022 report. 2023. https://www.cpsc.gov/s3fs-public/2022_Tip_Over_Report_Final.pdf
6. Lindner J. Television ownership statistics [fresh research]. Published 2023. https://gitnux.org/television-ownership-statistics/. Accessed 18 Apr 2024.
7. Marnewick J, Dansey R, Morreau P, Hamill J. Television tip-overs: the starship children's hospital experience and literature review. Injury. 2011;42(5):534–8. https://doi.org/10.1016/j.injury.2009.12.015.
8. Ferguson R, Mickalide A. A report to the nation on home safety: the dangers of TV tip-overs. Published online December 2012. https://www.safekids.org/sites/default/files/documents/ResearchReports/TV%20Tipovers%20Research%20Rpt.pdf. Accessed 18 Mar 2023.
9. Truong P, Truong L, Le T, Kuklova K. Orthopedic injuries from video games: a literature review and implications for the future. Int Arch Orthop Surg. 2020;3. https://clinmedjournals.org/articles/iaos/international-archives-of-orthopaedic-surgery-iaos-3-020.php?jid=iaos. Accessed 20 Mar 2023.
10. Jalink MB, Heineman E, Pierie JPEN, Hoedemaker C, Henk O. Nintendo related injuries and other problems: review. BMJ. 2014;349:g7267. https://doi.org/10.1136/bmj.g7267.
11. Kyriakou G, Glentis A. Skin in the game: video-game-related cutaneous pathologies in adolescents. Int J Pediatr Adolesc Med. 2021;8(2):68–75. https://doi.org/10.1016/j.ijpam.2019.09.002.
12. Povolotskiy R, Gupta N, Leverant AB, Kandinov A, Paskhover B. Head and neck injuries associated with cell phone use. JAMA Otolaryngol Head Neck Surg. 2020;146(2):122–7. https://doi.org/10.1001/jamaoto.2019.3678.
13. Lee LK, Douglas K, Hemenway D. Crossing lines: a change in the leading cause of death among U.S. children. N Engl J Med. 2022;386(16):1485–7. https://doi.org/10.1056/NEJMp2200169.
14. Quon P, Lahey K, Grisdale M, et al. Prevalence of distracted walking with mobile technology: an observational study of Calgary and Edmonton high school students. Can J Public Health. 2019;110(4):506–11. https://doi.org/10.17269/s41997-019-00200-9.
15. National Center for Statistics and Analysis. Driver Electronic Device Use in 2021 (Traffic Safety Facts Research Note. Report No. DOT HS 813 357). Published online August 2022. https://crashstats.nhtsa.dot.gov/Api/Public/ViewPublication/813357#:~:text=The%20percentage%20of%20passenger%20vehicle,Figure%201%20and%20Table%202. Accessed 8 Mar 2023.
16. Ehsani J, Ionides E, KLauer S, Perlus J, Gee B. Effectiveness of cell phone restrictions for young drivers: review of the evidence https://journals.sagepub.com/doi/abs/10.3141/2602-05?journalCode=trra. Accessed 8 Mar 2023.
17. Li L, Pope CN, Andridge RR, Bower JK, Hu G, Zhu M. Cellphone laws and teens' calling while driving:

analysis of repeated cross-sectional surveys in 2013, 2015, 2017, and 2019. Injury Epidemiol. 2020;7:65. https://doi.org/10.1186/s40621-020-00290-x.
18. Stavrinos D, McManus B, Beck H. Demographic, driving experience, and psychosocial predictors of adolescent distracted driving beliefs. Accid Anal Prev. 2020;144:105678. https://doi.org/10.1016/j.aap.2020.105678.
19. Strayer DL, Cooper JM. Driven to distraction. Hum Factors. 2015;57(8):1343–7. https://doi.org/10.1177/0018720815610668.
20. Creaser JI, Edwards CJ, Morris NL, Donath M. Are cellular phone blocking applications effective for novice teen drivers? J Saf Res. 2015;54:75–8. https://doi.org/10.1016/j.jsr.2015.06.014.
21. Tholl C, Bickmann P, Wechsler K, Froböse I, Grieben C. Musculoskeletal disorders in video gamers – a systematic review. BMC Musculoskelet Disord. 2022;23(1):678. https://doi.org/10.1186/s12891-022-05614-0.
22. Coenen P, van der Molen HF, Burdorf A, et al. Associations of screen work with neck and upper extremity symptoms: a systematic review with meta-analysis. Occup Environ Med. 2019;76(7):502–9. https://doi.org/10.1136/oemed-2018-105553.
23. Abdel-Aziem AA, Abdel-Ghafar MAF, Ali OI, Abdelraouf OR. Effects of smartphone screen viewing duration and body position on head and neck posture in elementary school children. J Back Musculoskelet Rehabil. 2022;35(1):185–93. https://doi.org/10.3233/BMR-200334.
24. Straker L, Smith A, Campbell A, O'Sullivan P. Are neck pain and posture related? Phys Ther Rev. 2010;1 https://doi.org/10.1179/174328810X12719009060029.
25. Brink Y, Louw QA. A systematic review of the relationship between sitting and upper quadrant musculoskeletal pain in children and adolescents. Man Ther. 2013;18(4):281–8. https://doi.org/10.1016/j.math.2012.11.003.
26. Gustafsson E, Johnson PW, Hagberg M. Thumb postures and physical loads during mobile phone use – a comparison of young adults with and without musculoskeletal symptoms. J Electromyogr Kinesiol. 2010;20(1):127–35. https://doi.org/10.1016/j.jelekin.2008.11.010.
27. Straker L, Maslen B, Burgess-Limerick R, Johnson P, Dennerlein J. Evidence-based guidelines for the wise use of computers by children: physical development guidelines. Ergonomics. 2010;53(4):458–77. https://doi.org/10.1080/00140130903556344.
28. Bedford R, Saez de Urabain IR, Cheung CHM, Karmiloff-Smith A, Smith TJ. Toddlers' fine motor milestone achievement is associated with early touchscreen scrolling. Front Psychol. 2016;7:1108. https://doi.org/10.3389/fpsyg.2016.01108.
29. Straker L, Abbott R, Collins R, Campbell A. Evidence-based guidelines for wise use of electronic games by children. Ergonomics. 2014;57(4):471–89. https://doi.org/10.1080/00140139.2014.895856.
30. Khasawneh A, Chalil Madathil K, Zinzow H, et al. Factors contributing to adolescents' and young adults' participation in web-based challenges: survey study. JMIR Pediatr Parent. 2021;4(1):e24988. https://doi.org/10.2196/24988.
31. Manganello JA, Chauhan AG. Car riding behavior in television programs watched by adolescents in the U.S. J Child Media. 2011;5(2):194–203. https://doi.org/10.1080/17482798.2011.558276.
32. Kriegel ER, Lazarevic B, Athanasian CE, Milanaik RL. TikTok, tide pods and Tiger king: health implications of trends taking over pediatric populations. Curr Opin Pediatr. 2021;33(1):170–7. https://doi.org/10.1097/MOP.0000000000000989.
33. Avery AH, Rae L, Summitt JB, Kahn SA. The fire challenge: a case report and analysis of self-inflicted flame injury posted on social media. J Burn Care Res. 2016;37(2):e161–5. https://doi.org/10.1097/BCR.0000000000000324.
34. Moran K. Jumping to (fatal) conclusions? An analysis of video film on a social networking web site of recreational jumping from height into water. Int J Inj Control Saf Promot. 2014;21(1):47–53. https://doi.org/10.1080/17457300.2012.755207.
35. Carter PN, Hall EE, Ketcham CJ, Ahmed OH. Not just for dancing? A content analysis of concussion and head injury videos on tiktok. Front Sports Active Living. 2021;3. https://www.frontiersin.org/articles/10.3389/fspor.2021.692613. Accessed 9 Feb 2023.
36. Defenderfer EK, Austin JE, Davies WH. The choking game on YouTube. Glob Pediatr Health. 2016;3:2333794X15622333. https://doi.org/10.1177/2333794X15622333.

# Introduction to the Section on Digital Media and Mental Health

Paul Weigle

"I have multiple personality disorder, just like my best friend and TikTokker 'Wonderland'," the bright-eyed 12-year-old girl told me matter-of-factly upon psychiatric admission for suicidality. She then proceeded to list off the *Diagnostic and Statistical Manual of Mental Disorders* (DSM) criteria, describe her several personalities in practiced detail, and reassure me that only one of them, in fact, wanted to die, and "he" refused to talk to me.

In 20 years of clinical practice, I have borne witness to a gradual shift by which more and more of my patients' mental health problems are wrapped up in their screen media habits and experiences, for better or worse. This change has brought unprecedented opportunities for youth suffering psychiatric illness, as well as new risks to mental health, transforming how I evaluate and treat them.

The most obvious change in the lives of children and teens is how they spend their day, now largely dominated by screen entertainment. Studies confirm that youth spend more time on entertainment media than any other activity besides sleep [1]. Former activities and pastimes have diminished or fallen away to make room for streaming videos, playing video games, and scrolling social media.

This massive shift in the daily habits of youth is accompanied by a number of other important changes, for better or worse. The doubling of screen media engagement over the past few decades has seen significant declines in teen pregnancy [2] and deaths by auto accidents [3], homicides [4], and illicit substance use [5]. Conversely, young people are spending less time socializing in person, doing chores, various other hobbies, and moving their bodies and are more likely than ever to suffer from regular deficient sleep [6].

Recent years have seen soaring rates of depression, anxiety, self-harm, and suicidality among youth, leading the American Academy of Pediatrics and the American Academy of Child and Adolescent Psychiatry to declare an unprecedented national emergency in child and adolescent mental health [7]. This crisis in the well-being of our youth demands a timely, commensurate response. However, such a response demands a full understanding of the problem. What is causing such mental suffering and impairment for so many of our nation's youth, and what can be done to help them? Popular opinion holds that increases in screen media engagement have caused the mental health crisis, but this theory is unproven. Youth on screens the most are also the most likely to have mental health problems, but not all heavy media users suffer in this way.

We rely on scientific inquiry to definitively reveal how screen media engagement affects mental health and consequently what we can do about it. Thousands of scientific studies have

P. Weigle (✉)
Department of Psychiatry, University of Connecticut School of Medicine, Farmington, CT, USA
e-mail: paul.weigle@hhchealth.org


D. A. Christakis, L. Hale (eds.), *Handbook of Children and Screens*,
https://doi.org/10.1007/978-3-031-69362-5_16

attempted to do just that by nearly as many means, and the evidence they provide sheds significant light on this vital question. In this handbook, groups of leading researchers, clinicians, and practitioners in their respective fields have gathered, evaluated, translated, and summarized findings of the existing body of scientific evidence regarding the relationships between screen media use and mental health. They have identified important gaps in our current knowledge to inform future research and used our current understanding to make actionable recommendations for parents, teachers, clinicians, and other stakeholders to safeguard the mental health of those growing up in an increasingly digital world.

The topic has been broken up into separate chapters regarding the interplay between various aspects of mental health and screen media, our ability to identify at-risk youth, and ways that digital media can be used to benefit mental health.

Although adolescents, especially children, spend more time engaging with streaming and video games than with social media, their interactions on social media seem to bear unique consequences for their mental health. During the 2020 pandemic quarantine, adolescents largely replaced in-person interactions with social media (and social gaming) with seemingly harmful results, given the mental health crisis that shortly followed. For many teens, time spent on social media has significant consequences for their well-being. Online contacts, response to posts, conflicts, and social comparison can have high psychological stakes unique to social media. Patients often present for mental health care following a crisis related to such social media interactions. In "Social Media and Youth Mental Health: A Departure From the Status Quo," Coyne et al. (see Chap. 17) summarize research on the interactions between mental health and social media habits and experiences. They find that the nature and valence of social media content and interactions to a large extent appear to influence mental health changes, for good or ill.

In "Youth Anxiety in the Digital Age: Present Status and Future Considerations," Ariefdjohan et al. (see Chap. 18) explore how media habits and experiences are connected to anxiety disorders, the most common psychiatric conditions in youth. Screen entertainment is typically a relief from everyday stressors and worries but can be harmful to those who overindulge. In my clinical practice, I often see socially anxious youth who prefer social interactions via social media or gaming to in-person get-togethers. Entertainment screen media may enable anxious youth to avoid in-person interactions with their peers and other anxiety-provoking experiences in a manner that progressively exacerbates their anxiety. In other cases, social media interactions may progress to in-person socializing in a therapeutic manner. Research to date has found mixed associations between screen media engagement and anxiety. Problematic, or excessive, screen media engagement is associated with symptoms of anxiety, but use of social media to facilitate meaningful social interactions or elicit social support may in some cases be beneficial. It has become increasingly important to understand how screen media affect anxiety and how to guide youth who suffer from it, but ultimately more evidence is needed for this endeavor.

I have observed clinically that overuse of entertainment screen media sometimes enables youth to avoid their important daily responsibilities and healthy behaviors such as schoolwork, chores, family interactions, and sufficient sleep. This avoidance, when habitual, can lead to feelings of inadequacy, which either cause or worsen depressive disorders. Ironically, those who appear most harmed by excessive screen media habits are typically those who value those habits the most and are the most resistant to change them. However, youth with depression often highly value screen media as a means of escapism and inspiration, to learn about their peers' experiences with depression and to share their own. Twenge et al. (see Chap. 19) review the relationship between electronic media and depressive disorders in "Social Media and Depressive Symptoms." They present evidence of unhealthy screen media habits as a controllable cause of depression, discuss possible mediating factors, and offer related recommendations regarding how to protect youth.

In recent years, the suicide rate among adolescents has tragically increased, even as referrals for evaluation of suicidality in teens have skyrocketed, overwhelming the capacity of emergency rooms and treatment providers and programs. The most common scenario for which adolescents are referred to my care occurs when the teen posts a depiction of their self-harm or suicidal ideation on social media. Many youth in crisis find it preferable to communicate such thoughts and behaviors online than by other means, often to elicit support. Such social media posts can prompt peers to express caring or alert adults who may facilitate needed professional care but also risks inviting criticism, maladaptive coping, and inspiring self-harm in others. In "Media Influences on Self-Harm, Suicidality, and Suicide," Kruzan et al. (see Chap. 20) describe what we know about how news and social media content related to self-harm and suicide can inspire or discourage self-directed violence. They also describe how specific gaming and social media habits and experiences may inform this risk. The authors make vital recommendations for reducing the risks of self-harm and suicidality by further research, family education, and interventions by clinicians and schools.

For many, the most significant effects of social media engagement have to do with the internalization of beauty standards and the inevitable comparison of one's own appearance to others. Adolescent girls in my practice often appear equally preoccupied with scrolling through the selfies posted on social media by their peers and cultivating, perfecting, and sharing their own. These patients typically enjoy learning about fashion trends via social media but are also most likely to be dissatisfied with their bodies and thus experiment with restrictive eating and self-induced vomiting. In "Social Media Use, Body Image Concerns, and Disordered Eating Among Adolescents," Choukas-Bradley et al. (see Chap. 21) review the current state of research on this vital topic, bolstered by a surprising amount of controlled experimental data. They convincingly argue that the effects of viewing idealized social media images interact with platform features, sociocultural pressures, and adolescent developmental processes, resulting in a "perfect storm" of negative appearance comparisons, self-esteem, and, ultimately, disordered eating for vulnerable youth.

My role as a child and adolescent psychiatrist leads me to focus on the lives of youth who are struggling and those who come to me for treatment of mental illness. I see little of their peers who are mentally well. Although the great majority of today's children and teens regularly engage with hours of entertainment screen media every day, not all are suffering from mental health problems. Despite the crisis of mental illness in youth, the majority are well, and a great many are thriving despite (or perhaps because of) their screen media habits. Determining which youth are more sensitive to the beneficial and harmful effects of screen experiences is vital. In "Who Is Most at Risk?: Identifying the Risks for Mental Health Problems Related to Social Media," Hamilton et al. (see Chap. 22) describe which demographic and individual factors make youth more susceptible to both positive and negative psychological sequelae of screen media exposures and suggest the next steps for clarifying and leveraging this information.

These chapters testify to the power of screen media as a tool to greatly affect mental health. Used in the correct manner, it has the power to greatly benefit psychological well-being. I have witnessed patients recover from depression by leveraging social media contacts into supportive in-person friendships, improve their self-esteem through cultivating popular social media posts, learn effective techniques to avoid self-harm from streaming videos, and practice their social skills after bonding with schoolmates over a beloved video game.

Mental health providers successfully treat mental illness with a combination of behavioral interventions, psychotherapies, and medication treatments. However, treatment-resistant illness is not uncommon. Science informs innovations creating more effective treatments. Tele-therapy and computerized mental health records have revolutionized how care is delivered and documented, but digital technology has been rarely used directly for treatment so far. In "Digital

Therapeutics in Child Psychiatry: Harnessing Technology to Treat Pediatric Mental Health," Gansner et al. (see Chap. 23) encapsulate the state of research into computer technology designed to treat mental illness, from ecological momentary intervention protocols to the Food and Drug Administration (FDA)-approved video games and online cognitive behavioral therapy programs. The authors describe the benefits and limits associated with these novel treatments and provide a glimpse and road map for the promise of more efficacious and equitable computerized treatments to come.

Indeed, a unique feature of growing up in modern times is that technology is both the cause and solution of many of life's problems. As long as childhood and adolescence continue to evolve, it is the responsibility and privilege of psychology and psychiatry to evaluate novel threats and avenues to well-being, and to continue to translate science into beneficial interventions. Evidence suggests that technology had a role in causing the mental health crisis in youth, and only understanding that role will enable us to overcome this crisis. Raising, teaching, and treating children to live healthy, balanced lives in the age of the Internet is challenging, but the understanding and recommendations provided in these chapters go a long way to making it easier.

**Conflict of Interest and Funding Disclosures** None.

## References


1. Rideout V, Peebles A, Mann S, Robb MB. Common sense census: media use by tweens and teens, 2021. San Francisco: Common Sense; 2022.
2. Tollestrup J. Teen birth trends. In Brief Congressional Research Service 2020.
3. Curtin S. Motor vehicle traffic death rates among adolescents and young adults aged 15–24, by urbanicity: United States, 2000–2018. Center for Disease Control and Prevention; 2020.
4. Statistical Research Team, Number of serious violent crimes committed by youth aged between 12 and 17 years in the U.S. from 1980 to 2021 https://www.statista.com/statistics/477466/number-of-serious-violent-crimes-by-youth-in-the-us/. Accessed 3/21/2024.
5. Miech RA, Johnston LD, Patrick ME, O'Malley PM, Bachman JG, Schulenberg JE. Monitoring the future National Survey Results on drug use, 1975–2022: Secondary school students. Ann Arbor: Institute for Social Research, The University of Michigan; 2023.
6. Centers for Disease Control and Prevention. 2021 Youth Risk Behavior Survey Data. Available at: www.cdc.gov/yrbs
7. AAP-AACAP-CHA Declaration of a National Emergency in Child and Adolescent Mental Health https://www.aap.org/en/advocacy/child-and-adolescent-healthy-mental-development/aap-aacap-cha-declaration-of-a-national-emergency-in-child-and-adolescent-mental-health/. Accessed 3/21/2024.

# Social Media and Youth Mental Health: A Departure from the Status Quo

Sarah M. Coyne, César Escobar-Viera, Mesfin A. Bekalu, Linda Charmaraman, Brian Primack, Reem M. A. Shafi, Patti M. Valkenburg, and Kofoworola D. A. Williams

## 1 Background

Mental health problems are increasingly common among adolescents, with depression, anxiety, and suicide all rising dramatically since the early 2000s. For example, the prevalence of anxiety disorders has almost doubled in the past 20 years [1]. During the same period of time, rates of suicide have increased by almost a third, making suicide the third leading cause of death among young people [2]. Rates of mental health problems for adolescents from marginalized backgrounds (sexual, gender, racial, or ethnic minorities) are disproportionately high compared to their White, cisgender, heterosexual peers [3].

Use of social media has also increased rapidly during the same period, leading many to speculate that social media use might have caused the current mental health crisis [4]. Some states are either considering or passing bills that restrict the use of social media among youth, whereas others are suing social media companies for knowingly engaging in practices that harm mental health [5]. Some suggest that social media might be beneficial in providing social connections, community, emotional, informational, instrumental, and appraisal support to youth, especially those with marginalized identities and during times of a crisis [6]. However, concerns about social media use and mental health remain high among adolescents themselves, parents, medical professionals,

Notes: Sarah M. Coyne and César Escobar-Viera are co-first authors. Co-authors are listed alphabetically after the first two authors.

S. M. Coyne (✉)
School of Family Life, Brigham Young University, Provo, UT, USA
e-mail: smcoyne@byu.edu

C. Escobar-Viera
Department of Psychiatry, University of Pittsburgh School of Medicine, Pittsburgh, PA, USA

M. A. Bekalu
Department of Social and Behavioral Sciences, Harvard T. H. Chan School of Public Health, Boston, MA, USA

L. Charmaraman
Wellesley Centers for Women, Wellesley College, Wellesley, MA, USA

B. Primack
College of Public Health and Human Sciences, Oregon State University, Corvallis, OR, USA

R. M. A. Shafi
Department of Psychiatry, Cairns and Hinterland Hospital and Health Services, Cairns, QLD, Australia

P. M. Valkenburg
Amsterdam School of Communication Research, University of Amsterdam, Amsterdam, Netherlands

K. D. A. Williams
Department of Community Health and Prevention, Drexel University Dornsife School of Public Health, Philadelphia, PA, USA


D. A. Christakis, L. Hale (eds.), *Handbook of Children and Screens*,
https://doi.org/10.1007/978-3-031-69362-5_17

educators, policymakers, and politicians, which has translated into several reports and advisories published over the last few years [7, 8]. This chapter will provide a summary of the academic research on social media use and youth mental health, suggest future directions for research, and highlight recommendations for parents, media professionals, and policymakers.

## 2 Current State

A comprehensive assessment of the hundreds of studies on social media use and youth is beyond the scope of this chapter. We focus on time spent on social media, problematic social media use (PSMU), the context and content of social media use, and recent neurological studies.

### 2.1 Time Spent on Social Media

Research on time spent on social media is mixed. A small number of longitudinal studies have been conducted, and, while some have found positive associations between social media use and negative mental health outcomes such as depression and anxiety [9, 10], others have found weak or no association [11]. While meta-analyses suggest that there is a small but significant effect of time spent on social media on mental health, scholars interpret the effect sizes in vastly different ways [12]. Indeed, the majority of included studies are cross-sectional, self-report surveys, thereby limiting their conclusions.

The link between time spent on social media and mental health also varies across individuals. A recent study focused on individual susceptibility has found that 92% of adolescents reported either neutral or positive effects of time spent on social media on their self-esteem (which is related to mental health) and 8% reported consistent negative effects [13]. Researchers have also begun to examine developmental sensitivities, with early adolescence (around age 11–13) representing a critical period, particularly for girls [14].

### 2.2 Problematic Social Media

Research has also examined problematic social media use (PSMU), defined as using social media in ways that interfere with the ability to function in daily life [15]. Estimates vary, but approximately 4–9% of adolescents report PSMU, which tends to be a better predictor of mental health struggles than time spent on social media alone [16]. Again, most research on PSMU and mental health is cross-sectional, rendering the directionality of effects unknown, although likely bidirectional [17]. Additionally, most measures of PSMU have items that specifically tap mental health, so there is likely a significant overlap when correlated with mental health outcomes [18].

### 2.3 Content and Context of Social Media Use

Beyond time and problematic use, an individual's experiences with social media likely depend on the content and the context of what they experience in a given interaction. The characteristics of the person posting, the audience, the message, and the platform all likely impact outcomes [19]. For example, empirical evidence demonstrates that asking participants what proportion of their social media use is "positive" or "negative" (without giving any explicit examples) can significantly predict mental health outcomes. For example, exposure to "positive" content is associated with lower levels of depression, and "negative" content is associated with higher levels of depression [20, 21]. However, negative content tends to be more potent and is more strongly related to depression than is positive content.

Additionally, the context of social media use likely influences user experience. For example, a recent scoping review has found that even though some research suggests that using social media actively (e.g., posting, commenting) compared to passively (e.g., scrolling) might be related to better outcomes for adolescents a majority of studies have not confirmed this hypothesis [18]. Given these findings, we believe that additional research and development of nuanced and objective measures of active and passive social media use will be useful. Other research suggests that youths turn to social media specifically to *address* their mental health concerns. For example, some youths might turn to social media to learn about mental illness, share their experiences, and get support during difficult times [22].

The way one interacts on social media and whom that person interacts with is also important. For example, positive feedback on social media might change the experience for individuals. Functional magnetic resonance imaging (fMRI) research suggests heightened neural activity in reward processing regions when viewing one's own posts with a higher number of likes, suggesting a neurobiological basis for the association between social media use and mental health outcomes [23]. Additionally, following celebrities on social media has been associated with depression and online social anxiety [24], and, while social media interactions with strangers is associated with negative mental health outcomes, social media interactions with close real-life friends is beneficial [25].

### 2.4 Intrinsic Characteristics of the Individual

Factors intrinsic to the user are also important. For example, associations between social media use and mental health differ among marginalized youth. A longitudinal study found that social media experiences of acceptance predicted lower symptoms of depression and anxiety among LGBTQ but not heterosexual participants [26]. Consistent with this, in a recent study of early adolescents, LGBTQ youths were significantly more likely to join online support groups to reduce feelings of isolation [27].

A prior diagnosis of mental illness is also relevant. Compared to healthy peers, adolescents with diagnosed preexisting depression tend to show heightened physiological reactions after engaging with social media, showing higher levels of stress than those without depression [28].

In summary, multiple factors are likely to influence the association between social media use and mental health, including those that relate to the content of social media exposures and the context of these. Whether content is positive or negative, passive vs. active use, with whom the individual interacts with, and intrinsic user characteristics might influence the association between social media use and mental health. These factors therefore represent potential targets for future interventions to promote well-being.

## 3 Future Research

Given inconsistent evidence related to the associations between time spent on social media and youth mental health, as well as the methodological limitations mentioned before, future research must address:

- *What is the influence of social media interactions/experiences on adolescent mental health? What are the protective and risky ways of interacting with social media?* Affordances of social media platforms allow different forms of user interactions: one-to-one, one-to-many, synchronous, asynchronous, positive, and negative, with a wide array of content ranging from text to short videos etc. [29] Therefore, intensive data collection methods such as ecological momentary assessments and social media data mining from consenting study participants should be leveraged. Studies using such methods are rapidly growing in number [30], facilitated by the widespread use of smartphones among youth. We believe that such studies are crucial to gain a better understanding of the effects of social media on mental health.
- *What is the temporality of the associations between social media interactions/experiences and adolescent mental health?* Prior research found that interactions such as online victimization have higher proximal impact on suicidal thoughts and behavior that decreases over the weeks that follow the interaction [31]. It is important to understand the temporal

association between other forms of social media interactions and different mental health outcomes as well as how these effects change over time. This will require a focus on longitudinal studies combined with intensive data collection methods.

- *Do social media-based interactions/experiences mimic those that are offline in their impact on youth mental health?* There are well-known protective (e.g., social support) and risk (e.g., victimization) experiences for adolescent mental health that occur in the offline environment. Similar interactions take place on social media, but we do not know how the effect of social media-based interactions compare to those that happen offline [32]. Such understanding would help identify novel targets for intervention development research focused on adolescent mental health. As our experience of the online and the offline worlds become more intertwined and is shaped by everchanging platform features, measurement instruments should be evaluated frequently regarding their purpose, validity, and reliability.
- *Who is most likely to benefit from social media interactions?* Qualitative research among marginalized groups (e.g., LGBTQ+, racially/ethnically diverse, people living with mental illness or chronic health conditions) suggests that social media interactions might enhance community/capacity building and be protective of emotional well-being [33]. Marginalized groups experience mental health disparities, mediated, in part, by minority stress, racial discrimination, stigma, and/or difficulty accessing mental health services [34]. While social media is a potential route to deliver services more effectively to these groups, we do not know what kinds of social media-based interventions (e.g., synchronous or asynchronous) or to whom these will be the most beneficial. Future research must specifically target these groups. This can be achieved via approaches to recruitment such as purposeful sampling, oversampling, n-of-1 studies, and longitudinal studies.
- *What are the ethical concerns related to social media research that leverages users' data?* We believe that it is crucial to engage research participants in studies that collect social media data, posing an important challenge to researchers in terms of handling the data of participants [35] and those users interacting with participants. Such data collection may include highly private content (e.g., discussion of personal struggles outside of the scope of the study, exchanges of a sexual nature) and problematic interactions (e.g., inappropriate exchanges between adolescents and adults). While machine learning and deep learning methods offer an opportunity for leveraging social media data to identify mental health problems at both individual and population levels, future research should continue incorporating user perspectives to triangulate, contextualize, and explain the results of automated analyses. Maximally leveraging social media research requires multiple methods, including qualitative, quantitative, and mixed-method studies focused on all adolescents (with a strong emphasis on those from marginalized backgrounds) in order to reach generalizable conclusions.

## 4 Recommendations

### 4.1 For Clinicians and Providers

- Professional organizations for preventive pediatric health care should standardize an evaluation of digital well-being as part of their wellness visits. This evaluation should cover areas like motivation for using social media (e.g., seeking support, finding a community), self-regulation of screen time, unhealthy social media interactions, prevention of online victimization, and coping skills for youth who have already experienced it. This should be offered to all youths.
- Clinicians that provide care to youths from marginalized backgrounds, those who identify as LGBTQ+, or who live with chronic health conditions should also prioritize preventive interventions (similar to recommendation 1) among their patients. The available evidence suggests that for these groups of adolescents,

social media is an important source for connecting with other youths living in similar situations and to seek support; therefore, recommending restrictive limitations on screens across the board may not be appropriate for all youths.

- For youths who have experienced in-person victimization, events of online victimization should be closely evaluated. These two forms of victimization often co-occur, and online victimization is proximally associated with an increase in suicidal thoughts and behaviors. Online aggressors should also be evaluated since both victimization and perpetration are associated with poor mental health outcomes. Even if no online victimization events are identified, preventive interventions should be included, with content similar to our recommendation 1.
- In all of the previous recommendations, parents/caregivers should receive similar educational interventions in order to appropriately support their child should the opportunity arrive.

## 4.2 For Policymakers

- Social media has the potential to promote positive youth development. Many adolescents turn to social media to make friends, build connections, find information, develop a sense of autonomy, seek support, or for entertainment. Social media companies must develop and implement tools that are developmentally appropriate to support this usage while providing a safe environment for adolescent users from all backgrounds. Policymakers can facilitate this process with regulations that incentivize social media companies to invest in developing these resources, specifically:

  - Require that companies adapt their privacy algorithms with the understanding that children under the age of 13 also use their platforms. This may take the form of suggesting features in order to protect their safety and reduce the potential for problematic scrolling.
  - Require companies to have their social media platforms evaluated by psychological experts to determine how to customize features and affordances to be more developmentally appropriate for young users.
  - Implement and enforce objective means for verifying the age of users and limiting the availability of certain features (e.g., connecting with adults without parental/caregiver consent) to youths below a certain age.

## 4.3 For Educators and Teachers

- Professional development for educators should include how social media is a relevant social context in normative adolescent development. Social media literacy aimed at mitigating mental health concerns in relation to social media, should be implemented in every classroom in the United States from a young age. To make this more feasible in schools, we recommend that this training could be tied to existing social and emotional learning, digital citizenship, or computer science programs in K–12th grade schools.
- Programs should be tailored to individual needs, recognizing that for some youths (especially those from marginalized backgrounds), social media might be one of few, if not the only way to be part of a community, connect with others with a similar experience, and seek support.

## 4.4 For Parents

- Talk to children about the complexities of social media, with an intent to help them become critical consumers of what they see online.
- Set limits and be highly involved when children get their first smartphone and join their first social media site. Rules and restrictions should decrease as children age and become

more confident and comfortable using social media. Parents should respect privacy and allow for autonomy where developmentally appropriate.

**Conflict of Interest and Funding Disclosures** CE-V is supported by a "Pathway to Independence Award," National Institute of Minority Health and Health Disparities [R00MD012813]. KDAW is supported by the Drexel FIRST (Faculty Institutional Recruitment for Sustainable Transformation) Program, National Institutes of Health [U54CA267735-02].

## References

1. Bitsko RH, Holbrook JR, Ghandour RM, et al. Epidemiology and impact of healthcare provider-diagnosed anxiety and depression among U.S. children. J Dev Behav Pediatr. 2018;39:395–403. https://doi.org/10.1097/DBP.0000000000000571.
2. American Foundation for Suicide Prevention. Suicide statistics. https://afsp.org/suicide-statistics/. Accessed Feb 2023.
3. The Trevor Project. National survey on LGBTQ+ mental health. https://www.thetrevorproject.org/survey-2022/. Accessed 7 Feb 2023.
4. Haidt J. Facebook's dangerous experiment on teenage girls. The Atlantic. Published November 21, 2021. https://www.theatlantic.com/ideas/archive/2021/11/facebooks-dangerous-experiment-teen-girls/620767/. Accessed 7 Feb 2023.
5. NPR. Encore: Seattle sues social media over youth mental health. Published January 16, 2023. https://www.npr.org/2023/01/16/1149423335/encore-seattle-sues-social-media-over-youth-mental-health. Accessed 7 Feb 2023.
6. Rosen AO, Holmes AL, Balluerka N, et al. Is social media a new type of social support? Social media use in Spain during the COVID-19 pandemic: A mixed methods study. Int J Environ Res Public Health. 2022;19(7):3952. https://doi.org/10.3390/ijerph19073952.
7. National Academies of Sciences, Engineering, and Medicine. Social media and adolescent health. Washington, DC: The National Academies Press; 2023. https://doi.org/10.17226/27396.
8. Burrow A, Hill P, Williams JL, Leve L, Dahl R, Fuligni A, Masten C, The National Scientific Council on Adolescence. Cultivating purpose in adolescence, Council Report No. 3 (2023). Retrieved from https://developingadolescent.org/
9. Twenge JM, Haidt J, Lozano J, Cummins KM. Specification curve analysis shows that social media use is linked to poor mental health, especially among girls. Acta Psychologica. 2022;224:103512. https://doi.org/10.1016/j.actpsy.2022.103512.
10. Primack BA, Shensa A, Sidani JE, Escobar-Viera CG, Fine MJ. Temporal associations between social media use and depression. Am J Prev Med. 2021;60(2):179–88. https://doi.org/10.1016/j.amepre.2020.09.014.
11. Coyne SM, Rogers AA, Zurcher JD, Stockdale L, Booth M. Does time spent using social media impact mental health?: An eight year longitudinal study. Comput Hum Behav. 2020;104:106160. https://doi.org/10.1016/j.chb.2019.106160.
12. Valkenburg PM, Meier A, Beyens I. Social media use and its impact on adolescent mental health: an umbrella review of the evidence. Curr Opin Psychol. 2022;44:58–68. https://doi.org/10.1016/j.copsyc.2021.08.017.
13. Valkenburg P, Beyens I, Pouwels JL, van Driel II, Keijsers L. Social media use and adolescents' self-esteem: heading for a person-specific media effects paradigm. J of Commun. 2021;71(1):56–78. https://doi.org/10.1093/joc/jqaa039.
14. Orben A, Przybylski AK, Blakemore SJ, Kievit RA. Windows of developmental sensitivity to social media. Nat Commun. 2022;13(1):1649. https://doi.org/10.1038/s41467-022-29296-3.
15. Huang C. A meta-analysis of the problematic social media use and mental health. Int J Soc Psychiatry. 2022;68(1):12–33. https://doi.org/10.1177/0020764020978434.
16. Shannon H, Bush K, Villeneuve PJ, Hellemans KGC, Guimond S. Problematic social media use in adolescents and young adults: systematic review and meta-analysis. JMIR Mental Health. 2022;9(4):1–12. https://doi.org/10.2196/33450.
17. Raudsepp L, Kais K. Longitudinal associations between problematic social media use and depressive symptoms in adolescent girls. Prev Med Rep. 2019;15:100925. https://doi.org/10.1016/j.pmedr.2019.100925.
18. Valkenburg PM. Social media use and well-being: What we know and what we need to know. Curr Opin Psychol. 2022;45:101294. https://doi.org/10.1016/j.copsyc.2021.12.006.
19. Weinstein E, James C. Behind their screens: what teens are facing (and adults are missing). MIT Press; 2022.
20. Primack BA, Bisbey MA, Shensa A, et al. The association between valence of social media experiences and depressive symptoms. Depress Anxiety. 2018;35(8):784–94. https://doi.org/10.1002/da.22779.
21. Skogen JC, Andersen AIO, Finserås TR, Ranganath P, Brunborg GS, Hjetland GJ. Commonly reported negative experiences on social media are associated with poor mental health and well-being among adolescents: results from the "LifeOnSoMe"-study. Front Public Health. 2023;2(11):1192788. https://doi.org/10.3389/fpubh.2023.1192788.

22. Williams KDA, Wijaya C, Stamatis CA, Abbott G, Lattie E. Insights into needs and preferences for mental health support on social media and through mobile apps among black male university students: exploratory qualitative study. JMIR Form Res. 2022;6(8):e38716. https://doi.org/10.2196/38716.
23. Sherman LE, Payton AA, Hernandez LM, Greenfield PM, Dapretto M. The power of the like in adolescence: effects of peer influence on neural and behavioral responses to social media. Psychol Sci. 2016;27(7):1027–35. https://doi.org/10.1177/0956797616645673.
24. Charmaraman L, Richer AM, Liu C, Doyle Lynch A, Moreno M. Early adolescent social media-related body dissatisfaction: associations with depressive symptoms, social anxiety, peers, and celebrities. J Dev Behav Pediatr. 2021;42(5):401–7. https://doi.org/10.1097/DBP.0000000000000911.
25. Shensa A, Sidani JE, Escobar-Viera CG, et al. Real-life closeness of social media contacts and depressive symptoms among university students. J Am Coll Health. 2018;66(8):747–53. https://doi.org/10.1080/07448481.2018.1440575.
26. Pellicane MJ, Cooks JA, Ciesla JA. Longitudinal effects of social media experiences on depression and anxiety in LGB+ and heterosexual young adults. J Gay Lesbian Mental Health. 2021;25(1):68–93. https://doi.org/10.1080/19359705.2020.1776805.
27. Charmaraman L, Zhang A, Wang K, Chen B. Sexual minorities and loneliness: exploring sexuality through social media and gender-sexuality alliance (GSA) supports. Int J Environ Res Public Health. 2024;21(3):300. https://doi.org/10.3390/ijerph21030300.
28. Shafi RMA, Nakonezny PA, Miller KA, et al. Altered markers of stress in depressed adolescents after acute social media use. J Psychiatr Res. 2021;136:149–56. https://doi.org/10.1016/j.jpsychires.2021.01.055.
29. Nesi J, Choukas-Bradley S, Prinstein MJ. Transformation of adolescent peer relations in the social media context: Part 1-A theoretical framework and application to dyadic peer relationships. Clin Child Fam Psychol Rev. 2018;21(3):267–94. https://doi.org/10.1007/s10567-018-0261-x.
30. Das Swain V, Chen V, Mishra S, Mattingly S, Abowd G, De Choudhury M. Semantic gap in predicting mental wellbeing through passive sensing. In: Proceedings of the 2022 CHI conference on human factors in computing systems, vol. 374; 2022. p. 1–16. https://doi.org/10.1145/3491102.3502037.
31. Marciano L, Schulz PJ, Camerini AL. Cyberbullying perpetration and victimization in youth: a meta-analysis of longitudinal studies. J Comput Mediat Comm. 2020;25(2):163–81. https://doi.org/10.1093/jcmc/zmz031.
32. Shensa A, Sidani JE, Escobar-Viera CG, Switzer GE, Primack BA, Choukas-Bradley S. Emotional support from social media and face-to-face relationships: associations with depression risk among young adults. J Affect Disord. 2020;260:38–44. https://doi.org/10.1016/j.jad.2019.08.092.
33. Escobar-Viera C, Shensa A, Hamm M, et al. "I don't feel like the odd one": utilizing content analysis to compare the effects of social media use on well-being among sexual minority and nonminority US young adults. Am J Health Promot. 2020;34(3):285–93. https://doi.org/10.1177/0890117119885517.
34. Hatzenbuehler ML. How does sexual minority stigma "get under the skin"? A psychological mediation framework. Psychol Bull. 2009;135(5):707–30. https://doi.org/10.1037/a0016441.
35. Fadda M, Sykora M, Elayan S, et al. Ethical issues of collecting, storing, and analyzing geo-referenced tweets for mental health research. Digit Health. 2022;8:20552076221092539. https://doi.org/10.1177/20552076221092539.

# Youth Anxiety in the Digital Age: Present Status and Future Considerations

Merlin Ariefdjohan, Jacqueline Nesi, Benjamin Mullin, Matthew Pesko, and Sandra Fritsch

## 1 Background

Anxiety disorders are the most common diagnosable psychiatric condition among youth, and it can progress in severity during childhood and adolescence [1]. The prevalence of youth anxiety has increased by approximately 29% from 2016 to 2019 (pre-pandemic years), a trend that has persisted in the years post-pandemic [2]. With an estimated 5.6 million children in the United States (US) affected by anxiety, anxiety disorders are more prevalent in childhood than asthma, attributing to a concerning public health trend [2, 3]. The American Academy of Pediatrics (AAP), the American Academy of Child and Adolescent Psychiatry (AACAP), and the Children's Hospital Association (CHA) voiced their concerns by declaring a national emergency in pediatric mental health in 2021, followed by the issuance of the US Surgeon General advisory titled "Protecting Youth Mental Health." [4, 5]

The increasing trend in mental health disorders among children and adolescents corresponds with the trajectory of screen media use in this population, igniting a public health debate regarding causality [6, 7]. Screens, such as smartphones, tablets, computers, and TVs, along with the Internet, social media, and virtual games, are now fully integrated into society as a means of information sharing, communication, education, telehealth, commerce, and social interactions. A recent study has shown that access to digital devices among youth is widespread, with 95% of teens having smartphones, 90% owning computers, and 80% having gaming consoles [8]. Nearly half of the participants in one study professed to be "almost constantly" online, and over half found it challenging to reduce screen time [8]. Screen media use has also increased by 3% for

The authors of this study would like to thank the editorial team of "Children & Screens" and Springer for coordinating this timely supplement and the invitation to submit an article.

M. Ariefdjohan
Department of Psychiatry, University of Colorado Anschutz Medical Campus, Aurora, CO, USA

J. Nesi
Department of Psychiatry and Human Behavior, Brown University, Providence, RI, USA

Bradley Hasbro Research Center, Rhode Island Hospital, Providence, RI, USA

B. Mullin · S. Fritsch (✉)
Department of Psychiatry, University of Colorado Anschutz Medical Campus, Aurora, CO, USA

Pediatric Mental Health Institute, Children's Hospital Colorado, Aurora, CO, USA
e-mail: Sandra.fritsch@childrenscolorado.org

M. Pesko
Department of Psychiatry, University of Colorado Anschutz Medical Campus, Aurora, CO, USA

Denver Health Medical Center, Denver, CO, USA


D. A. Christakis, L. Hale (eds.), *Handbook of Children and Screens*,
https://doi.org/10.1007/978-3-031-69362-5_18

tweens and by 11% for teens from 2015 to 2019, with a 17% rise from 2019 to 2021 [9]. Considerable attention has been devoted to investigating the influence of screen media use on the incidence of anxiety (as summarized in Glover et al. [10, 11]), yet current findings yield conflicting results. The recent Childhood to Adolescence Transition Study observed that teenage girls with high social media use as accessed through screens had significantly increased odds of anxiety symptoms (odds ratio (OR): 1.99; 95% confidence interval (95% CI): 1.32–3.00) than those with minimal use [12]. However, another study showed that acute reduction of social media screen time did not show any causal relationship with development of anxiety symptoms [13].

In consideration of this complex issue, this chapter aims to briefly review the current literature on the impacts (both adverse and beneficial) of screen media use on anxiety disorders among children and adolescents, to recommend strategies for managing screen media use to mitigate anxiety, and to suggest future research directions.

## 2 Current State

Several factors contribute to youth anxiety. Behavioral inhibition, characterized by a tendency to respond to novel experiences with fear and withdrawal, is identified as a temperamental risk factor for anxiety disorders in childhood [14]. Cognitive risk factors such as selective attention to potential threats (threat bias) and perceiving uncertain situations as threatening (intolerance of uncertainty) also play a role [15, 16]. Additionally, avoidance behaviors are consistently linked to the onset and persistence of anxiety disorders [17]. Recent research has suggested that neurobiological factors, including altered structural and functional connectivity in the emotion processing regions in the brain, can also contribute to anxiety risk (see review in Strawn et al. [18]). Overall, youths with a combination of these risk factors might be more emotionally vulnerable when exposed to unfiltered content on screen media affecting their mental well-being and potentially contributing to development of anxiety.

During adolescence, individuals navigate the development of their identity and social skills through managing relationships with their peers. Self-presentation (the process by which individuals selectively manage the image and identity they show to others) and self-disclosure (sharing their thoughts, feelings, and behaviors) are crucial processes during this period of exploration [19, 20]. Digital social platforms such as Instagram, TikTok, Facebook, and YouTube provide avenues for youths to actively engage in practicing and mastery of self-presentation and self-disclosure. A national survey of 1060 American teens that explored the nuances of friendship in the digital age noted that 83% of respondents indicated that social media made them feel more connected to their friends and that 68% endorsed reception of social support via digital technologies during challenging times [21]. These observations aligned with another study's key findings on the impact of screen-based social media use during the COVID-19 pandemic [22]. The authors emphasized that the social connections facilitated by screen use in this period positively influenced overall well-being and social sentiments [22].

Computer-mediated communication (CMC) offered by social media platforms allows text-based conversations, which bypass the vocal and visual cues of in-person interactions, as well as allows a delayed response. A cross-sectional study of Italian youths observed that socially anxious teens felt more comfortable interacting with their peers online via social media since it allowed them to pause and craft a response, rather than having direct face-to-face interactions that require an immediate response [23]. Excessive use of social media, however, can contribute to the fear of missing out (FOMO) syndrome among individuals, particularly youth. Constant exposure to idealized content and images on social media platforms such as Instagram and TikTok, which showcase peers engaging in fun activities or achieving milestones, can evoke feelings of exclusion, inadequacy, and loneliness [24, 25].

Prolonged immersion in CMC may also foster dependency on frequent validation (e.g., via "likes") and inhibit self-censorship while posting. Subsequently, tendencies of image-related self-comparison and perfectionism, and experiences of negative online interactions including cyberbullying, could elevate mental and emotional stress and exacerbate anxiety [10, 26–28]. Furthermore, a recent longitudinal study of teens in the United States has noted that daily social media use is linked to increased co-rumination, which, in turn, predicts a higher propensity for internalizing symptoms that could lead to anxiety [12].

A significant portion of ongoing research investigating the impact of screen media use on mental health is centered on examining the "displacement hypothesis." This theory suggests that the negative influence of screen media use is correlated with the duration of digital exposure that takes away time from non-screen activities [29]. Numerous studies indicate that excessive screen media use leads to lifestyle changes, including reduction in physical activity, decreased exposure to sunlight and the outside environment, increased in unhealthy snacking behaviors, and poor sleep quality [30–33]. The adoption of a combination of these lifestyle factors in favor of screen media use could subsequently pose an adverse impact on mental well-being, including the development or exacerbation of anxiety.

An alternative theory termed "the Goldilocks hypothesis," posits that, like Goldilocks determining the level of "just right" for porridge and mattress, there exists an optimum moderate level for screen media use that minimizes harm [34]. Essentially, in our digitally connected world, youths may lose out on valuable information and meaningful social interactions if they spend too little time on screens, but too much screen media use supplants important daily activities and causes adverse impacts [34]. Nonetheless, there remains a lack of consensus regarding the definition of "excessive" screen time. More studies are needed to further test this hypothesis, and it remains premature at this time to set guidelines for "moderate" use.

While our understanding of youth anxiety and screen media use has advanced, there are still limitations in the available evidence. Recent studies frequently depend on self-report measures that are prone to recall bias, utilize small samples that may not reflect the broader population, lack a prospective study design, and fail to account for pertinent covariates in their analyses [7, 31, 33, 35]. Furthermore, published studies often group anxiety with other proxies of mental health (e.g., depression, suicidality, loneliness, etc.) rather than as a standalone variable. Understanding the impact of screen media use on anxiety symptoms is multifaceted and requires examining *how* adolescents engage with screens, determining the type of screen activity (passive vs. active), and closely examining the specific features of commonly used screen media platforms. Furthermore, individual mental health status (e.g., preexisting anxiety or other mood disorders) may influence the extent to which screen media use could lead to adverse or beneficial effects [31, 36].

Resources and guidelines for monitoring screen media use are summarized in Table 1. Some are highlighted below with descriptions of potential clinical applications.

## 3 Future Research

Elucidating the relationship between screen media use and anxiety is an evolving area of study. Although the current body of work thus far has provided a good foundation, more research is needed. Here are several avenues that could be explored in future research:

- When and how do screen media serve as a useful and helpful tool for youths with anxiety disorders, and when do they cause, maintain, or exacerbate the symptoms? Studies have often failed to differentiate between specific activities in which the youth engage via screen media (e.g., streaming, social media, gaming). Focusing primarily on the overall "screen time" has limited our ability to disentangle

**Table 1** Resources for families, providers, and other stakeholders

| Resource | Link to resource | Potential use |
|---|---|---|
| Facts for Families Guide by the American Academy of Child & Adolescent Psychiatry (AACAP) | https://www.aacap.org/AACAP/Families_Youth/Facts-for-Families/ | Downloadable materials to guide families in matters related to youth anxiety and digital media use, including documents titled "Anxiety and Children," "Internet Use in Children," "Screen Time and Children," "Social Media and Teens," and "Video Games and Children: Playing with Violence" |
| HealthyChildren.org website by the American Academy of Pediatrics (AAP) | https://www.healthychildren.org/English/family-life/Media/ AND https://www.healthychildren.org/English/fmp/Pages/MediaPlan.aspx | Practical guidelines and support for families around youth digital media use, including the ability to create a customizable Family Media Plan |
| Age-Based Media Reviews for Families by Common Sense Media | https://www.commonsensemedia.org/ | Parent- and educator-focused youth digital media guide with age-based ratings of the appropriateness of games, apps, and YouTube channels |
| Youth Mental Health and Digital Media Priorities by the US Surgeon General's Office | https://www.hhs.gov/surgeongeneral/priorities/youth-mental-health/index.html | Advisory document and action items for youth mental health with significant sections on youth anxiety and social media and video game companies' responsibilities |
| Teens and Tech research compilation by the Winston National Center on Technology Use, Brain, and Psychological Development | https://www.teensandtech.org/ | Adolescent, researcher, and clinician guides for a more detailed research analysis on brain development as related to digital media use |

helpful versus harmful uses of digital technology for youths with anxiety.

- For which youths do screen media maintain or exacerbate anxiety disorders, and whom do they help? Evaluating individual differences, including by demographic factors (i.e., age, gender, race/ethnicity, culture) and individual characteristics (i.e., personality, preexisting psychiatric diagnoses), will be essential for a nuanced understanding of the relationship between media use and anxiety.
- Does the impact of screen media on youth anxiety differ depending on the severity of the symptoms, and, if so, how? Most studies in this area have been conducted with community samples of adolescents, which limit the generalizability of the key findings. More research is needed among clinical samples of youth to understand the impact of screen media use on those with more severe symptoms.
- How can clinicians, parents, and educators best support the youth in using technology in ways that prevent and alleviate anxiety disorders? Research into clinical and societal interventions that mitigate the harmful effects of screen media use is needed.
- How do secondary effects of excessive screen time on sleep, diet, and physical activity contribute to the development or worsening of youth anxiety? The current literature has mostly focused on the length of time spent using screens, but more work is needed to examine the potential mediators of these effects, such as displacement of sleep and exercise.

More importantly, future studies should broaden the investigation to explore the hypothesis that the relationship between screen media use and mental health, including anxiety, is nonlinear and multifactorial. Additionally, research should delve into the impacts of screen media use on brain health and consider the potential differential effects based on age and gender. This expanded approach will provide a more comprehensive understanding of the complex interplay between screen media use and mental well-being as well as informing tailored interventions and support strategies.

# 4 Recommendations

## 4.1 For Primary Care Providers

- Given the widespread use of screens and mental health concerns among today's youth, primary care providers should include discussing screen habits with patients and their parents during routine well-child visits. Simple questions such as "How do you think your screen media use impacts your day-to-day life?" or "What are some of the things you like and dislike about using screens?" may facilitate the conversation.

  - Standardized screening tools such as the Problematic and Risky Internet Use Screening Scale (PRIUSS) or the Adolescents' Digital Technology Interactions and Importance (ADTI) Scale can be helpful in understanding these behaviors [37, 38].
  - Daytime sleepiness can be considered a red flag for further screening since this behavior is consistently detected among youths with- or at-risk of excessive screen media use [32].
  - Relevant resources can be offered to address the concerns attributed to screen media habits. These resources may include techniques to promote healthy sleep habits, recommendations for activities that foster a balanced lifestyle such as participating in physical exercises, and other suggestions to manage screen media use (Table 1).

## 4.2 For Mental Health Providers

- Similar to the role of primary care providers outlined above, mental health providers can also support healthy screen media use habits. In this way, mental health providers could examine pre-existing mental health diagnoses, the types and frequency of online activities, the distinction between active versus passive screen time, the emotional impact of these activities, the balance between online activities and other important non-virtual activities, sleep patterns and routines, and the presence of positive or negative thoughts or coping skills associated with online activities [10].

– As an example, in one author's (BM) intensive outpatient program (IOP) for anxious adolescents, many of the patients habitually engage with screens in ways that appear to either maintain or exacerbate their anxiety. These include perseverating on negative self-comparisons while using social media apps, experiencing FOMO when viewing evidence of peer get-togethers via social media, or interacting with phones while in social settings to avoid direct interpersonal interactions (aka "phubbing"). In response, the program developed and implemented a treatment module that encouraged patients to explore the connection between their screen habits and levels of anxiety and then commit to a specific change for the duration of the program. Patients were asked to check their smartphone's internal record of daily and weekly screen time and report on emerging usage patterns. Examples of pertinent questions include: "Are you using your smartphone more than you thought?"; "When do you most frequently use your smartphone?"; "What apps do you spend the most time on?"; "Does your smartphone ever help you connect to people you would not have otherwise felt comfortable interacting with?"; "Do you often use your smartphone to avoid situations that make you feel anxious?". Rather than directly advising patients to reduce their screen time and smartphone usage, interventions rooted in acceptance and commitment therapy (ACT) were implemented in the program to help patients acknowledge their personal values, identify disparities between these values and their actions, and provide strategies promoting behaviors that better align with their values [39].

## 4.3 For Parents, Caregivers, and Families

- Parents, caregivers, and families play a vital role in monitoring youth screen media use and encouraging healthy habits.
- A caregiver of a youth with anxiety may consider whether their child's screen media use is detracting from or substituting for important activities (e.g., in-person socialization, exercise, sleep).
- A grassroots organization (https://www.waituntil8th.org/) encourages parents to wait until their children reach the eighth grade before giving them access to a smartphone to delay their exposure to screen media use, although this recommendation has not been backed by science.
- Recognizing the significant influence of caregivers and families, the AAP has recently released guidelines advising families to establish a structured approach to media use [40]. This includes setting clear boundaries such as limiting media access in teenagers' bedrooms at night and during study time, involving adolescents in selecting and viewing media content, and maintaining regular discussions on digital citizenship and online safety [40]. To assist with this process, the AAP has developed an interactive online tool called the Family Media Plan (Table 1), which parents and caregivers can utilize to create and implement these guidelines together with their children.

**Conflict of Interest and Funding Disclosures** JN is supported in part by Grant 5K23MH122669 from the National Institute of Mental Health (NIMH).

## References

1. Kessler RC, Ruscio AM, Shear K, Wittchen HU. Epidemiology of anxiety disorders. Curr Top Behav Neurosci. 2010;2:21–35.
2. Lebrun-Harris LA, Ghandour RM, Kogan MD, Warren MD. Five-year trends in US children's health and well-being, 2016–2020. JAMA Pediatr. 2022;176(7):e220056.
3. Bozzola E, Spina G, Agostiniani R, Barni S, Russo R, Scarpato E, et al. The use of social media in children

and adolescents: scoping review on the potential risks. Int J Environ Res Public Health. 2022;19(16)

4. Office of the U S. Surgeon General. Protecting youth mental health: The U.S. Surgeon General's Advisory. Washington (DC): US Department of Health and Human Services; 2021.
5. AAP, AACAP, CHA Declare National Emergency in Children's Mental Health [press release]. October 19, 2021.
6. Bell V, Bishop DVM, Przybylski AK. The debate over digital technology and young people. BMJ. 2015;351:h3064.
7. Odgers CL, Jensen MR. Annual research review: adolescent mental health in the digital age: facts, fears, and future directions. J Child Psychol Psychiatry Allied Discipl. 2020;61(3):336–48.
8. Vogels EA, Risa Gelles-Watnick R, Teens MN. Social media and technology 2022. Pew Research Center; 2022.
9. Rideout V, Peebles A, Mann S, Robb MB. Common sense census: media use by Tweens and Teens, 2021. San Francisco; 2022.
10. Glover J, Ariefdjohan M, Fritsch SL. #Kidsanxiety and the digital world. Child Adolesc Psychiatr Clin N Am. 2022;31(1):71–90.
11. Glover J, Fritsch SL. #Kidsanxiety and social media: a review. Child Adolesc Psychiatr Clin N Am. 2018;27(2):171–82.
12. Ohannessian CM, Fagle T, Salafia C. Social media use and internalizing symptoms during early adolescence: the role of co-rumination. J Affect Disord. 2021;280(Pt A):85–8.
13. Mahalingham T, Howell J, Clarke PJF. Assessing the effects of acute reductions in mobile device social media use on anxiety and sleep. J Behav Ther Exp Psychiatry. 2023;78:101791.
14. Beesdo K, Pine DS, Lieb R, Wittchen HU. Incidence and risk patterns of anxiety and depressive disorders and categorization of generalized anxiety disorder. Arch Gen Psychiatry. 2010;67(1):47–57.
15. Shihata S, McEvoy PM, Mullan BA, Carleton RN. Intolerance of uncertainty in emotional disorders: what uncertainties remain? J Anxiety Disord. 2016;41:115–24.
16. Waters AM, Craske MG, Bergman RL, Treanor M. Threat interpretation bias as a vulnerability factor in childhood anxiety disorders. Behav Res Ther. 2008;46(1):39–47.
17. Rapee RM. The development and modification of temperamental risk for anxiety disorders: prevention of a lifetime of anxiety? Biol Psychiatry. 2002;52(10):947–57.
18. Strawn JR, Lu L, Peris TS, Levine A, Walkup JT. Research review: pediatric anxiety disorders – what have we learnt in the last 10 years? J Child Psychol Psychiatry Allied Discipl. 2021;62(2):114–39.
19. Selkie E, Adkins V, Masters E, Bajpai A, Shumer D. Transgender adolescents' uses of social media for social support. J Adolesc Health. 2020;66(3):275–80.
20. Wood MA, Bukowski WM, Lis E. The digital self: how social media serves as a setting that shapes youth's emotional experiences. Adolesc Res Rev. 2015;1(2):163–73.
21. Lenhart A, Smith A, Anderson M, Duggan M, Teens PA. Technology and friendship. 2015; Contract No.: August
22. Midgley C, Lockwood P, Thai S. Can the social network bridge social distancing? Social media use during the covid-19 pandemic. Psychol Popular Media. 2024;13(1):44–54.
23. Angelini F, Gini G. Differences in perceived online communication and disclosing e-motions among adolescents and young adults: the role of specific social media features and social anxiety. J Adolesc. 2023:1.
24. Franchina V, Vanden Abeele M, van Rooij AJ, Lo Coco G, De Marez L. Fear of missing out as a predictor of problematic social media use and phubbing behavior among flemish adolescents. Int J Environ Res Public Health. 2018;15(10):1.
25. Papapanou TK, Darviri C, Kanaka-Gantenbein C, Tigani X, Michou M, Vlachakis D, et al. Strong correlations between social appearance anxiety, use of social media, and feelings of loneliness in adolescents and young adults. Int J Environ Res Public Health. 2023;20(5):1.
26. Charmaraman L, Richer AM, Liu C, Lynch AD, Moreno MA. Early adolescent social media-related body dissatisfaction: associations with depressive symptoms, social anxiety, peers, and celebrities. J Dev Behav Pediatr. 2021:1.
27. Hilty DM, Stubbe D, McKean AJ, Hoffman PE, Zalpuri I, Myint MT, et al. A scoping review of social media in child, adolescents and young adults: research findings in depression, anxiety and other clinical challenges. BJPsych Open. 2023;9(5):e152.
28. Molero MM, Martos Á, Barragán AB, Pérez-Fuentes MC, Gázquez JJ. Anxiety and depression from cybervictimization in adolescents: a metaanalysis and meta-regression study. Eur J Psychol Appl Legal Context. 2022;14(1):42–50.
29. Neuman SB. The displacement effect: assessing the relation between television viewing and reading performance. Read Res Q. 1988;23:414–40.
30. Taheri E, Heshmat R, Esmaeil Motlagh M, Ardalan G, Asayesh H, Qorbani M, et al. Association of physical activity and screen time with psychiatric distress in children and adolescents: Caspian-IV Study. J Trop Pediatr. 2019;65(4):361–72.
31. Tang S, Werner-Seidler A, Torok M, Mackinnon AJ, Christensen H. The relationship between screen time and mental health in young people: a systematic review of longitudinal studies. Clin Psychol Rev. 2021;86:102021.
32. Twenge JM, Hisler GC, Krizan Z. Associations between screen time and sleep duration are primarily driven by portable electronic devices: evidence from a population-based study of U.S. children ages 0–17. Sleep Med. 2019;56:211–8.

33. Zink J, Belcher BR, Imm K, Leventhal AM. The relationship between screen-based sedentary behaviors and symptoms of depression and anxiety in youth: a systematic review of moderating variables. BMC Public Health. 2020;20(1):472.
34. Przybylski AK, Weinstein N. A large-scale test of the goldilocks hypothesis: quantifying the relations between digital-screen use and the mental well-being of adolescents. Psychol Sci. 2017;28(2):204–15.
35. Shannon H, Bush K, Villeneuve PJ, Hellemans KGC, Guimond S. Problematic social media use in adolescents and young adults: systematic review and meta-analysis. JMIR Ment Health. 2022;9(4):e33450.
36. Kim S, Favotto L, Halladay J, Wang L, Boyle MH, Georgiades K. Differential associations between passive and active forms of screen time and adolescent mood and anxiety disorders. Soc Psychiatry Psychiatr Epidemiol. 2020;55(11):1469–78.
37. Jelenchick LA, Eickhoff J, Christakis DA, Brown RL, Zhang C, Benson M, et al. The Problematic and Risky Internet Use Screening Scale (PRIUSS) for adolescents and young adults: scale development and refinement. Comput Hum Behav. 2014;35
38. Moreno MA, Binger K, Zhao Q, Eickhoff J. Measuring interests not minutes: development and validation of the adolescents' digital technology interactions and importance scale (Adti). J Med Internet Res. 2020;22(2):e16736.
39. Coyne LW, McHugh L, Martinez ER. Acceptance and Commitment Therapy (Act): advances and applications with children, adolescents, and families. Child Adolesc Psychiatr Clin N Am. 2011;20(2):379–99.
40. Council on Communications and Media. Media use in school-aged children and adolescents. Pediatrics. 2016;138(5):1. https://doi.org/10.1542/peds.2016-2592.

# Social Media and Depressive Symptoms

Jean M. Twenge, Dale Peeples, Reem M. A. Shafi, Elroy Boers, Lauren Hale, and Paul Weigle

## 1 Background

Depression among children and adolescents is linked to a variety of short- and long-term negative outcomes, including an elevated risk of suicidal thoughts and behaviors as well as self-harm, an increased chance of depression in adulthood, lower educational attainment, and unemployment [1–3]. Many causes of depression are difficult or impossible to alter, including genetic predisposition, abuse, poverty, and discrimination. It is thus imperative to identify the possible causes of depression and depressive symptoms that are controllable, including how children and adolescents spend their time. In the last decade, one of the primary ways that youth spend their time is on screens, in particular social media. In 2023, Gallup reported that the average US teen spent 5 h a day on social media when video platforms such as YouTube and TikTok were included in the total along with platforms such as Instagram and Snapchat [4].

## 2 Current State

For decades, studies have documented associations between spending more time with screen media and higher rates of depression among children and adolescents [5, 6]. More recent studies using large samples have confirmed that heavy users of screen media are considerably more likely to suffer from symptoms of depression [7–10]. These links to depressive symptoms are often larger for time spent online and on social media and are smaller for gaming and TV time [11]. A recent meta-analysis found that the risk of depression is 13% higher with each hour of daily social media use [12]. These associations are often more pronounced among younger than older adolescents and more pronounced among girls than boys [13, 14].

Smartphones became widely used and social media nearly ubiquitous among teens in the early 2010s, coinciding with a sudden and pronounced rise in depression, self-harm, and suicide attempts in this population and a sudden decline in in-person social interactions [15–18]. Although this simultaneous rise cannot prove causation, the abrupt rise in adolescent loneliness around the world after 2012 seems difficult to explain via

J. M. Twenge (✉)
San Diego University, San Diego, CA, USA

D. Peeples
Augusta University, Augusta, GA, USA

R. M. A. Shafi
Mayo Clinic, Rochester, MN, USA

E. Boers
University of Montreal, Montreal, QC, Canada

L. Hale
Stony Brook University, Stony Brook, NY, USA

P. Weigle
University of Connecticut, Farmington, CT, USA


D. A. Christakis, L. Hale (eds.), *Handbook of Children and Screens*,
https://doi.org/10.1007/978-3-031-69362-5_19

another mechanism. Similarly, mental health problems among college students increased following the introduction of Facebook to their campuses, and mental health hospital admissions among adolescent girls rose in tandem with the rollout of high-speed Internet across regions of Spain [19]. These studies suggest that the impact of social media operates at both the group and individual levels, as social media changes social interactions among group members regardless of individual use.

Experimental evidence points to a causal role of social media use in depression. Adults who deactivated Facebook reported improved well-being [20]. College students who minimized social media use for a 3-week period became less depressed and less lonely than did those who continued their normal use [21].

Several theories may explain why social media time is linked to depression. First, social media time may displace time that could be spent on activities more beneficial to mental health such as in-person social interactions, especially at the group level as the norm for social interactions among young people moves away from in-person gatherings [22]. Second, social media use can exacerbate social comparison, appearance dissatisfaction, and body image issues, which, in turn, may lead to depressive symptoms [23]. Third, social media incurs the risk of cyberbullying, which is strongly linked to depressive symptoms [24]. Fourth, social media can exacerbate existing negative thinking as users seek out consistent content, which reinforces their emotions and cognitions, creating downward spirals popularly known as "rabbit holes." [7] Fifth, screen time in general and social media in particular can interfere with sleep. Multiple systematic literature reviews and meta-analyses have consistently shown that screen media use is associated with later bedtimes, shorter sleep duration, and poor-quality sleep, though effect sizes vary [25–27]. Light emitted from screens has an alerting effect on the brain, suppressing melatonin and making it harder to fall asleep [28]. Impaired sleep interferes with functioning and is associated with depressive symptoms, including among children and adolescents [29, 30].

## 3 Future Research

The most pressing research questions worthy of future research in this area include:

- *What is the causal link between social media time and depression among children and adolescents?* Most of the studies linking social media time to depression in youths are correlational, making causality difficult to infer. Although studies including young adults have provided some evidence that social media time causes depression, experimental studies on children and adolescents are scant. Future random assignment experimental studies should be conducted on children and adolescents. These should include examination of heavy social media users, as most previous studies have examined average users. Experiments involving groups—such as an entire school giving up social media—would be challenging to conduct but highly informative in discerning mechanisms operating at the group level.
- *Which types of screen time are most likely to cause depression?* More studies should examine the differences in the size of associations between screen time and depression based on the specific type of screen use (such as social media compared to gaming).
- *Which social media platforms and types of social media uses are most likely to lead to depression?* For example, is the use of Instagram, Snapchat, or TikTok most strongly linked to depression? Is there a difference between scrolling through social media and actively posting? Is there a difference between using social media primarily to see content from real-life friends or using it to see content from those who are otherwise strangers?
- *What interventions will minimize the effects of social media use on depressive symptoms in a sustainable manner?* How can social media be made healthier for children and teens? What changes to social media platforms will encourage more moderate use? How can parents help mitigate any negative effects of social media on their children?

- *Which populations are most at risk of experiencing the mental health effects of social media use?* Future research should examine moderators besides gender and age, including race, ethnicity, socioeconomic status, and LGBT identity.

## 4 Recommendations

Given the consistent links between social media use and depression and evidence of causality, actions to restrict social media use by children and adolescents should be considered.

- *Policymakers* should consider raising the minimum age for social media use to 16, a proposal with bipartisan support in the United States [31]. Age minimums for social media also need to be consistently enforced using effective age verification.
- *Parents* should take steps to ensure children aged 12 and under do not use social media (the minimum age for these platforms is currently set at 13) and might consider disallowing the platforms for those aged 13–15 given the stronger links to depression found for this age group.
- *Clinicians* should consider incorporating digital/social media habits and experiences within a psychiatric history as part of an initial assessment [32]. They should discuss healthy screen use and its parameters with patients and their parents (e.g., how sleep problems may result from screen time before bed). Providers can also share resources such as the American Academy of Pediatrics Family Media Plan and the American Academy of Child and Adolescent Psychiatry's Facts for Families.
- *Educators and leaders of extracurricular activities* (e.g., coaches) could eliminate any official use of social media platforms for communication with participants and their parents, as these uses then require that young participants have social media accounts even if they are not otherwise interested.
- *Parents* should restrict youths' use of devices in bedrooms at night and consider restricting use in the hour before bedtime.
- Face-to-face social interactions should be prioritized over online interactions given the latter's superiority for both mental health and developing social skills [33].
- *Parents* should strive to model behavior for their children by limiting their own use of screens in social situations and overnight.

Although technology is here to stay, benefits for mental health may accrue if families can be given tools to help manage screen time among children and adolescents.

**Conflict of Interest and Funding Disclosures** J.M.T. earns royalties from books, receives honoraria for speaking engagements, and has consulted and served as an expert witness for law firms on the topic of social media and mental health. She also writes Generation Tech, a psychology newsletter for which she receives subscription and sponsor payments.

## References

1. Fergusson DM, Woodward LJ. Mental health, educational, and social role outcomes of adolescents with depression. Arch Gen Psychiatry. 2002;59(3):225–31.
2. Fletcher JM. Adolescent depression and educational attainment: results using sibling fixed effects. Health Econ. 2010;19(7):855–71.
3. Mojtabai R, Stuart EA, Hwang I, et al. Long-term effects of mental disorders on employment in the National Comorbidity Survey ten-year follow-up. Soc Psychiatry Psychiatr Epidemiol. 2015;50(11):1657–68.
4. Rothwell J. Teens spend an average of 4.8 hours on social media per day. Gallup.
5. Messias E, Castro J, Saini A, Usman M, Peeples D. Sadness, suicide, and their association with video game and internet overuse among teens: results from the youth risk behavior survey 2007 and 2009. Suicide Life Threat Behav. 2011;41(3):307–15.
6. Primack BA, Swanier B, Georgiopoulos AM, Land SR, Fine MJ. Association between media use in adolescence and depression in young adulthood: a longitudinal study. Arch Gen Psychiatry. 2009;66(2):181–8.
7. Boers E, Afzali MH, Newton N, Conrod P. Association of screen time and depression in adolescence. JAMA Pediatr. 2019;173(9):853–9.
8. Kelly Y, Zilanawala A, Booker C, Sacker A. Social media use and adolescent mental health: findings from the UK millennium cohort study. EClinicalMedicine. 2018;6:59–68.
9. Li X, Buxton OM, Lee S, Chang AM, Berger LM, Hale L. Sleep mediates the association between ado-

lescent screen time and depressive symptoms. Sleep Med. 2019;57:51–60.
10. Neophytou E, Manwell LA, Eikelboom R. Effects of excessive screen time on neurodevelopment, learning, memory, mental health, and neurodegeneration: a scoping review. Int J Ment Heal Addict. 2021;19:724–44.
11. Twenge JM, Farley E. Not all screen time is created equal: associations with mental health vary by activity and gender. Soc Psychiatry Psychiatr Epidemiol. 2021;56(2):207–17.
12. Liu M, Kamper-DeMarco KE, Zhang J, Xiao J, Dong D, Xue P. Time spent on social media and risk of depression in adolescents: a dose–response meta-analysis. Int J Environ Res Public Health. 2022:19.
13. Orben A, Przybylski AK, Blakemore SJ, Kievit RA. Windows of developmental sensitivity to social media. Nat Commun. 2022;13(1):1649.
14. Twenge JM, Martin GN. Gender differences in associations between digital media use and psychological well-being: evidence from three large datasets. J Adolesc. 2020;79:91–102.
15. Mercado MC, Holland K, Leemis RW, Stone DM, Wang J. Trends in emergency department visits for nonfatal self-inflicted injuries among youth aged 10 to 24 years in the United States, 2001–2015. JAMA. 2017;318(19):1931–3.
16. Mojtabai R, Olfson M, Han B. National trends in the prevalence and treatment of depression in adolescents and young adults. Pediatrics. 2016;138(6):1.
17. Plemmons G, Hall M, Doupnik S, et al. Hospitalization for suicide ideation or attempt: 2008–2015. Pediatrics. 2018;141(6):1.
18. Twenge JM, Cooper AB, Joiner TE, Duffy ME, Binau SG. Age, period, and cohort trends in mood disorder indicators and suicide-related outcomes in a nationally representative dataset, 2005–2017. J Abnorm Psychol. 2019;128(3):185–99.
19. Braghieri L, Levy R, Makarin. Social media and mental health. Am Econ Rev. 2022;112:3660–93.
20. Allcott H, Braghieri L, Eichmeyter S, Gentzkow M. The welfare effects of social media. Am Econ Rev. 2020;110:629–76.
21. Hunt MG, Marx R, Lipson C, Young J. No more FOMO: limiting social media decreases loneliness and depression. J Soc Clin Psychol. 2018;37:751–68.
22. Stiglic N, Viner RM. Effects of screentime on the health and well-being of children and adolescents: a systematic review of reviews. BMJ Open. 2019;9(1):e023191.
23. Popat A, Tarrant C. Exploring adolescents' perspectives on social media and mental health and well-being – a qualitative literature review. Clin Child Psychol Psychiatry. 2023;28(1):323–37.
24. Hu Y, Bai Y, Pan Y, Li S. Cyberbullying victimization and depression among adolescents: a meta-analysis. Psychiatry Res. 2021;305:114198.
25. Alonzo R, Hussain J, Stranges S, Anderson KK. Interplay between social media use, sleep quality, and mental health in youth: a systematic review. Sleep Med Rev. 2021;56:101414.
26. Brautsch LA, Lund L, Andersen MM, Jennum PJ, Folker AP, Andersen S. Digital media use and sleep in late adolescence and young adulthood: a systematic review. Sleep Med Rev. 2023;68:101742.
27. Hale L, Guan S. Screen time and sleep among school-aged children and adolescents: a systematic literature review. Sleep Med Rev. 2015;21:50–8.
28. Chang AM, Aeschbach D, Duffy JF, Czeisler CA. Evening use of light-emitting eReaders negatively affects sleep, circadian timing, and next-morning alertness. Proc Natl Acad Sci USA. 2015;112(4):1232–7.
29. LeBourgeois MK, Hale L, Chang AM, Akacem LD, Montgomery-Downs HE, Buxton OM. Digital media and sleep in childhood and adolescence. Pediatrics. 2017;140(Suppl 2):S92–s96.
30. Lovato N, Gradisar M. A meta-analysis and model of the relationship between sleep and depression in adolescents: recommendations for future research and clinical practice. Sleep Med Rev. 2014;18(6):521–9.
31. Lima C. A new bill would ban anyone under 16 from using social media. Washington Post. 2023.
32. Carson NJ, Gansner M, Khang J. Assessment of digital media use in the adolescent psychiatric evaluation. Child Adolesc Psychiatr Clin N Am. 2018;27(2):133–43.
33. Twenge JM, Martin GN, Campbell WK. Decreases in psychological well-being among American adolescents after 2012 and links to screen time during the rise of smartphone technology. Emotion. 2018;18:765–80.

# Media Influences on Self-Harm, Suicidality, and Suicide

Kaylee P. Kruzan, Jacqueline Nesi, Jessica L. Hamilton, Carol Vidal, Jean M. Twenge, Dale Peeples, and Thomas Niederkrotenthaler

## 1 Background

Decades of empirical work demonstrate the influence of media on suicidal and self-injurious thoughts and behaviors (SSITBs).[1] At the population level, some media reports of suicide have been associated with subsequent increases in suicidal behaviors [1, 2], but, media coverage of, and the effects on, SSITBs are not uniform. Moreover, media platforms can offer unprecedented opportunities to extend the reach of prevention efforts [3, 4] and be a source of support and psychoeducation for young people with SSITBs [5]. Effective strategies to reduce the harm of media outlets, while building upon their benefits, are critical for prevention. Such efforts are especially salient given the sharp rise in media engagement, self-harm, suicidal ideation, and suicide among adolescents in the last decade [6, 7]. This chapter summarizes what we currently know about media and SSITBs, identifies limitations, and provides recommendations for future research, youths, families, and other stakeholders.

## 2 Current State

Media platforms and the interactions afforded between media and audiences have shifted and diversified substantially in the past decades. While earlier media formats (e.g., print, radio, television) were largely unidirectional, with platforms broadcasting messages to an audience, more recent media consist of bidirectional and mixed formats. These media allow for dynamic, synchronous, or asynchronous interactions between platforms and audiences and among audience members. Mirroring this high degree of variation, evidence on the effects of media on SSITBs also differs across platforms and circumstances. In this summary chapter, we review current evidence on SSITBs and three dominant forms of media: (1) entertainment/news or mass media coverage, (2) social media use, and (3) video games.

[1] Self-injurious thoughts and behaviors (SSITBs) describe thoughts and behaviors with (e.g., suicidal ideation, suicide plans, gestures, and behaviors) and without (e.g., NSSI) suicidal intent (Miller & Prinstein, 2019).

K. P. Kruzan (✉)
Northwestern University, Chicago, IL, USA
e-mail: kaylee.kruzan@northwestern.edu

J. Nesi
Brown University, Providence, RI, USA

J. L. Hamilton
Rutgers University, New Brunswick, NJ, USA

C. Vidal
Johns Hopkins University, Baltimore, MD, USA

J. M. Twenge
San Diego State University, San Diego, CA, USA

D. Peeples
Medical College of Georgia, Augusta, GA, USA

T. Niederkrotenthaler
Medical University of Vienna, Vienna, Austria


D. A. Christakis, L. Hale (eds.), *Handbook of Children and Screens*,
https://doi.org/10.1007/978-3-031-69362-5_20

### 2.1 Mass Media Coverage and SSITBs

The impact of mass media coverage of suicide on subsequent suicides has been studied extensively, dating back to the 1970s when the concept of the Werther effect was first introduced [8]. The Werther effect—an increase in suicides following media reports of suicide stories—is understood to be a form of social contagion whereby individuals imitate suicide-specific behaviors in reports. However, since the original publication of the Werther effect [8], studies have revealed more nuanced results. Evidence is strongest for the association between suicide rates and media coverage of celebrity suicides [9]. Historically, evidence for the effects of fictional suicide narratives on subsequent suicides has been less conclusive (aka the Werther effect) [10, 11], yet recent studies following the release of "13 Reasons Why"—a Netflix series narrated by a fictional protagonist who dies by suicide—have revealed related increases in youth suicide in both the United States and Canada at the population level [12, 13]. The show's release was also associated with a subsequent rise of emergency department visits for suicide attempts and self-harm [14].

Both the type and amount of media coverage of suicide narratives moderate suicide risk. Research has shown that sensationalized stories or stories that describe a particular method [9] are also associated with an increased risk of suicidal behaviors, particularly copycat behaviors in which youths use the same method as the narrative's subject. Extensive coverage is strongly associated with imitative suicidal behaviors [15].

In addition to the characteristics of media narratives and coverage, factors related to the individual audience members contribute to risk. Youths, especially those with preexisting mental health conditions, are particularly susceptible to media stories of suicide, potentially suffering greater harms [16]. Media effects may be amplified during adolescence since this developmental period is characterized by strong social orientation, heightened emotional sensitivity, risk-taking propensity, and a focus on forming one's identity. Research has shown that the risk is higher when the young media consumer perceives themselves to be similar to [17], or feels a sense of positive regard for, the individual described in the narrative [18].

Recent studies have shown that mass media can also play a protective role in promoting hopeful narratives or narratives of how people have managed and overcome SSITBs (aka the Papageno effect). In a meta-analysis of media narratives of hope and recovery from suicidal crises, six studies found a small reduction in suicidal ideation following exposure to hopeful messages [19]. For example, there was an increase in crisis line calls and a decrease in suicides in the month following the release of a song by the popular rap artist Logic, titled "1-800-273-8255," which is the number for the US suicide crisis line [20].

Based on the current evidence, media guidelines for safe reporting on suicide and self-harm have been developed [21–24]. Summarily, media outlets should provide information on where and how to seek help, educate public on facts, and report stories on how to cope. Conversely, media outlets should not oversimplify the reasons for suicide, provide details about the suicide (e.g., methods, location), use sensational language or photographs, or repeat or prominently feature suicide stories.

### 2.2 Social Media Use and SSITB Content

The recent rise in both social media use and rates of suicide-related behaviors among US adolescents has raised concerns about the effects of social media use on youth SSITBs [25]. While social media share qualities with traditional forms of mass media, in that SSITB narratives reach many young people quickly, they also enable greater interactions between users and their audiences and allow users to create and disseminate content. Social media use is associated with both benefits and risks. Tangible benefits of social media use that may reduce SSITB risk include connection to peers with similar experiences, social support, opportunities for self-expression, and information exchange [26]. Many young people engage in mental health-specific support groups through social media platforms. Exchanging support and information in these spaces can lead to reductions in social isolation and promote feelings of validation and being understood [27, 28]. Additionally, social media platforms are used to exchange information on coping techniques and ways to manage SSITBs [29]. However, social media use can also increase the risk of SSITBs. Research has shown that the amount, type, and content of social media use all moderate SSITB risk. A recent meta-analysis on the association between SSITBs and social media has pointed to several risks, including engagement with SSITB-related content, experiencing cybervictimization, and heavy and problematic social media use [30]. We describe each below.

### 2.2.1 Exposure to SSITB Content

Young people often communicate about SSITBs and other mental health concerns through social media. While social media can benefit youths (e.g., empowering social connectedness and social support) [5], exposure to SSITB social media content may increase SSITB risk. Teens are exposed to SSITB content frequently [31], with higher rates of exposure noted in clinical samples (43%) [32]. For example, in a longitudinal study controlling for preexisting SSITB vulnerability, exposure to self-harm content on Instagram was associated with increases in self-harm behaviors, suicidal ideation, and hopelessness 1 month later [33]. Moreover, SSITB content is so prevalent that most adolescent exposure to such content is unintentional [33], and well-intentioned moderation efforts may fail to prevent exposure.

### 2.2.2 Cyberbullying

The influence of cyberbullying on SSITB risk among youths is well-documented. Research suggests that youth victims of cyberbullying are over twice as likely to engage in self-harm, report a suicide attempt, and report suicidal thoughts, when compared to non-victims [34]. Perpetrators of cyberbullying are also at a heightened SSITB risk. Moreover, the risk of suicidal thoughts doubles for youths who both perpetrate cyberbullying and are victims when compared to those with either experience alone [34].

### 2.2.3 Heavy and Problematic Social Media Use

Heavy and problematic social media use has been associated with an increased risk of SSITBs. What constitutes "heavy use" varies across studies, but generally those who engage in social media use above a given threshold (e.g., >2 or >5 h a day across studies) are more likely to report SSITBs. In a review, seven out of nine relevant studies found a direct association between heavy social media and Internet use and suicide attempts [35]. Similarly, a large cross-sectional survey showed that adolescents reporting heavy digital media use were twice as likely to report suicidal thoughts, suicide plans, and suicide attempts when compared to light users [25]. However, other research studies paint a more nuanced picture. For example, one research study suggests that the risks of SSITB outcomes follow a curvilinear pattern, with benefits derived from some use, versus no use, and an increased risk most significantly from low or moderate to heavy use [25]. Other studies reveal a linear dose–response relationship with social media being protective. Among adolescents under treatment for depression and SSITBs, no social media use was associated with a greater risk of having suicidal thoughts with a plan, whereas more social media use was associated with less risk [36]. This underscores the need for future work to examine subgroups of youths, such as those already at risk of suicide, to better understand the risk dynamics.

## 2.3 Video Games and SSITBs

As with social media use, evidence shows an association between problematic gaming and suicidal ideation [37, 38]. Problematic gaming is operationalized differently across studies, with some studies examining time spent gaming and others looking at addictive symptoms. In general, time spent gaming has been associated with greater suicidality. Low levels of gaming have a mild association with suicide risk [38], but the risk increases with greater time spent gaming. In a 2022 meta-analysis of 12 studies focused on problem gaming and suicidality [39], 11 showed a positive association between problem gaming and suicidal ideation and 3 showed a positive association between problem gaming and suicide attempts. In addition, a research study has shown a relationship between *violent* video gaming and aggressive behavior [40]. However, these effects have been debated and evidence is mixed [41, 42]. Whether violent video games also increase the likelihood of violent self-directed behaviors, like suicide or self-injury, is a subject that merits further empirical attention.

### 2.4 Limitations to What We Know

Several important limitations should be considered:

1. Most evidence on the relationship between mass media coverage and SSITBs has focused on suicide attempts, with less data on suicidal ideation and non-suicidal self-injury. Evidence for social media and gaming has most often focused on suicide attempts and ideation, with less focus on non-suicidal self-injury. Given that treatment targets, functions, and frequency vary across these behaviors, ways of engaging with media for support and information and risks may also differ.
2. Irrespective of the media type, research has largely relied on cross-sectional designs, with less prospective work to investigate temporal associations. Future studies should aim to understand causality via longitudinal or experimental designs. As an example, newer studies of hope and recovery media stories use randomized controlled designs [43, 44].
3. Inconsistent operationalization of heavy and problematic social media use and gaming limits our ability to draw pooled conclusions.
4. Participation in social media and video games is often assessed as stable/static (once and over a general period) and does not account for dynamic exposure that may fluctuate with time, individual, familial, and other broader/ecological factors.
5. Research focused on minoritized populations to understand generalizability of existing findings is scarce.

## 3 Future Research

Based on current knowledge, we recommend that researchers consider the following questions:

- *How do media effects on SSITBs differ across youth populations?* There is a need for research that includes populations with predispositions to mental health conditions as well as work that compares different age cohorts to explore developmental differences in risk and resiliency.
- *How can we harness the power of mass media social contagion to promote behaviors that reduce SSITB risk and increase access to services for those in distress?* Research examining the effects of media narratives focused on hope, overcoming suicidal crises, and help-seeking as well as campaigns around safe social media use (e.g., #chatsafe) are needed.
- *What is the best way for lived experiences of SSITB narratives to be shared through media?* Research on the effects of various depictions of lived experiences of SSITBs across different media formats is needed.
- *What specific social media and gaming interactions or factors are most associated with increased risk, and which have protective value?* More research is needed to understand the effects of exposure to different content/genres. In addition, focused attention is needed on existing moderation efforts, like trigger warnings and filter screens that

require a user to opt in to seeing content on popular social media platforms.

# 4 Recommendations

## 4.1 For Youths

- Follow healthy use guidelines [45], including taking regular breaks from all media types, being mindful of how media consumption makes you feel, and minimizing exposure to, and engagement with, SSITB content.
- #chatsafe guidelines provide evidence-based strategies for engagement of suicide-related content on social media developed with and for young people: https://www.orygen.org.au/chatsafe

## 4.2 For Parents

- Maintain a regular, and open, dialogue with your child about their media consumption, including whether they have been exposed to (or are engaged with) any SSITB-related content or are experiencing cyberbullying.
- Watch for problematic use—media use that interferes with your child's daily routines including sleep—and, if concerned, have conversations around limiting when, how much, and what type of media use your child engages in. Empower them to contribute to limit-setting, and model these limits in your own media habits.

## 4.3 For Clinicians

- Speak with patients about their media consumption and engagement as part of regular checkups. Assess for problematic media consumption or use and ask whether and why they engage with content related to self-harm or suicide.
- Distribute informational handouts to patients and families regarding healthy media consumption practices in the office and via websites.

## 4.4 For Schools

- Implement training and protocols for school personnel on how to manage student social media posts regarding self-harm and suicide.
- Consider incorporating media literacy and digital citizenship programs into curricula so that youths can learn safe ways of navigating media platforms and associated risks and benefits.
- Distribute handouts to students and parents on healthy media habits and ways to manage and respond to social media posts regarding suicide or self-harm.

## 4.5 For Media Platforms

- Promote positive stories of hope and recovery following suicidal crisis, and limit or censor media reports on harmful narratives by following expert guidance (e.g., the Suicide Prevention Resource Center; Suicide Awareness Voices of Education).
- Establish clear and effective policies for handling suicide and self-harm related posts, and provide resources to at-risk users and those witnessing such content.

## 4.6 For Policymakers

- Enforce existing guidelines for media reporting on SSITBs with specifications for reporting and reposting in social media contexts.
- Establish regulations for the safe exchange of SSITB-related material through social media.

**Conflict of Interest and Funding Disclosures** JN writes *Techno Sapiens*, a psychology newsletter for which she receives subscription and sponsor payments. She is the co-owner of Tech Without Stress, LLC, which provides free and paid resources for parents raising children in the digital age. No other authors reported a conflict of interest.

J.M.T. earns royalties from books, receives honoraria for speaking engagements, and has consulted and served as an expert witness for law firms on the topic of social media and mental health. She also writes Generation Tech, a psychology newsletter for which she receives subscription and sponsor payments.

## References


1. Stack S. Media impacts on Suicide: a quantitative review of 293 findings. Soc Sci Q. 2000;81(4):957–71.
2. Sisask M, Värnik A. Media roles in Suicide prevention: a systematic review. Int J Environ Res Public Health. 2012;9(1):123–38. https://doi.org/10.3390/ijerph9010123.
3. Thorn P, Hill NT, Lamblin M, et al. Developing a Suicide prevention social media campaign with young people (the #Chatsafe project): co-design approach. JMIR Ment Health. 2020;7(5):e17520. https://doi.org/10.2196/17520.
4. Nathan NA, Nathan KI. Suicide, stigma, and utilizing social media platforms to gauge public perceptions. Front Psychiatry. 2020;10 https://doi.org/10.3389/fpsyt.2019.00947.
5. Biernesser C, Sewall CJR, Brent D, Bear T, Mair C, Trauth J. Social media use and deliberate self-harm among youth: a systematized narrative review. Child Youth Serv Rev. 2020;116:105054. https://doi.org/10.1016/j.childyouth.2020.105054.
6. Burstein B, Agostino H, Greenfield B. Suicidal attempts and ideation among children and adolescents in US emergency departments, 2007–2015. JAMA Pediatr. 2019;173(6):598–600. https://doi.org/10.1001/jamapediatrics.2019.0464.
7. Spiller HA, Ackerman JP, Smith GA, et al. Suicide attempts by self-poisoning in the United States among 10–25 year olds from 2000 to 2018: substances used, temporal changes and demographics. Clin Toxicol. 2020;58(7):676–87. https://doi.org/10.1080/15563650.2019.1665182.
8. Phillips DP. The influence of suggestion on suicide: substantive and theoretical implications of the Werther effect. Am Sociol Rev. 1974;39(3):340–54. https://doi.org/10.2307/2094294.
9. Niederkrotenthaler T, Braun M, Pirkis J, et al. Association between suicide reporting in the media and suicide: systematic review and meta-analysis. BMJ. 2020:m575. https://doi.org/10.1136/bmj.m575.
10. Ferguson CJ. 13 reasons why not: a methodological and meta-analytic review of evidence regarding Suicide contagion by fictional media. Suicide Life Threat Behav. 2019;49(4):1178–86. https://doi.org/10.1111/sltb.12517.
11. Niederkrotenthaler T, Kirchner S, Till B, et al. Systematic review and meta-analyses of suicidal outcomes following fictional portrayals of suicide and suicide attempt in entertainment media. EClinicalMedicine. 2021;36:100922. https://doi.org/10.1016/j.eclinm.2021.100922.
12. Sinyor M, Williams M, Tran US, et al. Suicides in young people in Ontario following the release of "13 reasons why". Can J Psychiatr. 2019;64(11):798–804. https://doi.org/10.1177/0706743719870507.
13. Niederkrotenthaler T, Stack S, Till B, et al. Association of increased youth suicides in the United States with the release of 13 reasons why. JAMA Psychiatry. 2019;76(9):933–40. https://doi.org/10.1001/jamapsychiatry.2019.0922.
14. Cooper MT, Bard D, Wallace R, Gillaspy S, Deleon S. Suicide attempt admissions from a single children's hospital before and after the introduction of Netflix series 13 reasons why. J Adolesc Health. 2018;63(6):688–93. https://doi.org/10.1016/j.jadohealth.2018.08.028.
15. Chen YY, Yip PSF, Chan CH, et al. The impact of a celebrity's suicide on the introduction and establishment of a new method of suicide in South Korea. Arch Suicide Res. 2014;18(2):221–6. https://doi.org/10.1080/13811118.2013.824840.
16. Niederkrotenthaler T, Stack S. Media and suicide: international perspectives on research, theory, and policy. Routledge; 2017.
17. Till B, Strauss M, Sonneck G, Niederkrotenthaler T. Determining the effects of films with suicidal content: a laboratory experiment. Br J Psychiatry. 2015;207(1):72–8. https://doi.org/10.1192/bjp.bp.114.152827.
18. Niederkrotenthaler T, Voracek M, Herberth A, et al. Role of media reports in completed and prevented suicide: Werther v. Papageno effects. Br J Psychiatry. 2010;197(3):234–43. https://doi.org/10.1192/bjp.bp.109.074633.
19. Niederkrotenthaler T, Till B, Kirchner S, et al. Effects of media stories of hope and recovery on suicidal ideation and help-seeking attitudes and intentions: systematic review and meta-analysis. Lancet Public Health. 2022;7(2):e156–68. https://doi.org/10.1016/S2468-2667(21)00274-7.
20. Niederkrotenthaler T, Tran US, Gould M, et al. Association of logic's hip hop song "1-800-273-8255" with lifeline calls and suicides in the United States: interrupted time series analysis. BMJ. 2021:e067726. https://doi.org/10.1136/bmj-2021-067726.
21. Westers NJ, Lewis SP, Whitlock J, et al. Media guidelines for the responsible reporting and depicting of non-suicidal self-injury. Br J Psychiatry. 2020;9:1–4. https://doi.org/10.1192/bjp.2020.191.
22. Preventing Suicide: A resource for media professionals, update 2017. World Health Organization; 2017.
23. Samaritans. Media Guidelines for Reporting Suicide; 2020. https://media.samaritans.org/documents/Media_Guidelines_FINAL.pdf
24. American Foundation for Suicide Prevention. Safe reporting guidelines for media; 2020. https://afsp.org/safereporting/. Accessed 18 Dec 2023.
25. Twenge JM, Campbell WK. Media use is linked to lower psychological well-being: evidence from three datasets. Psychiatry Q. 2019;90(2):311–31. https://doi.org/10.1007/s11126-019-09630-7.
26. Kruzan KP, Whitlock J. Digital media, suicide, and self-injury. In: Nesi J, Telzer EH, Prinstein M, editors. Handbook of adolescent digital media use and mental health. Cambridge University Press; 2022. p. 338–62.
27. Daine K, Hawton K, Singaravelu V, Stewart A, Simkin S, Montgomery P. The power of the web: a systematic review of studies of the influence of the internet on

self-harm and Suicide in young people. PLoS One. 2013;8(10):e77555. https://doi.org/10.1371/journal.pone.0077555.
28. Marchant A, Hawton K, Stewart A, et al. A systematic review of the relationship between internet use, self-harm and suicidal behaviour in young people: the good, the bad and the unknown. Choo KKR, ed. PLoS One. 2017;12(8):e0181722. https://doi.org/10.1371/journal.pone.0181722.
29. Duggan JM, Heath NL, Lewis SP, Baxter AL. An examination of the scope and nature of non-suicidal self-injury online activities: implications for school mental health professionals. School Ment Health. 2012;4(1):56–67. https://doi.org/10.1007/s12310-011-9065-6.
30. Nesi J, Burke TA, Bettis AH, et al. Social media use and self-injurious thoughts and behaviors: a systematic review and meta-analysis. Clin Psychol Rev. 2021;87:102038. https://doi.org/10.1016/j.cpr.2021.102038
31. Nesi J, Mann S, Robb MB. Teens and mental health: how girls really feel about social media. Common Sense; 2023.
32. Nesi J, Burke TA, Lawrence HR, MacPherson HA, Spirito A, Wolff JC. Online self-injury activities among psychiatrically hospitalized adolescents: prevalence, functions, and perceived consequences. Res Child Adolesc Psychopathol. 2021;49(4):519–31. https://doi.org/10.1007/s10802-020-00734-4.
33. Arendt F, Scherr S, Romer D. Effects of exposure to self-harm on social media: evidence from a two-wave panel study among young adults. New Media Soc. 2019;21(11–12):2422–42. https://doi.org/10.1177/1461444819850106.
34. John A, Glendenning AC, Marchant A, et al. Self-harm, suicidal behaviours, and cyberbullying in children and young people: systematic review. J Med Internet Res. 2018;20(4):e129. https://doi.org/10.2196/jmir.9044.
35. Sedgwick R, Epstein S, Dutta R, Ougrin D. Social media, internet use and suicide attempts in adolescents. Curr Opin Psychiatry. 2019;32(6):534–41. https://doi.org/10.1097/YCO.0000000000000547.
36. Hamilton JL, Biernesser C, Moreno MA, et al. Social media use and prospective suicidal thoughts and behaviors among adolescents at high risk for suicide. Suicide Life Threat Behav. 2021:sltb.12801. https://doi.org/10.1111/sltb.12801.
37. Jeong YW, Han YR, Kim SK, Jeong HS. The frequency of impairments in everyday activities due to the overuse of the internet, gaming, or smartphone, and its relationship to health-related quality of life in Korea. BMC Public Health. 2020;20(1):954. https://doi.org/10.1186/s12889-020-08922-z.
38. Roberston L, Twenge JM, Joiner TE, Cummins K. Associations between screen time and internalizing disorder diagnoses among 9- to 10-year-olds. J Affect Disord. 2022;311:530–7. https://doi.org/10.1016/j.jad.2022.05.071.
39. Erevik EK, Landrø H, Mattson ÅL, Kristensen JH, Kaur P, Pallesen S. Problem gaming and suicidality: a systematic literature review. Addict Behav Rep. 2022;15:100419. https://doi.org/10.1016/j.abrep.2022.100419.
40. Förtsch EMAD, Baumgart P, Teismann T, Ruscheweyh R, Hasenbring MI. No game, more pain – examining possible long term effects and underlying mechanisms of habitual violent video gaming on the acquired capability for suicide. Psychiatry Res. 2021;295:113512. https://doi.org/10.1016/j.psychres.2020.113512.
41. Bushman BJ, Huesmann LR. Twenty-five years of research on violence in digital games and aggression revisited. Eur Psychol. 2014;19(1):47–55. https://doi.org/10.1027/1016-9040/a000164.
42. Elson M, Ferguson CJ. Twenty-five years of research on violence in digital games and aggression. Eur Psychol. 2014;19(1):33–46. https://doi.org/10.1027/1016-9040/a000147.
43. Niederkrotenthaler T, Baumgartner J, Kautzky A, et al. Effects of media stories featuring coping with suicidal crises on psychiatric patients: randomized controlled trial. Eur Psychiatry. 2021;64(1):e70. https://doi.org/10.1192/j.eurpsy.2021.2244.
44. Braun M, Till B, Pirkis J, Niederkrotenthaler T. Effects of suicide prevention videos developed by and targeting adolescents: a randomized controlled trial. Eur Child Adolesc Psychiatry. 2023;32(5):847–57. https://doi.org/10.1007/s00787-021-01911-6.
45. American Psychological Association. Health Advisory on Social Media Use in Adolescence; 2023. https://www.apa.org/topics/social-media-internet/health-advisory-adolescent-social-media-use. Accessed 18 Dec 2023.

# Social Media Use, Body Image Concerns, and Disordered Eating Among Adolescents

Sophia Choukas-Bradley, Anne J. Maheux, Jennifer Stevens Aubrey, Linda Charmaraman, Megan K. Maas, Jacqueline Nesi, L. Monique Ward, and Chia-chen Yang

## 1 Background

In 2021, a *Wall Street Journal* exposé of Meta's internal research findings amplified public concern about the role of social media (SM) in adolescents' body image concerns and mental health, particularly for girls [1]. Subsequently, US congressional hearings and legislative proposals have focused on social media's potential mental health harms [2]. As public debate rages, academic research has also progressed—moving beyond a focus on overall screen time and toward a more nuanced perspective on how and why social media may affect adolescents' body image and mental health. In this chapter, we provide a brief overview of the existing literature on adolescent social media use, body image, and disordered eating. We focus on research on youth aged 12–18, drawing on studies from young adults (i.e., roughly aged 18–29) to fill in gaps when necessary. Our focus is on the broad spectrum of body image concerns and disordered eating,

The third through eighth listed authors (JSA, LC, MKM, JN, LMW, CCY) made equal intellectual contributions to this chapter and share third authorship; these names are listed alphabetically.

We are grateful to Savannah R. Roberts, whose prior work contributed to the thinking for this chapter.

S. Choukas-Bradley (✉)
Department of Psychology, University of Pittsburgh, Pittsburgh, PA, USA
e-mail: scb.1@pitt.edu

A. J. Maheux
Department of Psychology and Neuroscience, University of North Carolina at Chapel Hill, Chapel Hill, NC, USA

J. S. Aubrey
Department of Communication, University of Arizona, Tucson, AZ, USA

L. Charmaraman
Wellesley Centers for Women, Wellesley College, Wellesley, MA, USA

M. K. Maas
Department of Human Development & Family Studies, Michigan State University, East Lansing, MI, USA

J. Nesi
Department of Psychiatry & Human Behavior, Alpert Medical School of Brown University, Providence, RI, USA

Bradley-Hasbro Research Center, Rhode Island Hospital, Providence, RI, USA

L. M. Ward
Department of Psychology, University of Michigan, Ann Arbor, MI, USA

C. Yang
School of Educational Foundations, Leadership and Aviation, Oklahoma State University, Stillwater, OK, USA


D. A. Christakis, L. Hale (eds.), *Handbook of Children and Screens*,
https://doi.org/10.1007/978-3-031-69362-5_21

rather than clinical eating disorders. The role of social media in clinical eating disorders is reviewed elsewhere [3].

Long before the advent of highly visual social media (e.g., Instagram, Snapchat, TikTok), adolescents, especially girls, reported high rates of body image concerns and disordered eating [4]. Disordered eating refers to a range of maladaptive eating and weight-related behaviors usually aimed at altering one's body size and shape (e.g., restricting food intake, purging, excessive exercise). The single strongest predictor of adolescent girls' disordered eating is body dissatisfaction [4]. Highly visual social media may augment long-standing sociocultural and developmental risk factors for body image concerns, through processes outlined in Choukas-Bradley et al.'s (2022) "perfect storm" theoretical framework [5]. The features of social media (e.g., their provision of quantifiable peer feedback) intersect with the developmental features of adolescence (e.g., heightened attunement to peer feedback) and sociocultural gendered appearance pressures (e.g., ever-changing, largely unattainable beauty ideals) to predict body image concerns, which, in turn, may lead to disordered eating (Fig. 1) [5]. Consistent with this framework, we conceptualize body image concerns as including not only body dissatisfaction but also self-objectification (i.e., considering one's body and appearance from the perspective of an outside observer), body shame, and weight, shape, and other appearance concerns. The goal of this chapter is not to provide a systematic or exhaustive review but rather to offer a brief overview of the current state of the literature regarding adolescents' social media use, body image concerns, and disordered eating. We begin by discussing idealized appearance content and upward social comparisons on social media. Next, we address self-presentation and appearance-related social media consciousness. Third, we discuss "body-positive" content. We conclude by providing guidelines for future research as well as policy and clinical recommendations.

## 2 Current State

### 2.1 Idealized Appearance Content and Upward Social Comparisons on Social Media

According to Thompson et al.'s (1999) tripartite influence model [6], developed before the advent of modern social media, body dissatisfaction results when individuals perceive a discrepancy between their physical appearance and the beauty ideals transmitted by mass media, family, and peers. These beauty ideals are learned through upward social comparisons and become internalized. Social comparisons and idealized appearance internalization are two of the primary ways that social media use may promote body dissatisfaction and disordered eating [7–10]. Recent research has suggested that social media may lead adolescent girls and young women to engage in upward social comparisons with attractive peers, celebrities, and "influencers" (i.e., social media personalities who promote lifestyles and/or brands) and to internalize appearance ideals, leading to body image concerns [5]. Moreover, in the era of social media, beauty ideals have evolved, becoming increasingly specific and sexualized. For example, the contemporary "slim–thick" ideal refers to a thin waist and flat stomach, paired with larger or "thick" hips, buttocks, and thighs. A recent experiment by McComb and Mills, with a racially heterogeneous sample of Canadian undergraduate women (aged 18–25), has found that the slim–thick ideal was preferred across all racial groups and that comparisons with slim–thick social media imagery predicted more weight and appearance dissatisfaction than comparisons with thin-ideal images [11].

Evidence from experimental studies suggests that exposure to idealized images on social media can lead to or worsen body image concerns. A recent systematic review of 43 experimental studies by Fioravanti et al. has examined the effects of viewing idealized social media content among young people (aged 14–25; *M*age = 21.6) [12]. The key findings included: [1] viewing ide-

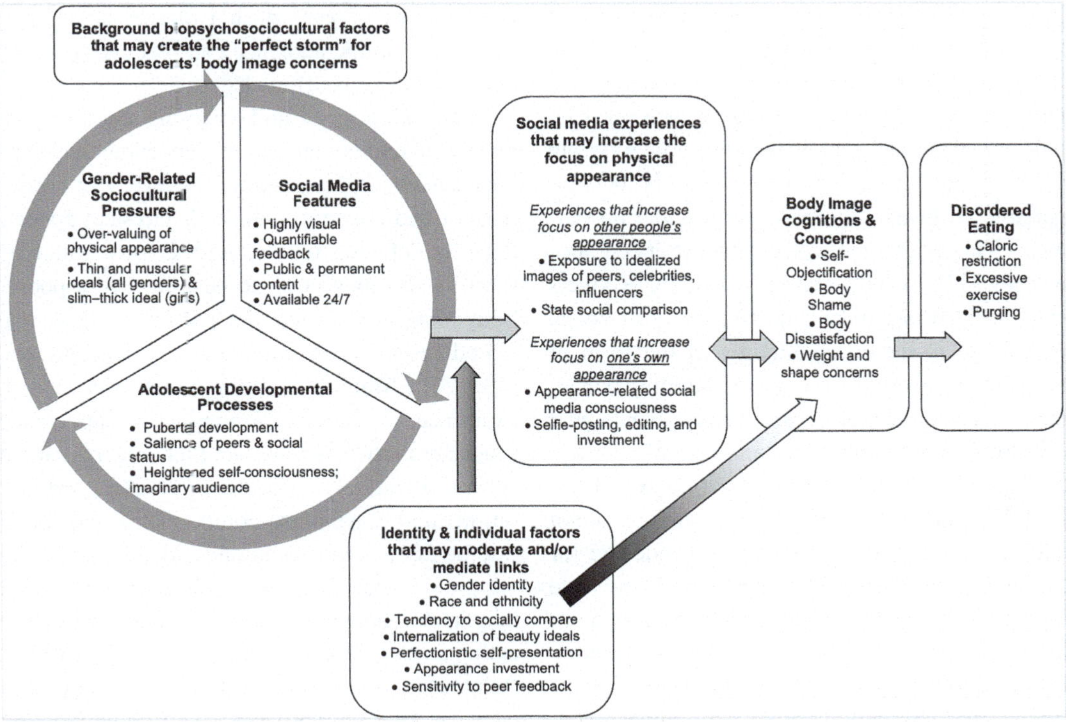


**Fig. 1** The "perfect storm" developmental–sociocultural framework of social media use, body image concerns, and disordered eating, adapted from the version first published in Choukas-Bradley et al. (2022) in *Clinical Child and Family Psychology Review* (Springer)

alized images directly led to body dissatisfaction among young women and men; [2] this effect was mediated by state appearance comparisons (i.e., engaging in social comparisons helped explain the link between idealized image exposure and body dissatisfaction); and [3] trait social comparisons moderated these effects (i.e., there were more body image concerns following exposure to idealized images among individuals with higher social comparison tendencies) [12]. For example, in one study among girls aged 14–18 in the Netherlands by Kleemans et al. (2018), exposure to Instagram images that had been edited, reshaped, and resized directly led to more body image concerns but only among girls with higher social comparison tendencies [13]. Moreover, participants did not recognize the extent to which these photos had been altered and preferred the edited photos, suggesting the powerful, insidious effects of online idealized images [13]. More than 90% of the studies in the experimental review were conducted in Anglophone, industrialized countries, with roughly half of participants identifying as White or Caucasian, consistent with the broader literature on social media and body image [12]. The vast majority of studies included young adult samples, with only two including younger participants, and more than 80% solely included women [12].

Research with other methodologies has also contributed to our understanding of these processes by identifying potential mediators and enhancing external validity. Many nonexperimental studies of adolescents have found social comparison and internalization of beauty ideals to mediate the association between highly visual social media use and body dissatisfaction across many nations [5]. For example, Roberts et al. (2022) examined social media appearance pressures (e.g., "I feel pressure from social media to look thinner") cross-sectionally among a racially and ethnically heterogeneous sample of US girls aged 13–18 [14]. In a structural equation model that accounted for appearance pressures from family, peers, and traditional media, social media use was the only source of appearance pressure that contributed to girls' lower appearance esteem via both thin-ideal internalization and body comparison. Girls also internalized muscular appearance ideals, without related changes in appearance esteem [14]. Another recent work by Rodgers et al. (2020) has linked the frequency of social media use to disordered eating, in the form of both dietary restraint and muscle-building behaviors, via internalization of beauty ideals and upward social comparisons, among early adolescent girls and boys in Australia (*M*age = 12.8) [15]. We note that cross-sectional studies cannot determine causality or temporal precedence; for example, it is possible that adolescents who have higher social comparison tendencies are more likely to seek out beauty-related social media. However, several recent longitudinal studies have suggested associations between appearance-related social media use and the development of self-objectification and body image concerns; for example, a study by Skowronski et al. with German adolescent girls and boys (*M*age = 15.1) found the use of sexualized Instagram images to predict increased body surveillance over time, via the mediator of valuing appearance [16].

## 2.2 Self-Presentation and Appearance-Related Social Media Consciousness

Highly visual social media sites and apps offer unique opportunities for presenting an idealized version of oneself—which aligns with key self-presentational goals that are salient during adolescence [5]. Adolescents are adept at using social media's affordances to craft a curated, photoshopped, and idealized self-presentation designed to maximize positive peer feedback [17]. The "imaginary audience" ideation, a social-cognitive aspect of development wherein adolescents feel as if they are in a spotlight with an audience of peers, is likely exacerbated by social media [18]. The constant possibility of peers' viewing one's posted images and videos means the online audience can feel ever-present, even when one is offline [5].

Many adolescents and emerging adults experience a phenomenon called "appearance-related social media consciousness" (ASMC) or awareness of and concern with one's physical appearance as depicted online. ASMC was found by Choukas-Bradley et al. to be linked to a poorer body image and greater disordered eating among US adolescents and young adult women and men [19, 20]. Similarly, Zimmer-Gembeck et al. examined "social media appearance preoccupation"—a construct that captures online self-presentation, appearance-related activity online, and appearance comparison—and found it to be more common among girls. Social media appearance preoccupation was associated with heightened appearance anxiety and disordered eating among both Australian boys and girls [21]. Related to this work, "selfie" behaviors have been described as a process of self-objectification that includes internalizing an observer's gaze on one's body and valuing one's physical appearance and sexual appeal over other skills or value-based qualities [5], in line with the original conception of self-objectification first proposed by Fredrickson and Roberts (1997) before the advent of modern social media [22]. Experimental studies with US undergraduate men and women, and self-report studies with adolescent girls in the United States and China, have found associations with selfie-related behaviors and self-objectification [5, 18, 23]. Taken together, these findings suggest a cross-cultural phenomenon of being conscious of one's appearance online as an indicator of broader self-objectification, even if beauty norms differ across cultures.

## 2.3 "Body-Positive" Content

The "body-positive" movement ostensibly promotes body acceptance through representation of diverse bodies and beauty norms—such as through showing images of larger bodies, women of color, and queer and gender-nonconforming people, accompanied by body-positive hashtags and captions. In theory, such content might be expected to reduce upward social comparisons and encourage a positive body image. However, reviews of experimental and nonexperimental studies of body-positive social media content suggest overall mixed effects [12, 24], which could be due in part to the frequently objectifying content of body-positive social media accounts [25]. Images that do not depict human figures at all, or that showcase average-sized and unmanipulated figures, are less detrimental to body image. In contrast, body acceptance text accompanying idealized images does not seem to mitigate the negative effects on body image [24]. Additionally, the work by Kvardova et al. with Czech adolescent girls and boys points to complex associations: findings from a survey-based study indicated that body-positive content may be associated with a positive body image among those who deliberately seek it out [26] (consistent with uses and gratifications theory) [27], whereas an experimental study revealed that positive appearance commentary intensified the effect of exposure to idealized bodies on body dissatisfaction, specifically among adolescent girls who perceived those images as highly attractive [28]. Collectively, both theoretical and empirical work suggest that the body-positive movement may lead to increased body image concerns among some young people via exacerbating the focus on physical appearance and increasing self-objectification [5]. Ultimately, nonappearance focused media may be most promotive of body satisfaction [24]. Consistent with this idea, "body neutrality" (i.e., appreciating a body's abilities rather than evaluating its appearance) has been identified as potentially valuable for mitigating body image concerns and disordered eating among diverse adolescents (e.g., gender-diverse populations) [29].

## 2.4 Conclusions

Overall, the current literature indicates that highly visual social media use is associated with adolescents' body dissatisfaction and disordered eating. Exposure to idealized and sexualized appearance content, social comparison, and preoccupation with one's self-presentation on social media appear to be the key drivers of this association. More research is needed to further understand in what context and for whom highly visual social media may pose the largest risk of body dissatisfaction and disordered eating as well as to identify efficacious tools for intervention and to develop policies to mitigate harm.

# 3 Future Research

A critical direction for future research is to investigate the appearance-related social media experiences of adolescents of color, youth in the Global South, boys and young men, and adolescents with LGBTQ+ identities. This work should begin with qualitative methods that allow a detailed exploration of lived experiences, followed by model building and testing to understand how youths' marginalized identities intersect with social media experiences to affect body image and disordered eating. For instance, further research is needed regarding how social media may affect other appearance norms besides the thin and muscular ideals among adolescents, such as those related to colorism, as well as other racialized or culturally relevant aspects of appearance [30–33].

Additionally, more research is needed on the opportunities for social media to be spaces of resistance and community, especially among marginalized youths, such as transgender youths and youths of color. Rather than focusing on between-group comparisons (e.g., racial disparities in body image concerns), it is important for researchers to focus on understanding the nuanced individual differences related to sociodemographic identities and cultural contexts, to better understand the moderators and mediators proposed by the "perfect storm" framework [5]. More attention to moderators and individual differences (e.g., identities, sensitivity to peer feedback) will be essential in understanding where, when, and with whom to intervene.

Furthermore, it is important to continue to build on the development and testing of prevention programming (e.g., social media literacy programs; school-based health and wellness programs) to promote healthy social media use [34]. Intervention and prevention programming should integrate a focus on structural and culturally relevant factors, rather than positioning social media-related body image concerns as solely individual-level problems. A focus on social media must also be integrated into the evaluation and therapeutic interventions for adolescents struggling with body image and/or disordered eating.

## 4 Recommendations

The following are policy and clinical recommendations:

- Greater investment is needed to support research on adolescent social media use and body image concerns. Although body image concerns have historically been viewed by funders as a niche issue, they are in fact a potent risk factor for a broad range of mental health problems [4, 5].
- Further development, evaluation, and dissemination of evidence-based prevention and intervention programming is needed. The promise of single-session interventions (i.e., structured and targeted programs that intentionally include one sole session), recently developed by Schleider et al., should be further investigated [35, 36]. Clinicians may also consider adapting approaches that are empirically supported for other distressing behaviors (e.g., from cognitive behavioral therapy), as in the digital well-being resources recently developed by the Center for Digital Thriving and Common Sense Education [37].
- Recommending abstinence from social media may be unrealistic or developmentally maladaptive for some adolescents. For adolescents struggling with body image concerns or disordered eating, parents, educators, and clinicians should assess for uses of social media that may exacerbate the problem (e.g., following beauty-focused influencers or spending excessive time taking and modifying selfies) [5]. In this case, the interventions discussed in the second recommendation may be useful.
- Rather than supporting blanket interventions to curb adolescents' social media use, policymakers should focus their efforts on incentivizing social media companies to implement humane and human-centered technology designs that address developmental considerations, promote adolescent health, and mitigate harm. Recent efforts by social media companies to alter their platforms to improve user well-being, particularly for youth and their families [38], should be expanded. This positive trend would be strengthened by collaborations between these companies and researchers who could independently monitor and assess the effectiveness of intervention strategies, such as training algorithms to avoid showing negative content to minors.

**Conflict of Interest and Funding Disclosures** This material is based upon work supported by the National Science Foundation (NSF) Graduate Research Fellowship under Grant No. 1940700 awarded to AJM. JN is partially supported by a grant from the National Institute of Mental Health (NIMH; K23-MH122669). JN writes Techno Sapiens, a psychology newsletter for which she receives subscription and sponsor payments. She is co-owner of Tech Without Stress, LLC, which provides free and paid resources for parents raising children in the digital age. Any opinion, findings, and conclusions or recommendations expressed in this material are those of the authors and do not necessarily reflect the views of the NSF or NIMH.

## References

1. The Facebook Files. Wall Street Journal. https://www.wsj.com/articles/the-facebook-files-11631713039. Published October 1, 2021. Accessed 11 Feb 2022.
2. Blumenthal and Blackburn introduce comprehensive kids' online safety legislation. Published online 2022. https://www.blumenthal.senate.gov/newsroom/press/release/blumenthal-and-blackburn-introduce-comprehensive-kids-online-safety-legislation
3. Padín PF, González-Rodríguez R, Verde-Diego C, Vázquez-Pérez R. Social media and eating disorder psychopathology: A systematic review. Cyberpsychology. 2021;15(3) https://doi.org/10.5817/CP2021-3-6.
4. Stice E, Marti CN, Durant S. Risk factors for onset of eating disorders: evidence of multiple risk path-

ways from an 8-year prospective study. Behav Res Ther. 2011;49(10):622–7. https://doi.org/10.1016/j.brat.2011.06.009.

5. Choukas-Bradley S, Roberts SR, Maheux AJ, Nesi J. The perfect storm: a developmental–sociocultural framework for the role of social media in adolescent girls' body image concerns and mental health. Clin Child Fam Psychol Rev. 2022;25:681–701. https://doi.org/10.1007/s10567-022-00404-5.
6. Thompson JK, Heinberg LJ, Altabe M, Tantleff-Dunn S. Exacting beauty: theory, assessment, and treatment of body image disturbance. American Psychological Association; 1999. https://doi.org/10.1037/10312-000.
7. Holland G, Tiggemann M. A systematic review of the impact of the use of social networking sites on body image and disordered eating outcomes. Body Image. 2016;17:100–10. https://doi.org/10.1016/j.bodyim.2016.02.008.
8. Roberts SR, Maheux AJ, Ladd BA, Choukas-Bradley S. The role of digital media in adolescents' body image and disordered eating. In: Nesi J, Telzer EH, Prinstein MJ, editors. Handbook of adolescent digital media use and mental health. 1st ed. Cambridge University Press; 2022. p. 242–63. https://doi.org/10.1017/9781108976237.014.
9. Rodgers RF. The relationship between body image concerns, eating disorders and internet use, Part II: An integrated theoretical model. Adolesc Res Rev. 2016;1(2):121–37. https://doi.org/10.1007/s40894-015-0017-5.
10. Perloff RM. Social media effects on young women's body image concerns: theoretical perspectives and an agenda for research. Sex Roles. 2014;71(11-12):363–77. https://doi.org/10.1007/s11199-014-0384-6.
11. McComb SE, Mills JS. The effect of physical appearance perfectionism and social comparison to thin-, slim-thick-, and fit-ideal Instagram imagery on young women's body image. Body Image. 2022;40:165–75. https://doi.org/10.1016/j.bodyim.2021.12.003.
12. Fioravanti G, Bocci Benucci S, Ceragioli G, Casale S. How the exposure to beauty ideals on social networking sites influences body image: a systematic review of experimental studies. Adolesc Res Rev. 2022;7(3):419–58. https://doi.org/10.1007/s40894-022-00179-4.
13. Kleemans M, Daalmans S, Carbaat I, Anschütz D. Picture perfect: the direct effect of manipulated Instagram photos on body image in adolescent girls. Media Psychol. 2018;21(1):93–110. https://doi.org/10.1080/15213269.2016.1257392.
14. Roberts SR, Maheux AJ, Hunt RA, Ladd BA, Choukas-Bradley S. Incorporating social media and muscular ideal internalization into the tripartite influence model of body image: towards a modern understanding of adolescent girls' body dissatisfaction. Body Image. 2022;41:239–47. https://doi.org/10.1016/j.bodyim.2022.03.002.
15. Rodgers RF, Slater A, Gordon CS, McLean SA, Jarman HK, Paxton SJ. A biopsychosocial model of social media use and body image concerns, disordered eating, and muscle-building behaviors among adolescent girls and boys. J Youth Adolesc. 2020;49(2):399–409. https://doi.org/10.1007/s10964-019-01190-0.
16. Skowronski M, Busching R, Krahé B. Predicting adolescents' self-objectification from sexualized video game and Instagram use: a longitudinal study. Sex Roles. 2021;84:584–98. https://doi.org/10.1007/s11199-020-01187-1.
17. Chua THH, Chang L. Follow me and like my beautiful selfies: Singapore teenage girls' engagement in self-presentation and peer comparison on social media. Comput Hum Behav. 2016;55:190–7. https://doi.org/10.1016/j.chb.2015.09.011.
18. Zheng D, Ni X, Luo Y. Selfie posting on social networking sites and female adolescents' self-objectification: the moderating role of imaginary audience ideation. Sex Roles. 2019;80(5–6):325–31. https://doi.org/10.1007/s11199-018-0937-1.
19. Choukas-Bradley S, Nesi J, Widman L, Galla BM. The Appearance-Related Social Media Consciousness Scale: development and validation with adolescents. Body Image. 2020;33:164–74. https://doi.org/10.1016/j.bodyim.2020.02.017.
20. Maheux AJ, Roberts SR, Nesi J, Widman L, Choukas-Bradley S. Psychometric properties and factor structure of the Appearance-Related Social Media Consciousness Scale among emerging adults. Body Image. 2022;43:63–74. https://doi.org/10.1016/j.bodyim.2022.08.002.
21. Zimmer-Gembeck MJ, Hawes T, Pariz J. A closer look at appearance and social media: measuring activity, self-presentation, and social comparison and their associations with emotional adjustment. Psychol Pop Media. 2021;10(1):74–86. https://doi.org/10.1037/ppm0000277.
22. Fredrickson BL, Roberts TA. Objectification theory: toward understanding women's lived experiences and mental health risks. Psychol Women Q. 1997;21(2):173–206. https://doi.org/10.1111/j.1471-6402.1997.tb00108.x.
23. Terán L, Yan K, Aubrey JS. "But first let me take a selfie": U.S. adolescent girls' selfie activities, self-objectification, imaginary audience beliefs, and appearance concerns. J Child Media. 2020;14(3):343–60. https://doi.org/10.1080/17482798.2019.1697319.
24. Rodgers RF, Paxton SJ, Wertheim EH. #Take idealized bodies out of the picture: a scoping review of social media content aiming to protect and promote positive body image. Body Image. 2021;38:10–36. https://doi.org/10.1016/j.bodyim.2021.03.009.
25. Cohen R, Irwin L, Newton-John T, Slater A. #bodypositivity: a content analysis of body positive accounts on Instagram. Body Image. 2019;29:47–57. https://doi.org/10.1016/j.bodyim.2019.02.007.
26. Kvardova N, Machackova H, Smahel D. A moderated mediation model for body-positive online

content and body image among adolescents. Body Image. 2022;42:370–4. https://doi.org/10.1016/j.bodyim.2022.07.002.
27. Rubin AM. Media uses and effects: a uses-and-gratifications perspective. In: Media effects: advances in theory and research. Lawrence Erlbaum Associates; 1994. p. 417–36.
28. Kvardova N, Machackova H, Gulec H. 'I wish my body looked like theirs!': how positive appearance comments on social media impact adolescents' body dissatisfaction. Body Image. 2023;47:101630. https://doi.org/10.1016/j.bodyim.2023.101630.
29. Perry M, Watson L, Hayden L, Inwards-Breland D. Using body neutrality to inform eating disorder management in a gender diverse world. Lancet Child Adolesc Health. 2019;3(9):597–8. https://doi.org/10.1016/S2352-4642(19)30237-8.
30. Ladd BA, Maheux AJ, Roberts SR, Choukas-Bradley S. Black adolescents' appearance concerns, depressive symptoms, and self-objectification: exploring the roles of gender and ethnic-racial identity commitment. Body Image. 2022;43:314–25. https://doi.org/10.1016/j.bodyim.2022.09.008.
31. Landor AM, Ramseyer Winter VL, Thurston IB, et al. The Sociostructural-Intersectional Body Image (SIBI) framework: understanding the impact of white supremacy in body image research and practice. Body Image. 2024;48:101674. https://doi.org/10.1016/j.bodyim.2023.101674.
32. Romo LF, Mireles-Rios R, Hurtado A. Cultural, media, and peer influences on body beauty perceptions of Mexican American adolescent girls. J Adolesc Res. 2016;31(4):474–501. https://doi.org/10.1177/0743558415594424.
33. Rosario RJ, Minor I, Rogers LO. "Oh, you're pretty for a dark-skinned girl": black adolescent girls' identities and resistance to colorism. J Adolesc Res. 2021;36(5):501–34. https://doi.org/10.1177/07435584211028218.
34. Gordon CS, Jarman HK, Rodgers RF, et al. outcomes of a cluster randomized controlled trial of the SoMe Social Media Literacy Program for improving body image-related outcomes in adolescent boys and girls. Nutrients. 2021;13(11):3825. https://doi.org/10.3390/nu13113825.
35. Schleider JL, Beidas RS. Harnessing the Single-Session Intervention approach to promote scalable implementation of evidence-based practices in healthcare. Front Health Serv. 2022;2:997406. https://doi.org/10.3389/frhs.2022.997406.
36. Schleider JL, Smith AC, Ahuvia I. Realizing the untapped promise of single-session interventions for eating disorders. Int J Eat Disord. 2023;56(5):853–63. https://doi.org/10.1002/eat.23920.
37. Weinstein E, Tench B, Choukas-Bradley S, James C, Buch E, Nesi J. Teaching digital well-being: evidence-based resources to help youth thrive. Published online 2023. centerfordigitalthriving.org
38. Keenan C. New features for teens and families on TikTok. https://newsroom.tiktok.com/en-us/new-features-for-teens-and-families-on-tiktok-us. Published online March 1, 2023.

# Who Is Most at Risk?: Identifying the Risks for Mental Health Problems Related to Social Media

Jessica L. Hamilton, Kaylee P. Kruzan, Hannah Szlyk, Jazmin Reyes-Portillo, Candice Biernesser, Michaeline Jensen, Jamie Zelazny, Brian Primack, John Torous, and Paul Weigle

## 1 Background

Since the launch of Facebook in February 2004, there has been concern around social media exposure and mental health outcomes in youths. The rates of mental health problems have increased in recent years, alongside social media use, further driving debate. Empirical research on this topic is mixed [1]. Nearly all youths engage with social media on a daily basis [2], but not all are negatively affected. Theory suggests that youths may experience differential susceptibility to (social) media effects [3]. The differential susceptibility to media effects model proposes that some individuals are more susceptible to media effects (e.g., based on dispositional, developmental, and social variables) and their susceptibility is then either reduced or enhanced based on cognitive, emotional, and excitative response states [3]. Indeed, large research studies in youths, as well as recent reviews, suggest that on average one-third of youths find social media helpful to their mental health, one-third neutral, and one-third harmful [1, 4]. In reality, most youths likely experience both their negative and positive impacts. This leads to the central question: Which youths are most likely to have negative mental health outcomes related to social media?

J. L. Hamilton (✉)
Rutgers University, New Brunswick, NJ, USA
e-mail: jessica.hamilton@rutgers.edu

K. P. Kruzan
Northwestern University, Chicago, IL, USA

H. Szlyk
Washington University in St Louis, St Louis, MO, USA

J. Reyes-Portillo
Montclair University, Montclair, NJ, USA

C. Biernesser · J. Zelazny
University of Pittsburgh, Pittsburgh, PA, USA

M. Jensen
University of North Carolina- Greensboro, Greensboro, NC, USA

B. Primack
Oregon State University, Corvallis, OR, USA

J. Torous
Harvard University, Cambridge, MA, USA

P. Weigle
University of Connecticut School of Medicine, Farmington, CT, USA

## 2 Current State

This chapter reviews the current state of research identifying what factors heighten the risk for mental health problems related to social media among youths, with a focus on individual characteristics (demographic, mental health history) and social media behaviors (e.g., type of engagement). While it is outside of the scope of this chapter, it is worth noting that youths at risk of negative experiences may also reap benefits from social media use (for reviews, see Choukas-


D. A. Christakis, L. Hale (eds.), *Handbook of Children and Screens*,
https://doi.org/10.1007/978-3-031-69362-5_22

Bradley et al. [5] and Marchant et al. [6]). Current limitations and key directions for future research are identified. Based on the current state of the field, preliminary recommendations are provided for young people and their families, clinicians and educators, policymakers, and industry.

## 2.1 Which Teens May Be Most at Risk for the Negative Mental Health Effects of Media?

Although social media use that is extremely heavy or problematic (i.e., difficult to control and interferes with daily life) has been associated with negative mental health effects for most populations, it is currently impossible to accurately predict *which* individuals are at the greatest risk. Yet, there is existing research on this topic focusing on individual characteristics, such as youth identity based on demographics (e.g., sex, gender, sexual orientation, race/ethnicity, and socioeconomic status) and preexisting mental health problems. Beyond individual factors, how youths engage with media (e.g., problematic use) also considerably impacts which youths may be most at risk. Research to date on this topic is summarized below.

## 2.2 Cisgender Females

Girls have a higher baseline risk for depression and suicidality during adolescence relative to boys [7]. Some studies find that higher levels of social media use are associated with symptoms of depression or poorer well-being among girls but not boys [8–10]. A recent research has suggested that there may be "windows of vulnerability" to social media exposure that differs by sex, with the greatest risk in cisgender females between 11 and 13 years of age and also at 19 years and in males between 14 and 15 years of age and at 19 years [11], which may align with periods of transition. However, similar studies have failed to confirm sex differences [12]. Sex differences in social media effects may vary based on mental health outcomes, such that cisgender boys may suffer from more related behavioral problems [13].

Offline vulnerabilities may explain the sex differences in how social media use affects mental health. Girls are more likely than are boys to experience social comparison and interpersonal stress offline, an effect that may be mirrored online (e.g., via cyberbullying) [2]. Developmental changes increase the salience of social relationships and networks, especially for girls, which may heighten mental health problems in the context of social media's unique features (e.g., quantifiable metrics and comments) [14].

## 2.3 Minoritized Identities

Youths who hold minoritized identities, including LGBTQIA+, youths of color, and gender-diverse youths, may be at a heightened risk for the negative effects of social media and other online activities. They are more likely to experience online identity-based victimization, including being directly and indirectly targeted by verbal and sexual harassment and threats of physical harm [15] and experiencing vicarious exposure to discrimination based on race [16], sexual orientation, and gender identity [17]. Such experiences are linked to a range of negative mental health outcomes, such as depression, substance use [18], and suicidal thoughts and behaviors [19]. Exposure to content that stigmatizes minoritized identities or videos of violence toward those with a shared identity may contribute to unique risks among youths of color [20] and LGBTQIA+ youths [17].

## 2.4 Socioeconomic Disadvantage

Youths who are economically disadvantaged spend, on average, 1.5–3 hours or more per day using digital technology and receive less supervision and support [1]. Teens from low-income households also report more spillover of negative online experiences. For instance, economically disadvantaged adolescents perceive more negative offline experiences (e.g., arguments, physical fights) resulting from their technology use compared with their peers [21]. The same cross-sectional study found a stronger association between having a social media account and both conduct problems and psychological distress among persistently economically disadvantaged adolescents [21].

### 2.5 Preexisting Mental Health Problems

Youths with mental health problems may be more likely to experience the negative effects of social media [22]. Youths who have depression or are at risk for suicide engage with media in ways that exacerbate mental health problems [23], such as problematic use [24]. Depressed teens share more dysphoria, anhedonia, and suicidal thoughts via social media than do their peers who are not depressed, which, in turn, may worsen depression [25]. Youths with mental health problems may have more negative online experiences (e.g., cybervictimization, exposure to self-harm content) [19]. A mixed methods study among adolescents who interacted with depression-related content on social media found that individuals endorsing mental issues (e.g., symptoms of depression, a history of suicidal behavior) were more likely to describe negative sequelae (e.g., adverse social repercussions, feeling triggered) compared with peers who did not report these mental health issues [24]. One experimental study found that adolescents with depression experience greater physiological reactivity after social media use compared with healthy adolescents [26], which may mediate vulnerability to media-related effects. A recent systematic review has found that adolescents with a range of preexisting mental health problems experience similar negative experiences on social media [22]. However, they concluded that the existing literature is too limited to identify the disorder-specific effects of social media, with few studies drawing comparisons between conditions [22].

### 2.6 Problematic Engagement with Social Media

Youths who use media in problematic ways (e.g., characterized by loss of control, neglecting other hobbies or responsibilities) are more likely to experience the negative effects of social media, including depression [27], cyberbullying, upward social comparison [27], and disordered eating [28]. It is worth noting that youths that engage in problematic use of social media often have some of the dispositional traits discussed above. Although it is difficult to parse out the extent to which use itself contributes to risk, evidence for the relationship between problematic use and mental health is strong. Historically, it was found that youths who use social media more passively (e.g., scrolling without engaging, posting, or commenting) may suffer from more negative outcomes (e.g., social disconnection, stress, anxiety, depression, and lower well-being) [29]. This relationship may be more pronounced for those with more extensive or problematic use and complex at an individual level [30]. More extensive and passive use of media may be associated with greater exposure to negative experiences (e.g., cyberbullying) [31] and online discrimination [14, 16]. Yet, some scholars suggest that this dichotomy of passive use being negative and active use being positive has too many exceptions to truly understand youths' experiences online and outcomes for well-being. Instead, an extended model of active–passive social media use may provide a better insight into the relationship between social media use and mental health. Future research may apply this model to identify how youth characteristics intersect with different types of social media uses and youth reasons for use.

### 2.7 Key Limitations and Summary

Youths with offline vulnerabilities for mental health problems, due to individual characteristics, developmental changes, or environmental experiences, may be more likely to suffer from the negative effects of social media. Such individual or contextual vulnerabilities include female (cisgender) sex, minoritized identities, lower socioeconomic households, preexisting mental health problems, and problematic engagement with media. Youths at the intersection of these vulnerabilities may be at the greatest risk and warrant special consideration. For instance, girls who identify as LGBTQIA+ are "socially vulnerable" and have depressive symptoms, appear more likely to engage in problematic use, focus more on social media metrics, and have negative experiences on social media (though they may also benefit more from positive experiences) [32]. Yet, most existing research studies are limited by their use of cross-sectional designs, their focus on only usage patterns compared to social–emotional experiences, and their reliance upon self-reported measures. Furthermore, most studies examining direct effects find small effect sizes, within sufficient examination of potential moderators to better understand who is most at risk.

## 3 Future Research

Critical future directions to advance identification of youths at the greatest risk for negative mental health effects of media and to guide recommendations include the following:

- *Who is most affected and when?* Systematic inclusion of potential moderating factors, including demographic and other individual characteristics, and broader environmental factors, is needed to differentiate who is most affected, how, and under what circumstances. Research is needed to further consider the diverse experiences of youths with minoritized identities, including intersecting identities, on social media and mental health, especially given research highlighting the unique risks and benefits of social media in these populations. Longitudinal studies with nationally representative samples and cohort studies may be particularly useful in probing these relationships, with sufficient power to detect effects. A focus on modifiable factors that can be actively identified and targeted in clinical and educational settings (where teens are) is critical, beyond focus on only identity-based characteristics.
- *What is working well and for whom?* Most teens are *both* negatively and positively affected by specific aspects of their media engagement. Idiographic and mixed method studies are needed to better understand within-person effects, which would move beyond identifying who is most at risk, but also *when* media are conferring risk or protection at an individual level. Furthermore, studies using mixed methods and ambulatory assessment (e.g., ecological momentary assessment) monitoring of social media may offer a more accurate assessment of the temporal dynamics of engagement in media use and mental health [33]. A focus on applying strength-based or resiliency frameworks will better clarify risks and benefits, particularly when focusing on youths with minoritized identities.
- *What shared or unique mechanisms link media use and mental health outcomes for youth?* Identifying the potential mediators linking social media and mental health would move beyond the direct effects of the relationships currently explored. For instance, to what extent and for whom do social media drive social comparison, disruption of healthy habits and relationships, or effects on attention, memory, and social cognition? Additionally, emerging research suggests that the frequency of using certain platforms may be linked to specific mental health and behavioral health outcomes [34]. Exploring the mechanisms linking social media and different types of mental health problems, and the moderators of these relationships (e.g., moderated mediation frameworks), are critical to better identify the risks and prevent mental health problems.

## 4 Recommendations

Based on the current state of the field, recommendations for various stakeholders follow. Of note, recommendations may apply to more types of media uses than only social media, though social media remain the focus. Overall, recommendations center on the importance of assessment and ongoing dialogue about social media use among youths and their parents/guardians, clinicians, pediatricians, and researchers as part of mental health check-ins for all youths.

- Parents should become informed to effectively supervise and scaffold their teen's social media use and engage in open and ongoing dialogue about related health effects.
  - Seek out education to understand teens' positive and negative uses of social media, the types of social media with which your teen engages, and sample them yourself.
  - Social media's impact on mental health changes across development, and each young person will have a different relationship with media based on their individual characteristics and vulnerabilities. Tailor parental mediation of youth technology use to the teen's unique profile, including maturity, degree of responsibility shown in online behaviors, positive uses (e.g., for social support), and individual risk and protective factors.
  - Engage teens in ongoing dialogue about how media choices affect mental health, recognizing negative and positive effects. Invite youths to participate in setting expectations and limits around media use. Such active parental mediation, in combination with age- and individual-appropriate limit setting, may mitigate media's negative effects.
  - Engage in limit setting of social media to ensure healthy engagement in offline activities, particularly given the potential for problematic use to occur within this population.
  - Parental modeling of healthy media engagement, considering impacts on parents' own mental health, is critical to instill healthy use among teens.
- For teens with existing mental health problems, clinicians and parents should conduct more thorough assessments of media use via ongoing dialogue to identify the effects of media.
  - Clinicians should routinely inquire about social media use at regular intervals, ideally assessing overall experience and interactions, frequency and duration, problematic use, and the nature of content. Adolescents have expressed discomfort sharing openly about social media experiences, even those they find distressing, unless clinicians ask about this directly [35].
  - It is important to evaluate how such teens are using social media to understand influences on mental health, including both risks and benefits. Posting about mental health, exposure to negative content (e.g., suicide, self-harm, and alcohol use), negative interactions, extent of use, and investment in social media use may exacerbate mental health problems.
  - Recognize the potential for social media to offer mental health support and resources. Determine the veracity of online sources that teens use to learn about mental health and the nature of online communities with which they interact, which can offer teens a source of information and support when accurate (e.g., evidence-based).
- For teens who hold minoritized identities or from lower income households, clinicians and parents should regularly assess identity-based experiences and provide resources as needed.
  - Assess the experiences of cyberbullying and exposure to online identity-based victimization (i.e., vicarious and direct discrimination based on race, gender, sexual orientation, etc.). Online discrimination can negatively affect mental health, so it is especially important to check in with youth with minoritized identities to understand how such experiences impact them. Recognize that there is heterogeneity in the online experiences of such youths.
  - Recognize that youths from lower socioeconomic households may need more scaffolding and support around media,

particularly in moderating use, if this is a challenge given their individual environment.
- Teens should be encouraged to monitor and self-regulate their own media use. Usage may be evaluated via objective (e.g., "screen time" reports) and subjective measures (e.g., intermittent assessment of how media experiences make them feel) to identify interactions that affect well-being. Identify when media use has both negative and positive impacts on mental health for the individual to inform self-regulation.
- Researchers should include measures of media use in youth-focused mental health research to learn about how media influences teen mental health. Improve knowledge of this relationship through improved measurement (e.g., objective measures) and longitudinal design.
- Industry should partner with key informants (e.g., researchers, teens, clinicians, educators) to provide data to help better identify which youths are most vulnerable to the negative effects of media use on mental health and subsequently limit identified features that exacerbate these effects.

**Conflict of Interest and Funding Disclosures** None.

## References


1. Odgers CL, Jensen MR. Annual Research Review: adolescent mental health in the digital age: facts, fears, and future directions. J Child Psychol Psychiatry. 2020;61(3):336–48. https://doi.org/10.1111/jcpp.13190.
2. Vogels E, Gelles-Watnick R, Teens MN. Social Media and Technology 2022. Pew Research Center: Internet, Science & Tech. Published August 10, 2022. https://www.pewresearch.org/internet/2022/08/10/teens-social-media-and-technology-2022/.
3. Valkenburg PM, Peter J. The differential susceptibility to media effects model: differential susceptibility to media effects model. J Commun. 2013;63(2):221–43. https://doi.org/10.1111/jcom.12024.
4. Rideout V, Fox S. Digital health practices, social media use, and mental well-being among teens and young adults in the U.S. Artic Abstr Rep. 2018;1093. https://digitalcommons.psjhealth.org/publications/1093.
5. Choukas-Bradley S, Kilic Z, Stout CD, Roberts SR. Perfect storms and double-edged swords: recent advances in research on adolescent social media use and mental health. Adv Psychiatry Behav Health. 2023;3(1):149–57. https://doi.org/10.1016/j.ypsc.2023.03.007.
6. Marchant A, Hawton K, Stewart A, et al. A systematic review of the relationship between internet use, self-harm and suicidal behaviour in young people: the good, the bad and the unknown. Choo KKR, ed. PLoS One. 2017;12(8):e0181722. https://doi.org/10.1371/journal.pone.0181722.
7. CDC. U.S. Teen girls experiencing increased sadness and violence. Centers for Disease Control and Prevention. Published February 13, 2023. Accessed March 30, 2023. https://www.cdc.gov/media/releases/2023/p0213-yrbs.html.
8. Booker CL, Kelly YJ, Sacker A. Gender differences in the associations between age trends of social media interaction and well-being among 10–15 year olds in the UK. BMC Public Health. 2018;18(1):321. https://doi.org/10.1186/s12889-018-5220-4.
9. Kreski N, Platt J, Rutherford C, et al. Social media use and depressive symptoms among United States adolescents. J Adolesc Health. 2021;68(3):572–9. https://doi.org/10.1016/j.jadohealth.2020.07.006.
10. Nesi J, Prinstein MJ. Using social media for social comparison and feedback-seeking: gender and popularity moderate associations with depressive symptoms. J Abnorm Child Psychol. 2015;43(8):1427–38. https://doi.org/10.1007/s10802-015-0020-0.
11. Orben A, Przybylski AK, Blakemore SJ, Kievit RA. Windows of developmental sensitivity to social media. Nat Commun. 2022;13(1):1649. https://doi.org/10.1038/s41467-022-29296-3.
12. Jensen M, George MJ, Russell MR, Odgers CL. Young adolescents' digital technology use and mental health symptoms: little evidence of longitudinal or daily linkages. Clin Psychol Sci. 2019;7(6):1416–33. https://doi.org/10.1177/2167702619859336.
13. Kim S, Colwell SR, Kata A, Boyle MH, Georgiades K. Cyberbullying victimization and adolescent mental health: evidence of differential effects by sex and mental health problem type. J Youth Adolesc. 2018;47(3):661–72. https://doi.org/10.1007/s10964-017-0678-4.
14. Nesi J, Choukas-Bradley S, Prinstein MJ. Transformation of adolescent peer relations in the social media context: part 1—A theoretical framework and application to dyadic peer relationships. Clin Child Fam Psychol Rev. 2018;21(3):267–94. https://doi.org/10.1007/s10567-018-0261-x.
15. Saha K, Kim SC, Reddy MD, et al. The language of LGBTQ+ minority stress experiences on social media. Proc ACM Hum Comput Interact. 2019;3(CSCW):1–22. https://doi.org/10.1145/3361108.
16. Tynes BM, English D, Del Toro J, Smith NA, Lozada FT, Williams DR. Trajectories of online racial discrimination and psychological functioning among

African American and Latino adolescents. Child Dev. 2020;91(5):1577–93. https://doi.org/10.1111/cdev.13350.
17. Berger MN, Taba M, Marino JL, Lim MSC, Skinner SR. Social media use and health and well-being of lesbian, gay, bisexual, transgender, and queer youth: systematic review. J Med Internet Res. 2022;24(9):e38449. https://doi.org/10.2196/38449.
18. Tao X, Fisher CB. Exposure to social media racial discrimination and mental health among adolescents of color. J Youth Adolesc. 2022;51(1):30–44. https://doi.org/10.1007/s10964-021-01514-z.
19. Nesi J, Burke TA, Bettis AH, et al. Social media use and self-injurious thoughts and behaviors: a systematic review and meta-analysis. Clin Psychol Rev. 2021;87:102038. https://doi.org/10.1016/j.cpr.2021.102038.
20. Maxie-Moreman AD, Tynes BM. Exposure to online racial discrimination and traumatic events online in Black adolescents and emerging adults. J Res Adolesc. 2022;32(1):254–69. https://doi.org/10.1111/jora.12732.
21. George MJ, Jensen MR, Russell MA, et al. Young adolescents' digital technology use, perceived impairments, and well-being in a representative sample. J Pediatr. 2020;219:180–7. https://doi.org/10.1016/j.jpeds.2019.12.002.
22. Kostyrka-Allchorne K, Stoilova M, Bourgaize J, Rahali M, Livingstone S, Sonuga-Barke E. Review: digital experiences and their impact on the lives of adolescents with pre-existing anxiety, depression, eating and nonsuicidal self-injury conditions – a systematic review. Child Adolesc Ment Health. 2023;28(1):22–32. https://doi.org/10.1111/camh.12619.
23. Vidal C, Lhaksampa T, Miller L, Platt R. Social media use and depression in adolescents: a scoping review. Int Rev Psychiatry Abingdon Engl. 2020;32(3):235–53. https://doi.org/10.1080/09540261.2020.1720623.
24. Szlyk HS, Li X, Kasson E, et al. How do teens with a history of suicidal behavior and self-harm interact with social media? J Adolesc. 2023:1–14. https://doi.org/10.1002/jad.12154.
25. Akkın Gürbüz HG, Demir T, Gökalp Özcan B, Kadak MT, Poyraz BÇ. Use of social network sites among depressed adolescents. Behav Inf Technol. 2017;36(5):517–23. https://doi.org/10.1080/0144929X.2016.1262898.
26. Shafi RMA, Nakonezny PA, Miller KA, et al. An exploratory study of clinical and physiological correlates of problematic social media use in adolescents. Psychiatry Res. 2021;302:114020. https://doi.org/10.1016/j.psychres.2021.114020.
27. Boer M, Stevens GWJM, Finkenauer C, de Looze ME, van den Eijnden RJJM. Social media use intensity, social media use problems, and mental health among adolescents: Investigating directionality and mediating processes. Comput Hum Behav. 2021;116:106645. https://doi.org/10.1016/j.chb.2020.106645.
28. Jiotsa B, Naccache B, Duval M, Rocher B, Grall-Bronnec M. Social media use and body image disorders: association between frequency of comparing one's own physical appearance to that of people being followed on social media and body dissatisfaction and drive for thinness. Int J Environ Res Public Health. 2021;18(6):2880. https://doi.org/10.3390/ijerph18062880.
29. Frison E, Eggermont S. Toward an integrated and differential approach to the relationships between loneliness, different types of Facebook use, and adolescents' depressed mood. Commun Res. 2020;47(5):701–28. https://doi.org/10.1177/0093650215617506.
30. Valkenburg PM, van Driel II, Beyens I. The associations of active and passive social media use with well-being: a critical scoping review. New Media Soc. 2022;24(2):530–49. https://doi.org/10.1177/14614448211065425.
31. Fredrick SS, Nickerson AB, Livingston JA. Adolescent social media use: pitfalls and promises in relation to cybervictimization, friend support, and depressive symptoms. J Youth Adolesc. 2022;51(2):361–76. https://doi.org/10.1007/s10964-021-01561-6.
32. Teens and Mental Health: How Girls Really Feel About Social Media | Common Sense Media. Accessed March 30, 2023. https://www.commonsensemedia.org/research/teens-and-mental-health-how-girls-really-feel-about-social-media.
33. Gansner M, Nisenson M, Lin V, Carson N, Torous J. Piloting smartphone digital phenotyping to understand problematic internet use in an adolescent and young adult sample. Child Psychiatry Hum Dev. 2022; https://doi.org/10.1007/s10578-022-01313-y.
34. Vassey J, Galimov A, Kennedy CJ, Vogel EA, Unger JB. Frequency of social media use and exposure to tobacco or nicotine-related content in association with E-cigarette use among youth: a cross-sectional and longitudinal survey analysis. Prev Med Rep. 2022;30:102055. https://doi.org/10.1016/j.pmedr.2022.102055.
35. Biernesser C, Zelazny J, Brent D, Bear T, Mair C, Trauth J. Automated monitoring of suicidal adolescents' digital media use: qualitative study exploring acceptability within clinical care. JMIR Ment Health. 2021;8(9):e26031. https://doi.org/10.2196/26031.

# Digital Therapeutics in Child Psychiatry: Harnessing Technology to Treat Pediatric Mental Health

Meredith Gansner, Nicholas C. Jacobson, Lisa A. Marsch, and Randy Kulman

## 1 Background

Digital media have become an integral part of youths' everyday lives, encompassing recreation, extracurricular activities, and academics. The ease with which children and adolescents have readily adapted to using digital technologies, and the amount of time they spend engaging with screens, has prompted a growing interest in use of these technologies in pediatric health care. Similar to how digital innovations like smartphone-based ecological momentary assessment have improved existing methods of data collection in pediatric research [1], digital therapeutics such as smartphone applications and video games have the potential to improve treatment outcomes in pediatric mental health.

Novel treatment modalities in child and adolescent psychiatry are becoming increasingly important. Higher rates of childhood anxiety and depression internationally [2] have resulted in overburdened mental health-care systems unable to meet the growing demands for psychiatric treatment. Early recognition and treatment of psychiatric illness in childhood is imperative and requires a multipronged approach [3]. Untreated chronic mental illness can impair employment, interpersonal relationships, and physical health. Evidence-based digital therapeutics could alleviate some of the pressure experienced by pediatric mental health systems while also improving patient outcomes.

By leveraging widespread ownership of digital devices and the ability to gather and integrate diverse streams of sensor-based data from smartphones and wearables (e.g., smartwatches), digital therapeutics could help address significant limitations of existing mental health systems [4, 5]. First, they could make evidence-based mental health treatments more accessible. National implementation of telepsychiatry was accelerated by the COVID-19 pandemic, but it failed to address the shortage of pediatric mental health providers. Digital tools that help patients manage their psychiatric conditions outside the clinical setting could enable a reduced frequency of clinical visits, thus increasing the overall number of patients who can be seen by a practitioner. Furthermore, pediatric patients often struggle to practice the skills they learn during treatment sessions, delaying symptom improvement and pro-

M. Gansner (✉)
Department of Psychiatry, Boston Children's Hospital, Boston, MA, USA

N. C. Jacobson · L. A. Marsch
Center for Technology and Behavioral Health, Dartmouth College, Lebanon, NH, USA

R. Kulman
LearningWorks for Kids, Wakefield, RI, USA


D. A. Christakis, L. Hale (eds.), *Handbook of Children and Screens*,
https://doi.org/10.1007/978-3-031-69362-5_23

longing the treatment course. An interactive digital interface that is able to provide real-time feedback could offer users a more granular understanding of their psychiatric symptoms [6], as well as an engaging modality to reinforce self-regulatory techniques between clinical sessions, thus bolstering treatment efficacy and efficiency.

Unfortunately, the rapidly growing number of publicly available digital products claiming to benefit mental health (including thousands of mental health apps) has created market confusion. The efficacy of each digital intervention is often evaluated differently (if evaluated at all), and it is challenging for both patients and clinicians to become knowledgeable about each new digital intervention and the evidence-based research that supports its use in treatment. This chapter of existing digital therapeutics targeting child mental health symptoms examines both commercially available interventions and those not yet readily accessible. Rather than providing a comprehensive list of all existing interventions, this chapter focuses on those digital treatments with a more robust body of research evidence supporting their use; interventions are grouped by the category of psychiatric disorder, and a broad overview of the technologies featured here can be found in Table 1.

## 2 Current State

Recent years have seen significant progress in the development of digital therapeutics for pediatric mental health, including the publication of dozens of studies investigating the efficacy of various digital approaches [7–20]. Most existing digital therapeutics are designed to augment existing treatment modalities and can be categorized into either: (1) treatments that use gamification to improve symptom management or (2) therapeutics that rely on repeated temporal assessments of symptoms and behavioral patterns to manage interactions between an individual's thoughts, symptoms, and behaviors (i.e., ecological momentary intervention or EMI). Some applications incorporate elements of both EMI and gaming, and interventions in both groups process active data input by the patient in order to provide individualized feedback. While each therapeutic may differ in terms of its symptom target and user interface, all digital interventions must be easy to use, accessible, cost-effective, and efficacious.

Digital interventions have been designed to address a wide variety of pediatric psychiatric disorders and symptoms. However, the majority of existing digital interventions target the symptoms of more prevalent psychiatric illnesses in children and adolescents (e.g., depression,

**Table 1** Summary of the digital interventions discussed in this chapter

| Name | Maker | Treatment target | Treatment modality |
|---|---|---|---|
| EndeavorRx | Akili Interactive | ADHD-related inattention | Video game-based platform for cognitive training |
| Joon | Joon Care Inc. | ADHD-related executive dysfunction | Gamified CBT |
| PlayAttention | Unique Logic + Technology, Inc. | ADHD-related inattention, executive dysfunction and mood dysregulation | Neurofeedback, Cognitive training exercises |
| SparkRx | Limbix Health | Addiction, Substance use disorder (SUD) | CBT and Behavioral activation protocols |
| MoodGYM | The Australian National University | Depression and Anxiety | CBT |
| Mission: Amygdala | Calmsie Health | Anxiety and stress management | Video game-based CBT |
| CopeSmart | CopeSmart Technologies, Inc | Stress, Anxiety | EMI to teach increased emotional awareness and regulation |
| Mightier | Neuromotion Labs | Emotional regulation | Biofeedback-based gaming intervention |

anxiety, and attention-deficit/hyperactivity disorder (ADHD)), whereas few studies explore the efficacy of digital treatments for uncommon, high-risk diagnoses such as eating, psychotic or personality disorders [7].

## 2.1 Digital Therapeutics Targeting ADHD

The comorbidity between ADHD and problematic gaming is well-known [21], making ADHD and its associated symptoms prime targets for gamified treatment options that utilize neurofeedback techniques. In 2020, EndeavorRx became the first and only video game to receive Food and Drug Administration (FDA) approval as a "prescription digital therapeutic" for treatment of ADHD-related inattention based on its performance in 5 clinical studies in more than 600 children [16]. Similar to medication treatments, EndeavorRx is only available via prescription and may be covered by insurance. The therapeutic game uses an algorithm to provide individualized treatment for each patient's unique profile, with the goal of improving patient focus and the ability to avoid distractions. However, outstanding concerns remain regarding the potential of EndeavorRx. For example, it is unclear to what extent the improvement seen in clinical trials translates to ADHD-related inattention in the real-world setting. Other commercially available digital treatment options for pediatric ADHD include Joon, a gamified smartphone application for iPhone or android that also purports to improve focus as well as assist with time management and task completion [22], and the computer-based attention-training system by Play Attention [23], which, similar to EndeavorRx, offers individualized feedback to optimize executive functioning and behavioral regulation. Randomized controlled trials (RCTs) exist to support the use of other video game treatments for ADHD, but these interventions are presently only available for research, and few have been studied in more than one or two clinical trials [24].

## 2.2 Digital Therapeutics Targeting Anxiety and Depression

Across studies of digital mental health interventions for children and adolescents, depression and anxiety appear to be the most commonly targeted symptoms [7]. These interventions frequently adapt evidence-based cognitive behavioral therapy (CBT) protocols for anxiety and depression in a computerized format. Marketing itself as "the first digital treatment for adolescent depression," Limbix Health's SparkRx is a 5-week digital program that borrows from both CBT and behavioral activation protocols; while SparkRx is commercially available as long as the user is under a doctor's care, it is still in pursuit of FDA approval based on the initial results from a virtual RCT in 121 adolescents and subsequent studies [25]. MoodGYM is another multi-session, CBT-based online program that has been assessed in the adolescent population; three school-based RCTs indicated a reduction in both anxiety and depressive symptoms in adolescents, although with a range of effect sizes [9, 17, 18]. Innovative digital interventions for these disorders also include the packaging of CBT techniques into less traditional vehicles; Mission: Amygdala, a video game developed by Calmsie, incorporates avatars to help youths learn CBT for anxiety and depression [26]. This intervention engages patients in a video game-based space journey that requires them to manage their challenging emotions while video-bot avatars engage in real-time conversations with the patients, helping them develop strategies to gain better control over their negative thoughts, emotions, and actions [26].

## 2.3 Digital Therapeutics Targeting Substance Use

Given the difficulties with treatment access and adherence for patients who struggle with substance use disorders (SUDs), digital interventions for substance use disorders (SUDs) have the potential to provide enormous benefits. ReSET and ReSET-O (for opioid use disorder) are the first FDA-approved digital therapeutics that can be prescribed for adjunctive treatment of adult SUDs, with authorization based on a multisite, unblinded 12-week clinical trial [27]. ReSET and ReSET-O offer Internet-based cognitive behavioral therapy with additional emphasis on those specific evidence-based techniques used when treating individuals with SUDs, like contingency management. Preliminary research suggests that digital interventions may also be beneficial for pediatric SUDs. For example, mindfulness-based interventions may be suitably administered via EMI to reduce cravings [28], and some studies on digital treatments for other conditions have demonstrated benefit for youth substance use as well [29].

## 2.4 Digital Therapeutics Targeting Nonspecific Psychiatric Symptoms and Overall Wellness

Rather than focusing on a specific psychiatric diagnosis, some digital interventions aim to reduce symptoms common to multiple psychiatric diagnoses (e.g., executive functioning or emotional regulation). Studied in an RCT of more than 200 adolescents, CopeSmart is a digital therapeutic that uses EMI to teach increased emotional awareness and regulation [14, 15]. Mightier is a series of video games that use biofeedback via a wireless heart rate monitor to help children and adolescents develop and practice emotional regulation skills, improving outburst frequency and long-term regulation skills in two double-blinded randomized sham-control trials and anger in another open-label study [13, 30]. Additionally, a 2022 meta-analysis found evidence to suggest that digital CBT for insomnia (CBT-i) could be a moderately effective therapeutic for adolescent insomnia based on data from four RCTs [31]. Recently, FDA-approved NightWare and Somryst, prescription digital interventions that operationalize behavioral therapies for the treatment of adult post-traumatic stress disorder (PTSD)-related nightmares [32] and insomnia [33], respectively, have been able to provide some guidance regarding what such therapeutics could look like in the pediatric population.

## 2.5 Limitations of the Current Research and Application

Despite a number of studies evaluating digital interventions for treatment of disorders like ADHD, anxiety, or depression, the heterogeneity of study design makes it challenging to compare findings across studies. In general, few digital tools are supported by data from multiple clinical trials, with numerous mental health applications commercially available without a single RCT. Even when a specific therapeutic has been scrutinized in multiple studies, these studies may vary in terms of the quality of study design or may use different clinical assessment scales or outcome measures to determine clinical efficacy [7, 29, 34]. Additionally, while intervention acceptability (e.g., ease of use) tends to be good, many studies recruit pediatric patients with only mild or moderate psychiatric symptoms, so it is difficult to generalize such findings to a whole clinical population [7]. Digital health interventions for pediatric mental health that adopt CBT techniques appear most effective, but the degree to which an intervention requires participant self-direction can impact adherence and therefore efficacy [7].

Even if an intervention appears acceptable and effective, additional barriers limit the widespread adoption of digital therapeutics. For the minor patient and family, significant privacy concerns persist regarding the collection and handling of personal mental health information. For example, disclosures regarding data-sharing practices appear particularly inadequate or inconsistent for commercially available smartphone applications for mental health [35]. Lack of accessibility to a reliable Internet connection, high cost, and low digital literacy can also limit a patient's ability to benefit from digital tools. A clinician's own digital literacy can impact whether they recommend any digital therapeutic to a patient, and a lack of knowledge about the data supporting available digital treatment options may make clinicians feel poorly equipped to discuss a tool's potential risks and benefits.

## 3 Future Research

In order to take advantage of novel technological advancements, digital therapeutic development moves quickly, particularly within industry. Public enthusiasm surrounding new cutting-edge technologies like virtual reality or artificial intelligence-assisted treatments [36] fuels rapid creation of new digital therapeutics that outpaces the performance of independently funded randomized control trials to assess each new intervention [7]. Therefore, efficacy studies are frequently funded (and performed) by the companies that developed the technology being evaluated, thus creating a potential conflict of interest. More unbiased replication studies are needed for the overwhelming majority of digital interventions in order to establish efficacy and compare with that of existing mental health treatments.

"Non-digital" CBT and other behavioral therapies have been shown to improve treatment outcomes for numerous psychiatric diagnoses, but treatment nonadherence is a frequent limitation. Studies piloting digital CBT for youth anxiety and depression evaluate participant adherence differently, making it difficult to draw conclusions about to what degree protocol adherence impacts intervention outcomes [37]. For the many digital interventions based on CBT protocols or including components of CBT, research is needed to investigate acceptability and effectiveness for patients of various demographics and with psychiatric comorbidities. This lack of population-specific data leads to uncertainty regarding which patients might benefit from newer neurotechnologies, further limiting access to appropriate mental health care for understudied populations.

Finally, more research is needed to establish the long-term effectiveness of those interventions for which short-term efficacy has been established. Existing studies are typically short in duration and cannot address how long symptom improvement will last. Children and adolescents may struggle to maintain their engagement with an intervention in the long term, and there is no consensus regarding the optimal study protocol length to test long-term adherence in this novel field. Follow-up studies are also needed to assess how skills gained via these digital technologies effectively translate to real-world settings. For example, a child who learns to control their emotional reactivity in a video game may or may not be able to operationalize that skill in a chaotic classroom environment.

## 4 Recommendations

As the field of digital therapeutics continues to expand, collaboration between researchers, clinicians, technology developers, and policymakers will be critical. Each of the above has distinct responsibilities to address the important questions that remain surrounding the development and implementation of effective, ethical, and equitable digital therapeutics.

- *How can we ensure that new interventions are subjected to unbiased testing?* Regulatory approval for new pediatric digital health interventions should require full transparency regarding funding sources and clear policies related to data sharing.
- *How can we ensure that these technologies are accessible to **all** youth?* Racial and ethnic minority individuals are less likely to access mental health care, including digital treatments like video televisits [38, 39]. It is imperative that we build not only effective digital treatments but also infrastructure to help underserved communities access these treatments. Local governments should ensure that these communities have reliable Internet access and options for affordable ownership of Internet-capable devices. Federally funded health insurance programs like Medicaid and Medicare should ensure coverage of novel digital treatments.
- *How can we ensure that these technologies offer effective treatments to **all** youth?* There

should also be greater incentive for innovators, particularly those in the private sector, to ensure that their technologies do not perpetuate existing inequities in access to mental health care. Federal funding should be prioritized for projects that outline plans for diverse subject recruitment and assess acceptability and feasibility in racial and ethnic minority populations. For example, Black men in the United States are experiencing disproportionate rates of fatal opioid overdoses compared to other races and ethnicities [27]. Thus, it is critical that interventions designed to treat adolescent SUDs assess intervention efficacy specifically in Black adolescents as well as other populations.

- *How should clinicians incorporate these technologies into patient care?* The rapid pace at which new digital therapeutics are developed makes it increasingly challenging for clinicians to be up to date with all available digital treatment options. Thus, clinicians should prioritize guiding patients and their families toward a consistent framework to use when evaluating a new digital therapeutic. While the choice of any treatment option should always be a personal decision, it is recommended that each tool be evaluated in at least five areas: background information about the tool (e.g., cost, developer, compatible phone operating systems), privacy/safety, evidence/clinical foundation, usability, and therapeutic target [40]. Clinicians also need to feel comfortable discussing issues of data privacy, if they will be accessing a patient's data (and if so, how frequently), and how the therapeutic might affect their existing treatment relationship with the patient.
- *How do we ensure that clinicians remain up to date on these new treatment interventions?* Medical societies should offer education about digital therapeutics in continuing medical education (CME) activities. Clinician training programs must develop and provide curricula pertaining to the use of digital therapeutics in the treatment of pediatric psychiatric illness. State licensing boards could also make learning about digital therapeutics a requisite part of CME, and individual hospital systems can invite educational speakers who are able to provide related education. Educational activities about digital therapeutics should review treatment options, teach attendees how to assess a new intervention, and discuss ethical implications of the use of digital therapeutics in clinical treatment.

**Conflict of Interest and Funding Disclosures** MG and NJ have no conflicts of interest or disclosures related to this content. LM has affiliations with Pear Therapeutics, Square2 Systems, and Click Therapeutics, and these relationships are extensively managed by LM's institution, Dartmouth College. RK has previously done consulting work for Akili Interactive Labs, the developer of EndeavorRx.

## References

1. Russell MA, Gajos JM. Annual research review: ecological momentary assessment studies in child psychology and psychiatry. J Child Psychol Psychiatry. 2020;61(3):376–94. https://doi.org/10.1111/jcpp.13204.
2. Benton TB, Boyd RC, Njoroge WFM. Addressing the global crisis of child and adolescent mental health. JAMA Pediatr. 2021;175(11):1108–10.
3. Colizzi M, Lasalvia A, Ruggeri M. Prevention and early intervention in youth mental health: is it time for a multidisciplinary and trans-diagnostic model for care? Int J Ment Health Syst. 2020;14(23):1–14.
4. Torous J, Baker JT. Why psychiatry needs data science and data science needs psychiatry: connecting with technology. JAMA Psychiatry. 2016;73(1):3. https://doi.org/10.1001/jamapsychiatry.2015.2622.
5. Insel TR. Digital phenotyping: a global tool for psychiatry. World Psychiatry. 2018;17(3):276–7. https://doi.org/10.1002/wps.20550.
6. Nisenson M, Lin V, Gansner M. Digital phenotyping in child and adolescent psychiatry: a perspective. Harv Rev Psychiatry. 2021; Publish Ahead of Print. https://doi.org/10.1097/HRP.0000000000000310
7. Hollis C, Falconer CJ, Martin JL, et al. Annual Research Review: digital health interventions for children and young people with mental health problems – a systematic and meta-review. J Child Psychol Psychiatry. 2017;58(4):474–503. https://doi.org/10.1111/jcpp.12663.
8. Byrne S, Kotze B, Ramos F, Casties A, Starling J, Harris A. Integrating a mobile health device into a community youth mental health team to manage severe mental illness: protocol for a randomized controlled trial. JMIR Res Protoc. 2020;9(11):e19510. https://doi.org/10.2196/19510.

9. Calear AL, Christensen H, Mackinnon A, Griffiths KM, O'Kearney R. The YouthMood Project: a cluster randomized controlled trial of an online cognitive behavioral program with adolescents. J Consult Clin Psychol. 2009;77(6):1021–32. https://doi.org/10.1037/a0017391.
10. Casella CB, Zuccolo PF, Sugaya L, et al. Brief internet-delivered cognitive-behavioural intervention for children and adolescents with symptoms of anxiety and depression during the COVID-19 pandemic: a randomised controlled trial protocol. Trials. 2022;23(1):899. https://doi.org/10.1186/s13063-022-06836-2.
11. Dietvorst E, Aukes MA, Legerstee JS, et al. A smartphone serious game for adolescents (Grow It! App): development, feasibility, and acceptance study. JMIR Form Res. 2022;6(3):e29832. https://doi.org/10.2196/29832.
12. Domhardt M, Messner EM, Eder AS, et al. Mobile-based interventions for common mental disorders in youth: a systematic evaluation of pediatric health apps. Child Adolesc Psychiatry Ment Health. 2021;15(1):49. https://doi.org/10.1186/s13034-021-00401-6.
13. Ducharme P, Kahn J, Vaudreuil C, et al. A "Proof of Concept" randomized controlled trial of a video game requiring emotional regulation to augment anger control training. Front Psychiatry. 2021;12:591906. https://doi.org/10.3389/fpsyt.2021.591906.
14. Kenny R, Dooley B, Fitzgerald A. Ecological momentary assessment of adolescent problems, coping efficacy, and mood states using a mobile phone app: an exploratory study. JMIR Ment Health. 2016;3(4):e51. https://doi.org/10.2196/mental.6361.
15. Kenny R, Dooley B, Fitzgerald A. Feasibility of "CopeSmart": a telemental health app for adolescents. JMIR Ment Health. 2015;2(3):e22. https://doi.org/10.2196/mental.4370.
16. Kollins SH, DeLoss DJ, Cañadas E, et al. A novel digital intervention for actively reducing severity of paediatric ADHD (STARS-ADHD): a randomised controlled trial. Lancet Digit Health. 2020;2(4):e168–78. https://doi.org/10.1016/S2589-7500(20)30017-0.
17. O'Kearney R, Kang K, Christensen H, Griffiths K. A controlled trial of a school-based Internet program for reducing depressive symptoms in adolescent girls. Depress Anxiety. 2009;26(1):65–72. https://doi.org/10.1002/da.20507.
18. O'Kearney R, Gibson M, Christensen H, Griffiths KM. Effects of a cognitive-behavioural internet program on depression, vulnerability to depression and stigma in adolescent males: a school-based controlled trial. Cogn Behav Ther. 2006;35(1):43–54. https://doi.org/10.1080/16506070500303456.
19. Pramana G, Parmanto B, Kendall PC, Silk JS. The SmartCAT: an m-Health platform for ecological momentary intervention in child anxiety treatment. Telemed J E Health. 2014;20(5):419–27. https://doi.org/10.1089/tmj.2013.0214.
20. Pramana G, Parmanto B, Lomas J, Lindhiem O, Kendall PC, Silk J. Using mobile health gamification to facilitate cognitive behavioral therapy skills practice in child anxiety treatment: open clinical trial. JMIR Serious Games. 2018;6(2):e9. https://doi.org/10.2196/games.8902.
21. Sugaya N, Shirasaka T, Takahashi K, Kanda H. Bio-psychosocial factors of children and adolescents with internet gaming disorder: a systematic review. Biopsychosoc Med. 2019;13:3. https://doi.org/10.1186/s13030-019-0144-5.
22. Brenner B, Bunarjo K, Eaves I. Joon. Published online 2021. https://www.joonapp.io/
23. Play Attention. https://www.playattention.com/.
24. Peñuelas-Calvo I, Jiang-Lin LK, Girela-Serrano B, et al. Video games for the assessment and treatment of attention-deficit/hyperactivity disorder: a systematic review. Eur Child Adolesc Psychiatry. 2022;31(1):5–20. https://doi.org/10.1007/s00787-020-01557-w.
25. Limbix Health, Inc. A CBT-based mobile intervention as first line treatment for adolescent depression during COVID-19. 2020. https://clinicaltrials.gov/ct2/show/NCT04524598.
26. Calmsie. Mission: Amygdala. Published online 2021. https://missionamygdala.com/
27. Pear Therapeutics. ReSET. Published online 2023. https://www.resetforrecovery.com/reset
28. Shrier LA, Harris SK. Associations of momentary mindfulness with affect and cannabis desire in a trial of cannabis use interventions with and without momentary assessment. J Adolesc Health. 2023;72(1):126–9. https://doi.org/10.1016/j.jadohealth.2022.09.002.
29. Grist R, Porter J, Stallard P. Mental health mobile apps for preadolescents and adolescents: a systematic review. J Med Internet Res. 2017;19(5):e176. https://doi.org/10.2196/jmir.7332.
30. Mightier. Published online 2016. https://www.mightier.com.
31. Tsai HJ, Yang AC, Zhu JD, Hsu YY, Hsu TF, Tsai SJ. Effectiveness of digital cognitive behavioral therapy for insomnia in young people: preliminary findings from systematic review and meta-analysis. J Pers Med. 2022;12(3):481. https://doi.org/10.3390/jpm12030481.
32. Davenport ND, Werner JK. A randomized sham-controlled clinical trial of a novel wearable intervention for trauma-related nightmares in military veterans. J Clin Sleep Med. 2023;19(2):361–9. https://doi.org/10.5664/jcsm.10338.
33. Morin CM. Profile of Somryst prescription digital therapeutic for chronic insomnia: overview of safety and efficacy. Expert Rev Med Devices. 2020;17(12):1239–48. https://doi.org/10.1080/17434440.2020.1852929.
34. Reyes-Portillo JA, Mufson L, Greenhill LL, et al. Web-based interventions for youth internalizing problems: a systematic review. J Am Acad Child Adolesc Psychiatry. 2014;53(12):1254–1270.e5. https://doi.org/10.1016/j.jaac.2014.09.005.

35. Huckvale K, Torous J, Larsen ME. Assessment of the data sharing and privacy practices of smartphone apps for depression and smoking cessation. JAMA Netw Open. 2019;2(4):e192542. https://doi.org/10.1001/jamanetworkopen.2019.2542.
36. Götzl C, Hiller S, Rauschenberg C, et al. Artificial intelligence-informed mobile mental health apps for young people: a mixed-methods approach on users' and stakeholders' perspectives. Child Adolesc Psychiatry Ment Health. 2022;16(1):86. https://doi.org/10.1186/s13034-022-00522-6.
37. Li SH, Achilles MR, Werner-Seidler A, Beames JR, Subotic-Kerry M, O'Dea B. Appropriate use and operationalization of adherence to digital cognitive behavioral therapy for depression and anxiety in youth: systematic review. JMIR Ment Health. 2022;9(8):e37640. https://doi.org/10.2196/37640.
38. Eberly LA, Kallan MJ, Julien HM, et al. Patient characteristics associated with telemedicine access for primary and specialty ambulatory care during the COVID-19 pandemic. JAMA Netw Open. 2020;3(12):e2031640. https://doi.org/10.1001/jamanetworkopen.2020.31640.
39. Cauce AM, Domenech-Rodríguez M, Paradise M, et al. Cultural and contextual influences in mental health help seeking: a focus on ethnic minority youth. J Consult Clin Psychol. 2002;70(1):44–55. https://doi.org/10.1037/0022-006X.70.1.44.
40. Torous J, Luo J, Chan SR. Mental health apps: what to tell patients: an evaluation model created specifically for such apps can help guide your discussions. Curr Psychiatry. 2018;17(3):21–5.

# Introduction to the Section on Problematic Use of the Internet in Childhood and Adolescence

Don Grant and Hans-Jürgen Rumpf

## 1 Background

Global utilization of the Internet through various devices (computers, smart/mobile phones, and other electronics), which deliver its exponentially growing legions of myriad programs, websites, applications, gaming opportunities, social media, commerce, and communication platforms, has vigorously and dynamically increased over recent decades. While truly wonderful benefits of Internet engagement have been identified for users [1], there have also been cogent concerns expressed by experts, researchers, legislators, parents, and mental health professionals surrounding how excessive Internet use may also be correlated to seriously negative consequences for children and adolescents [2, 3]. While no country or global health organization has yet to sanctify "Internet Addiction" per se as a legitimate "diagnosis," several have targeted specific Internet-based behaviors (i.e., gaming) as such, while a significant number are also currently either in the process of considering its consecration, discussing or implementing guardrail legislation to reduce any risks potentially associated with it (especially in terms of child and adolescent online protection, health, and safety), and/or working in partnership with researchers and accredited advocates to discuss pragmatic strategies, regulations, recommendations, and solutions for the future [4–6].

Following a series of six subsequent annual expert meetings organized by the World Health Organization (WHO) focused on the public health implications of addictive behaviors within the conceptual framework of disorders due to addictive behaviors and the context of the *11th revision of the International Classification of Diseases* (ICD-11), the WHO officially adopted "Gaming Disorder" (GD) to be included in the ICD-11 [7]. The global expert group also continued its dedicated work by developing GD screening and diagnostic instruments [8]. The decision for the inclusion of GD was based on the scientific evidence for this condition to be regarded as a behavioral addiction, as well as the clear clinical and public health need [9]. Although the official diagnosis acceptance of any Internet-only behavior beyond those surrounding online gaming has not yet been acknowledged, the inclusion

*On behalf of all our authors, we also extend our sincerest appreciation to Children and Screens: Institute of Digital Media and Child Development and Springer Publishing, for the opportunity to contribute to this distinct, momentous, and important work.*

D. Grant (✉)
Center for Research and Innovation, Newport Healthcare, Nashville, Tennessee, USA

H.-J. Rumpf
University of Lübeck, Department of Psychiatry and Psychotherapy, Lübeck, Germany


D. A. Christakis, L. Hale (eds.), *Handbook of Children and Screens*,
https://doi.org/10.1007/978-3-031-69362-5_24

of GD in the ICD-11 provided a strong foothold in support of further research and discussion across the world regarding the potential validity of several others.

Toward that objective, and for the purposes, intent, and goals of the chapters included in this section, we invited global experts from the research, academic, media psychology, and clinical disciplines to examine and discuss four specific Internet-centric areas that we believe potentially pose the most significant risks for children and adolescents: *Problematic Internet Use (PIU)*, *GD*, *Dysregulated use of Mobile/Smartphone*, and *Treatment Considerations in Problematic Screen Use*.

## 2 Chapters

Each chapter included in this section details a specific Internet-driven behavior background (i.e. explaining why this issue is important and what its implications are/may be), current state (i.e., where we currently are with respect to this issue; what is known about it; why is it a problem; how might a solution; what are the limitations of our knowledge regarding it), the authors' suggestions for future research, and finally their recommendations for scientists, investigators, policymakers, educators, media technology creators and producers, treatment providers, clinicians, and mental health practitioners (i.e., pediatricians, educators, mental health professionals, and practitioners), and the general public moving forward.

### 2.1 Problematic Internet Use

In their chapter exploring *PIU*, the authors (see chapter "Problematic Internet Use: A General Perspective") annotate its defined background, various forms of symptomatic manifestations, recent improvements in specific instruments of assessment, epidemiology, underpinning mechanisms, the current state of both evidenced effective and emerging interventions, existent research, and finally their recommendations for stakeholders to consider. They also propose identifier correlations to impairment or distress across biological, psychological, sociological, and/or academic functioning and note that adolescents with vulnerabilities across developmental or sociological domains may be at higher risk of susceptibility for PIU.

### 2.2 Gaming Disorder

Although "Internet Gaming Disorder" remains classified as a "Condition for Further Study" in the *Diagnostic and Statistical Manual of Mental Disorders, Fifth Edition* (*DSM*-5) (published in 2013 by the American Psychiatric Association) [10], "Gaming Disorder" (as mentioned above) was recognized by the WHO as a formal diagnosis in 2019 and included in the *11th revision of the International Classification of Diseases* (ICD-11) [11]. With that global disparity in play, the authors (see chapter "Gaming Disorder Among Children and Adolescents") of our *GD* chapter offer an erudite examination of online gaming and GD, beginning with its pre-Internet roots in adolescent obsessions with amusement arcade video games, then chronicle its evolution to the massive and only expected to expand-online gaming opportunities available today. GD prevalence, etiology, and individualized biological, sociological, psychological, and environmental factors that may play a contributory role in the development of GD are discussed within this chapter, as are future research proposals. Recommendations for new screening instruments created especially for adolescent populations, country-specific regulatory oversight, gaming awareness programs for schools, parents, and educators, GD prevention programs, industry-funded treatment interventions, and data sharing obliged by governments (with the consensual goal of protecting the health and safety of adolescent gamers), are other suggestions of the globally respected GD expert authors of this chapter.

## 2.3 Dysregulated Use of Mobile/Smartphone

With the acknowledgment that though once primarily used for verbal communication, the mobile/smartphones of today have evolved into sophisticated devices that deliver (and by many individuals are substantially employed in the pursuit of) so much more, the authors (see chapter "Dysregulated Use of Mobile/Smartphone") of the *Dysregulated Use of Mobile/Smartphone* chapter provide a full review of the current state of mobile/smartphone research, identify gaps in the existent literature, and outline future directions for investigation and healthier mobile/smartphone practices by children and adolescents. Although not yet a recognized diagnosis, (and sometimes referred to in the literature as either "Smartphone Addiction" or "Problematic Smartphone Use" (PSU)), this chapter acknowledges the myriad functions our modern mobile/smartphones offer, including access to Internet applications, online platforms, content-based communication, educational opportunities, media streaming, pornography viewing, commerce, gaming, entertainment, and even lifestyle support. The chapter further catalogs mobile/smartphone measurements, dysregulated use of mobile/smartphone prevalence, risk factors, and correlates of use. Recommendations for new adolescent-focused assessments, healthy and safe mobile/smartphone use partnerships between children, their parents, educational environments, and technology producers, further considerations of protective mobile/smartphone design features for adolescents experiencing dysregulation or exacerbation of pre-existing struggles due to their mobile/smartphone use, and additional funding for research designed to better delineate criteria for distinguishing between normal (even if somewhat excessive) and dysregulated smartphone use to prevent further or future harm at the literal hands of adolescent users, are just a few of the authors' suggestions moving forward.

## 2.4 Treatment Considerations in Problematic Screen Use

The increase in screen-based struggles has, of course, equally positively correlated to the need and demand for evidence-based treatment across almost all Internet-driven behaviors. In this chapter, experts (see chapter "Treatment and Prevention of Internet Use Disorders in Children and Adolescents") with long-term experience in the treatment of PSU discuss its diagnostic nosology, identify biological pathways, and share the historical course of effective PSU treatment development over the past 2+ decades. They explain how the PSU treatment approach has historically often been guided by the standardized modalities and practices utilized to treat other behavioral addictions, including a significant focus on instant gratification, reward, reconditioning, and variable ratio reinforcement models. The authors further describe PSU prevalence, current and proposed standard models and modalities of treatment, and medication-assisted treatment through psychopharmacological support when/if appropriate. The early-age introduction of PSU intervention and prevention strategies is suggested. The authors note, however, that the evidence of prevention measures is premature and that specific treatments for young age groups have rarely been studied. While the authors agree that the standard addiction model can be useful in positively influencing the treatment process, they also outline current limitations. Due in part to the relative recency of this now profoundly emerging behavior, inadequate treatment subject numbers, patient noncompliance, and incongruent outcome measures are some of the more frustrating variables the authors identify as impediments to research study interpretations. They do believe that in the current culture of PSU treatment, a customized approach including the entire family, and utilizing multiple treatment modalities and settings, appears to offer the best opportunities for successful outcomes and rebalanced screen use recovery and sustainability. Finally, considerations for variances in the individualities of patients and their family situations, barriers to adaptive functioning, contexts, goals of screen use, and author proposals for future research are acknowledged.

## 3 Discussion

Although each chapter differs in terms of topic-focused content, an overall "takeaway" shared by all our authors is their strong, unanimous, and ardent recommendation for more research lensed toward adolescents and children across all the subjects explored through their individual works. Due in large part to the very nascent nature of these phenomena, there obviously has not been enough time to create an ideally robust library of conclusive investigative literature on just about any digital-based behavior, with some areas even demonstrating a clear paucity of externally valid or consensually agreed beliefs, proposals, or even consensual study outcomes.

While vigorously expanding interest, experts' expressed concerns, and growing public awareness have generated a tremendous surge in the contribution of both published and in-progress studies to the existent literature [8], the same lack of time dimension, as well as reasonable attribution to other reasons, (i.e. deficiencies in longitudinal studies, depth of diversity in research subject populations, inequities of opportunities/source material/data/funding/governmental support in certain geographic regions, and a dearth in legitimate investigations of specific Internet-driven behaviors), currently leaves our Internet research catalogs still somewhat anemic compared to other, more established, and psychometrically targeted subject areas.

In terms of the existing literature on our selected section topics (and again with the awareness of the lack of longitudinal studies and the relatively adolescent stage of widespread global Internet use itself), there is also some controversy regarding certain theories, beliefs, investigation outcomes, and even expert expressed concerns regarding some specific areas of adolescent and child Internet use and utilization. Scientists and investigators currently positing polarized hypotheses surrounding specific online behaviors such as social media use [1, 3, 12, 13], for example, demonstrate not only our lack of full understanding of their potential long-term impact but also the limits imposed by the immaturity of the Internet age itself. Sophisticated and evidence-based established theories of behavioral addictions have been developed, however, and are guiding both basic research as well as the design of promising interventions [14]. Such theories are of particular importance to future work. Thus, the chapters included within this section give clear guidance on what we already know and also what still needs to be studied surrounding each topic. Hopefully, this combined knowledge blueprint will further support the quick development of clear evidence to help us overcome, or even avoid, any impending controversies.

What we do know for certain is that the Internet (or its future evolutionary progeny) has already established itself as an (and dare we even say "the") increasingly significant, influential, and symbiotic partner in our daily lives. This trend is only expected to continue to proliferate. It is with this understanding that our authors have each dedicated their scholarship, research, and even careers (as well as the chapters they so generously contributed to this section) to the pursuit of investigating various aspects of the Internet, its perpetually fluid and expanding power, and how our interactions with it—and the devices that deliver it—potentially influence us, both positively and negatively.

During their organic stages of development, children are especially vulnerable to the impact of external variables across, arguably all areas and stages [15]. For our current generations of adolescents, this fact, layered with the timing of their births and maturation in exact synchronicity with those of the Internet, also means that they have been unwittingly positioned and will historically be remembered as having not only been its proverbial guinea pigs but also our metaphorical virtual canaries in the digital coal mines.

How might the current Internet-based behaviors of our children and adolescents today impact, alter, influence, or even forwardly forever change the biological, psychological, and/or sociological bases across not only their own life span trajectories but also those of child and adolescent users in the future? These are crucial and critical questions, which, of course, only time will reveal. With that unchangeable given variable in place, our only choice is to prioritize research, utilizing our current knowledge base to investigate hypotheses dedicated to increasing it now. Perhaps only then will we have a chance to prophylactically prevent any incubating or even currently emergent Internet behavior-driven risks or harms to both our children today and theirs tomorrow.

We dedicate this section to that goal and offer our deepest respect and appreciation to the phenomenal scholars who have contributed their knowledge, reflections, discussions, and future recommendations to the chapters included within it.

**Conflict of Interest and Funding Disclosures** No funding was secured for this report. The work of HJR on this article was carried out in the context of the Research Unit ACSID, FOR2974, funded by the Deutsche Forschungsgemeinschaft (DFG, German Research Foundation) and the German Innovation Fund (01NVF19031).

## References

1. Bekalu MA, McCloud RF, Viswanath K. Association of social media use with social well-being, positive mental health, and self-rated health: disentangling routine use from emotional connection to use. Health Educ Behav. 2019;46(2 suppl):69–80. https://doi.org/10.1177/1090198119863768.
2. Boniel-Nissim M, van den Eijnden RJJM, Furstova J, et al. International perspectives on social media use among adolescents: implications for mental and social well-being and substance use. Comput Hum Behav. 2022;129:107144. https://doi.org/10.1016/j.chb.2021.107144.
3. Bozzola E, Spina G, Agostiniani R, et al. The use of social media in children and adolescents: scoping review on the potential risks. Int J Environ Res Public Health. https://www.ncbi.nlm.nih.gov/pmc/articles/PMC9407706/.
4. Chung S, Lee J, Lee HK. Personal factors, internet characteristics, and environmental factors contributing to adolescent internet addiction: a public health perspective. Int J Environ Res Public Health. 2019;16(23):4635. https://doi.org/10.3390/ijerph16234635.
5. Holly L, Wong BL, van Kessel R, Awah I, Agrawal A, Ndili N. Optimising adolescent wellbeing in a digital age. BMJ. 2023; https://doi.org/10.1136/bmj-2021-068279.
6. Shah J, Das P, Muthiah N, Milanaik R. New age technology and social media. Curr Opin Pediatr. 2019;31(1):148–56. https://doi.org/10.1097/mop.0000000000000714.
7. Carragher N, Billieux J, Bowden-Jones H, et al. Brief overview of the who collaborative project on the development of new international screening and diagnostic instruments for gaming disorder and gambling disorder. Addiction. 2022;117(7):2119–21. https://doi.org/10.1111/add.15780.
8. Saunders JB, Hao W, Long J, et al. Gaming disorder: its delineation as an important condition for diagnosis, management, and prevention. J Behav Addict. 2017;6(3):271–9. https://doi.org/10.1556/2006.6.2017.039.
9. Rumpf H-J, Achab S, Billieux J, et al. Including gaming disorder in the ICD-11: the need to do so from a clinical and public health perspective. J Behav Addict. 2018;7(3):556–61. https://doi.org/10.1556/2006.7.2018.59.
10. In: Diagnostic and statistical manual of mental disorders: DSM-5. American Psychiatric Association; 2013, p. 795–8.
11. Gaming disorder. World Health Organization. https://www.who.int/standards/classifications/frequently-asked-questions/gaming-disorder.
12. Prinstein M. Written testimony of Mitch Prinstein, PhD, ABPP chief science officer... Written Testimony of Mitch Prinstein, PhD, ABPP Chief Science Officer American Psychological Association Protecting Our Children Online Before the U.S. Senate Committee on Judiciary (PDF). https://www.help.senate.gov/imo/media/doc/Prinstein.pdf. Published February 14, 2023.
13. Oberle E, Ji XR, Kerai S, Guhn M, Schonert-Reichl KA, Gadermann AM. Screen Time and extracurricular activities as risk and protective factors for mental health in adolescence: a population-level study. Prev Med. 2020;141:106291. https://doi.org/10.1016/j.ypmed.2020.106291.
14. Brand M, Wegmann E, Stark R, et al. The interaction of person-affect-cognition-execution (I-PACE) model for addictive behaviors: update, generalization to addictive behaviors beyond internet-use disorders, and specification of the process character of addictive behaviors. Neurosci Biobehav Rev. 2019;104:1–10. https://doi.org/10.1016/j.neubiorev.2019.06.032.
15. Goldstein S, Naglieri JA, editors. Encyclopedia of child behavior and development, vol. 1-3. Heidelberg: Springer; 2011.

# Problematic Internet Use: A General Perspective

Naomi A. Fineberg, Don Grant, Zsolt Demetrovics, Matthias Brand, Julius Burkauskas, Ornella Corazza, Meredith Gansner, Douglas A. Gentile, Biljana Gjoneska, Mark D. Griffiths, Orsolya Király, Marc N. Potenza, and Aviv M. Weinstein

## 1 Background

Digitalization brings both benefits and risks for individuals and civil society. For children and adolescents using digital technologies, benefits include opportunities for transitioning from families to wider peer communities, harvesting positive support, expanding social consciousness, gaining new coping mechanisms, and communicating. Challenges include problems balancing time spent online and offline, negative biological, psychological, and sociological impacts, vulnerability to cyberaggression, and other digital risks. While some studies associate the frequency of Internet use with poor mental health, others find associations with positive well-being, with outcomes overall depending not simply on the amount of time spent online but on the specific motivation, quality, and pattern of use (normative vs. "addictive") [1].

Problematic Internet Use (PIU) involves diverse forms of maladaptive online activities. PIU implies diminished control over Internet use or hazardous use patterns that create unfavorable consequences for health and well-being, including neglect of normative behaviors and relationships. Children and adolescents, especially those with vulnerabilities in affective, cognitive, motivational, and interpersonal domains, have immature cognitive control and may be particularly susceptible to, and disproportionately affected by, PIU. The impact of PIU may be particularly damaging to youth by disrupting developmental steps in transition to adulthood [1, 2].

N. A. Fineberg (✉)
School of Life and Medical Sciences, University of Hertfordshire, Hatfield, UK

D. Grant
Center for Research and Innovation, Newport Healthcare, Newport, RI, USA

Z. Demetrovics
Institute of Psychology, ELTE Eötvös Loránd University, Budapest, Hungary

Centre of Excellence in Responsible Gaming, University of Gibraltar, Gibraltar, Gibraltar

College of Education, Psychology and Social Work, Flinders University, Adelaide, Australia

M. Brand
General Psychology: Cognition and Center for Behavioral Addiction Research (CeBAR), University of Duisburg-Essen, Duisburg, Germany

Erwin L. Hahn Institute for Magnetic Resonance Imaging, Essen, Germany

J. Burkauskas
Lithuanian University of Health Sciences Neuroscience Institute, Kaunas, Lithuania

O. Corazza
Department of Psychology and Cognitive Science, University of Trento, Trento, Italy

University of Hertfordshire, Hatfield, UK


D. A. Christakis, L. Hale (eds.), *Handbook of Children and Screens*,
https://doi.org/10.1007/978-3-031-69362-5_25

## 2 Current State

### 2.1 Forms of PIU

PIU involves frequent online activity associated with marked functional impairment and/or distress. Activities can include online gaming, gambling, shopping, video-streaming, cybersex, the use of pornography, and social media [1]. Two main subtypes of PIU, generalized and specific, have been proposed. Some specific forms may be more *impulsive* (online gaming, gambling, buying/shopping, cybersex/online pornography use, social media use, video streaming) and others more compulsive (cyberchondria, cyberstalking, digital hoarding), although there is debate and overlap of addictive, impulsive, and compulsive features [2, 3]. The concept of PIU, however, remains controversial. Some have suggested that the Internet constitutes a channel for problematic or addictive behaviors [4], whereas others propose that digital platforms play active roles [5].

Balancing research evidence with public health needs, the World Health Organization introduced two specific PIU-related diagnoses into the ICD-11 category of Disorders due to Addictive Behaviors; the online forms of Gambling Disorder and Gaming Disorder [6]. Other PIU-related addictive disorders can conditionally be given an ICD-11 diagnosis as Other Specified or Unspecified Disorders due to Addictive Behaviors (sic), with online activity named as a diagnostic specifier. Such specific behaviors may include problematic online pornography viewing, shopping/buying, and social media use [7]. Definitions of other possible PIU-related disorders not yet defined in the ICD-11, such as cyberchondria and cyberbullying, have also been proposed [1].

### 2.2 Assessment

Recent progress has been made in refining and simplifying assessment instruments, which historically relied upon forms of the Internet Addiction Test (IAT) [8]. The Compulsive Internet Use Scale (CIUS) and its short versions are also up-to-date instruments possessing established psychometric properties validated in many languages [9]. Over 30 screening instruments have additionally been developed to assess problematic online gaming. Among them, the IGDT-10 and the IGDS9-SF present advantages, including reference to an identified nosography, robust psychometric properties, cross-cultural validation, and available cut-off points. Additional WHO efforts are presently active [10].

However, validated assessment instruments for many forms of PIU are lacking and there are methodological concerns with many existing assessment tools, including insufficient attention

M. Gansner
Department of Psychiatry, Boston Children's Hospital, Boston, MA, USA

D. A. Gentile
Iowa State University, Ames, IA, USA

B. Gjoneska
Macedonian Academy of Sciences and Arts, Skopje, North Macedonia

M. D. Griffiths
International Gaming Research Unit, Psychology Department, Nottingham Trent University, Nottingham, UK

O. Király
Institute of Psychology, ELTE Eötvös Loránd University, Budapest, Hungary

M. N. Potenza
Department of Psychiatry, Yale University School of Medicine, New Haven, CT, USA

Child Study Center, Yale University School of Medicine, New Haven, CT, USA

Connecticut Mental Health Center, New Haven, CT, USA

Connecticut Council on Problem Gambling, Wethersfield, CT, USA

Department of Neuroscience, Yale University, New Haven, CT, USA

Wu Tsai Institute, Yale University, New Haven, CT, USA

A. M. Weinstein
Ariel University, Ariel, Israel

to item-response theory, validation against appropriate measures of functional impairment, and *measurement variance* across different countries and cultures [10]

## 2.3 Epidemiology

According to a meta-analysis, around 7% of the global population shows signs of PIU [11]. While it is too early to determine if the increased time on the Internet during the COVID-19 pandemic has resulted in a higher global PIU prevalence [12], a greater burden of PIU was found for those living in low/lower–middle-income countries, for whom higher prevalence estimates during the pandemic compared with earlier estimates have been reported [13]. Young people with existing mental health problems and specific neurodevelopmental disorders (e.g., attention deficit hyperactivity disorder (ADHD), autism spectrum disorder (ASD)) show increased vulnerability to PIU, linked not only to increased digital media use, but also to isolation, loneliness, financial hardship, substance misuse, anxiety, and depression, although there is considerable heterogeneity in study findings [1, 12]. However, given the heterogeneity and the relative lack of consistency in terms of the diagnostic criteria for PIU and the diversity of assessment instruments, samples, and sampling designs, prevalence estimates of PIU vary widely across different studies and should be approached with caution [12].

PIU also appears to differ between males and females. Problematic/excessive use and greater severity of *smartphone* use, social media use, and online buying–shopping have generally been associated with the female gender, whereas males may be more prone to problematic online gaming, online gambling, and online pornography use, although heterogeneity exists across studies and jurisdictions [14].

PIU is associated with co-occurring disorders, including among younger and older pediatric samples [15]. ADHD, depression, aggressive behaviors, social anxiety, obsessive-compulsive disorder (OCD), and ASD have been implicated both as candidate predictors and as consequences of PIU [16]. Other associations have variously been reported with *suicidality* [17], self-injurious behaviors [18], somatization, eating disorders, *psychoticism*, poor life skills, poor well-being, poor self-esteem, decreased physical activity and fitness, poor dietary hygiene, problems in family relationships, and loneliness [19, 20]. Problematic use of social media has also been associated with aggression, cyberbullying, fear of missing out (FOMO), and poor sleep [21].

## 2.4 Underpinning Mechanisms

The Interaction of Person-Affect-Cognition-Execution (I-PACE) model [3] describes potential vulnerabilities driving the risk of PIU, their interactions with urges, impulses, and self-control, and consequences for mental health. Individual and relational factors include neurodevelopmental (ASD, ADHD), mental health (anxiety, depression, OCD, addiction), personality (affect regulation), and inhibitory control (and other executive functions) features. Societal factors include changing communication patterns and platform features, including advertising and regulation policies (e.g., minimum age limits, parental control).

For young people with ADHD and conduct disorders, *impulsivity* and positive reinforcement motivations may represent key factors, while for those with OCD and ASD, attentional inflexibility may result in difficulties disconnecting. For those with internalizing symptoms such as anxiety and depression, online activities (e.g., social media use) may be used to escape from distressing emotions (negative reinforcement motivations). However, fear of failure and body image disturbances generated by exposure to social comparisons may also induce anxiety, depressive symptoms [22], dysmorphophobia, and eating disorders, as well as an increased use (especially during the COVID-19 pandemic) of certain substances such as performance and image-enhancing drugs and related *psychopathology* [23].

Digital platforms may influence PIU via interplays between diverse social factors and types of human interactions to which young people may be particularly attracted, including socialization, support, and entertainment [2, 4]. This is especially relevant for platforms that provide intermittent positive reinforcement, to which repeated exposure may result in increasingly compulsive online use with negative consequences. Attention-focused designs intended to generate, or possibly exploit, potentially addictive features (e.g., "likes") and conditioned responses (e.g., notifications) alongside powerful algorithm-based technologies may lead youth to stay online longer than either intended or recommended [2, 4]. These "tools" operationalized by digital platform designers may pose risks to a youth's self-management of their online behaviors by influencing/manipulating choices, opinions, or behaviors, potentially exposing them to human rights violations (e.g., risk of addictions, undermining autonomous free will, abuse of minors, trafficking, and connected liberties) [1]. Investigating the interactions of these factors over time should be prioritized to identify potentially causal relationships and risk determinants as a basis for preventative or therapeutic interventions and health and social policy changes [1, 2, 4].

Functional brain mechanisms at cognitive/affective levels, and/or changes in brain structure, may also contribute significantly to the etiology of PIU and to early identification and intervention. A meta-analysis of case-controlled studies of cognition demonstrated that PIU (broadly defined) was associated with significant reductions in inhibitory control, decision-making, and working memory. Age, gender, geographical area of reporting, or the type of predominant online behavior did not significantly moderate the observed relationships [24]. Another meta-analysis of changes in structural brain measures in PIU detected significantly reduced gray matter in the anterior *cingulate cortex* (ACC), dorsolateral prefrontal cortex (DLPFC), and *supplementary motor area* (SMA), regions linked to reward processing, habit learning, and inhibitory control [25]. Data suggests reduced functional connectivity in brain networks involved in cognitive control, executive function, motivation, and reward [26]. Taken together, findings further suggest specific brain structures and functions related to cortical inhibition of the generation and execution of reward-based responses, both in generalized PIU and specific forms like gaming disorder [2].

Because existing studies are largely cross-sectional, it remains uncertain whether these neuro-cognitive features represent a cause or consequence of PIU or both. Longitudinal studies following the progression from vulnerability to full PIU may help identify cognitive and affective risk factors and clarify the extent to which these changes can be used to discriminate against an individual at high risk of PIU, for future screening aids. The scarcity of studies employing robust controls for confounding variables such as psychiatric comorbidities [24, 25] and the limitations of standardization and validation of existing assessment tools and PIU definitions highlight the need for additional research to delineate the contributions of specific variables to the underpinning mechanisms of PIU.

## 2.5 Effective and Emerging Interventions for PIU

Interventional research is steadily developing but remains at an early stage, with most studies conducted in adults and few in youth. Most studies have focused on problematic gambling and gaming. Various forms of psychotherapy (mainly cognitive behavior therapy [CBT]) and to a lesser extent pharmacotherapy (mainly antidepressants and *stimulants*) have been tested in acute-phase trials, with some promising findings, particularly in relation to the short-term effects of CBT. However, while a recent study demonstrated that CBT may reduce PIU symptom severity among "at-risk" youth, reductions in the incidence of new cases have not been established [27]. Non-invasive *neurostimulation* targeting cortical brain regions involved in cognitive control and craving, using techniques such as *transcranial magnetic stimulation* and *transcranial direct current stimulation*, is also emerging as another promising area of study [28]. Overall, there is a need for higher-quality research, including large, preregistered, randomized clinical trials, to determine efficacious and cost-effective options in PIU treatment.

## 3 Future Research

Many important gaps in knowledge about PIU remain outstanding, including a qualitative and quantitative understanding of the scale and impact of PIU on youth health and well-being. Child and adolescent screen time is increasing annually, but the long-term health consequences of this increase remain poorly understood [1]. Several studies associate PIU with negative biological, health, psychological, and sociological outcomes across diverse groups [2]. Reduced general quality of life in adolescence was also found to be "dose dependently" linked to PIU severity [29]. However, an accurate estimation of the global burden of PIU in general or that related to specific internet-use disorders is also sorely lacking. Few longitudinal studies exist, and most identified associations are based on cross-sectional data. As health and well-being issues can be seen as risk factors as well as outcomes of PIU, causal relationships are likely complicated [30]. To bridge existing knowledge gaps, future studies should include improved interpretation of causal relationships (with insight from longitudinal data and investigations of bi-directional relationships), address methodological weaknesses with a more unified approach to the conceptualization and assessment of PIU, include qualitative data and use of convenience sampling, and account for the wide variety of behaviors performed on the Internet.

Other key research goals include improved insight into the dynamics of PIU with reliable methods for early identification of individuals at risk for PIU, a better understanding of the course and evolution of PIU-related problems across different age groups, genders, and specific vulnerable groups, and efficacious and cost-effective preventative and therapeutic interventions that can be successfully implemented at scale.

Considering that PIU occurs within the digital environment and can be captured using digital tools, the ubiquity of smart technology, and the considerable amounts of "real-time" information they may gather through behavioral tracking techniques, which may potentially be used to make Internet use more addictive [31], (and which may also be used in online gambling and gaming disorder research to improve prevention efforts), future research harnessing smart devices is anticipated to hold promise for addressing specific research questions. Given the amount of time spent on smartphones and inaccuracies in recalling personal digital media use, the use of digital technologies to identify PIU may prove of particular benefit to adolescents. By enabling the characterization of "digital phenotypes" underlying one or more forms of PIU (and thereby those individuals at elevated risk), digital technologies may also offer new opportunities for remote interventions at scale.

## 4 Recommendations

- Given the convergence of changing digital industries, widespread use, and youth vulnerability, it is vital to support the impetus for change to address and prevent online harms through ethical health and social policy changes.
- Developments in diagnostic criteria for PIU should be grounded in reliable data [32].
- Children's and adolescents' well-being should be central to such interventions and strategies, including improved digital literacy programs.
- Dialogue among key players (including the government and technology companies), new policy standards involving increased corporate responsibility, re-evaluation of the business models steering digital services provision, and potential regulation, including that of transnational technology companies, are also needed to ensure a nurturing digital environment.
- Globally, wide variations exist in the range and scope of regulatory, public, and clinical health policies and models. As observed with

other potentially health-harming industries (e.g., gambling), increased regulation or perceived market penetration in some jurisdictions may result in greater commercial exploitation of low- and middle-income countries. Therefore, pragmatic, equitable, and inclusive global solutions are needed.

- Stakeholders have called for governmental regulation underpinned by international law vis-a-vis children's rights in the digital environment, requiring technology companies to ensure age-appropriate design safeguards for all services likely to be accessed by children [33], and including clear criteria for enforcement. While some regulatory initiatives are underway (e.g., the European Commission Digital Services Act), the extent to which young people at risk of PIU can be safeguarded will depend on international standards governing the day-to-day practices of digital service providers, the transparency of corporate behavior, and the effectiveness of available remedies, including digital literacy programming.

**Conflict of Interest and Funding Disclosure** ZD's contribution was supported by the Hungarian National Research, Development, and Innovation Office (KKP126835). ZD also acknowledges that the University of Gibraltar receives funding from the Gibraltar Gambling Care Foundation, an independent, not-for-profit charity, and the ELTE Eötvös Loránd University receives funding from Szerencsejáték Ltd. (the gambling operator of the Hungarian government) to maintain a telephone helpline service for problematic gambling. NF has held research grants paid to her institution by UK Research and Innovation, UK National Institute for Health Research, COST Action, Orchard, received payment for lecturing from the Global Mental Health Academy and participated as an investigator in a study supported by Compass Pathways.

## References

1. Fineberg NA, Menchón JM, Hall N, et al. Advances in problematic usage of the internet research – A narrative review by experts from the European network for problematic usage of the internet. Compr Psychiatry. 2022;118:152346. https://doi.org/10.1016/j.comppsych.2022.152346.
2. Brand M. Can internet use become addictive? Science. 2022;376:798–9. https://doi.org/10.1126/science.abn4189.
3. ICD-11. n.d. https://icd.who.int/en (accessed August 17, 2022).
4. Starcevic V, Aboujaoude E. Internet addiction: reappraisal of an increasingly inadequate concept. CNS Spectr. 2017;22(1):7–13.
5. Flayelle M, Brevers D, King DL, Maurage P, Perales JC, Billieux J. A taxonomy of technology design features that promote potentially addictive online behaviours. Nat Rev Psychol. 2023:1–15.
6. Brand M, Rumpf H-J, Demetrovics Z, Müller A, Stark R, King DL, et al. Which conditions should be considered as disorders in the international classification of diseases (ICD-11) designation of "other specified disorders due to addictive behaviors"? J Behav Addict. 2020; https://doi.org/10.1556/2006.2020.00035.
7. Young KS. Caught in the net: how to recognize the signs of Internet addiction – and a winning strategy for recovery. New York: J. Wiley; 1998.
8. Lopez-Fernandez O, Griffiths MD, Kuss DJ, Dawes C, Pontes HM, Justice L, et al. Cross-cultural validation of the compulsive internet use scale in four forms and eight languages. Cyberpsychol Behav Soc Netw. 2019;22:451–64. https://doi.org/10.1089/cyber.2018.0731.
9. Carragher N, Billieux J, Bowden-Jones H, et al. Brief overview of the who collaborative project on the development of new international screening and diagnostic instruments for gaming disorder and gambling disorder. Addiction. 2022;117(7):2119–21. https://doi.org/10.1111/add.15780.
10. Pan Y-C, Chiu Y-C, Lin Y-H. Systematic review and meta-analysis of epidemiology of internet addiction. Neurosci Biobehav Rev. 2020;118:612–22. https://doi.org/10.1016/j.neubiorev.2020.08.013.
11. Burkauskas J, Gecaite-Stonciene J, Demetrovics Z, Griffiths MD, Király O. Prevalence of problematic Internet use during the coronavirus disease 2019 pandemic. Curr Opin Behav Sci. 2022;46:101179. https://doi.org/10.1016/j.cobeha.2022.101179. Epub 2022 Jun 15. PMID: 35719702; PMCID: PMC9197820.
12. Gjoneska B, Potenza MN, Jones J, Sales CM, Hranov G, Demetrovics Z. Problematic use of the Internet in low- and middle-income countries before and during the COVID-19 pandemic: a scoping review. Curr Opin Behav Sci. 2022;48:101208. https://doi.org/10.1016/j.cobeha.2022.101208. Epub 2022 Jul 29. PMID: 35919788; PMCID: PMC9334935.
13. Mohler-Kuo M, et al. Stress and mental health among children/adolescents, their parents, and young adults during the first COVID-19 lockdown in Switzerland. J Environ Res Public Health. 2021;18:4668.
14. Baloğlu M, Sahin R, Arpaci I. A review of recent research in problematic internet use: gender and cultural differences. Curr Opin Psychol. 2020;36:124–9. https://doi.org/10.1016/j.copsyc.2020.05.008.
15. Jeong H, Yim HW, Lee S-Y, Lee HK, Potenza MN, Park M. Joint effects of children's emotional problems and parental depressive symptoms on the occurrence of internet gaming disorder among children and adolescents: a longitudinal study. J Behav Addict. 2021;10:244–52. https://doi.org/10.1556/2006.2021.00030.

16. Murray A, Koronczai B, Király O, Griffiths MD, Mannion A, Leader G, et al. Autism, problematic internet use and gaming disorder: a systematic review. Rev J Autism Dev Disord. 2021; https://doi.org/10.1007/s40489-021-00243-0.
17. Marchant A, Hawton K, Stewart A, Montgomery P, Singaravelu V, Lloyd K, et al. A systematic review of the relationship between internet use, self-harm and suicidal behaviour in young people: the good, the bad and the unknown. PLoS One. 2017;12:e0181722. https://doi.org/10.1371/journal.pone.0181722.
18. Greenberg NR, Zhai ZW, Hoff RA, Krishnan-Sarin S, Potenza MN. Difficulties in impulse control in adolescents with problematic use of the internet and self-injurious behaviors. Psychiatry Res. 2022;317:114919.
19. Alimoradi Z, Lin CY, Broström A, Bülow PH, Bajalan Z, Griffiths MD, Ohayon MM, Pakpour AH. Internet addiction and sleep problems: a systematic review and meta-analysis. Sleep Med Rev. 2019;47:51–61. https://doi.org/10.1016/j.smrv.2019.06.004. Epub 2019 Jul 4. PMID: 31336284.
20. Wacks Y, Weinstein AM. Excessive smartphone use is associated with health problems in adolescents and young adults. Front Psychol. 2021;12:669042. https://doi.org/10.3389/fpsyt.2021.669042.
21. Weinstein A. Problematic social networking site use- effects on mental health and the brain. Front Psychiatry. 2023;13:1106004. https://doi.org/10.3389/fpsyt.2022.1106004.
22. Cataldo I, Billieux J, Esposito G, Corazza O. Assessing problematic use of social media: where do we stand and what can be improved? Curr Opin Behav Sci. 2022;45:101145.
23. Cataldo I, Burkauskas J, Dores AR, Carvalho IP, Simonato P, De Luca I, et al. An international cross-sectional investigation on social media, fitspiration content exposure, and related risks during the COVID-19 self-isolation period. J Psychiatr Res. 2022;148:34–44.
24. Ioannidis K, Hook R, Goudriaan AE, Vlies S, Fineberg NA, Grant JE, et al. Cognitive deficits in problematic internet use: meta-analysis of 40 studies. Br J Psychiatry. 2019;215:639–46. https://doi.org/10.1192/bjp.2019.3.
25. Solly JE, Hook RW, Grant JE, et al. Structural gray matter differences in Problematic Usage of the Internet: a systematic review and meta-analysis. Mol Psychiatry. 2022;27:1000–9. https://doi.org/10.1038/s41380-021-01315-7.
26. Weinstein A, Lejoyeux M. Neurobiological mechanisms underlying Internet and Gaming Disorder (IGD). Dialogues Clin Neurosci. 2020;22(2):113–26.
27. Lindenberg K, Kindt S, Szász-Janocha C. Effectiveness of cognitive behavioral therapy-based intervention in preventing gaming disorder and unspecified internet use disorder in adolescents: a cluster randomized clinical trial. JAMA Netw Open. 2022;5(2):e2148995. https://doi.org/10.1001/jamanetworkopen.2021.48995. PMID: 35179587; PMCID: PMC8857686.
28. Xu LX, Geng XM, Zhang JL, Guo XY, Potenza MN, Zhang JT. Neuromodulation treatments of problematic use of the internet. Curr Opin Behav Sci. 2022;48:101215.
29. Machimbarrena JM, González-Cabrera J, Ortega-Barón J, Beranuy-Fargues M, Álvarez-Bardón A, Tejero B. Profiles of problematic internet use and its impact on adolescents' health-related quality of life. Int J Environ Res Public Health. 2019;16(20):3877. https://doi.org/10.3390/ijerph16203877. PMID: 31614899; PMCID: PMC6843246
30. Rumpf HJ, Brandt D, Demetrovics Z, Billieux J, Carragher N, Brand M, et al. Epidemiological challenges in the study of behavioral addictions: a call for high standard methodologies. Curr Addict Rep. 2019;6:331–7. https://doi.org/10.1007/s40429-019-00262-2.
31. King DL, Delfabbro PH, Gainsbury SM, Dreier M, Greer N, Billieux J. Unfair play? Video games as exploitative monetized services: an examination of game patents from a consumer protection perspective. Comput Hum Behav. 2019;101:131–43.
32. Billieux J, Flayelle M, King DL. Addiction: expand diagnostic borders with care. Nature. 2022;611(7937):665.
33. Hainsworth J. Baroness Beeban Kidron Chair 5Rights Foundations n.d.:2. https://5rightsfoundation.com/uploads/joint-ngo-letter-to-council-on-childrens-rights-in-dsa.pdf.

# Gaming Disorder Among Children and Adolescents

Mark D. Griffiths, Vasileios Stavropoulos, Halley M. Pontes, Xavier Carbonell, Daniel L. King, Chung-Ying Lin, Zsolt Demetrovics, and Orsolya Király

## 1 Background

Research examining problematic video game playing dates back to the early 1980s when the first reports started appearing concerning adolescents being 'obsessed' with or 'addicted' to the playing of arcade video games such as *Space Invaders* [1]. The playing of video games (i.e., 'gaming') has evolved during this time from playing video games in amusement arcades in the 1980s to playing video games on dedicated gaming consoles and personal computers in the 1990s, to playing video games online in the 2000s [1]. More recently, technology has advanced so that gaming can be engaged from almost anywhere through smartphones and Wi-Fi-enabled mobile handheld devices, as well as in virtual reality [2]. Historically, gaming has traditionally been an activity predominantly engaged in by children and adolescents, but gaming has now become a popular activity among adults [1]. However, children and adolescents, appear to be a vulnerable group when it comes to experiencing the negative consequences of gaming excessively which can adversely affect their educational performance, mental health, and/or personal relationships [1]. Consequently, this has become an important issue of concern for many different stakeholder groups (e.g., parents, teachers, treatment providers, healthcare practitioners, policymakers, government bodies, and the gaming industry).

M. D. Griffiths (✉)
International Gaming Research Unit, Psychology Department, Nottingham Trent University, Nottingham, UK
e-mail: mark.griffiths@ntu.ac.uk

V. Stavropoulos
RMIT University, School of Health and Biomedical Sciences, Melbourne, VIC, Australia

H. M. Pontes
University of London, Department of Organizational Psychology, Birkbeck, London, UK

X. Carbonell
Ramon Llull University, Department of Psychology, Barcelona, Spain

D. L. King
Flinders University, College of Education, Psychology, & Social Work, Adelaide, SA, Australia

C.-Y. Lin
Institute of Allied Health Sciences, College of Medicine, National Cheng Kung University, Tainan, Taiwan

Z. Demetrovics
Centre of Excellence in Responsible Gaming at the University of Gibraltar, Gibraltar, Gibraltar

Institute of Psychology, ELTE Eötvös Loránd University, Budapest, Hungary

College of Education, Psychology and Social Work, Flinders University, Adelaide, SA, Australia

O. Király
Institute of Psychology, ELTE Eötvös Loránd University, Budapest, Hungary


D. A. Christakis, L. Hale (eds.), *Handbook of Children and Screens*,
https://doi.org/10.1007/978-3-031-69362-5_26

Despite the many positives of gaming, a small minority of individuals appear to engage in gaming to such an extent that it disrupts and compromises many areas of their everyday lives. Therefore, problematic gaming has become a topic of increasing research interest. However, there are multiple debates about terminology, with many terms being used interchangeably in the extant literature (e.g., 'excessive', 'problematic', 'disordered', 'dependent', 'compulsive', 'addictive', and 'pathological') [1]. For the sake of consistency, the present review uses the term 'disorder(ed)', given that this is the term used in psychiatric diagnostic manuals.

This marked increase in research from many different perspectives (e.g., epidemiological, clinical, developmental, neurobiological, etc.), led the American Psychiatric Association (APA) to introduce 'internet gaming disorder' (IGD) as a tentative disorder in the fifth edition of the *Diagnostic and Statistical Manual of Mental Disorders* (DSM-5) in 2013 [3]. The APA describes IGD as a behavioral addiction like gambling disorder, defining it as *'persistent and recurrent use of the internet to engage in games, often with other players, leading to clinically significant impairment or distress'* (p. 795) [3]. More recently, the World Health Organization (WHO) included 'gaming disorder' (GD) as a formal diagnosis in the 11th revision of the International Classification of Diseases (ICD-11) in 2019 [4]. The criteria for both of these are shown in Table 1.

## 2 Current State of Knowledge

### 2.1 Prevalence of Gaming Disorder

In the past three decades, many studies have attempted to determine the prevalence of disordered gaming. However, given the existing various definitions, screening instruments, and/or self-selected samples used, there has been a varied number of prevalence estimates across studies. To date, three meta-analyses have been published. Fam [5] examined the prevalence estimates of IGD among adolescents in 28 studies ($N$ = 61,737; 20 studies in Europe, four in Australia; two in Asia, and one in North America). There was wide variability in prevalence rates (0.5–19.9%) with a pooled prevalence rate of 4.6% of GD among adolescents (with male adolescents having higher GD prevalence rates [6.8%] than female adolescents [1.3%]). A meta-analysis by Stevens et al. [6] comprised 53 studies ($N$ = 226,247; 17 coun-

**Table 1** Definitions and criteria for internet gaming disorder and gaming disorder as proposed in the DSM-5-TR and ICD-11 (DSM-5-TR: Diagnostic and Statistical Manual of Mental Disorders, Fifth Edition, Text Revision; ICD-11: International Classification of Diseases 11th Revision)

| | DSM-5-TR Internet Gaming Disorder | ICD-11 Gaming Disorder |
|---|---|---|
| Definition | 'Persistent and recurrent use of the internet to engage in games, often with other players, leading to clinically significant impairment or distress'. (Also includes non-internet computerized games as well as internet games)'. | 'The behavior pattern is of sufficient severity to result in significant impairment in personal, family, social, educational, occupational or other important areas of functioning'. |
| Criteria endorsement and duration of the condition | An individual should endorse five (or more) out of nine criteria over a 12-month period. | An individual should endorse all the criteria over a 12-month period or more, although the required duration may be shortened if all diagnostic requirements are met, and symptoms are severe. |

(continued)

**Table 1** (continued)

| | DSM-5-TR Internet Gaming Disorder | ICD-11 Gaming Disorder |
|---|---|---|
| Criteria | Being excessively preoccupied with gaming | Impaired control over gaming |
| | Having withdrawal symptoms when not gaming | Elevated priority given to gaming |
| | Spending more and more time gaming | Increased time spent on gaming despite problems |
| | Failed attempts to reduce or quit gaming | |
| | Losing interest in hobbies due to gaming | |
| | Engaging in gaming despite its adverse consequences | |
| | Deceiving others about gaming duration | |
| | Achieving a positive mood by gaming | |
| | Risking, jeopardizing, or losing a job or relationship because of gaming | |

tries). The prevalence of GD was 3.05% but lower in high-quality studies (1.96%). Males had a higher GD prevalence rate (6.31%) than females (2.54%). The most recent meta-analysis by Kim et al. [7] comprised 61 studies ($N$ = 227,665; 29 countries). The prevalence rate of GD was 3.3% but lower when only including data from 28 representative samples (2.4%). Males had a higher GD prevalence rate (8.5%) than females (3.5%). The study also estimated prevalence rates for six different age categories. The pooled prevalence rates were 6.6% for children and adolescents (based on five studies), 6.3% for adolescents and young adults (five studies), 3.4% for young adults (nine studies), 3.3% for adolescents (38 studies), 1.9% for all adults (six studies), and 1.3% for adolescents and adults (five studies). All three of the meta-analyses reported high heterogeneity in their reported GD prevalence rates. These were influenced by both methodological variables (e.g., screening instrument used, terminology regarding problematic gaming use, study design, type of sample surveyed, type of sampling method used) and participant variables (e.g., sample size, country/region of participants, age of participants).

## 2.2 Etiology of Gaming Disorder

One of the key topics in the GD field is etiology. A recent comprehensive review of the etiology of GD [8] outlined the three overarching interacting factors that are involved in the acquisition, development, and maintenance of GD. These are the: (i) individual factors (i.e., person-based characteristics such as genetic/biological predispositions, personality factors, motivations for playing, etc.), (ii) gaming-related factors (e.g., structural characteristics of the video games themselves, the medium in which the video games are played), and (iii) environmental factors (i.e., the situational characteristics such as peer, family, and cultural influences in video game playing) [8].

## 2.3 Individual Factors

Individual factors that play a contributory role in the etiology of GD (among others) include genetic/biological predispositions, personality traits, demographic risk factors, motivations, and comorbid psychopathologies. The neural mechanisms associated with GD appear to resemble those of other addictions [9]. The cognitive-affective alterations found in GD include impaired executive functioning, impaired emotional regulation, impaired decision-making, and impulsivity related to different functioning in prefrontal areas and the front-limbic, temporoparietal, and subcortical regions [10], as well structural changes in several brain regions including altered white-matter density and reduced grey matter volume (controlling emotional regulation, cognitive/motor control, decision-making, and behavioral inhibition). Studies have also indicated that compared to controls, those with GD show activation in the (i) orbitofrontal cortex (indicating a lower level of punishment sensitivity), and (ii) dorsolateral prefrontal cortex (associated with a higher level of craving) [11].

Many studies have explored the association between GD and the 'Big Five' personality traits. Two meta-analyses have been published [12, 13]. These have shown a very consistent positive relationship between GD and neuroticism. Given that neurotic individuals are more prone to depression, stress, and anxiety, they may use gaming as an escape because virtual worlds feel (or are perceived as) safer than their real-life personal environments. The meta-analyses also found negative associations with conscientiousness. Given that individuals with low conscientiousness are more careless, impulsive, and disorganized, the finding that they are more likely to experience GD is unsurprising. Another very consistent finding in the literature is the positive relationship between GD and impulsivity. One recent systematic literature review reported a positive relationship between impulsivity in 32 out of 33 studies [14].

As noted in the meta-analyses concerning the prevalence of GD, the literature has consistently shown that males are much more likely to experience GD than females and this also includes children and adolescents. Age also seems to be important, with adolescents and emerging adults being at higher risk of GD than other age cohorts. Various explanations have been provided in the literature from cultural perspectives (e.g., males have both a much greater affinity to, and enjoyment of, playing video games), evolutionary perspectives (e.g., males have a greater inclination towards competition, aggression), and neurobiological perspectives (e.g., males demonstrating higher cue-elicited craving-related neural responses). Other factors have been examined but are less consistent and/or contradictory in findings related to increased risk of GD (e.g., ethnicity, relationship status, employment status, income, educational level, etc.) [8].

In the case of GD, comorbidity tends to be the norm rather than the exception [8]. Research has consistently found a positive association between GD and (i) depression [15], (ii) anxiety [16], (iii) ADHD (hyperactivity and inattention) [8], (iv) comorbid polysubstance use [17], (v) autism [18], and (v) risk for suicidal ideation [8]. However, given that the majority of studies examining these associations with comorbid conditions are cross-sectional, longitudinal research is needed because the directions of the associations are uncertain. However, in many, the associations may well be reciprocal.

## 2.4 Gaming-Related Factors

To facilitate habitual and rewarding video game playing, game design plays a role in exploiting psychological mechanisms (e.g., operant conditioning) [8]. For vulnerable and susceptible individuals (such as those who experience social anxiety or who have low self-esteem), such design features may facilitate excessive and (and among a minority of individuals) disordered gaming. GD [19]. For instance, although GD has been reported among offline gamers, it is much more prevalent among online gamers [8]. Among adolescents who are socially anxious and/or who have poor social skills, online gaming environments can help meet their social needs if they find face-to-face interactions anxiety-inducing.

The genre of video games may also contribute to GD. For instance, research has consistently found that massively multiplayer online role-playing games (MMORPGs) are most associated with GD. Other genres have been associated with GD including multiplayer online battle arena (MOBA) games, real-time strategy (RTS) games, and shooter games (both first-person and third-person [8]. These types of video game tend to be far more immersive than other video game genres and appear to be an important factor in the maintenance of GD.

The structural characteristics of the video games themselves may also contribute to GD. Given that virtual in-game rewards can result in the release of dopamine [8], such features are critical in reinforcement and game continuance [8, 20]. The unpredictability of when a reward will occur, particularly in video games such as MMORPGs, can result in individuals playing for hours and hours in single gaming sessions. Game designers can exploit the principles of operant conditioning and players can find themselves locked into variable-ratio reinforcement schedules, which result in habitual gaming patterns. Players designing their in-game avatars can create extensions of themselves which may be psychologically rewarding and/or act as a compensatory mechanism for those with low body satisfaction to overcome their social anxiety, and thus boost their self-esteem [21]. Complimenting this, GD has been shown to increase when gamers experience their avatars as themselves (i.e., identification), their avatar's needs as their own (often prioritized to their offline needs [immersion]), their avatar being able to behave in ways that they cannot in their real lives (i.e., repression), and their avatar as the person/character they would like to have been (i.e., idealization) [19].

Research in media psychology-inspired concepts further reinforces the significance of structural game features for GD [19, 21]. These refer to the extent gamers are absorbed by (i) the virtual world, experiencing the latter as real (i.e., as if they were there [presence/telepresence]) [19] and (ii) their in-game activity, due to the gradual increase of in-game challenges, at a rate that matches the increase of the player's in-game skills. For gamers to be challenged and completely engaged with their in-game action, these challenges need to slightly exceed their current skill level. If game demands are significantly higher than players' skills, gamers become distressed and disengage. Similarly, if players' demands are significantly lower than their skills, they will experience boredom and disengage. As players keep engaging with the game, their skills concurrently increase, requiring the game developer to increase the level of game challenges at a similar pace (i.e., level-up process) to maintain sustained game content consumption and process/state ('flow') [19].

Finally, the past few years have seen the introduction of arguably 'predatory' monetization techniques by the gaming industry in the form of micro-transactions (e.g., loot boxes where players spend real money to open virtual crates or boxes to win something that might help them in the progression of the games). A number of scholars have noted the similarities between loot boxes and gambling. Given that loot boxes are available to minors, it has raised concerns that loot-box buying may be a 'gateway' to gambling [8, 22]. Based on the empirical research to date, there appears to be a consensus that loot-box buying and expenditure are indeed associated with both problematic gaming and problematic gambling among adolescents and adults [8, 23].

## 2.5 Environmental Factors

Excluding cultural factors (which are beyond the remit of this chapter), research has consistently shown that early life experiences (e.g., familial relationships) can be risk factors for acquiring GD. Systematic reviews examining family factors associated with GD among adolescents have consistently shown that specific factors in relationship quality (e.g., single-parent families, family/marital conflicts, poor family functioning, poor parenting styles [neglectful, authoritarian, permissive], childhood maltreatment, violent disciplining, etc.) are positively associated with GD severity [24, 25]. Other environmental factors that have been associated with adolescent GD include having difficulty in making friends and having low levels of school-related well-being [8, 26].

## 3 Future Research

Despite the marked increase in research examining GD in child and adolescent samples and given that the majority of studies have used cross-sectional convenience sampling, further research is needed with large-scale representative samples using longitudinal designs. Also, more cross-cultural comparisons are needed - especially between Southeast Asia and Europe given the large cultural differences in these regions and variances in how parents and policymakers view gaming in the countries within them. Further research is additionally needed from a neurobiological perspective, including whether GD may be influenced by inherited biological and/or genetic factors. There is also a dearth of data concerning clinical samples given the large reliance on community sample data. There also needs to be research into the growing area of esports (i.e., professional gaming) because playing video games professionally can take up lots of time and resources if adolescents have aspirations to have a career in gaming [27].

Research is also needed to help design a taxonomy relevant to current video games and that contributes to identifying which structural characteristics and game mechanics affect the behaviors of the players, especially because some of these characteristics may have age-sensitive effects. The impact of loot-box buying, for example, maybe more detrimental to adolescents than adults. Finally, those in the field could also collaborate with cognate areas (such as the gambling disorder field) and try to acquire datasets from gaming operators, with the goal of identifying online gaming profiles using behavioral tracking data (e.g., using tidy classification algorithms to predict GD risk, based on engagement game mechanics [presence, flow, user-avatar bond]).

## 4 Recommendations

- One of the limitations in the field of GD field is the lack of screening instruments specifically developed for use within child and adolescent populations. Although there are a few psychometric instruments (e.g., Gaming Addiction Scale for Adolescents [28], Videogame Addiction Scale for Children) [29] most of the screens were developed and validated with adult samples. More recent screens have relied on DSM-5 and ICD-11 criteria, which are arguably designed for adults. Therefore, bespoke age-appropriate screening instruments are vital and needed in terms of both research integrity and best clinical practices.
- As with other consumptive products that can cause problems when engaged in excessively (e.g., alcohol, gambling), there should be independent regulators in each country that oversee the video game industry, to ensure that player protection and harm minimization are dedicated core components of their commercial practices and goals.
- Unlike gambling and alcohol use which are adult-only activities, gaming is freely available to children and adolescents, therefore social responsibility initiatives for players need to be introduced in the same way that has happened in the gambling industry (e.g., limit setting, mandatory breaks, real-time personalized feedback, pop-up messaging on-screen, etc.) [30].
- Research, educational awareness (for schools, parents, teachers), prevention programs, and treatment interventions should be funded by the gaming industry.
- Governments could also oblige the gaming industry to share behavioral data for research purposes.
- Countries could introduce a levy where (say) 1% of all profits are donated to an independent body for closely monitored, legitimately, and inclusively distributed funding towards these aforementioned areas and initiatives.

**Conflict of Interest and Funding Disclosures** MDG has received research funding from *Norsk Tipping* (the gambling operator owned by the Norwegian government). MDG has received funding for a number of research projects in the area of gambling education for young people, social responsibility in gambling, and gambling treatment from Gamble Aware (formerly the Responsibility in

Gambling Trust), a charitable body that funds its research program based on donations from the gambling industry. MDG undertakes consultancy for various gambling companies in the area of player protection and social responsibility in gambling. The University of Gibraltar receives funding from the Gibraltar Gambling Care Foundation, an independent, not-for-profit charity, and the ELTE Eötvös Loránd University receives funding from Szerencsejáték Ltd. (the gambling operator of the Hungarian government) to maintain a telephone helpline service for problematic gambling. C-YL was supported by the Ministry of Science and Technology, Taiwan (MOST 110-2410-H-006-115; MOST 111-2410-H-006-110). VS is supported by the Australian Research Council Discovery Early Career Researcher Award DE210101107. ZD's and OK's contribution was supported by the Hungarian National Research, Development and Innovation Office (KKP126835).

## References

1. Griffiths MD, Kuss DJ, King DL. Video game addiction: past, present and future. Curr Psychiatr Rev. 2012;8:308–18.
2. Lopez-Fernandez O, Männikkö N, Kääriäinen M, et al. Mobile gaming and problematic smartphone use: a comparative study between Belgium and Finland. J Behav Addict. 2018;7:88–99.
3. American Psychiatric Association. Diagnostic and statistical manual of mental disorders (fifth edition, text revision). American Psychiatric Publishing; 2022.
4. World Health Organization. Gaming disorder. 2019. Available at: https://www.who.int/standards/classifications/frequently-asked-questions/gaming-disorder. Accessed April 20, 2023.
5. Fam JY. Prevalence of internet gaming disorder in adolescents: a meta-analysis across three decades. Scand J Psychol. 2018;59(5):524–31.
6. Stevens MW, Dorstyn D, Delfabbro PH, King DL. Global prevalence of gaming disorder: a systematic review and meta-analysis. Aust N Z J Psychiatry. 2021;55(6):553–68.
7. Kim HS, Son G, Roh EB, et al. Prevalence of gaming disorder: a meta-analysis. Addict Behav. 2022;126:107183.
8. Király O, Koncz P, Griffiths MD, Demetrovics Z. Gaming disorder: a summary of its characteristics and aetiology. Compr Psychiatry. 2023;122:152376.
9. von Deneen KM, Hussain H, Waheed J, et al. Comparison of frontostriatal circuits in adolescent nicotine addiction and internet gaming disorder. J Behav Addict. 2022;11:26–39.
10. Schettler L, Thomasius R, Paschke K. Neural correlates of problematic gaming in adolescents: a systematic review of structural and functional magnetic resonance imaging studies. Addict Biol. 2022;27:e13093.
11. Cho TH, Nah Y, Park SH, Han S. Prefrontal cortical activation in Internet Gaming Disorder Scale high scorers during actual real-time internet gaming: a preliminary study using fNIRS. J Behav Addict. 2022;11:492–505.
12. Akbari M, Seydavi M, Spada MM, Mohammadkhani S, Jamshidi S, Jamaloo A, et al. The Big Five personality traits and online gaming: a systematic review and meta-analysis. J Behav Addict. 2021;10:611–25.
13. Chew PK. A meta-analytic review of internet gaming disorder and the Big Five personality factors. Addict Behav. 2022;126:107193.
14. Şalvarlı Şİ, Griffiths MD. The association between internet gaming disorder and impulsivity: a systematic review of literature. Int J Ment Heal Addict. 2022;20:92–118.
15. Ostinelli EG, Zangani C, Giordano B, et al. Depressive symptoms and depression in individuals with internet gaming disorder: a systematic review and meta-analysis. J Affect Disord. 2021;284:136–42.
16. Wang C-Y, Wu Y-C, Su C-H, Lin P-C, Ko C-H, Yen J-Y. Association between Internet gaming disorder and generalized anxiety disorder. J Behav Addict. 2017;6:564–71.
17. Burleigh TL, Griffiths MD, Sumich A, Stavropoulos V, Kuss DJ. A systematic review of the co-occurrence of Gaming Disorder and other potentially addictive behaviors. Curr Addict Rep. 2019;6:383–401.
18. Murray A, Koronczai B, Király O, et al. Autism, problematic internet use and gaming disorder: a systematic review. Rev J Autism Dev Disord. 2021;9:120–40.
19. Stavropoulos V, Motti-Stefanidi F, Griffiths MD. Being young in the digital era: mental health risks and opportunities. Eur Psychol. 2022;27(2):86–101.
20. King D, Delfabbro P, Griffiths M. Video game structural characteristics: a new psychological taxonomy. Int J Ment Heal Addict. 2010;8:90–106.
21. Szolin K, Kuss D, Nuyens F, Griffiths M. Gaming disorder: a systematic review exploring the user-avatar relationship in videogames. Comput Hum Behav. 2022;128:107124.
22. Király O, Zhang J, Demetrovics Z, Browne DT. Gambling features and monetization in video games creates challenges for young people, families, and clinicians. J Am Acad Child Adolesc Psychiatry. 2021;61:854–6.
23. Gibson E, Griffiths MD, Calado F, Harris A. The relationship between videogame micro-transactions and problem gaming and gambling: a systematic review. Comput Hum Behav. 2022;131(107):219.
24. Schneider LA, King DL, Delfabbro PH. Family factors in adolescent problematic Internet gaming: a systematic review. J Behav Addict. 2017;6:321–33.
25. Nielsen P, Favez N, Rigter H. Parental and family factors associated with problematic gaming and problematic internet use in adolescents: a systematic literature review. Curr Addict Rep. 2020;7:365–86.
26. Rehbein F, Baier D. Family-, media-, and school-related risk factors of video game addiction. J Media Psychol. 2013;25:118–28.

27. Lemmens JS, Valkenburg PM, Peter J. Development and validation of a game addiction scale for adolescents. Media Psychol. 2009;12(1):77–95.
28. Czakó A, Király O, Koncz P, et al. Safer esports for players, spectators, and bettors: issues, challenges, and policy recommendations. J Behav Addict. 2023;12:1–8.
29. Yilmaz E, Griffiths MD, Kan A. Development and validation of Video Game Addiction Scale for Children (VASC). Int J Ment Heal Addict. 2017;15:869–82.
30. Griffiths MD, Pontes HM. The future of gaming disorder research and player protection: what role should the video game industry and researchers play? Int J Ment Heal Addict. 2020;2020(18):784–90.

# Dysregulated Use of Mobile/Smartphone

Sarah E. Domoff, Jon D. Elhai, Jiang Long, Olatz Lopez-Fernandez, Christian Montag, Vladan Starcevic, Attila Szabo, Mariek M. P. Vanden Abeele, Zsolt Demetrovics, and Joel Billieux

## 1 Background

Mobile device ownership (e.g., mobile phones, cell phones, smartphones, or tablets) is prevalent among children and adolescents living in industrialized societies. In the United States, for example, nearly 90% of 13 to 18-year-olds and 40% of 8 to 12-year-olds have their own smartphone [1]. Children use or interact with smartphones in their early years. Csibi et al. [2] demonstrated that preschool children, along with young adults, are at the highest risk for dysregulated smartphone use. Given the ability to use the internet and applications (apps) that are both immediately accessible and highly rewarding to users (e.g., social media, gaming, pornography, streaming content), con-

S. E. Domoff (✉)
Department of Psychology, University at Albany, State University of New York, Albany, NY, USA
e-mail: sdomoff@albany.edu

J. D. Elhai
Department of Psychology, and Department of Psychiatry, University of Toledo, Toledo, OH, USA

J. Long
Shanghai Mental Health Center, Shanghai Jiao Tong University School of Medicine, Shanghai, China

O. Lopez-Fernandez
Faculty of Psychology, Campus de Somosaguas, Universidad Complutense de Madrid, Madrid, Spain

Universidad Francisco de Vitoria, Psychology, Madrid, Spain

Centro de Estudios Universitarios Cardenal Cisneros, University College, Department of Psychology, Madrid, Spain

Hospital Universitario Fundación Jiménez Díaz, Servicio de Psiquiatría, Madrid, Spain

C. Montag
Department of Molecular Psychology, Institute of Psychology and Education, Ulm University, Ulm, Germany

V. Starcevic
FRANZCP, Discipline of Psychiatry, Sydney Medical School, Nepean Clinical School, Faculty of Medicine and Health, University of Sydney, Sydney, NSW, Australia

A. Szabo
Faculty of Education and Psychology, ELTE Eötvös Loránd University, Budapest, Hungary

M. M. P. Vanden Abeele
imec-mict, Ghent University, Ghent, Belgium

Z. Demetrovics
Institute of Psychology, ELTE Eötvös Loránd University, Budapest, Hungary

Centre of Excellence in Responsible Gaming, University of Gibraltar, Gibraltar, Gibraltar

College of Education, Psychology and Social Work, Flinders University, Adelaide, SA, Australia

J. Billieux
Institute of Psychology, University of Lausanne, Lausanne, Switzerland


D. A. Christakis, L. Hale (eds.), *Handbook of Children and Screens*,
https://doi.org/10.1007/978-3-031-69362-5_27

cern exists regarding the development of excessive and dysregulated smartphone use, also often referred to as 'smartphone addiction.'

Children and adolescents are developing their self-regulatory capacities (e.g., executive and inhibitory control, emotion regulation) and are therefore vulnerable to potential harm due to dysregulated use of digital devices across childhood [3]. Research on dysregulated smartphone use in these age groups has thus far examined excessive phone use and its associated risk factors and correlates. Understanding contributors to dysregulated smartphone use in childhood is essential for tailoring prevention of this type of problematic use and its consequences; further, identifying mechanisms maintaining dysregulated phone use in children is necessary to inform clinical management with affected youth and families.

## 2 Current State

Most research on dysregulated smartphone use has surveyed samples of young adults or college students, with varying terminology used to capture the construct (e.g., problematic/addictive phone use or the smartphone or specific types of app). For the purpose of this chapter, research specific to dysregulated smartphone use in children under 18 years will be discussed. While this chapter focuses on what we know about children's dysregulated and excessive smartphone use from a general standpoint, it should be noted that this use can manifest in different forms, including in the excessive use of mobile social media, video games, pornography, or other online activities (e.g., streaming, online gambling).

### 2.1 Measurement and Prevalence of Dysregulated Smartphone Use

There is a sizeable consensus among scholars that to be considered dysregulated, smartphone use needs to be associated with a (1) significant loss of control over the behavior, resulting in (2) severe and persistent functional impairment in daily life. There are noted limitations in the conceptualization, and hence in operationalizing dysregulated smartphone use during childhood, it is thus important to outline some of these concerns when considering the strength of the evidence.

In particular, different terms have been used to define the construct, and existing measures do not necessarily assess the same construct. Although most assessment tools target excessive or addictive usage generically (e.g., Smartphone Addiction Scale [4]; Smartphone Application-Based Addiction Scale) [5], some measures focus more specifically on risky or antisocial patterns of smartphone use, such as smartphone use while driving, that could impair functioning (Problematic Mobile Phone Use Questionnaire) [6]. There also is a debate as to whether the term smartphone addiction itself—which we do not use in the current chapter—is a misnomer [7]. First, several criteria used to define substance use disorders, such as *tolerance* or *withdrawal*, have been criticized when applied to smartphone overuse [8], of which are devices increasingly involved in daily living and tasks. Second, smartphone users are not dependent on the device per se—rather it is a problematic involvement in specific activities facilitated by a smartphone (e.g., social media, gaming, pornography consumption) [8]. To clarify these distinctions, we refer readers to the comprehensive framework proposed by Billieux et al. [9] which theorizes different pathways (e.g., impulsive pathway, reassurance pathway) leading to various types of problematic usage patterns (e.g., addictive, risky, or antisocial use). Given the discrepancies in conceptualization and measurement of dysregulated smartphone use, prevalence rates vary widely across studies.

### 2.2 Risk Factors and Correlates of Dysregulated Smartphone Use

Most research conducted among children and adolescents is cross-sectional, using self-report surveys of dysregulated smartphone use (with varying clusters of symptoms) and potential correlates. Regarding risk factors, early adolescents (i.e., between 11 and 14 years old) tend to display increased dysregulated use [10]. Concerning gender, a review of the literature suggests female adolescents may have higher rates of dysregulated smartphone use compared to male adolescents [11]. Primarily using social media or gaming apps appears to also increase the risk for dysregulated smartphone use [12]. Further, poorer emotion and behavioral regulation has been identified as a risk factor for dysregulated smartphone use [13–15].

The most consistent correlates of dysregulated smartphone use include psychiatric symptoms and poor sleep health. In particular, youth reporting greater dysregulated use also endorse more internalizing symptoms (e.g., depression symptoms and anxiety symptoms) [16, 17]. Further, excessive mobile device use, including dysregulated smartphone use, has been associated with poorer indicators of sleep health, such as poorer sleep quality and shorter sleep duration [18]. Evidence also indicates that dysregulated smartphone use is associated with lower academic achievement [19].

Because there are few longitudinal studies with rigorous methodology (e.g., behavioral observations, mobile phone usage tracking, multi-informant or multimethod approaches), it is not clear whether the correlates precede, co-occur with, or follow the onset of dysregulated smartphone use. Consistent conceptualization suggests that mental health problems could drive or precede dysregulated smartphone use [20]. One exception is an examination of problematic smartphone use among late adolescents over 3 years, which found that dysregulated phone use predicted later symptoms of depression [16]. Thus, conducting longitudinal research is imperative to assess temporality, and to clarify causal relationships, if any, between dysregulated smartphone use, psychopathology, and other health concerns. Such research could be especially attentive to the potential of bi-directional causality, which could trigger a downward co-morbidity spiral in children.

### 2.3 Limitations of Research on Dysregulated Smartphone Use

First and foremost, most of the research based on dysregulated smartphone use has been gathered in adult samples. Evidence collected in children and adolescents remains scarce, while the age of smartphone acquisition and use is diminishing at the worldwide level. Moreover, in addition to the limited research that uses longitudinal designs, a major weakness in the literature entails the sample characteristics. Convenience samples further limit what we know about dysregulated smartphone use in children who are racially and ethnically diverse, in children from lower-income households, and among youth with co-occurring mental health concerns. A few notable exceptions include research among adolescents who have been psychiatrically hospitalized, wherein smartphones have been removed during treatment [21].

As has been suggested with younger children, it is critical to consider how the settings and environments in which a child develops may influence a child's risk for problematic media use [22]. Examining parent- (e.g., parental mediation) and family-level influences [23], as well as individual risk factors (facets of self-regulation), could be particularly illustrative for prevention efforts [14]. To elaborate, future research needs to explore the embedding of children's dysregulated smartphone use within the peer group, and within the broader social organization of society. As for the peer group, young individuals are part of a mobile youth culture in which they are socialized in relation to particular values, norms, and behaviors, as well as in relation to smartphone use. Peer group involvement may lead teenagers to engage in risky and dysregulated smartphone use, as such behaviors may be 'currency' to achieve peer popularity and acceptance [24]. As for the broader social organization of society, future research needs to further scrutinize the role of the tech industry in fostering 'addictive design' principles to reap the rewards of our attention economy [25].

Finally, we lack research examining ways in which specific design features of smartphone-mediated activities (e.g., likes, repost, or forward functions in social media, or random loot boxes in video games) promote dysregulated smartphone use in children and adolescents [25]. Beyond this, most studies in the field do not investigate how smartphone use influences human neurobiology, and evidence—mostly from magnetic resonance imaging studies—is scarce (in particular when children and adolescents are the focus of the research) [26]. This is a critical gap in the literature because children and adolescents are in a phase of brain maturation, where self-regulation abilities still need to evolve. Finally, research about dysregulated smartphone use needs to be supplemented by objective recording of actual behavior [27]. Hence digital phenotyping and mobile sensing principles might help to obtain a deeper understanding of dysregulated smartphone use [28].

## 3 Future Research

- How can dysregulated smartphone use be better distinguished from dysregulated use of social media, gaming, pornography watching, or other excessive involvement in activities via smartphones?
- What is the nature of the relationship and interaction between various mental health problems (i.e., internalizing and externalizing symptoms) and dysregulated smartphone use across childhood?
- How can parents and clinicians recognize early problematic smartphone use in children, and what are the effective ways to handle it?
- What kinds of technology design features [25] promote dysregulated smartphone use in children and adolescents?
- What are the neurobiological effects of smartphone use and dysregulated smartphone use in children and adolescents?

## 4 Recommendations

- Considering the widespread and ever-increasing use of smartphones among the youth, research needs to delineate better criteria for distinguishing between normal (even if somewhat excessive) and dysregulated smartphone use. *For this reason, it is crucial to validate psychometrically sound screening instruments for dysregulated smartphone use in children and adolescents.* Parents' appraisal of their children's smartphone use could complement and validate subjective data obtained from children and adolescents.
- *Funding dedicated to research on the longitudinal trajectories of dysregulated smartphone use and psychopathology, as well as physical health outcomes, is recommended.* Given the high rates of smartphone ownership among children and young adolescents, clarifying how, and for whom, smartphone use interferes with functioning is critical. Funding is needed especially given the *costs for time-intensive, multimethod, and observational longitudinal or randomized controlled clinical trial studies.*
- Regardless of whether dysregulated smartphone use co-occurs with physical and mental health symptoms or is a contributing factor to poorer health (or both), *youth need support in learning how to use smartphones safely and develop skills to regulate their use. Those who are already experiencing negative consequences of smartphone use require support around harm reduction strategies.* In this context, *empirical research is needed to help answer at what age children should ideally receive a smartphone—often being accompanied by unregulated access.* In answering this question, researchers will have to account for the person-specific nature of digital media effects, however, as recent studies show vast among children in terms of vulnerabilities, uses, and effects of digital media [29].

- Importantly, given the links between dysregulated smartphone use and academic achievement, *schools may seek to evaluate multi-tiered systems of support (MTSS) for healthy/adaptive phone use*. Initial research suggests that at least some students could benefit from smartphone bans at schools in terms of better academic performance [30], which have been introduced in countries such as France and China at the moment of writing. Hence, in addition to universal prevention programming on healthy digital media use, targeted practices to support youth experiencing concerns related to smartphone use could be implemented. Since an MTSS framework has not been systematically tested as it relates to smartphone (or social media) overuse, *schools should evaluate strategies and their impact on student engagement, achievement, and well-being*.
- Finally, research needs to *explore whether the recent trend to 'digitally disconnect' from technology offers opportunities for children and teenagers to better regulate their smartphone use, both through the development of non-technological strategies for setting limits to connectivity*. These trends include banning the phone from the bedroom or generally practicing mindfulness in relation to one's smartphone use, to technological strategies, such as removing 'addictive' apps from the phone or using apps that create 'friction' between the user and their smartphone. *Clarifying which strategies have a strong evidence base will help clinicians, parents, and policymakers determine ways to prevent or reduce dysregulated phone use in childhood.*

**Conflict of Interest and Funding Disclosures** SED receives honoraria to present research on problematic media use at non-profit organizations, schools, and hospital/health systems. She has consulted with health systems and private practice clinics on problematic media use and mental health. In 2023, SED consulted with Pixel Digital Health, LLC, on their school-based prevention curriculum. She is on the board of the SmartGen Society. JDE receives royalties for several books published on posttraumatic stress disorder (PTSD); occasionally serves as a paid, expert witness on PTSD legal cases; and receives grant research funding from the U.S. National Institutes of Health. JL was a consultant to the WHO Department of Mental Health and Substance Use (Geneva, Switzerland) and worked on projects regarding disorders due to addictive behaviors from 2020 to 2021. OLF has no conflicts of interest relevant to this chapter to disclose. CM reports no conflict of interest. However, for reasons of transparency CM mentions that he has received (to Ulm University and earlier University of Bonn) grants from agencies such as the German Research Foundation (DFG). CM has performed grant reviews for several agencies; has edited journal sections and articles; has given academic lectures in clinical or scientific venues or companies; and has generated books or book chapters for publishers of mental health texts. For some of these activities, he received royalties, but never from gaming or social media companies. CM mentions that he was part of a discussion circle (Digitalität und Verantwortung: https://about.fb.com/de/news/h/gespraechskreis-digitalitaet-und-verantwortung/) debating ethical questions linked to social media, digitalization, and society/democracy at Facebook. In this context, he received no salary for his activities. Finally, he mentions that he currently functions as an independent scientist on the scientific advisory board of the Nymphenburg group (Munich, Germany). This activity is financially compensated. Moreover, he is on the scientific advisory board of Applied Cognition (Redwood, CA, USA), an activity which is also compensated. VS reports no conflict of interest. AS has no conflicts of interest relevant to this chapter to disclose. MVA has no conflicts of interest relevant to this chapter to disclose. ZD acknowledges that the University of Gibraltar receives funding from the Gibraltar Gambling Care Foundation, an independent, not-for-profit charity, and the ELTE Eötvös Loránd University receives funding from Szerencsejáték Ltd. (the gambling operator of the Hungarian government) to maintain a telephone helpline service for problematic gambling. None of these funding sources aren't related to this study, however. JB reports no conflict of interest. JL states this research was supported by the Institutional Grant of Shanghai Mental Health Center (2021-YJ15). ZD's contribution was supported by the Hungarian National Research, Development, and Innovation Office (KKP126835).

## References

1. Rideout V, Peebles A, Mann S, Robb M. Common Sense census: media use by tweens and teens, 2021. Common Sense; 2022.
2. Csibi S, Griffiths MD, Demetrovics Z, Szabo A. Analysis of problematic smartphone use across different age groups within the 'components model of addiction'. Int J Ment Heal Addict. 2021;19:616–31.
3. Radesky JS, Schumacher J, Zuckerman B. Mobile and interactive media use by young children: the good, the bad, and the unknown. Pediatrics. 2015;135(1):1–3.

4. Kwon M, Kim D-J, Cho H, Yang S. The smartphone addiction scale: development and validation of a short version for adolescents. PLoS One. 2013;8(12):e83558.
5. Csibi S, Griffiths MD, Cook B, Demetrovics Z, Szabo A. The psychometric properties of the smartphone application-based addiction scale (SABAS). Int J Ment Heal Addict. 2018;16(2):393–403.
6. Lopez-Fernandez O, Kuss DJ, Pontes HM, et al. Measurement invariance of the short version of the Problematic Mobile Phone Use Questionnaire (PMPUQ-SV) across eight languages. Int J Environ Res Public Health. 2018;15(6):1213. https://doi.org/10.3390/ijerph15061213.
7. Montag C, Wegmann E, Sariyska R, Demetrovics Z, Brand M. How to overcome taxonomical problems in the study of Internet use disorders and what to do with "smartphone addiction"? J Behav Addict. 2021;9(4):908–14.
8. Billieux J. Problematic use of the mobile phone: a literature review and a pathways model. Curr Psychiatr Rev. 2012;8(4):299–307.
9. Billieux J, Maurage P, Lopez-Fernandez O, Kuss DJ, Griffiths MD. Can disordered mobile phone use be considered a behavioral addiction? An update on current evidence and a comprehensive model for future research. Curr Addict Rep. 2015;2(2):156–62.
10. Lopez-Fernandez O, Honrubia-Serrano L, Freixa-Blanxart M, Gibson W. Prevalence of problematic mobile phone use in British adolescents. Cyberpsychol Behav Soc Netw. 2014;17(2):91–8.
11. Fischer-Grote L, Kothgassner OD, Felnhofer A. Risk factors for problematic smartphone use in children and adolescents: a review of existing literature. Neuropsychiatrie. 2019;33(4):179.
12. Chang F-C, Chiu C-H, Chen P-H, et al. Children's use of mobile devices, smartphone addiction and parental mediation in Taiwan. Comput Hum Behav. 2019;93:25–32. https://doi.org/10.1016/j.chb.2018.11.048.
13. Lee J, Sung M-J, Song S-H, et al. Psychological factors associated with smartphone addiction in South Korean adolescents. J Early Adolesc. 2018;38(3):288–302.
14. Meeus A, Eggermont S, Beullens K. Constantly connected: the role of parental mediation styles and self-regulation in pre- and early adolescents' problematic mobile device use. Hum Commun Res. 2019;45(2):119–47. https://doi.org/10.1093/hcr/hqy015.
15. Yang H, Wang Z, Elhai JD, Montag C. The relationship between adolescent emotion dysregulation and problematic technology use: systematic review of the empirical literature. J Behav Addict. 2022;11(2):290–304. https://doi.org/10.1556/2006.2022.00038.
16. Coyne SM, Stockdale L, Summers K. Problematic cell phone use, depression, anxiety, and self-regulation: evidence from a three year longitudinal study from adolescence to emerging adulthood. Comput Hum Behav. 2019;96:78–84.
17. Lee J, Ahn J-S, Min S, Kim M-H. Psychological characteristics and addiction propensity according to content type of smartphone use. Int J Environ Res Public Health. 2020;17(7):2292.
18. Sohn SY, Rees P, Wildridge B, Kalk NJ, Carter B. Prevalence of problematic smartphone usage and associated mental health outcomes amongst children and young people: a systematic review, meta-analysis and GRADE of the evidence. BMC Psychiatry. 2019;19(1):356. https://doi.org/10.1186/s12888-019-2350-x.
19. Sunday OJ, Adesope OO, Maarhuis PL. The effects of smartphone addiction on learning: a meta-analysis. Comput Hum Behav Rep. 2021;4:100114. https://doi.org/10.1016/j.chbr.2021.100114.
20. Kardefelt-Winther D, Heeren A, Schimmenti A, et al. How can we conceptualize behavioural addiction without pathologizing common behaviours? Addiction. 2017;112(10):1709–15.
21. Burke TA, Domoff SE, Croarkin PE, et al. Reactions to naturalistic smartphone deprivation among psychiatrically hospitalized adolescents. J Psychiatr Res. 2022;155:17–23.
22. Domoff SE, Borgen AL, Radesky JS. Interactional theory of childhood problematic media use. Hum Behav Emerg Technol. 2020;2(4):343–53.
23. Lai X, Huang S, Nie C, Yan JJ, Li Y, Wang Y, Luo Y. Trajectory of problematic smartphone use among adolescents aged 10–18 years: the roles of childhood family environment and concurrent parent–child relationships. J Behav Addict. 2022;11(2):577–87. https://doi.org/10.1556/2006.2022.00047.
24. Vanden Abeele MM. Mobile youth culture: a conceptual development. Mobile Media Commun. 2016;4(1):85–101.
25. Flayelle M, Brevers D, King DL, Maurage P, Perales JC, Billieux J. A taxonomy of technology design features that promote potentially addictive online behaviours. Nat Rev Psychol. 2023:1–15.
26. Montag C, Becker B. Neuroimaging the effects of smartphone (over-) use on brain function and structure—a review on the current state of MRI-based findings and a roadmap for future research. Psychoradiology. 2023;3(1):kkad001.
27. Ellis DA, Davidson BI, Shaw H, Geyer K. Do smartphone usage scales predict behavior? Int J Hum-Comput Stud. 2019;130:86–92.
28. Montag C, Rumpf H-J. The potential of digital phenotyping and mobile sensing for psychodiagnostics of internet use disorders. Curr Addict Rep. 2021;8:422–30.
29. Valkenburg P, Beyens I, Pouwels JL, van Driel II, Keijsers L. Social media use and adolescents' self-esteem: heading for a person-specific media effects paradigm. J Commun. 2021;71(1):56–78.
30. Beland L-P, Murphy R. Ill communication: technology, distraction & student performance. Labour Econ. 2016;41:61–76.

# Treatment and Prevention of Internet Use Disorders in Children and Adolescents

Clifford Sussman, Michael Tsappis, David Greenfield, Paul Weigle, and Hans-Jürgen Rumpf

## 1 Background

Internet-connected digital media provide an increasingly powerful, and engaging vehicle for entertainment, competition, creativity, commerce, social contact, and more. As Internet access and use increased over time, so did the recognition of IUDs [1, 2]. By the 2013 publishing of the Diagnostic and Statistical Manual, fifth edition (DSM-5), problematic video game use—"Internet Gaming Disorder"—was listed as a condition requiring further research [1]. In 2019, the World Health Organization (WHO) included "Gaming Disorder" as a recognized mental, behavioral, or neurodevelopmental disorder in the 11th revision of the International Classification of Diseases (ICD-11) [3]. Supported by the scientific evidence, formal recognition of this new condition was an important step toward meeting the growing IUD public health and clinical needs [4]. For those who struggle with IUDs in ways other than gaming, similar recognition and definition by diagnostic criteria is still needed [5].

Nearly three decades have passed since IUDs emerged as new mental disorders. During that time, scientific research and clinical investigation have focused on defining diagnostic nosology, identifying risk and protective factors, and developing effective treatments. Treatment approaches have often been based upon the framework of IUDs as behavioral addictions. This framework emphasizes the instant gratification and variable ratio reinforcement present in all Internet-delivered content [6].

An evolving understanding of the various forms of problematic screen use has led to debate among experts as to the validity of the initially adopted addiction model of IUDs; and whether the addiction model of IUDs is useful and adequate in influencing the treatment process [7]. Those struggling with IUDs represent a heterogenous population who develop the condition in the context of various combinations of biopsychosocial risk factors. Language devoid of refer-

In loving memory of David Greenfield, a pioneer in the study and treatment of digital use disorders. Your knowledge, passion, and contributions to the field will be missed but forever celebrated.

C. Sussman (✉)
George Washington University School of Medicine, Washington, DC, USA

M. Tsappis
Boston Children's Hospital, Boston, MA, USA

Harvard Medical School, Boston, MA, USA

D. Greenfield
The Center for Internet and Technology Addiction, West Hartford, CT, USA

P. Weigle
University of Connecticut School of Medicine, Farmington, CT, USA

H.-J. Rumpf
University of Lübeck, Department of Psychiatry and Psychotherapy, Lübeck, Germany


D. A. Christakis, L. Hale (eds.), *Handbook of Children and Screens*,
https://doi.org/10.1007/978-3-031-69362-5_28

ence to presumed psychopathology allows for a more nuanced understanding of IUDs as experienced by any individual presenting for care [8].

As we approach a formally agreed-upon definition and conceptual understanding of IUDs, demand for effective treatment already exists. While reported prevalence rates have varied significantly across time, methods, and geography, currently available research indicates that IUDs are common. A recent meta-analysis reported a prevalence of Generalized Internet Addiction of 4.6% in Western nations and 8.9% in Eastern nations and an Internet Gaming Disorder prevalence of 2.19% in Western nations and 3.1% in Eastern nations [9]. IUDs result in significant suffering and impairment and are associated with depression, anxiety, suicidality, aggression, relationship problems, sleep disruption, and academic underachievement [10]. The purpose of this chapter will be to explore the current research evidence on the treatment of IUDs, to propose questions for future research on treatment, and to recommend a course for the future of IUD treatment development.

## 2 Current State

### 2.1 Psychosocial Treatments

Most of the currently available evidence on treating IUDs is limited to treatment for Internet Gaming Disorder (IGD) [11] and, to a lesser extent, online pornography or social media addiction [12–14]. A few studies investigated other variables in treatment groups such as gender [15] or geographic factors [16]. The majority of studies on treatment are based on samples of adolescents and (young) adults.

In a recent systematic review of randomized controlled trials (RCTs) of 126 studies on IGD treatments, only seven met the proposed standard modeled after the Oxford Center for Evidence-Based Medicine (OCEBM) [17]. Three of these used group counseling, two employed manualized cognitive behavioral therapy (CBT), one utilized an Acceptance and Cognitive Restructuring Intervention Program (ACRIP) based on a cognitive behavioral and mindfulness model, and the last employed Craving Behavioral Intervention (CBI) [17]. All seven demonstrated positive findings. A CBT approach covering not only IGD but IUDs more generally reduced IGD symptoms (effect size $d = 1.19$), time spent online ($d = 0.88$), depression ($d = 0.67$), and increased psychosocial functioning ($d = 0.64$) [18].

Successful studies on the treatment of IUDs and IGD have also utilized modalities such as Motivational Interviewing (MI) [19–21], mindfulness [17, 19], and family interventions [19, 22]. Successful treatment outcomes were achieved in various reported therapeutic formats and settings: individual therapy, group therapy [19], specialty camps [23], inpatient [24], and school settings [25], but treatment setting is often not reported [19, 24]. In some studies, successful IUD treatment using the modalities above was related to improvement in comorbid conditions as well, such as ADHD, depression, and social anxiety [15, 26, 27].

The prevalence of IUDs among Eastern countries is reportedly equal to or greater than that of Western countries [9]. In light of potential sociocultural differences in risk exposures, the conceptualization of behavioral health problems, and healthcare delivery, it is informative to consider the similarities and differences between IUD treatment development in Eastern versus Western countries.

The majority of IUD treatments studied in Eastern countries overlap with those investigated in the West. For example, numerous Chinese trials of CBT have demonstrated benefits for IUDs. In a 2017 meta-analysis of treatment interventions in China and Korea, CBT was shown to have a large, significant effect on IUDs and improvements in co-occurring mental conditions. The benefits of CBT for IUDs were demonstrated in both individual and group treatment formats [28]. Another Chinese study demonstrated the effectiveness of CBT with Motivational Interview (MI) provided through online assessment and intervention modules based on psychotherapeutic principles [29]. Also consistent with treatment development in the West, family therapy has been evaluated as a treatment for IUDs. In one study, a group of Chinese adolescents and their families participated in multi-family group therapy for adolescent Internet addiction. Participants in the treatment group experienced significantly reduced Internet use time as well as improvement in parent-child communication, and relationships [30].

A notable example of differences between Eastern and western IUD treatment development is the emphasis on exercise as an intervention. A 2023 meta-analysis by Zhang included 39 randomized controlled trials of exercise for the treatment of IUDs and associated conditions. Studies analyzed not only the benefits of exercise, but also the relative strength of effects based on the categorization of exercise as single, double, or team sport. Exercise significantly reduced IUD symptoms as well as loneliness, anxiety, depression, and interpersonal sensitivity [31].

## 2.2 Abstinence and Restricting Screen Time

Because the studies above usually describe treatment modalities more than specific protocols, the question remains of how much direct regulation of screen time as a behavioral intervention should play a role in various forms of treatment. Fortunately, a few studies specifically examined the idea of temporary abstinence from all or specific types of screen use. A review of studies on voluntary temporary abstinence from digital devices, or "digital detoxes," found that while the benefits varied, these interventions usually resulted in reduced use following the period of abstinence [32]. One such study found that an 84-hour period of Internet gaming abstinence improved outcomes in an IGD group [33]. While temporary abstinence is just one way of moderating use, a 2024 workshop examined multiple self-regulatory interventions for reducing screen time and screen distractions in Oxford University students. These interventions, which included time-limiting apps and other motivational techniques to voluntarily place restrictions on screen time, led most students in the study to continue to benefit from controlling their digital device use after the workshop was completed [34].

## 2.3 Pharmacotherapy

The dopaminergic and noradrenergic antidepressant medication bupropion has been shown effective for IGD in multiple trials, comorbid with or independent of depression [27]. Medications used to treat ADHD such as methylphenidate and atomoxetine are effective for IGD, as well as decreasing impulsivity and inattentiveness in patients with comorbid ADHD. A recent meta-analysis of 124 studies on the treatment of all types of IUDs suggested combining CBT or multi-level counseling with medication management was more effective than either approach alone [28].

## 2.4 Prevention

The increased demand for treatment of IUDs during the pandemic led one international group of leading researchers to publish consensus guidance on preventing problematic Internet use in the home setting where youth were quarantined [35]. Recommendations included an emphasis on routine, structure, and scheduling, frequent off-screen social and stress-reducing activities, use of analog technical tools, physical activity, and parental role modeling of moderate Internet use. The school setting is of outstanding value in reaching children and adolescents to provide universal as well as selective and indicative prevention for IUDs. A systematic review and meta-analysis on the effectiveness of primary prevention approaches for PUI in adolescents and youths found five studies in which the single studies showed effectiveness, but the pooled results did not [30], which leads to the conclusion that additional research is needed. A meta-analysis in 2021 suggested that prevention begins when children are quite young by "establishing healthy online habits" [36] (p. 12).

### 2.5 Limitations

Interpreting the results of these studies is limited by problems such as inadequate subject numbers, patient noncompliance, and varying outcome measures, making it difficult to determine which of these treatments is the most effective [15, 17, 25]. Although the various forms of IUDs all theoretically involve the same limbic reward neurocircuitry [1], the lack of uniformity concerning inclusion criteria and treatment protocols also makes the interpretation of findings a challenge [15, 17, 25]. Treatments are typically defined in the literature as "effective" based on a reduction of scores on various scales assessing symptoms, without necessarily establishing long-term outcomes [15]. A frustrating confounding variable in the studies referenced in this chapter is the lack of treatment details provided by investigators, such that it is often unclear whether temporary abstinence from Internet use was a requirement to participate in either the treatment or the control group, and if so, whether this contributed to the success of treatments. Finally, various treatments of different behavioral disorders used in studies are sometimes administered online [21], therefore, it must be examined how such interventions can be used as stand-alone approaches or might be combined in blended treatments.

Regarding treatment recommendations specified for children and adolescents, current evidence is inadequate. Since most of the samples have included adolescents or (young) adults, there is at least partial evidence that some of the approaches work in younger age groups. However, there is a need for treatment studies testing specifically designed treatments for younger age groups. In addition, effective prevention and early intervention studies are of special importance and still not fully developed within high-quality studies.

## 3 Future Research

### 3.1 Clinical Treatments

Which therapeutic interventions are most useful across different IUDs, patient populations, including children and adolescents, and treatment settings? How can researchers obtain more comparative data on efficacy among treatments using similar settings and admission criteria? How does successful treatment of IUDs impact common comorbidities such as depression and social anxiety? Should treatment protocols include a stepwise progression, from evaluation, to establishment of therapeutic alliance and motivation, to skill building, and finally maintenance, upon return to adaptive functioning? Should screening for IUDs become a standard part of all pediatric or mental health evaluations?

### 3.2 Addressing IUDs Outside of the Clinic

How do we best reach and motivate children and adolescents with IUDs to participate in treatment? What are the most effective specific strategies and interventions for their parents? What consideration should be given to limits on screen time and developmentally inappropriate content, independence, privacy, and supporting self-regulation? How should strategies be adjusted for differences in culture and family values? Under what circumstances and for what duration is voluntary or enforced abstinence effective for IUDs?

### 3.3 Prevention

What specific strategies can families use to weigh the benefits of screen media use with the risk of excessive use? What simple interventions, such as programming more off-screen activities into a child's day, can prevent IUDs? Which other risk factors are modifiable in the course of developing IUDs? How will preventive measures change as digital technology and its impact on humans change?

## 4 Recommendations

### 4.1 For Clinicians

- Despite the greater demand than supply of care for IUDs, providers in all child and adolescent care settings must be able to identify available treatment options and levels of care currently available to patients with IUDs. For now, we recommend obtaining a detailed biopsychosocial assessment of the factors involved in the development and persistence of IUDs and a customized treatment approach that may utilize multiple treatment modalities and multiple settings and include the entire family.
- Young people entering treatment for IUDs have often experienced interpersonal conflict with parents and authority figures and often respond with opposition to any effort for change. A priority for clinicians is to build and maintain a therapeutic alliance with the youth, their parent(s), and other treatment providers while supporting cooperation between these parties. Motivational enhancement approaches should be utilized in the process of goal setting.
- Lifelong abstinence from screen media use is impractical because of the ubiquitous nature of online interactions in contemporary society. Sustained abstinence may even conflict with the ultimate goal of treatment: a balance of immediately gratifying screen media and activities requiring delayed gratification. Such a balance may foster self-regulation via inhibitory prefrontal cortical functioning, improving mindful and sustainable media use [7]. As referenced above, however, some experts recommend an initial period of enforced abstinence from screen media, or "digital detoxification," to address tolerance, withdrawal, and cravings in a manner similar to detoxification from substances. Others warn such an intervention risks damage to treatment alliances. Regardless, residential centers, wilderness programs, and therapeutic summer camps typically utilize enforced abstinence as an initial treatment phase, and some outpatient providers advise brief periods of abstinence, such as those enabled by a family camping trip.
- As a young person achieves greater regulation of screen media use, treatment efforts should include efforts to address remaining barriers to adaptive functioning, such as school truancy and erratic sleep patterns. Processing instances of failure to achieve treatment goals helps identify personal and family system vulnerabilities underlying IUDs. For example, IUDs driven by inhibitory control weakness may result in a different treatment barrier than that driven by a need for social connection.

### 4.2 For Parents

- Parents and caregivers may recognize screen media as a set of tools requiring skills to properly operate. From a child's first screen media exposure, skill development requires active, intentional parental involvement. As they mature and demonstrate the ability to use responsibly, children may be allowed greater screen media access to support independence.
- Parents and caregivers should understand the functionality and features of devices and applications before granting access and should consider privacy and content settings for children and young adolescents.
- Parents should maintain open dialogue to guide their children on media content choices, experiences, online interpersonal communications (including the sharing of personal information), time management, and balance. During adolescence, parent guidance may facilitate increasing autonomy, privacy, and control as needed to foster a successful transition to adulthood with the skills needed to

self-regulate electronic screen media and adjust to future technological advancements.
- Parents of children with IUDs often find themselves drawn towards unhelpful extremes of micromanagement or enabling and require more effective strategies. Parents should work with clinicians and community resources to set appropriate screen use intervals, help children disengage from screen media, use positive and negative consequences to incentivize healthy use, and encourage diverse leisure and entertainment activities offline in addition to screen activities, adjusting environmental cues and Internet access accordingly. Successful treatment usually requires consistent family investment, including therapy attendance as needed and the adoption of adaptive screen use patterns for all.

**Conflict of Interest and Funding Disclosures** No funding was secured for this report. The work of HJR on this chapter was carried out in the context of the Research Unit ACSID, FOR2974, funded by the Deutsche Forschungsgemeinschaft (DFG, German Research Foundation) and the German Innovation Fund (01NVF19029).

## References

1. Sussman CJ, Harper JM, Stahl JL, Weigle P. Internet and video game addictions: diagnosis, epidemiology, and neurobiology. Child Adolesc Psychiatr Clin N Am. 2018;27(2):307–26. https://doi.org/10.1016/j.chc.2017.11.015.
2. Greenfield DN. Psychological characteristics of compulsive internet use: a preliminary analysis. Cyberpsychol Behav. 1999;2(5):403–12. https://doi.org/10.1089/cpb.1999.2.403.
3. ICD-11 for mortality and morbidity statistics. https://icd.who.int/browse11/l-m/en#/http%3a%2f%2fid.who.int%2ficd%2fentity%2f1448597234.
4. Saunders JB, Hao W, Long J, et al. Gaming disorder: its delineation as an important condition for diagnosis, management, and prevention. J Behav Addict. 2017;6(3):271–9. https://doi.org/10.1556/2006.6.2017.039.
5. Brand M, Rumpf H-J, Demetrovics Z, et al. Which conditions should be considered as disorders in the International Classification of Diseases (ICD-11) designation of "other specified disorders due to addictive behaviors"? J Behav Addict. Published online June 30, 2020. https://doi.org/10.1556/2006.2020.00035.
6. Greenfield DN. Clinical considerations in internet and video game addiction treatment. Child Adolesc Psychiatr Clin N Am. 2022;31(1):99–119. https://doi.org/10.1016/j.chc.2021.09.003.
7. Starcevic V. Is internet addiction a useful concept? Aust N Z J Psychiatry. 2013;47(1):16–9. https://doi.org/10.1177/0004867412461693.
8. Starcevic V. Internet gaming disorder: inadequate diagnostic criteria wrapped in a constraining conceptual model. J Behav Addict. 2017;6(2):110–3.
9. Pan YC, Chiu YC, Lin YH. Systematic review and meta-analysis of epidemiology of internet addiction. Neurosci Biobehav Rev. 2020;118:612–22. https://doi.org/10.1016/j.neubiorev.2020.08.013.
10. Poorolajal J, Ahmadpoor J, Mohammadi Y, Soltanian AR, Asghari SZ, Mazloumi E. Prevalence of problematic internet use disorder and associated risk factors and complications among Iranian university students: a national survey. Health Promot Perspect. 2019;9(3):207–13. https://doi.org/10.15171/hpp.2019.29.
11. Zajac K, Ginley MK, Chang R. Treatments of internet gaming disorder: a systematic review of the evidence. Expert Rev Neurother. 2020;20(1):85–93. https://doi.org/10.1080/14737175.2020.1671824.
12. Fernandez DP, Kuss DJ, Griffiths MD. The pornography "rebooting" experience: a qualitative analysis of abstinence journals on an online pornography abstinence forum. Arch Sex Behav. 2021;50(2):711–28. https://doi.org/10.1007/s10508-020-01858-w.
13. Turel O, Cavagnaro DR. Effect of abstinence from social media on time perception: differences between low- and at-risk for social media "addiction" groups. Psychiatry Q. 2019;90(1):217–27. https://doi.org/10.1007/s11126-018-9614-3.
14. Zhou X, Rau PLP, Yang CL, Zhou X. Cognitive Behavioral therapy-based short-term abstinence intervention for problematic social media use: improved well-being and underlying mechanisms. Psychiatry Q. 2021;92(2):761–79. https://doi.org/10.1007/s11126-020-09852-0.
15. Stevens MWR, King DL, Dorstyn D, Delfabbro PH. Cognitive–behavioral therapy for internet gaming disorder: a systematic review and meta-analysis. Clin Psychol Psychother. 2019;26(2):191–203. https://doi.org/10.1002/cpp.2341.
16. Ko CH, Yen JY, Lin PC. Association between urbanization and internet addiction. Curr Opin Psychiatry. 2022;35(3):219–25. https://doi.org/10.1097/YCO.0000000000000780.
17. Chen Y, Lu J, Wang L, Gao X. Effective interventions for gaming disorder: a systematic review of randomized control trials. Front Psychiatry. 2023:14. https://doi.org/10.3389/fpsyt.2023.1098922.
18. Wölfling K, Müller KW, Dreier M, et al. Efficacy of short-term treatment of internet and computer game addiction: a randomized clinical trial. JAMA Psychiatry. 2019;76(10):1018. https://doi.org/10.1001/jamapsychiatry.2019.1676.

19. Xu L, Wu LL, Geng XM, et al. A review of psychological interventions for internet addiction. Psychiatry Res. 2021;302:114016. https://doi.org/10.1016/j.psychres.2021.114016.
20. Schmidt H, Brandt D, Meyer C, et al. Motivational brief interventions for adolescents and young adults with internet use disorders: a randomized-controlled trial. J Behav Addict. 2022;11(3):754–65. https://doi.org/10.1556/2006.2022.00049.
21. Bottel L, Brand M, Dieris-Hirche J, Herpertz S, Timmesfeld N, Wildt BTT. Efficacy of short-term telemedicine motivation-based intervention for individuals with internet use disorder-a pilot-study. J Behav Addict. 2021;10(4):1005–14. https://doi.org/10.1556/2006.2021.00071.
22. Bonnaire C, Liddle HA, Har A, Nielsen P, Phan O. Why and how to include parents in the treatment of adolescents presenting internet gaming disorder? J Behav Addict. 2019;8(2):201–12. https://doi.org/10.1556/2006.8.2019.27.
23. Sakuma H, Mihara S, Nakayama H, et al. Treatment with the self-discovery camp (SDiC) improves internet gaming disorder. Addict Behav. 2017;64:357–62. https://doi.org/10.1016/j.addbeh.2016.06.013.
24. King DL, Delfabbro PH, Wu AMS, et al. Treatment of internet gaming disorder: an international systematic review and CONSORT evaluation. Clin Psychol Rev. 2017;54:123–33. https://doi.org/10.1016/j.cpr.2017.04.002.
25. Lindenberg K, Kindt S, Szász-Janocha C. Effectiveness of cognitive behavioral therapy-based intervention in preventing gaming disorder and unspecified internet use disorder in adolescents: a cluster randomized clinical trial. JAMA Netw Open. 2022;5(2):e2148995. https://doi.org/10.1001/jamanetworkopen.2021.48995.
26. Seo EH, Yang HJ, Kim SG, Park SC, Lee SK, Yoon HJ. A literature review on the efficacy and related neural effects of pharmacological and psychosocial treatments in individuals with internet gaming disorder. Psychiatry Investig. 2021;18(12):1149–63. https://doi.org/10.30773/pi.2021.0207.
27. Chang CH, Chang YC, Yang L, Tzang RF. The comparative efficacy of treatments for children and young adults with internet addiction/internet gaming disorder: an updated meta-analysis. Int J Environ Res Public Health. 2022;19(5):2612. https://doi.org/10.3390/ijerph19052612.
28. Liu J, Nie J, Wang Y. Effects of group counseling programs, cognitive behavioral therapy, and sports intervention on internet addiction in East Asia: a systematic review and meta-analysis. Int J Environ Res Public Health. 2017;14(12):1470. https://doi.org/10.3390/ijerph14121470.
29. Su W, et al. Internet-based intervention for the treatment of online addiction for college students in China: a pilot study of the healthy online self-helping center. Cyberpsychol Behav Soc Netw. 2011;14(9):497–503. https://doi.org/10.1089/cyber.2010.0167.
30. Liu Q-X, et al. Multi-family group therapy for adolescent internet addiction: exploring the underlying mechanisms. Addict Behav. 2015;42:1–8. https://doi.org/10.1016/j.addbeh.2014.10.021.
31. Zhang X, Yang H, Zhang K, et al. Effects of exercise or tai chi on internet addiction in college students and the potential role of gut microbiota: a randomized controlled trial. J Affect Disord. 2023;327:404–15. https://doi.org/10.1016/j.jad.2023.02.002.
32. Radtke T, et al. Digital Detox: An effective solution in the smartphone era? A systematic literature review. Mobile Media Commun. 2021;10(2):190–215. https://doi.org/10.1177/20501579211028647.
33. King DL, et al. Effectiveness of brief abstinence for modifying problematic internet gaming cognitions and behaviors. J Clin Psychol. 2017;73(12):1573–85. https://doi.org/10.1002/jclp.22460.
34. Lyngs U, Lukoff K, Slovak P, et al. "I finally felt I had the tools to control these urges": empowering students to achieve their device use goals with the reduce digital distraction workshop. 2024.
35. Király O, Potenza MN, Stein DJ, et al. Preventing problematic internet use during the COVID-19 pandemic: consensus guidance. Compr Psychiatry. 2020;100:152180. https://doi.org/10.1016/j.comppsych.2020.152180.
36. Romero Saletti SM, Van Den Broucke S, Chau C. The effectiveness of prevention programs for problematic internet use in adolescents and youths: a systematic review and meta-analysis. Cyberpsychol J Psychosoc Res Cyberspace. 2021;15(2). https://doi.org/10.5817/CP2021-2-10.

# Introduction to the Section on Youth Digital Wellbeing

Katie Davis and Linda Charmaraman

Recent years have marked a growing societal worry about technology's negative impact on young people. This worry is largely fueled by alarming increases in youth mental health concerns that coincide with the rise of smartphones and social media. As a result, school districts are bringing lawsuits against big tech companies for alleged damage to their students' well-being. Governments across the globe are introducing legislation to compel tech companies to prioritize youth mental health and well-being in their designs. And the people in youth's lives, from parents to pediatricians, are looking for guidance on how to provide the best support around digital experiences.

Observing that the harms of social media—including problematic social media use, cyberbullying, and negative mental and physical health effects—are well-addressed in other parts of the handbook, the authors of the chapters in this section focus more on the positive dimensions of young people's social media experiences. The six chapters in this section paint a nuanced picture of technology's role in young people's lives, focusing primarily (but not exclusively) on adolescents and emerging adults, and often underscoring the unique experiences of marginalized youth. By examining positive dimensions alongside the negative, the authors bring a measured approach to the current state of knowledge and present targeted recommendations to guide stakeholders going forward. In this introduction, we provide an executive summary of each chapter, pulling out notable themes that address the section's overarching focus on youth well-being, kindness, social communication, and connection in online environments.

Uhls et al. (see Chapter "Adolescents' Online Communication Practices in a Digital World") examine youth's experiences with online communication through three common modalities: direct messaging, video-mediated communication, and social gaming. They describe current knowledge about how adolescents use each modality and the social mechanisms underlying their motivations for use. Direct messaging, for instance, provides a private and intimate setting for adolescents to build social connections and receive social support. Video-mediated communication, which rose in popularity during the COVID-19 pandemic, affords adolescents opportunities for social connection especially when in-person contact is not possible. Social gaming supports online connections through shared gaming experiences and can sometimes lead to offline friendships. The authors point out that, across these modalities, self-disclosure and

K. Davis (✉)
Information School, University of Washington, Seattle, WA, USA
e-mail: kdavis78@uw.edu

L. Charmaraman
Wellesley Centers for Women, Wellesley College, Wellesley, MA, USA



D. A. Christakis, L. Hale (eds.), *Handbook of Children and Screens*,
https://doi.org/10.1007/978-3-031-69362-5_29

emotional connection are two important mechanisms driving adolescents' successful online communication.

Uhls et al. pay particular attention to the critical role that online communication plays in the well-being of many marginalized youth. They observe that for some youth, such as adolescents struggling with mental or physical health issues, queer youth, and adolescent girls, online environments offer support and understanding that is missing offline. However, the authors note that the use of online communication tools can also pose risks for some vulnerable youth. For instance, some adolescents can get caught in a negative reinforcing spiral through their participation in communities that glorify harmful behavior such as self-injury.

Charmaraman et al. (see Chapter "Youth Digital Wellbeing and Social Connectedness") explore how adolescents' participation in online environments—especially social media platforms—impacts their well-being and opportunities for social connection. The authors place this exploration in a developmental context, emphasizing the critical roles that peer relationships and social connectedness play during adolescence. Consistent with Uhls et al., the authors observe that social connectedness online is a double-edged sword. On the one hand, social media platforms offer adolescents opportunities to connect with similar youth and find social support, particularly for vulnerable populations that do not have strong offline support. On the other hand, negative peer feedback, including peer victimization, can be harmful to adolescents' well-being. The authors observe that murky methodology is another factor, and they call for clearer, more consistent definitions, as well as more nuanced research approaches that move beyond cross-sectional studies that measure "screen time" or aggregate measures together that approximate "wellbeing."

The lack of a singular research narrative is partially due to the multi-dimensional and contextual nature of adolescents' social media engagement. The authors caution against parents, educators, clinicians, and policymakers perpetuating a narrative that portrays social media as entirely negative, which can backfire and undermine youth wellbeing. They propose that future research focuses on identifying peer norms and technology designs that support rather than undermine youth well-being. This knowledge can be used to inform policies that incentivize tech companies to take youth wellbeing into account and research practices that are strengths-based and center youth's perspectives.

James et al. (see Chapter "Empathy, Kindness, and Dignity in a Connected World") similarly embrace a nuanced view of youth's engagement with digital technologies in the context of empathy, kindness, and dignity. For instance, the authors point to research showing a correlation between narcissism and social media use, but they observe other research showing that teens who use more social media have higher empathy 1 year later. James et al. acknowledge the legitimacy of concerns about toxic disinhibition and bullying behavior in digital exchanges, but they also provide examples of youth engaging with digital technologies in empathic and prosocial ways. These examples include interventions that make use of text messages and smartphone apps to increase empathy in youth, and research showing a correlation between social media engagement and online donations.

The authors emphasize that promoting empathy, kindness, and prosocial behavior in online settings is not simply an individual-level challenge. Design and policy play key roles. As one example, they observe the tendency for algorithmic design to spread racist, sexist, and other hate-filled content, as well as the role that policy can play in curtailing the spread of such content. Drawing on the United Nations Convention on the Rights of the Child, which asserts that children have the right to protection and participation in digital environments, James et al. discuss the dignity framework as a promising approach for designing and regulating rights-based online environments.

Bond et al. (see Chapter "Parasocial Relationships in Children and Teens") consider social connection in online environments through the lens of parasocial relationships (PSR), fandom, and popular culture. Pointing to the ubiquity of entertainment media—and the characters and celebrities associated with them—in youth's lives, the authors explore how children and adolescents relate to media personalities and form interpersonal connections with them. Their investigation looks across development, from toddlers who can name their favorite TV character to adolescents' parasocial relationships with pop stars. They observe how changes in technology change the scope and nature of youth's PSRs. For example, the introduction of conversational agents (e.g., Siri, Alexa) has expanded the concept of a parasocial relationship, and the advent of social media has provided a degree of reciprocity with parasocial others.

PSRs can play an important role in youth's wellbeing and identity development. Identification with a media personality or fictional character can be particularly valuable for youth who lack others like them in their daily lives. Identification can also support social development, such as by providing opportunities to practice taking on another person's perspective. The authors warn, however, that extreme forms of identification, such as celebrity worship, have been linked with lowered wellbeing. In addition, some youth may also identify with harmful messages, such as when adolescents internalize unrealistic beauty standards that are promoted by celebrities they admire.

Yang et al. (see Chapter "Online Self-Presentation and Identity: Insights from Diverse and Marginalized Youth") explore the topic of identity and its relationship to wellbeing by taking stock of current research relating to online self-presentation and its connection to adolescent identity development, body image, and the experiences of marginalized youth. They observe that adolescents and emerging adults are motivated to put forward a positive self-presentation online, yet they also value self-authenticity. Existing research suggests these motivations are not necessarily at odds. Studies of emerging adults showed either a positive or null correlation between positive and authentic self-presentation. Moreover, research suggests that both forms of self-presentation are generally associated with positive identity outcomes.

Exceptions to this positive association include identity issues related to body image and marginalized youth. Yang et al. observe that body concerns increase during adolescence, especially among girls. With respect to marginalized youth, the authors focus on sexual and gender minority (SGM) youth, youth from underrepresented cultural and racial/ethnic backgrounds, and migrant youth. For each of these groups, they identify identity-related opportunities and challenges. For example, social media can be a place for SGM youth to share their authentic self without stigma if they can find supportive online communities. At the same time, sharing their authentic self can place SGM youth at risk for cyberbullying and discrimination in less supportive online communities. The authors call for future research that explores youth's experiences with and understanding online self-presentation in the context of intersecting identities.

Moving from an individual to a collective focus, Middaugh et al. (see Chapter "Youth Participatory Politics: Understanding and Supporting Civic Engagement in the Social Media Era") examine youth civic engagement in the social media era. The authors focus on the concept of participatory politics, which they define as "decentralized practices through which individuals and groups seek to exert voice and influence on issues of public concern, often by using digital tools and networks to access, circulate, and produce media and to engage with others and mobilize action." Participatory politics centers on youth agency, participation, and social connectedness. The authors connect these elements of participatory politics to positive youth development.

Middaugh et al. describe both benefits and risks associated with youth engagement in participatory politics. Benefits include opportunities to develop an empowering narrative around one's identity—especially for identities that have been historically marginalized—and connect that identity to collective political expression. They also cite research showing a connection between youth's engagement in participatory politics and positive social–emotional development, including empathy. Risks include exposure to discrimination, racism, and enabling radicalization through participation in online communities that promote extreme views. The authors observe the challenges that many youth face in navigating online conflict, as well as misinformation and disinformation. Surveillance, censorship, and self-censorship represent additional risks associated with participatory politics.

Looking to future research on youth civic engagement, Middaugh et al. present a set of promising strategies aimed at promoting the benefits and minimizing the risks of participatory politics. These strategies are intended to contribute to youth's "civic media literacy," which refers to the capacity to access, analyze, and communicate information for civic goals. Among these strategies, the authors emphasize the value of providing youth opportunities to practice engaging in difficult political conversations in the context of trusting relationships.

Collectively, these chapters provide an important contribution to our current understanding of factors affecting youth wellbeing, kindness, social communication, and connection in online environments. Reflecting on the complexity of the research landscape, the authors observe the value of taking a nuanced view of youth's online experiences, one that accounts for the multifaceted relationships among individual, contextual, and technological factors. The chapters in this section also underscore the need to attend to the developmental context of youth's online interactions. A developmental lens helps advance our understanding of young people's motivations, experiences, and vulnerabilities as they interact with digital technologies. Lastly, the chapters argue for the need to look beyond individual-level dimensions of youth wellbeing and online connection, including a collective framework that recognizes the basic human need for social connection and interaction. Discussions of government policy and technology design point to key system-level factors that can play a crucial role in supporting youth's positive digital experiences.

**Conflict of Interest and Funding Disclosures** None.

# Adolescents' Online Communication Practices in a Digital World

Yalda T. Uhls, Amber van der Wal, Nicole Ellison, Anne Collier, Kaveri Subrahmanyam, and Patti M. Valkenburg

## 1 Background

Online communication, the exchange of messages via computers or mobile devices, has evolved significantly over the last few decades. Changes encompass features such as video, image, audio, geolocation, and various communication modes (e.g., one-on-one, groups, etc.). The advent of mobile technology has further facilitated asynchronous and nearly instant real-time communication, allowing users to connect with others at any time and place, as long as they have cellular or internet access. It is believed that the constant mobile connectivity provided by smartphones has resulted in unique developmental experiences for contemporary adolescents, which differ from those of previous generations [1–3]. As one teen aptly put it, "I don't have an addiction to technology, I have an addiction to my friends" [4].

Author "Yalda T. Uhls" designates first authorship

Y. T. Uhls (✉)
Center for Scholars & Storytellers, University of California Los Angeles, Los Angeles, CA, USA
e-mail: yalda@scholarsandstorytellers.com

A. van der Wal · P. M. Valkenburg
University of Amsterdam, Amsterdam, Netherlands

N. Ellison
University of Michigan, Ann Arbor, MI, USA

A. Collier
The Net Safety Collaborative, Salt Lake City, UT, USA

K. Subrahmanyam
University of North Florida, Jacksonville, FL, USA

This chapter aims to highlight research on how adolescents use digital media for communication, along with the positive and negative implications for their social well-being, defined as experiencing high levels of interpersonal connection and low levels of loneliness [5]. First, we discuss recent advancements in modalities that support online communication. Next, we review some of the social mechanisms that may underlie adolescents' motivation to use digital communication tools. Importantly, we review the critical role online communication plays in the social well-being of many marginalized youth who may be at risk for isolation and rely on these tools for connection with like-minded peers. Finally, we offer suggestions for future research and provide recommendations for stakeholders.

Our focus is on adolescents, defined by the National Academy of Sciences as being between the ages of 10 and 25 [6]. Furthermore, our attention is directed outside of school, where adolescents choose their own methods for digital communication, especially with peers.

## 2 Current State

### 2.1 Social Media

Social media are internet-based channels of masspersonal communication in which value is primarily derived from user-generated content [7]. Adolescents connect with others through


D. A. Christakis, L. Hale (eds.), *Handbook of Children and Screens*,
https://doi.org/10.1007/978-3-031-69362-5_30

using social media for one-to-one or group communication. Types of communication practices vary, with adolescents using tools that allow for direct messaging, video chat, and interaction while gaming, etc. The chapter reviews these particular modalities and their social affordances [8].

### 2.1.1 Direct Messaging

Instant or direct messaging has been popular since the 1990s. This mode of communication is still widely used, in particular by adolescent girls who report spending on average nearly 2 hours per day on messaging apps such as Instagram and Snapchat [9]. Direct messaging may encourage stronger social connections, possibly due to its private and intimate setting. For example, a mixed-methods study of approximately 1000 Austrian early adolescents found that instant messaging was perceived as the most helpful tool for building friendships compared to other digital tools [10]. Furthermore, in a 2022 focus group study—although large differences existed between adolescents—many adolescents indicated that when they were feeling bad, they would message their friend(s) directly for social support [11]. Direct online communication is also associated with the ability to initiate offline friendships [12]. However, adolescents may also experience a downside of the direct messaging modality. That is, some adolescents, particularly girls, can receive unwanted messages from strangers, such as inappropriate requests and pictures [9, 11].

### 2.1.2 Video-Mediated Communication (VMC)

The COVID-19 pandemic led to a rapid increase in the adoption of VMC tools, such as Zoom, WhatsApp, and FaceTime. Today, a significant percentage of US adolescents report using VMCs [13]. VMCs offer real-time socially contingent interaction, providing many opportunities to connect with peers.

*How does VMC compare to in-person interaction?* A pre-pandemic study of over 1700 adolescents, which used experience sampling to measure online versus in-person interaction, found that in-person communication had more social and emotional benefits, yet respondents also reported experiencing more positive affect when interacting online than when being alone [14]. A study with 2000 participants showed that VMCs, used during the COVID-19 pandemic, were associated with positive social well-being among young people [15]. Thus, when in-person contact is unavailable, as during this pandemic, but also when adolescents are at home or otherwise prohibited from seeing their friends in person [11], VMC can be an important source of social and emotional support.

### 2.1.3 Social Gaming

While popular media paint a typical videogamer as a 12-year-old boy playing on a console alone in his basement, gaming has become a community sport, where players can communicate as they play [16]. This kind of gaming encourages social connections and can meet developmental needs for interaction with peers. Furthermore, online gaming may lead to offline friendships. For example, researchers interviewed 21 pairs of adult gamers who met on Twitch channels to determine whether they became friends and met in person at a later date and found several dyads did indeed develop close relationships [17]. Similarly, over 10 years, researchers followed the development of friendship ties between Nintendo DS players. The relationships of these gamers went from total strangers to online acquaintances, to online friends, to offline friends [18]. Thus, some adolescents can overcome physical barriers and build relationships through meaningful social interactions while gaming [18]. Moreover, in-person interactions were helpful in validating and maintaining the connections made online. Yet researchers also showed that when the gaming community is larger, fewer opportunities exist for interpersonal connection [17]. Although online communication can facilitate perceived trust and intimacy, in-person interactions gave authenticity to these perceptions and contributed to sustaining the relationships [18].

## 2.2 Drivers and Consequences of Adolescents' Online Communication

Two important mechanisms seem to drive adolescents' successful use of online communication to form and strengthen both online and offline friendships: self-disclosure and emotional connection. Adolescents' mobile connectivity may also lead to negative consequences, such as feeling overwhelmed, jealous, or left out and "cyberbullying" or online harassment. This chapter now reviews research on these mechanisms and some of the potential benefits and risks.

### 2.2.1 Self-disclosure

Self-disclosure, which refers to the act of sharing personal information about oneself, is an important mechanism for building social relationships. Research finds that the ability to disclose information about oneself through digital channels can support adolescents' social needs [12]. In a longitudinal study, Valkenburg and colleagues investigated intimate online and offline self-disclosure using self-reports. Results showed that online self-disclosure improved offline communication skills, demonstrating a transfer of developmentally important skills [19]. A recent literature review compared online and offline self-disclosure, revealing that in-person self-disclosure is more beneficial for enhancing relationship quality. Interestingly, the same review reported that some adolescents, such as highly anxious individuals and boys ages 12–13, gain more benefits from online self-disclosure than offline self-disclosure [12]. For these youth, the ability to seek out more information about peers and to respond asynchronously was helpful. Additionally, a systematic review of digital media and adolescents during the COVID-19 pandemic found that online self-disclosure, when conducted with friends, had a positive impact on mental wellness [20].

### 2.2.2 Emotional Connection

Adolescents often use social media to emotionally connect with others. This is especially true for those adolescents who struggle to establish connections offline. As one 16-year-old girl said: "I usually find it challenging to make contact with others, but social media makes it easier for me" [11]. Additionally, many adolescents report feeling emotionally connected to their friends by keeping in touch with them throughout the day. In this manner, rather than replacing in-person interaction, social media can add a layer of emotional connectivity to many adolescents' lives [11].

Furthermore, many adolescents use online communication with their peers to attempt to understand and work out emotional responses. A study by Uhls and colleagues [21] found that 6th-grade students in 2017 were better able to read nonverbal emotional cues in photographs than 6th-grade students in 2012. These findings may be explained because online communication shifted from text-based to photo-based applications that enable adolescents to share pictures, often with emotional expressions, with friends [22].

Nevertheless, while online communication could increase emotional understanding and connections for some, it can also result in feelings of distress. A longitudinal study found that adolescents who used online communication to cope with emotional stressors reported more overtly negative emotions 1 week later, mainly related to worry and jealousy [23]. Relatedly, some adolescents reported feeling left out or jealous, particularly when they received messages about friends hanging out without them. Finally, many adolescents appear to feel pressure to be constantly available or responsive to peers via online communication [9, 11].

### 2.2.3 Cyberbullying

While a review of cyberbullying is beyond the scope of this chapter, much of the literature on the negative consequences of online communication focuses on cyberbullying. Nearly half of US teens reported experiencing some form of cyberbullying in a recent Pew study [24]. The literature also shows that cyberbullying—both perpetration and victimization—is a complex issue that involves both individual and contextual factors [25]. For example, individual predictors of cyberbullying perpetration and victimization include low self-esteem and empathy, as well as factors such as age, gender, and poor psychosocial adjustment [26]. Contextual factors that may predict cyberbullying are peer influence and parental monitoring [25].

Complicating this issue, Marciano and colleagues conducted a meta-analysis of longitudinal studies and found that cyberbullying perpetration and victimization were related to each other over time, indicating a bidirectional relationship between the two, meaning that victims may become perpetrators of cyberbullying and vice versa [27]. Other research found that individuals who engage in offline bullying are also likely to engage in online cyberbullying [28]. Similarly, individuals who are victimized offline are also at an increased risk of being victimized online. As such, it is important to recognize that online and offline bullying are often interrelated, just as victimization and perpetration are, and effective prevention and intervention strategies should take this into account.

### 2.2.4 Vulnerable Groups

In this chapter, we want to pay special attention to the role of online communication in the lives of adolescents from different vulnerable or marginalized groups, such as adolescents struggling with mental or physical health issues, queer[1] youth, and adolescent girls. For some of these groups, there seem to be substantial benefits to online communication, which provides possibilities, support, and understanding that may not be available offline [29]. Research shows that queer youth are more likely to have close supportive online friendships compared to offline friendships (50% versus 19%) [29, 30]. Similarly, adolescents who have Autism Spectrum Disorder or a chronic illness find online spaces and communication helpful for building relationships with others who have similar experiences [31].

Moreover, online communication can provide an anonymous way for individuals to disclose personal information [32]. This can be particularly useful for some types of support and information-seeking, such as asking about stigmatized health conditions or for sexual minority youth who may not feel comfortable discussing their sexuality with others in person [32].

The use of online communication tools also poses risks for vulnerable adolescents [9]. Girls and queer youth, in particular, may be at higher risk for online harassment and cyberstalking. Other research find that harmful behavior can be normalized. For example, in an anonymous online communication setting where they feel understood, some adolescents can share self-injury-related content, with the consequent risk of possibly instigating such harmful behaviors for others [33]. This could also result in a negative reinforcing spiral among the members of a particular subgroup. In conclusion, while online communication tools can provide valuable support and resources for vulnerable groups, it is essential to be aware of the potential risks and to take steps to mitigate them.

## 3 Future Research

While the corpus of scholarship on this topic is much more robust than 20 years ago, more work is needed to account for the nuances of online communication tools and the myriad and constantly evolving set of social media practices adolescents engage in. Future research should expand in several critical areas:

1. *Comparative studies across different cultures and socioeconomic backgrounds*: While much of the current research focuses on adolescents from WEIRD (White, Educated, Industrialized, Rich, and Democratic) populations, a need exists to understand how online communication impacts youth in diverse environments globally.
2. *Individual differences in adolescents' online communication and social well-being:* Research increasingly recognizes the signifi-

[1] The word "queer" is a term that is being reclaimed by many people, particularly those in younger generations. It is meant to describe sexual or gender orientation that is not heterosexual or cisgender.

cant variability in how adolescents engage with online communication tools and the resulting impacts on their social well-being. Future studies should delve deeper into the factors contributing to these individual differences. This approach will enhance our comprehension of why certain adolescents thrive in digital environments while others may struggle. Understanding these nuances can help in tailoring interventions that support healthy online interactions tailored to individual needs and circumstances.

3. *Role of artificial intelligence and emerging technologies*: As AI becomes increasingly integrated into social media platforms, understanding its influence on social interactions and their consequences becomes crucial. Future research should investigate how AI-based technologies might alter interpersonal dynamics and self-perception among adolescents. For instance, algorithmically-generated recommendations on platforms like TikTok can feel to users as if they are reflecting elements of their own identity and help users find like-minded communities [34], but these systems can also privilege content from some users, leading to users with marginalized social identities feeling stigmatized or invisible [35].

## 4 Recommendations

### 4.1 For Youth

- *Critical thinking and decision-making:* Adolescents should be educated on strategic online communication choices, helping them evaluate the best settings, people, and communication modes (private vs. public) based on their own needs and circumstances.
- *Digital literacy enhancement:* Adolescents should learn to become savvy digital citizens, understanding both the functionality of digital tools and the broader implications of their online actions, including privacy concerns and the permanence of online footprints.

### 4.2 For Parents and Guardians

- *Active participation in digital activities:* Parents should engage with their children's online activities to better understand their social interactions and guide them in managing online relationships.
- *Promotion of open communication:* An environment should be fostered where children feel free to discuss their online experiences and challenges without fear of parental judgment or undue restriction.

### 4.3 For Tech Companies

- *Promote positive online experiences:* Platforms should be designed to encourage positive interactions and discourage negative behaviors by using algorithms that prioritize promoting positive communication and demote harmful content such as cyberbullying and misinformation.
- *Collaborate with adolescent researchers:* Platforms should engage with adolescent researchers to design tools that safeguard young users while fostering innovation and freedom of expression.
- *Implement ethical AI practices:* Platforms should ensure that AI systems used on social platforms do not perpetuate biases and are regularly audited for ethical compliance, particularly to prevent unfair treatment of specific groups of users.

### 4.4 For Policymakers

- *Regulations that protect young users:* Regulations should compel social media platforms to prioritize the safety and wellbeing of adolescent users. These regulations should include robust measures to protect against online sexual exploitation and data exploitation. Simultaneously, such regulations must also uphold the rights of young users to free and open communication and consider individual differences and both positive and negative use. The recent implementation of the Digital Services Act in Europe serves as a promising example of such protective measures.

- *Promote public education campaigns:* Implement national campaigns to raise awareness about the benefits of online communication for adolescents as well as the risks, and in addition educate the public on how to support young people in navigating these spaces safely.

**Conflict of Interest and Funding Disclosures** None.

## References

1. Uhls Y, Subrahmanyam K, Third A. Digital media and social connection in the lives of children, adolescents and families. Published online November 29, 2022. https://play.google.com/store/books/details?id=yFKeEAAAQBAJ
2. Uhls YT. Media Moms & Digital Dads: a fact-not-fear approach to parenting in the digital age. Routledge; 2015.
3. Uhls YT, Ellison NB, Subrahmanyam K. Social media in adolescence: selected benefits and costs. Pediatrics. 2017;140(Supplement 2):S67–70.
4. Common Sense Media Focus Group. Published online 2014.
5. Hall J, Pennington N, Holmstrom A. Connecting through technology during COVID-19. Human Commun Technol. 2021;2(1) http://journals.ku.edu/hct/article/view/15026
6. National Academies of Sciences, Engineering, and Medicine; Health and Medicine Division; Division of Behavioral and Social Sciences and Education; Board on Children, Youth, and Families; Committee on the Neurobiological and Socio-behavioral Science of Adolescent Development and Its Applications. Backes EP, Bonnie RJ, editors. The promise of adolescence: realizing opportunity for all youth. National Academies Press (US).
7. Carr CT, Hayes RA. Social media: defining, developing, and divining. Atlantic J Commun. 2015;23(1):46–65. https://www.tandfonline.com/doi/abs/10.1080/15456870.2015.972282
8. Moreno MA, Uhls YT. Applying an affordances approach and a developmental lens to approach adolescent social media use. Digit Health. 2019;5:2055207619826678.
9. Teens and mental health: How girls really feel about social media. Common Sense Media. Accessed 4 April 2023. https://www.commonsensemedia.org/research/teens-and-mental-health-how-girls-really-feel-about-social-media
10. Mittmann G, Woodcock K, Dörfler S, Krammer I, Pollak I, Schrank B. "TikTok Is My Life and Snapchat Is My Ventricle": a mixed-methods study on the role of online communication tools for friendships in early adolescents. J Early Adolesc. 2022;42(2):172–203.
11. van der Wal A, Valkenburg PM, van Driel II. In their own words: how adolescents differ in their social media use and how it affects them. Soc Med Soc. 2024;
12. Towner E, Grint J, Levy T, Blakemore SJ, Tomova L. Revealing the self in a digital world: a systematic review of adolescent online and offline self-disclosure. Curr Opin Psychol. 2022;45:101309.
13. Rideout V, Peebles A, Mann S, Robb MB. Common sense census: media use by tweens and teens, 2021. Common Sense. Published online 2022.
14. Achterhof R, Kirtley OJ, Schneider M, et al. Adolescents' real-time social and affective experiences of online and face-to-face interactions. Comput Human Behav. 2022;129(107159):107159.
15. Brown G, Greenfield PM. Staying connected during stay-at-home: communication with family and friends and its association with well-being. Human Behav Emerg Technol. 2021;3(1):147–56.
16. Granic I, Lobel A, Engeles RCM. The benefits of playing video games. Am Psychol. Published online 2013.
17. Sheng JT, Kairam SR. From virtual strangers to IRL friends: relationship development in livestreaming communities on twitch. Proc ACM Hum-Comput Interact. 2020;4(CSCW2):1–34.
18. Lai G, Fung KY. From online strangers to offline friends: a qualitative study of video game players in Hong Kong. Media Cult Soc. 2020;42(4):483–501.
19. Valkenburg PM, Peter J. Online communication among adolescents: an integrated model of its attraction, opportunities, and risks. J Adolesc Health. 2011;48(2):121–7.
20. Marciano L, Ostroumova M, Schulz PJ, Camerini AL. Digital media use and adolescents' mental health during the Covid-19 pandemic: a systematic review and meta-analysis. Front Public Health. 2022:9. https://doi.org/10.3389/fpubh.2021.793868.
21. Uhls YT, Broome J, Levi S, Szczepanski-Beavers J, Greenfield P. Mobile technologies and their relationship to children's ability to read nonverbal emotional cues: a cross-temporal comparison. Cyberpsychol Behav Soc Netw. 2020;23(7):465–70.
22. Cigelske T. The highest form of like: Snapchat, college students and hyperpersonal communication. Marquette University; 2018. https://www.proquest.com/dissertations-theses/highest-form-like-snapchat-college-students/docview/2087772856/se-2.
23. Duvenage M, Correia H, Uink B, Barber BL, Donovan CL, Modecki KL. Technology can sting when reality bites: adolescents' frequent online coping is ineffec-

tive with momentary stress. Comput Human Behav. 2020;102:248–59.
24. Vogels EA. Teens and cyberbullying 2022. Pew Research Center: Internet, Science & Tech. Published December 15, 2022. Accessed 4 April 2023. https://www.pewresearch.org/internet/2022/12/15/teens-and-cyberbullying-2022/
25. Chen L, Ho SS, Lwin MO. A meta-analysis of factors predicting cyberbullying perpetration and victimization: from the social cognitive and media effects approach. New Media Soc. 2017;19(8):1194–213.
26. Kowalski RM, Giumetti GW, Schroeder AN, Lattanner MR. Bullying in the digital age: a critical review and meta-analysis of cyberbullying research among youth. Psychol Bull. 2014;140(4):1073–137.
27. Marciano L, Schulz PJ, Camerini AL. Cyberbullying perpetration and victimization in youth: a meta-analysis of longitudinal studies. J Comput Mediat Commun. 2020;25(2):163–81.
28. Juvonen J, Gross EF. Extending the school grounds? - bullying experiences in cyberspace. J Sch Health. 2008;78(9):496–505.
29. Devito MA, Walker AM, Birnholtz J, et al. Social technologies for digital wellbeing among marginalized communities. In: Conference companion publication of the 2019 on computer supported cooperative work and social computing. CSCW '19. Association for Computing Machinery; 2019. p. 449–54.
30. Selkie E, Adkins V, Masters E, Bajpai A, Shumer D. Transgender adolescents' uses of social media for social support. J Adolesc Health. 2020;66(3):275–80.
31. Wolf CT, Faucett H, Dombrowski L, Hayes GR. "Will I always be not social?" Re-Conceptualizing Sociality in the Context of a Minecraft Community for Autism. *of the 2016 CHI* .... Published online 2016. https://dl.acm.org/doi/abs/10.1145/2858036.2858038?casa_token=T98KEkLlLggAAAAA:cdcgo6F1p8hILTCipfKOxUKAF0Gh6eZihx4EmdaOSw0UHXpLS8GeNeEUYH-bRiMG6GdWoQ7TbmmUyzY
32. Ellison NB, Blackwell L, Lampe C, Trieu P. "The question exists, but you don't exist with it": strategic anonymity in the social lives of adolescents. Soc Media Soc. 2016;2(4):2056305116670 67.
33. Cataldo I, Lepri B, Neoh MJY, Esposito G. Social media usage and development of psychiatric disorders in childhood and adolescence: a review. Front Psych. 2020;11:508595.
34. Lee AY, Mieczkowski H, Ellison NB, Hancock JT. The algorithmic crystal: conceptualizing the self through algorithmic personalization on TikTok. Proc ACM Human-Comput Interact. 2022;6(CSCW2):1–22.
35. Algorithmic Folk Theories and identity: how TikTok users co-produce knowledge of identity and engage in algorithmic Res.... Accessed 19 April 2024. https://ouci.dntb.gov.ua/en/works/9Zj68nv9/

# Youth Digital Wellbeing and Social Connectedness

Linda Charmaraman, Jacqueline Nesi, Stephen M. Schueller, Sophia Choukas-Bradley, J. Maya Hernandez, and Katie Davis

## 1 Background

A widely agreed-upon definition of wellbeing is elusive. The World Health Organization (WHO) defines mental health as not just the absence of mental illness, but also a state of wellbeing in which an individual realizes their own abilities, can cope with the normal stresses of life, and can work productively and make a contribution to their community [1]. This definition involves both hedonic (e.g., feeling good) and eudaimonic (e.g., doing good) perspectives. Most psychological research on wellbeing tends to focus on hedonic wellbeing, operationalizing wellbeing as a measurement of such constructs as life satisfaction, happiness, or positive affect [2]. Youth wellbeing and social connectedness are intricately tied concepts. In hedonic perspectives, relationships contribute strongly to positive emotions and life satisfaction. In eudaimonic perspectives, relationships, and social connectedness are important ingredients of the good life.

Regardless of the perspective, these conceptualizations agree that relationships play a central role in promoting wellbeing, which is especially true in the adolescent years. Increasingly, these social interactions are unfolding over networked platforms. Through curated online communities, social media is shaping and influencing youth wellbeing and social connectedness in complex and interconnected ways. Recent years have seen an increase in not only the amount of time youth are spending on digital media, but also changes to the types of things youth can do on social media platforms, including creating content, connecting with others, and curating experiences.

Social connection is especially developmentally salient and important during adolescence due to social and biological changes that occur during this period [3]. Because of these changes, adolescents are highly attuned to social status and peer feedback [4]. Negative peer relationships (e.g., victimization, peer rejection, loneli-

We are grateful to Carolyn Bacaj for copyediting and formatting assistance.

L. Charmaraman (✉)
Wellesley Centers for Women, Wellesley College, Wellesley, MA, USA
e-mail: lcharmar@wellesley.edu

J. Nesi
Department of Psychiatry and Human Behavior, Brown University, Providence, RI, USA

Bradley-Hasbro Research Center, Rhode Island Hospital, Providence, RI, USA

S. M. Schueller
Psychological Science and Informatics, University of California, Irvine, Irvine, CA, USA

S. Choukas-Bradley
Psychology, University of Pittsburgh, Pittsburgh, PA, USA

J. M. Hernandez
Social Ecology, University of California, Irvine, Irvine, CA, USA

K. Davis
Information School, University of Washington, Seattle, WA, USA


D. A. Christakis, L. Hale (eds.), *Handbook of Children and Screens*,
https://doi.org/10.1007/978-3-031-69362-5_31

ness) are strong predictors of maladaptive developmental trajectories, while positive peer relationships (e.g., strong social connection, reciprocal friendships) can promote wellbeing and buffer against the effects of interpersonal stressors [5]. Unfortunately, loneliness is currently a worldwide epidemic among adolescents [6]. This chapter will highlight the current state of the field in research regarding youth digital wellbeing and social connectedness, including limitations to this knowledge, future directions, and recommendations for key stakeholders.

## 2 Current State

### 2.1 Mixed Findings Due to Measurement Variability

Despite media reports of an overall negative impact of social media on today's youth, the state-of-the-field findings have been mixed when it comes to associations between media use and social factors, such as social connection, loneliness, and peer relationships. While some prior meta-analyses and reviews have revealed associations between greater use of social media and heightened feelings of social connection, access to social support, and social capital, others point to associations with greater loneliness and lower wellbeing [7]. Large-scale, aggregate studies seem to point to a small, negative relationship between social media use and social connection, but there are methodological challenges due to inconsistent definitions and measures (e.g., lumping together "wellbeing" constructs that should be investigated separately) [2], cross-sectional studies, and other limitations. Increasingly, studies are moving beyond overall measures of "screen time," and emphasizing specific social experiences (e.g., self-presentation, social comparison, peer feedback), and examining how these experiences may differentially impact different adolescents [8].

### 2.2 Movement Toward Embracing Methodological Diversity

As digital peer connections are increasingly ubiquitous among diverse populations of youth, how we understand associations between digital technology use and wellbeing requires updated methodological approaches. There remains an overreliance on cross-sectional correlative studies; however, recent studies of longitudinal links between frequent social technology use for communication and lower depressive symptoms indicate the importance of digital social connection to wellbeing [9, 10]. Additionally, emerging qualitative work [11, 12] and youth-centered approaches [13, 14] may help to further identify unique online features that promote positive youth connections linked to identity formation and improved social capital.

### 2.3 Context Is Key

Theoretical work [15] suggests that adolescents' peer experiences are fundamentally shaped by the social media environment, which offers unprecedented opportunities for interactions that are more public, immediate, and "quantifiable" than ever before. Recent experimental work has found that adolescents who receive negative peer feedback (i.e., fewer "likes") on social media report more negative affect and feelings of rejection and that youth with prior experiences of "offline" peer victimization may be especially sensitive to this negative feedback [16]. Negative social comparisons may also be facilitated by the online environment, with meta-analytic evidence linking heightened social comparisons on social media, particularly upward comparisons, with greater depressive symptoms [17].

## 2.4 Debunking the Popular Myth That Social Media Is the Enemy of Social Connection

At the same time, social media platforms may provide powerful opportunities for youth to connect with similar peers and access social support. Nationally-representative survey data in the U.S. highlight that more than two-thirds (68%) of adolescents report they have people on social media who support them through tough times, and 81% feel that social media allows them to feel more connected to friends [18]. A 2020 nationally representative survey of 14- to 22-year-olds found that one in five respondents (21%) reported that social media was very important for helping them feel less alone, an increase from 15% 2 years earlier [19]. This demonstrates that digital technology's role in social connection may have been even further amplified during periods of isolation associated with the COVID-19 pandemic [20, 21]. Recent work using daily diary methods finds that frequent texters tend to be less depressed [9] and on days when girls used video-chatting and text messaging to talk to peers (but not social media), they reported higher feelings of closeness [22].

Digital technologies, and especially social media, can provide critically important sources of social support and connection for youth with marginalized identities. Although racial/ethnic minorities are the most active users of social media sites, most research in this area utilizes predominantly white samples; thus little is known about how youth of different racial/ethnic backgrounds use these platforms in unique ways to connect around their identities [23]. In contrast, more research on marginalized subgroups has revealed that adolescents with sexual minority identities—and especially those living in rural areas, who may feel socially isolated and without in-person access to LGBTQ+ communities—may use social media to connect with other LGBTQ+ youth [24–26]. Social media may promote wellbeing among LGBTQ+ adolescents and other youth with marginalized identities if it helps improve social connections and/or affirms one's identity [26, 27]. On the other hand, social media experiences may negatively impact the wellbeing of LGBTQ+ youth and other youth with marginalized identities if they involve harassment, victimization, and exposure to hate speech [24, 26, 28]. Collectively, these findings suggest pathways through which identity may shape the social media experiences that youth seek out, while these experiences reciprocally influence youths' identity development processes and wellbeing, consistent with transactional models of media use [29]. Notably, research on social media use among LGBTQ+ youth has primarily relied on qualitative studies with small samples; future research with larger samples and longitudinal designs will be important for continuing to understand the connection between social media use and wellbeing among youth with marginalized identities.

## 2.5 Limitations of Our Current Knowledge

Because the vast majority of funded studies and measures used to study social media use focus on risk variables, fewer studies are published about normative, non-problematic, or prosocial uses of social media to connect with others; therefore, less is known about the concept of "digital wellbeing" and socially connective, socially supportive, resilient users of social media. There seems to be no consensus about for whom and under what circumstances social media can enhance wellbeing and social connectedness. The field needs studies large enough to look at moderation and personalization of effects; we need analytic techniques that focus on idiographic findings rather than mean levels and group averages [30]. We need more longitudinal studies (e.g., Tang et al., 2021) [31] focused on online content consumed and social context, rather than the quantity of time spent [8, 32]. Furthermore, although qualitative research suggests that social media may be especially important for social connection among LGBTQ+ youth (as discussed above), longitudinal and quantitative research is lacking within research focused on marginalized youth.

There is still an overreliance on examining a limited view of social media use (e.g., time spent; active vs. passive). More nuanced investigations should examine such factors as specific content consumed while passively lurking; motivations behind social media use; and the influence of online and offline communities on wellbeing. Furthermore, the question of whether online connections are actually as beneficial as in-person connections for youth wellbeing remains unanswered.

### 2.6 Conclusion

Although digital media can involve maladaptive uses and effects on adolescents' mental health, evidence supports its potential to harness the power of social connection and enhance wellbeing, particularly when offline support is lacking. Future applied research and practice should capitalize on the potential of digital spaces to improve socially connective features, and to center youth voices as key stakeholders at the forefront of clinical, curriculum, policy, and technology design.

## 3 Future Research

- *In what ways and for whom do different social contexts and content on social media influence effects on wellbeing?* Given that there is no one-size-fits-all approach to enhancing wellbeing in the context of social media use, more research should focus on identified vulnerable populations, whether based on offline social difficulties, marginalized identities, or mental health symptoms. Such work should examine whether these youth might be experiencing both more of the risks of digital technology, as well as more of the benefits, in terms of connection.
- *When do the benefits of online spaces outweigh their risks and vice versa?* Systematic reviews have demonstrated that there are both adaptive and maladaptive elements of social media use, at times even within the same person, depending on the social context. More research is needed regarding any critical developmental markers or social environments that can help or hinder the benefits of social connectedness and wellbeing on these platforms.
- *What specific tech designs affect differential youth outcomes?* This is needed to understand when social media is and is not supporting social connectedness, with implications for tech companies and government regulation [33].
- *How do young people's momentary and long-term feelings of connectedness and belonging parallel their use of social media and overall wellbeing?* Research involving different phases of adolescent development will help illuminate any critical markers or stages that can help or hinder wellbeing.

## 4 Recommendations

### 4.1 For Clinicians (e.g., Pediatricians, Social Workers, Mental Health Counselors, Psychiatrists)

- Assessment is a critical first step to understanding the role these technologies play in adolescents' lives and asking them directly about it.
- Framing digital media as all good or all bad is unlikely to be helpful. If done appropriately, social media may provide important growth opportunities to support youth wellbeing and may allow exploration of aspects of identity in safe ways.

### 4.2 For Educators (e.g., K-12 Teachers, Media/Tech Specialists, Digital Librarians, Afterschool Youth Workers)

- Avoid framing digital media use as "purely negative" or "unproductive," as this contrasts with youths' actual experiences and makes future conversations more difficult. This framing is also at odds with the need to prepare adolescents to be digital citizens in our connected world. Promote the attitudes and online behaviors that lead to greater digital wellbeing and connectedness, rather than a sole focus on what NOT to do.

- Incorporate media literacy lessons that harness the power of collaboration and communication by encouraging youth to be co-creators and innovators of these technologies.

## 4.3 For Policymakers (e.g., Community-Based, State/Federal Level)

- With the recent WHO global framework for achieving wellbeing [34], governments can introduce regulations that require companies to show how they are or are not supporting youth wellbeing. A growing number of governments around the globe are passing legislation to this effect, with immediate responses from tech companies (e.g., changes to default privacy settings for teen accounts).
- News media companies can support their own journalists and press staff to present more balanced, nuanced views of the benefits and challenges of social media for youth digital wellbeing and connection rather than leaning into the default narrative portraying social media as entirely negative.
- Basic protections can be put into place to make digital media safe social spaces where youth can maximize opportunities to promote their wellbeing.

## 4.4 For Industry (e.g., Social Media Platforms, Mental Health Apps)

- Creating digital ecosystems that facilitate positive social connectedness, while minimizing risks for youth, cannot be done without industry stakeholders. The technology industry can make further efforts with experts in academic settings to implement developmentally appropriate and theoretically driven designs for future social technology platforms. For instance, social media companies could work with academic experts to determine whether certain features (e.g., endless scrolling, autoplay) serve to co-opt attention rather than to actually support connection, and to investigate how best to support social connection in the context of these platforms.
- Social media companies should be aware of policies that create barriers to youth connection due to privacy policies or changes to user agreements (e.g., algorithms limiting "pornographic" content that blocks LGBTQ+ users from connecting). More collaborative research with marginalized youth who are primary users of social media apps is recommended. We encourage industry to consider youth as critical stakeholders and diverse communities in their policy practices in order to promote inclusivity and a more supportive online space [14].

**Conflict of Interest and Funding Disclosures** JN is supported in part by a grant from the National Institute of Mental Health (NIMH; K23-MH122669). JN writes Techno Sapiens, a psychology newsletter for which she receives subscription and sponsor payments. She is co-owner of Tech Without Stress, LLC, which provides free and paid resources for parents raising children in the digital age. Other authors have indicated that they have no potential conflicts of interest to disclose.

## References

1. Mental health fact sheet. WHO; 2022. https://www.who.int/news-room/fact-sheets/detail/mental-health-strengthening-our-response.
2. Valkenburg PM. Social media use and well-being: what we know and what we need to know. Curr Opin Psychol. 2022;45:101294. https://doi.org/10.1016/j.copsyc.2021.12.006.
3. Somerville LH. The teenage brain: sensitivity to social evaluation. Curr Dir Psychol Sci. 2013;22(2):121–7. https://doi.org/10.1177/0963721413476512.
4. Brechwald WA, Prinstein MJ. Beyond Homophily: a decade of advances in understanding peer influence processes: BEYOND HOMOPHILY. J Res Adolesc. 2011;21(1):166–79. https://doi.org/10.1111/j.1532-7795.2010.00721.x.

5. Bukowski MW, Laursen B, Rubin KH, editors. Handbook of peer interactions, relationships, and groups. 2nd ed. The Guilford Press; 2018.
6. Twenge JM, Haidt J, Blake AB, McAllister C, Lemon H, Le Roy A. Worldwide increases in adolescent loneliness. J Adolesc. 2021;93(1):257–69. https://doi.org/10.1016/j.adolescence.2021.06.006.
7. Orben A. Teenagers, screens and social media: a narrative review of reviews and key studies. Soc Psychiatry Psychiatr Epidemiol. 2020;55(4):407–14. https://doi.org/10.1007/s00127-019-01825-4.
8. Odgers CL, Schueller SM, Ito M. Screen time, social media use, and adolescent development. Ann Rev Dev Psychol. 2020;2(1):485–502. https://doi.org/10.1146/annurev-devpsych-121318-084815.
9. Jensen M, George MJ, Russell MR, Odgers CL. Young adolescents' digital technology use and mental health symptoms: little evidence of longitudinal or daily linkages. Clin Psychol Sci. 2019;7(6):1416–33. https://doi.org/10.1177/2167702619859336.
10. Schacter HL, Margolin G. When it feels good to give: depressive symptoms, daily prosocial behavior, and adolescent mood. Emotion. 2019;19(5):923–7. https://doi.org/10.1037/emo0000494.
11. Brough M, Literat I, Ikin A. "Good social media?": underrepresented youth perspectives on the ethical and equitable design of social media platforms. Soc Media Soc. 2020;6(2):205630512092848. https://doi.org/10.1177/2056305120928488.
12. Itō M, Baumer S, Bittanti M, Antin J, editors. Hanging out, messing around, and Geeking out: kids living and learning with new media. MIT Press; 2010.
13. Delcourt CG, Charmaraman L, Durrani S, Gu Q, Xiao LF. Innovating novel online social spaces with diverse middle school girls: ideation and collaboration in a synchronous virtual design workshop. In: CHI conference on human factors in computing systems. ACM; 2022. p. 1–16. https://doi.org/10.1145/3491102.3517576.
14. Hernandez JM, Ahumada-Newhart V. Latine health and development in the digital age: assets-based inclusive design as a social movement for equitable distributions of power. Interactions. 2022;29(5):39–43. https://doi.org/10.1145/3550199.
15. Nesi J, Choukas-Bradley S, Prinstein MJ. Transformation of adolescent peer relations in the social media context: part 1—a theoretical framework and application to dyadic peer relationships. Clin Child Fam Psychol Rev. 2018;21(3):267–94. https://doi.org/10.1007/s10567-018-0261-x.
16. Lee HY, Jamieson JP, Reis HT, et al. Getting fewer "likes" than others on social media elicits emotional distress among victimized adolescents. Child Dev. 2020;91(6):2141–59. https://doi.org/10.1111/cdev.13422.
17. Yoon S, Kleinman M, Mertz J, Brannick M. Is social network site usage related to depression? A meta-analysis of Facebook–depression relations. J Affect Disord. 2019;248:65–72. https://doi.org/10.1016/j.jad.2019.01.026.
18. Jiang J, Anderson M. Teens' Social Media Habits and Experiences. November, 2018. Pew Research Center; 2018. https://www.pewresearch.org/internet/2018/11/28/teens-social-media-habits-and-experiences/.
19. Rideout V, Fox S, Peebles A, Robb MB. How young people use digital media to manage their mental health. Common Sense Hopelab. 2021; pp. 9, 30. https://www.commonsensemedia.org/research/coping-with-covid-19-how-young-people-use-digital-media-tomanage-their-mental-health
20. Charmaraman L, Lynch AD, Richer AM, Zhai E. Examining early adolescent positive and negative social technology behaviors and well-being during the COVID-19 pandemic. Tech Mind Beh. 2022;3(1) https://doi.org/10.1037/tmb0000062.
21. Pitt C, Hock A, Zelnick L, Davis K. The kids are / not / sort of all right*. In: Proceedings of the 2021 CHI conference on human factors in computing systems. Association for Computing Machinery; 2021. p. 1–14. Accessed October 28, 2021. https://doi.org/10.1145/3411764.3445541.
22. James KM, Silk JS, Scott LN, et al. Peer connectedness and social technology use during COVID-19 lockdown. Res Child Adolesc Psychopathol Published online. 2023; https://doi.org/10.1007/s10802-023-01040-5.
23. Charmaraman L, Hernandez JM, Hodes R. Marginalized and understudied populations using digital media. In: Nesi J, Telzer EH, Prinstein MJ, editors. Handbook of adolescent digital media use and mental health. 1st ed. Cambridge University Press; 2022. https://doi.org/10.1017/9781108976237.
24. Berger MN, Taba M, Marino JL, et al. Social media's role in support networks among LGBTQ adolescents: a qualitative study. Newman C, ed. Sex Health. 2021;18(5):421–31. https://doi.org/10.1071/SH21110.
25. Karim S, Choukas-Bradley S, Radovic A, Roberts SR, Maheux AJ, Escobar-Viera CG. Support over social media among socially isolated sexual and gender minority youth in rural U.S. during the COVID-19 pandemic: opportunities for intervention research. IJERPH. 2022;19(23):15611. https://doi.org/10.3390/ijerph192315611.
26. Selkie E, Adkins V, Masters E, Bajpai A, Shumer D. Transgender adolescents' uses of social media for social support. J Adolesc Health. 2020;66(3):275–80. https://doi.org/10.1016/j.jadohealth.2019.08.011.
27. Paceley MS, Goffnett J, Sanders L, Gadd-Nelson J. "Sometimes you get married on Facebook": the use of social media among nonmetropolitan sexual and gender minority youth. J Homosex. 2022;69(1):41–60. https://doi.org/10.1080/00918369.2020.1813508.
28. Wike TL, Bouchard LM, Kemmerer A, Yabar MP. Victimization and resilience: experiences of rural LGBTQ+ youth across multiple contexts. J Interpers Violence. 2022;37(19-20):NP18988-NP19015. https://doi.org/10.1177/08862605211043574.

29. Valkenburg PM. Theoretical foundations of social media uses and effects. In: Nesi J, Telzer EH, Prinstein MJ, editors. Handbook of adolescent digital media use and mental health. 1st ed. Cambridge University Press; 2022. p. 39–60. https://doi.org/10.1017/9781108976237.004.
30. Fisher AJ, Medaglia JD, Jeronimus BF. Lack of group-to-individual generalizability is a threat to human subjects research. Proc Natl Acad Sci USA. 2018;115(27) https://doi.org/10.1073/pnas.1711978115.
31. Tang S, Werner-Seidler A, Torok M, Mackinnon AJ, Christensen H. The relationship between screen time and mental health in young people: a systematic review of longitudinal studies. Clin Psychol Rev. 2021;86:102021. https://doi.org/10.1016/j.cpr.2021.102021.
32. Prinstein MJ, Nesi J, Telzer E. Commentary: an updated agenda for the study of digital media use and adolescent development – future directions following Odgers & Jensen. J Child Psychol Psychiatr. 2020;61:349–352. https://doi.org/10.1111/jcpp.13219.
33. Davis K. Technology's child: digital media's role in the ages and stages of growing up. The MIT Press; 2023.
34. World Health Organization. Achieving well-being: a global framework for integrating well-being into public health utilizing a health promotion approach. Geneva: World Health Organization; 2024. https://www.who.int/publications/i/item/9789240084858

# Empathy, Kindness, and Dignity in a Connected World

Carrie James, Anne Collier, Katie Davis, Sara Konrath, Tijana Milosevic, Elizabeth Milovidov, Elisabeth Staksrud, and Emily Weinstein

## 1 Background

Wonders and worries abound about how today's hyper-connected world is shaping human kindness, empathy, and dignity. Even among researchers, genuine debates ensue about the human impacts of living in a networked world. News reports about cyberbullying can fuel concerns that, on balance, technology is a net negative for human compassion. And the very design of technologies—including social media sites and emerging AI technologies—raises wider ethical concerns. Tech affordances (the "possibilities for action" that a technology offers, such as content visibility and spreadability) [1] can amplify digital acts of kindness but also of hate. App-specific features like private stories can be spaces for empathy and support, yet they can also fuel the dynamics of exclusion. Algorithms can tailor content to users' interests but also propagate systemic oppression [2]. This chapter describes what is currently known about the implications of smartphones and social media for empathy, kindness, and dignity; names open or understudied questions; and suggests recommendations.

## 2 Current State

### 2.1 Empathy and Kindness in a Connected World

New technologies often spark concerns about implications for empathy; digital technologies are no exception. Empathy involves cognitive perspective-taking and feeling compassion for others [3]. Humans have a powerful empathic capacity, fueled by their motivation and imagination. Digital technologies have features that can make it difficult to connect empathically (e.g., limited emotional cues, information overload), yet they can also facilitate genuine empathic exchanges. Empathy is an important motivator of kindness, including online [4]. Kindness includes formal prosocial behaviors (e.g., donating, volunteering) and informal actions to support

C. James (✉) · E. Weinstein
Harvard Graduate School of Education, Cambridge, MA, USA
e-mail: carrie_james@harvard.edu

A. Collier
The Net Safety Collaborative, Salt Lake City, UT, USA

K. Davis
University of Washington, Seattle, WA, USA

S. Konrath
Indiana University, Bloomington, IN, USA

University of Michigan, Ann Arbor, MI, USA

T. Milosevic
University College Dublin, Dublin, Ireland

E. Milovidov
The LEGO Group, Digitalem S.A.S, Paris, France

E. Staksrud
University of Oslo, Oslo, Norway


D. A. Christakis, L. Hale (eds.), *Handbook of Children and Screens*,
https://doi.org/10.1007/978-3-031-69362-5_32

friends, relatives, and strangers. Existing evidence is contributing to our understanding of relevant questions about technology, empathy, and kindness.

*When youth are face-to-face, does the presence of digital technologies compromise empathic connection?* A meta-analysis found that having smartphones nearby during conversations does not in itself impair feelings of connection and empathy for in-person conversation partners. However, actively using the phone during face-to-face interactions ("phubbing" or "technoference") can potentially lead to these negative effects [5, 6]. Importantly, there is virtually no research on how social usage of smartphones (e.g., watching funny videos together) affects social connectedness.

*How are digital technologies used in empathic ways?* Despite longstanding and legitimate concerns about toxic disinhibition in digital exchanges, newer research also finds that technology-facilitated interactions can support empathic exchanges. One study found that patients undergoing minor surgical procedures needed four times less pain medication after texting with a friend or stranger [7]. And interventions that use text messages [8] and smartphone apps [9] can increase empathy in youth. Teaching mindful and prosocial strategies can improve social media interactions (e.g., thinking before posting can reduce cyber harassment) [10], and empathic responses can reduce hate speech [11].

*How is digital technology use related to empathy?* Research has found a link between narcissism and social media usage [12]; however, the correlation does not mean social media use increases narcissism. Perhaps narcissistic people are simply drawn to social media. Fewer studies focus specifically on empathy and social media, with mixed results. Teens who use more social media actually have higher empathy one year later [13]. Newer research also finds that the link between empathy and social media usage may depend on age and country [14]. The impacts of newer technologies are being studied. A meta-analysis of 43 studies found that, overall, virtual reality can increase empathic feelings but not cognitive empathy [15]. This may be because virtual reality makes empathy too easy and does not let the user flex and strengthen their empathy muscles. In addition, VR does not necessarily translate to more prosocial behavior [16].

*How does online prosocial behavior benefit youth?* Research consistently finds that youth who engage in online prosocial behaviors—even brief, low-cost online prosocial actions (likes, supportive sharing)—are more likely to engage in offline prosocial behaviors [17, 18]. Compared to in-person actions, digital prosocial behaviors (civic posting, donating money) have fewer barriers and are often more permanent and public [19].

Contrary to fears that time spent on social media reduces prosociality, young people who are more active on social media are also more likely to engage in prosocial behaviors [20]. Indeed, 42% of Gen Z donors were influenced to give by social media requests; 76% of U.S. Gen Z donors made online donations in 2022, and nearly half (48%) of these gave via smartphone or tablet [21]. "Stunt philanthropy" is a popular emerging form of digital giving that sidesteps traditional nonprofits and gives directly to recipients [22].

As for informal prosocial behaviors, two-thirds (67%) of U.S. teens say social media makes them feel like they have people who can provide support during tough times [23]. Indeed, giving and receiving informal acts of digital kindness are highly correlated among teens [17]. Digital prosocial engagement can empower teens, facilitate identity development, and meet needs to belong and contribute [19]. Yet, a hidden toll of empathy for friends in an always-on world: teens can feel pressure to be constantly available and responsive to others, and may face social support burdens when peers share struggles on social media or reach out digitally for help [24].

*How is low empathy related to cyberbullying?* Concerns about cyber aggression and cyberbullying are widespread. While there is disagreement among scholars regarding cyberbullying definitions, the phenomenon can be broadly described as a digital form of peer-based aggression [27]. Cyberbullying definitions do not always capture the complexity of the phenomenon as experienced by children and young people. Many digital situations that young people find hurtful can fly under the radar of adults when they do not meet the definitional criteria of cyberbullying [28].

Despite the prosocial findings described above, high social media usage can also be associated with digital antisocial behavior. Low empathy and moral disengagement have been linked with cyberbullying perpetration [25]; and a recent review found that perpetrators score lower on cognitive and emotional empathy [26].

We also need attention to how dignity might inform understandings of cyberbullying incidents and subsequent intervention and prevention mechanisms. As an ethical framework, dignity emphasizes respect for the inherent worth of every human being [29].

## 2.2 Dignity in a Connected World

Supporting empathy and kindness in the context of youth technology use requires consideration of individual and relationship-level factors and behaviors (such as narcissism and bullying), but also broader factors, including technology design and moderation, and state-level policies that monitor ethical concerns and advocate prioritization of rights and well-being over profits. As examples, algorithmic design can help spread uncivil content, meanness, and disinformation [30] and can promote biased, stereotypical, racist, and sexist views [2]; the business model of online platforms is based on extractive data and surveillance practices that can violate children's privacy [31]; and while artificial intelligence can be used to proactively detect and remove harmful online content, such behavioral monitoring can nonetheless violate children's privacy [32].

As per the United Nations Convention on the Rights of the Child (UNCRC),[1] which applies in digital environments, children have the right to protection, which includes harm from risks ranging from grooming, privacy infringements, and cyberbullying, but also rights to participation, such as engaging in social media and having a say in decisions concerning them, and provision rights (to quality content, policies, and digital infrastructures that benefit their development and well-being). This means that in countries where the treaty has been ratified, the state has an obligation to ensure the balance of children's digital rights, including the regulation of relevant stakeholders, including online platforms and content providers [33]. To date, 196 countries have ratified the treaty; the United States is the only United Nations member that has not ratified it.

*How can the state, industry stakeholders, and educators contribute to the creation of online environments that facilitate children's well-being?* A relevant framework for designing rights-based online environments is the dignity framework. It proposes that one's actions be informed by understanding the inherent worth of every human being, which, unlike respect, need not be earned [32]. This implies a recognition that dignity and self-worth are not derived from one's social status, wealth, academic achievement, appearance, or any other conventional symbol of success. A culture of dignity (online and offline) is one where everyone can feel safe to participate as what they perceive to be their authentic selves and to contribute with their talents [34].

The dignity framework has implications for educational interventions, especially ones aimed at countering cyberbullying, online hate, and sexual harassment. Yet, in the context of such dignity violations, recent research suggests that many adolescents expect to encounter meanness online and believe that one needs to develop thick skin to be on social media [33]. Experiences of cruelty can be amplified by digital features, including publicity, spreadability, and permanence of content [35].

Thus, it is crucial that technological platforms engage in effective content moderation that enables and facilitates dignity-upholding behaviors (e.g., prosocial behaviors described above), and does not enhance harmful behavior and content—without infringing on children's participatory rights. Beyond ensuring that offensive content is taken down, this also means creating *safety-by-design* tools that actively promote perspective-taking before posting toward the cre-

[1] The Convention has been ratified by 196 countries worldwide, but not by the United States government.

ation of dignified online environments. Examples include reflective messaging with automatic prompts to nudge reconsideration before posting something potentially hurtful [10].

## 3 Future Research

Existing research signals ways technology can both support and undercut empathy and kindness, yet also points to meaningful areas of opportunity. Thus, one important area for future research is how digital technologies—including their design, content, and uses—can support prosociality. What features and affordances contribute to or undercut empathy? What kinds of interventions effectively nudge youth toward kind digital interactions, and how can they be scaled? When do prosocial experiences have the most enduring positive impacts?

### 3.1 Empathy and Kindness

Future research should also aim to examine how specific factors affect empathy, kindness, and dignity development in digital contexts. Specific research questions include: What kinds of social media content facilitate prosocial behaviors (including upstanding behaviors), in which digital contexts, and why? What kinds of online behaviors and/or design features promote more empathy, kindness, and prosociality in others? Who is most likely to engage in empathic and kind online behaviors, and why? How do contextual factors in young people's lives affect their online prosociality? What are the mental and physical health implications of digital prosocial behaviors in youth? (e.g., does "joy of giving" happen online/at a distance?)

### 3.2 Dignity

From the dignity framework perspective, it would be helpful if future research examined how dignity and dignity-informed behaviors could be taught to children and young people in a manner that resonates with them rather than preaching dignity to them (moralizing, patronizing, top-down approach). It would also be important to understand how technological design reflects dignity principles. For example, a type of algorithmic design that might reflect dignity principles and merits further research is *bridging-based ranking*, which rewards content that leads to positive interactions across groups rather than promoting divisive behavior that receives a lot of attention [36].

## 4 Recommendations

Digital technologies can facilitate both prosocial behaviors and social harms; supporting the former and mitigating the latter requires actions by multiple stakeholder groups.

### 4.1 For Educators and Peer Mentors

Schools and out-of-school learning contexts are crucial spaces for supporting social-emotional skills and dispositions for treating others with empathy, kindness, and dignity, both online and offline:

- Educators are encouraged to tap research-based curricula and high-quality professional learning experiences that equip them to support students' social/emotional skill building in a complicated landscape.
- Youth-led and peer mentorship contexts can also powerfully support teens' dispositions by facilitating "collective agency" or mutual support to navigate the challenges of growing up in a technology-rich world [24].

Suggested resources include: Common Sense Education's Digital Citizenship Curriculum (https://www.commonsense.org/education/digital-citizenship/curriculum), CyberWise's Cyber Civics Curriculum (https://www.cybercivics.com/), and the Center for Digital Thriving's resource collection (https://digitalthriving.gse.harvard.edu/resources/).

### 4.2 For Clinicians, Including Mental Health Providers

- When discussing media use with patients and families, providers should be mindful of the prosocial, well-being-supportive aspects of young people's media lives—while staying alert to signs that social media experiences are a net negative for some teens.

### 4.3 For Parents

- Parents can encourage their children to pay attention to how features of digital technologies can be supportive of and/or work against empathy, kindness, and respect for the dignity of others, as well as encouraging self-respect and self-care.

### 4.4 For Tech Designers

Technology is not neutral. How a technology is designed and by whom will shape the kinds of actions that are possible and encouraged:

- Technology designers and their companies can adopt a youth-centered approach to design that prioritizes well-being and prosocial behaviors from the start, drawing on research evidence and young people's own digital practices to guide their efforts.
- Technology companies can partner with youth (and adult) users to track how specific features are used and to take responsibility for unanticipated uses that support and/or undercut empathy, kindness, dignity, and well-being.

Relevant resources include Design It for Us (https://designitforus.org/) and Digital Futures for Children's report, "The Best Interests of the Child in the Digital Environment" (https://www.digital-futures-for-children.net/best-interests).

### 4.5 For Policymakers

Policymakers need to ensure that measures implemented balance children's rights for provision, protection, and participation in digital environments.

- Policymakers need to advocate for changes in the incentives that currently drive the tech industry. The business model of the internet feeds an attention economy that prioritizes time spent on apps above value to users and implications for their well-being. Regulation can induce tech companies to shift their focus from user care to legal compliance, even as their business model compels them to prioritize user engagement over well-being.

**Conflict of Interest and Funding Disclosures** CJ and EW were supported by grants from the Susan Crown Exchange and Pivotal Ventures. CJ, SK, and EW were supported by a grant from the Mind & Life Institute.

## References

1. Evans SK, Pearce KE, Vitak J, Treem JW. Explicating affordances: a conceptual framework for understanding affordances in communication research. J Comput Mediat Commun. 2017;22(1):35–52.
2. Noble SU. Algorithms of oppression: how search engines reinforce racism. NYU Press; 2018.
3. Davis MH. Measuring individual differences in empathy: evidence for a multidimensional approach. J Pers Soc Psychol. 1983;44(1):113–26.
4. Guo Y, Shachat J, Walker MJ, Wei L. Viral social media videos can raise pro-social behaviours when an epidemic arises. J Econ Sci Assoc. 2021;7(2):120–38.
5. Courtright J, Caplan S. A meta-analysis of mobile phone use and presence. Human Commun Technol. 2020;1(2):20–35.
6. Mackay LJ, Komanchuk J, Hayden KA, Letourneau N. Impacts of parental technoference on parent-child relationships and child health and developmental outcomes: a scoping review protocol. Syst Rev. 2022;11(1):45.
7. Guillory JE, Hancock JT, Woodruff C, Keilman J. Text messaging reduces analgesic requirements during surgery. Pain Med. 2015;16(4):667–72.
8. Konrath S, Falk E, Fuhrel-Forbis A, Liu M, Swain J, Tolman R, et al. Can text messages increase empathy and prosocial behavior? The development and

initial validation of text to connect. PLoS One. 2015;10(9):e0137585.
9. Konrath S, Martingano AJ, Tolman R, Winslow M, Bushman B. Random App of Kindness (RAKi): evaluating the potential of a smartphone intervention to increase adolescents' empathy and change their behavior. Psychol Pop Media. 2023; (in press)
10. Van Royen K, Poels K, Vandebosch H, Adam P. "Thinking before posting?" reducing cyber harassment on social networking sites through a reflective message. Comput Human Behav. 2017;66:345–52.
11. Hangartner D, Gennaro G, Alasiri S, Bahrich N, Bornhoft A, Boucher J, et al. Empathy-based counterspeech can reduce racist hate speech in a social media field experiment. Proc Natl Acad Sci. 2021;118(50):e2116310118.
12. McCain JL, Campbell WK. Narcissism and social media use: a meta-analytic review. Psychol Pop Media Cult. 2018;7(3):308–27.
13. Vossen HG, Valkenburg PM. Do social media foster or curtail adolescents' empathy? A longitudinal study. Comput Human Behav. 2016;63:118–24.
14. Martingano AJ, Konrath S, Zarins S, Okaomee AA. Empathy, narcissism, alexithymia, and social media use. Psychol Pop Media; 2022.
15. Martingano AJ, Hererra F, Konrath S. Virtual reality improves emotional but not cognitive empathy: a meta-analysis. Technol Mind Behav. 2021;2(1). https://tmb.apaopen.org/pub/vr-improvesemotional-empathy-only/release/2.
16. Martingano AJ, Konrath S, Henritze E, Brown AD. The Limited Benefits of Using Virtual Reality 360° Videos to Promote Empathy and Charitable Giving. Nonprofit and Voluntary Sector Quarterly. Published online November 23, 2021.
17. Erreygers S, Vandebosch H, Vranjes I, Baillien E, De Witte H. Development of a measure of adolescents' online prosocial behavior. J Child Media. 2018:1–17. https://doi.org/10.1080/17482798.2018.1431558.
18. Lane DS, Dal Cin S. Sharing beyond slacktivism: the effect of socially observable prosocial media sharing on subsequent offline helping behavior. Inf Commun Soc. 2018;21(11):1523–40.
19. Armstrong-Carter E, Telzer EH. Advancing measurement and research on youths' prosocial behavior in the digital age. Child Dev Perspect. 2021;15(1):31–6.
20. Lee YJ. Social media capital and civic engagement: does type of connection matter? Int Rev Public Nonprofit Mark. 2022;19(1):167–89.
21. Giving USA. The role of technology. In: Giving by generation: examining the shifts in giving among donor generations. Giving USA special report; 2023. p. 15–21.
22. Miller V, Hogg E. 'If you press this, I'll pay': MrBeast, YouTube, and the mobilisation of the audience commodity in the name of charity. Convergence. 2023;0(0)
23. Anderson M, Vogels E, Perrin A, Rainie L. Connection, creativity and drama: teen life on social media in 2022. Pew Research Center Report. Published November 16, 2022. Accessed 7 April 2023. https://www.pewresearch.org/internet/2022/11/16/connection-creativity-and-drama-teen-life-on-social-media-in-2022/
24. Weinstein E, James C. Behind their screens: what teens are facing (and adults are missing). MIT Press; 2022.
25. Giumetti GW, Kowalski RM. Cyberbullying via social media and Well-being. Curr Opin Psychol. 2022;45:101314.
26. Zych I, Baldry AC, Farrington DP, Llorent VJ. Are children involved in cyberbullying low on empathy? A systematic review and meta-analysis of research on empathy versus different cyberbullying roles. Aggress Violent Behav. 2019;45:83–97.
27. Espelage DL, Hong JS, Valido A. Cyberbullying in the United States. In: International perspectives on cyberbullying; 2018. p. 65–99.
28. Kofoed J, Staksrud E. 'We always torment different people, so by definition, we are no bullies': the problem of definitions in cyberbullying research. New Media Soc. 2018;21(4):1006–20.
29. Milosevic T, Collier A, Norman JO. Leveraging dignity theory to understand bullying, cyberbullying, and children's rights. Int J Bullying Prev. 2022; https://doi.org/10.1007/s42380-022-00120-2.
30. Carmi E, Yates SJ, Lockley E, Pawluczuk A. Data citizenship: rethinking data literacy in the age of disinformation, misinformation, and malinformation. Internet. Pol Rev. 2020;9(2)
31. Mascheroni G, Siibak A. Datafied childhoods. Peter Lang Incorporated, International Academic Publishers; 2021.
32. Milosevic T, Verma K, Carter M, Vigil S, Laffan D, Davis B, O'Higgins NJ. Effectiveness of artificial intelligence–based cyberbullying interventions from youth perspective. Soc Med Soc. 2023;9(1):205630512211473.https://doi.org/10.1177/20563051221147325.
33. Staksrud E. Children in the online world. Routledge; 2016.
34. Fuller RW, Gerloff P. Dignity for all: how to create a world without rankism. Berrett-Koehler Publishers; 2008.
35. Nesi J, Choukas-Bradley S, Prinstein MJ. Transformation of adolescent peer relations in the social media context: part 2-application to peer group processes and future directions for research. Clin Child Fam Psychol Rev. 2018;21(3):295–319.
36. Council on Technology and Social Cohesion. Designing Tech for Social Cohesion. 2023. https://techandsocialcohesion.org/conference/.

# Parasocial Relationships in Children and Teens

Bradley J. Bond, Karen E. Dill-Shackleford,
Jayson L. Dibble, Tracy R. Gleason,
Nancy Jennings, Sarah Rosaen,
and Rebecca Tukachinsky Forster

## 1 Background

Young people have easy access to an array of fictional characters and celebrities, many of whom exist across platforms (e.g., protagonists from the graphic novel *Heartstopper* now appear in live-action on Netflix) and are manifested in toys and other merchandise. Children and adolescents often create powerful, socioemotional connections with fictional characters and celebrities called parasocial relationships (PSRs). Preschoolers clutching Elmo dolls, tweens fantasizing about interactions with TikTok influencers, and queer teens finding affirmation in a gay couple on *Schitt's Creek* all hint at possible PSRs. These one-sided, imagined social ties might raise concerns for parents and other stakeholders; however, PSRs are generally normative and adaptive and provide many social affordances. Children and adolescents relate to media personalities in varied ways, and these connections can lead to a variety of outcomes ranging from improving school readiness to enhancing psychological well-being.

### 1.1 How Do Children Relate to Media Personalities?

PSRs are a primary way in which children and adolescents relate to media personalities. Those who engage in PSRs imagine social connections between the self and a character or media figure. Although they are imagined, PSRs are meaningful interpersonal connections that are psychologically similar to the social ties that people form with real others in their immediate social network [1]. Social needs can also be fulfilled through parasocial experiences [2]. Many PSRs offer social provisions such as affiliative attachments, security, and trust [1, 3, 4] and for adolescents, romance [5]. The unidirectional nature of these ties allows for low-risk simulations of various kinds of close relationships. Negative aspects of relationships, such as rejection, insensitivity, and enmity, are only part of these relationships if a person chooses to imagine them so; dislike of a

B. J. Bond (✉)
University of San Diego, San Diego, CA, USA
e-mail: bond@SanDiego.edu

K. E. Dill-Shackleford
Fielding Graduate University,
Santa Barbara, CA, USA
e-mail: kshack@fielding.edu

J. L. Dibble
Hope College, Holland, MI, USA

T. R. Gleason
Wellesley College, Wellesley, MA, USA

N. Jennings
University of Cincinnati, Cincinnati, OH, USA

S. Rosaen
University of Michigan-Flint, Flint, MI, USA

R. T. Forster
Chapman University, Orange, CA, USA


D. A. Christakis, L. Hale (eds.), *Handbook of Children and Screens*,
https://doi.org/10.1007/978-3-031-69362-5_33

media character tends to decrease the development of PSRs [6].

The nature of PSRs changes with maturation, but strong parasocial bonds with a variety of media figures are found across development [3]. Children as young as two can name their favorite media figures and report PSRs with them [4]. Among preschool-aged and older children, stronger parasocial connections occur with socially realistic media personae [7] and children cite attractiveness, having human-like needs, and providing friendships as central characteristics of PSR partners [4]. In general, children's favorite characters tend to be the same sex [3] and tweens tend to relate with YouTubers of the same gender that are funny, attractive, and successful [8].

When research into PSRs began in the mid-twentieth century, interactions or relationships with media figures were never directly reciprocated. However, social media platforms, chats, and comments, especially during a livestream, now afford media fans some degree of reciprocity in their PSRs. The expansion of the PSR concept to encompass such interactive phenomena also offers insight into the emotional connections that elementary-aged children develop with virtual voice assistants, like Siri and Alexa [9].

PSRs are conceptualized as similar to, but distinct from, other experiences with media figures like identification, liking, and similarity. For example, an audience member might move fluidly from identifying with a character to thinking of them as a friend (i.e., developing a PSR). In the case of identification, individuals "try on" what it would be like to be someone else by imagining that person's thoughts, feelings, and goals from a first-person perspective. Early in development, identification typically occurs with parents, but soon thereafter children experiment by identifying with peers. However, identities are not shaped by lived experiences alone. Fictional characters and celebrities also provide alternative viewpoints and lifestyles worthy of exploration [10].

According to identification theory [10], identification with fictional characters is vital to the socialization of children. For example, we read fictional stories to children with the goal that they will internalize some of the positive attributes of the characters and apply the lessons of the story, adopting parts of the character's identity (e.g., attitudes and values) into their own. Identifying with characters in stories allows children to simulate how they might feel and react in the situations in the stories from a position of safety. These experiences may foster personal growth and help children expand beyond their own perspective to understand and empathize with others [11], but unlike PSR, they are not associated with social affordances.

## 2 Current State

PSRs have been linked to outcomes in the cognitive and social development of youth. Specifically, researchers have explored whether and how children might learn through PSRs, the extent to which PSRs relate to emulating media figures, how PSRs affect intergroup relationships, and the relation between PSRs and psychological well-being. In each case, the implications for development are significant given the impact of media during early life.

### 2.1 Learning

The relationship between PSRs and learning in early childhood in many ways resembles that of young children's learning from others in their face-to-face environment given that children learn better from characters that they find socially meaningful [3]. Characters become meaningful to children when they are familiar, likable, and seem to engage in experiences that resemble those of the real world [1]. Characters that address children directly, elicit participation (e.g., a character asks, "What is 4 + 4?" and the child says "8" to the screen), and engage in contingent replies (e.g., artificially intelligent characters that can reply to the child) also facilitate learning [12]. Consider PBS Kids' 2024 debut *Lyla in the Loop*, a children's program that will feature AI-assisted interactive content allowing the titular character to interact with children. A sense of trust, emotional attachment, and friendship is particularly conducive to children's learning from media [3]. Moreover, facilitating preschool children's PSRs with an educational TV character (such as PBS Kids' Daniel Tiger or characters from *Sesame Street*) boosts children's learning from that show [13].

## 2.2 Modeling and Persuasion

Across development, individuals tend to emulate media figures with whom they have PSRs, internalize the values of their parasocial others, and embrace persuasive messages coming from those media figures. For example, adolescents' PSRs with social media celebrities, especially those that are attractive and similar, lead to greater materialism and purchase intention [14]. Consider Matilda Djerf, who within 4 years built a multi-million-dollar fashion and beauty business stemming from her massive following on Instagram via her conventional attractiveness, relatable personality, focus on sustainability, and size inclusiveness. More broadly, PSRs with media personalities that are morally ambiguous or make unhealthy choices can lead to reinforcement or replication of these problematic behaviors. Children with strong PSRs, for example, tend to see those characters as moral and likable, which can lead to accepting problematic behavior [15]. Engagement with attractive role models such as superheroes similarly correlates with later physical aggression in preschool children [16] and adolescent girls who have strong PSRs with the characters on MTV's *16 and Pregnant* hold more favorable attitudes towards teen pregnancy [17].

PSRs can promote internalization of beauty standards, which can operate both to hinder or help the development of healthy body images. PSRs with celebrities representing an excessively thin body ideal can hurt adolescents' body image (especially among girls) [18]. PSRs can also buffer against these effects in young adults [19], as PSRs with celebrities that do not embody the thin ideal can promote body positivity/neutrality. For example, social media influencers like Megan Jayne Crabbe and Chessie King have significant youth followings and regularly post body-affirming and self-love content.

The importance of PSRs for inducing particular behaviors has not been lost on the developers of tech platforms. Some developers appear to engineer their products deliberately to harness the influence of PSRs. For example, an examination of the smartphone apps used by three- to five-year-old children (as reported by parents) revealed that approximately one-quarter facilitated PSRs with in-game characters to keep the children playing. At times, characters even expressed disappointment if the child stopped playing [20].

## 2.3 Improving Intergroup Relationships

Media narratives can introduce their audiences to people from social groups with whom they may lack direct contact in their daily lives. Exposure to positive, diverse media figures can reduce stereotypes towards various social groups, such as LGBTQA+ individuals, people who struggle with stigmatized health issues, or ethnic and racial minorities [21]. These effects are largely explained by the PSRs that the audience members form with the outgroup media figures as well as identification with the ingroup characters whose onscreen behavior models harmonious intergroup relationships [22].

## 2.4 Psychological Well-Being

Involvement with media personalities can be important for adolescents' social and emotional well-being in many ways. Engagement with fictional characters and celebrities can have implications for identity development among adolescents by playing a part in how they develop autonomy, psychologically differentiating themselves from their parents [23]. Adolescent boys, in particular, see media figures as role models and discuss their favorite media figures with their peers, whereas adolescent girls' PSRs with celebrities provide a sense of affiliation and belonging [24]. These relationships might be particularly attractive for individuals with low self-concept clarity [25], however, the direction of these effects is unclear. Moreover, adolescents with marginalized group identities describe fandom communities as safe spaces that foster their self-acceptance and self-validation [26].

PSRs can also serve as surrogates for social relationships and provide media users with connections that they are lacking in their immediate environments. For example, PSRs can be particularly important to LGBTQIA+ adolescents [27] or at times of social isolation, such as during the COVID-19 lockdown [28].

Romantic PSRs (e.g., celebrity crushes) allow adolescents to safely explore their sexuality and consolidate romantic identity without the risks involved in actual dating. Romantic fantasies focusing on media figures enable adolescents to mentally simulate romantic scripts and prepare them for actual romantic relationships. However, the fanciful nature of these relationships may foster unrealistic romantic expectations and be detrimental to teens' satisfaction with their future romantic relationships and partners [5].

While PRSs and other forms of engagement are generally healthy and adaptive, extreme forms of celebrity worship have been linked to lower self-esteem and poorer markers of psychological well-being [29]. Pathological levels of celebrity worshipping (e.g., stalking or over-identification with the celebrity) are rare and are probably a symptom of underlying mental health issues rather than normal fandom leading to psychopathology. However, emerging literature links normative levels of parasocial engagement and nonclinical levels of anxiety in relationships. For example, adolescent girls who engage in PSRs experience more intense preoccupied attachment and anxiety in close relationships compared to their peers [30], but PSRs do not correlate with self-esteem or depressive symptoms in early adolescence [31].

## 3 Future Research

- What are the social affordances of PSRs for children of various ages? How do the content and purpose of PSRs change longitudinally, particularly across the transitions into adolescence and into young adulthood?
- How can young audiences' PSRs with media figures be used to promote psychological and emotional health and well-being?
- Could PSRs with fictional characters and celebrities across new and evolving media (e.g., virtual reality, AI chatbots) provide important lessons about social issues, and even help expose children and teens to marginalized groups or communities with whom they would otherwise lack contact?
- How can PSRs be used in embedded advertising and when might such a practice be considered problematic or unethical? Should policy regulate how advertisers harness PSRs in persuasive media messages aimed at promoting products, services, and ideas to children?
- Should there be media literacy training to help children understand PSRs? Should teachers or pediatricians incorporate media literacy into their interactions with children?
- What are the mechanisms through which identification and PSRs with marginalized (e.g., LBGTQ+) media figures might mitigate feelings of loneliness and isolation among marginalized youth?
- How are PSRs that afford reciprocity on new media platforms unique from traditional PSRs on traditional media that lack mutuality? At what point does the parasocial become social? Under what conditions do these episodic interactions intensify or mitigate media influence?

## 4 Recommendations

- Have open conversations with children and teens about who they admire in the media and why, and particularly for older children, the difference between reality and a curated public image.

- Understand that identifying with and relating to others (including fictional characters and celebrities) is an important and normal social developmental process that extends from children's identification with parents and is part of one's identity formation, including the development of autonomy.
- Encourage the development of PSRs for youth who may perceive that they lack like-others in their real lives, such that they may compensate through identification and validation from media figures.
- Approach adolescents' celebrity crushes with the understanding that they are developmentally normal and can have benefits. However, note signs of a possibly unhealthy crush such as (1) if the romantic PSR interferes with the development or maintenance of real-life relationships with peers, or (2) if the teen shows lack of understanding that their romantic PSR is fanciful and unidimensional.
- Be mindful that connecting with fictional characters and celebrities means connecting to popular culture; this helps young people relate to each other.
- Know that being entirely cut off from connections with popular media figures could be isolating and make relating to peers more difficult.
- Be aware that PSRs can help children understand themselves and others and learn things about their world.
- Encourage children to develop PSRs with characters that promote learning and desirable effects, but be vigilant about PSRs with characters that can have negative influences. Be mindful of ways in which various platforms and technologies promote PSRs.

**Conflict of Interest and Funding Disclosures** None.

## References

1. Bond BJ, Calvert SL. Parasocial breakup among young children in the United States. J Child Media. 2014;8(4):474–90. https://doi.org/10.1080/17482798.2014.953559.
2. Paravati E, Naidu E, Gabriel S, Wiedemann C. More than just a tweet: the unconscious impact of forming parasocial relationships through social media. Psychol Conscious. 2020;7(4):388–403. https://doi.org/10.1037/cns0000214.
3. Aguiar NR, Richards MN, Bond BJ, Brunick KL, Calvert SL. Parents' perceptions of their children's parasocial relationships: the recontact study. Imagin Cogn Pers. 2019;38(3):221–49. https://doi.org/10.1177/0276236618771537.
4. Richards MN, Calvert SL. Parent versus child report of young children's parasocial relationships in the United States. J Child Media. 2016;10(4):462–80. https://doi.org/10.1080/17482798.2016.1157502.
5. Tukachinsky R, Dorros SM. Parasocial romantic relationships, romantic beliefs, and relationship outcomes in USA adolescents: rehearsing love or setting oneself up to fail? J Child Media. 2018;12(3):329–45. https://doi.org/10.1080/17482798.201801463917.
6. Jennings N, Alper M. Young children's positive and negative parasocial relationships with media characters. Commun Res Rep. 2016;33(2):96–102. https://doi.org/10.1080/08824096.2016.1154833.
7. Rosaen SF, Dibble JL. Investigating the relationships among child's age, Parasocial interactions, and the social realism of favorite television characters. Commun Res Rep. 2008;25:145–54. https://doi.org/10.1080/08824090802021806.
8. Tolbert AN, Drogos KL. Tweens' wishful identification and parasocial relationships with YouTubers. Front Psychol. 2019:10. https://doi.org/10.3389/fpsyg.2019.02781.
9. Hoffman A, Owen D, Calvert SL. Parent reports of children's parasocial relationships with conversational agents: trusted voices in children's lives. Hum Behav Emerg Technol. 2021;3(4):606–17. https://doi.org/10.1002/hbe2.271.
10. Cohen J. Defining identification: a theoretical look at the identification of audiences with media characters. Mass Commun Soc. 2001;4(3):245–64. https://doi.org/10.1207/S15327825MC0403_01.
11. Dill-Shackleford KE, Vinney C, Hopper-Losenicky K. Connecting the dots between fantasy and reality: the social psychology of our engagement with fictional narrative and its functional value. Soc Personal Psychol Compass. 2016;10(11):634–46. https://doi.org/10.1111/spc3.12274.
12. Putnam MM, Ryan RM, Barba E, Nissen J, Calvert SL. Young children's mathematics learning from same-gender and other-gender intelligent character prototypes. Tech Mind Behav. 2022;3(2) https://doi.org/10.1037/tmb0000069.
13. Jennings NA, Hooker SD, Linebarger DL. Educational television as mediated literacy environments for preschoolers. Learn Media Technol. 2009;34(3):229–42. https://doi.org/10.1080/17439880903141513.
14. Lou C, Kim HK. Fancying the new rich and famous? Explicating the roles of influencer content, credibility, and parental mediation in adolescents' parasocial

relationship, materialism, and purchase intentions. Front Psychol. 2019:10. https://doi.org/10.3389/fpsyg.2019.02567.
15. Jennings NA, Rosaen SF, Banjo O, McCoy V. Honesty, morality, and parasocial relationships in U.S. children's media. J Child Media. 2022;16(4):575–86. https://doi.org/10.1080/17482798.2022.2079695.
16. Coyne SM, Stockdale L, Linder JR, et al. Pow! Boom! Kablam! Effects of viewing superhero programs on aggressive, prosocial, and defending behaviors in preschool children. J Abnorm Child Psychol. 2017;45:1523–35. https://doi.org/10.1007/s10802-016-0253-6.
17. Behm-Morawitz E, Aubrey JS, Pennell H, Kim KB. Examining the effects of MTV's 16 and pregnant on adolescent girls' sexual health: the implications of character affinity, pregnancy risk factors, and health literacy on message effectiveness. Health Commun. 2019;34(2):180–90. https://doi.org/10.1080/10410236.2017.1399506.
18. Ho SS, Lee EW, Liao Y. Social network sites, friends, and celebrities: the roles of social comparison and celebrity involvement in adolescents' body image dissatisfaction. Soc Med Soc. 2016;2016:2(3). https://doi.org/10.1177/2056305116664216.
19. Young AF, Gabriel S, Hollar JL. Batman to the rescue! The protective effects of parasocial relationships with muscular superheroes on men's body image. J Exp Soc Psychol. 2013;49(1):173–7. https://doi.org/10.1016/j.esp.2012.08.003.
20. Radesky J, Hiniker A, McLaren C, et al. Prevalence and characteristics of manipulative design in mobile applications used by children. JAMA Netw Open. 2022;5(6):e2217641. https://doi.org/10.1001/jamanetworkopen.2022.17641.
21. McGuire L, Marshall TE, Nilson MA, Palmer SB, Rutland A. Indirect contact and adolescents' intentions as bystanders to LGBTQ+ microaggressions. J Appl Dev Psychol. 2023;84:101485. https://doi.org/10.1016/j.appdev.2022.101485.
22. Ortiz M, Harwood J. A social cognitive theory approach to the effects of mediated intergroup contact on intergroup attitudes. J Broadcast Electron. 2007;51(4):615–31. https://doi.org/10.1080/08838150701626487.
23. Giles DC, Maltby J. The role of media figures in adolescent development: relations between autonomy, attachment, and interest in celebrities. Pers Individ Dif. 2004;36(4):813–22. https://doi.org/10.1016/S0191-8869(03)00154-S.
24. Gleason TR, Theran SA, Newberg EM. Parasocial interactions and relationships in early adolescence. Front Psychol. 2017;8:255. https://doi.org/10.3389/fpsyg.2017.00255.
25. Dajches L. Finding the self through others: exploring fandom, identification, and self-concept clarity among US adolescents. J Child Media. 2022;16(1):107–16. https://doi.org/10.1080/17482798.2021.1922474.
26. McInroy LB, Craig SL. "It's like a safe haven fantasy world": online fandom communities and the identity development activities of sexual and gender minority youth. Psychol Pop Media. 2020;9(2):236. https://doi.org/10.1037/ppm0000234.
27. Bond BJ. The development and influence of parasocial relationships with television characters: a longitudinal experimental test of prejudice reduction through parasocial contact. Commun Res. 2021;48(4):573–93. https://doi.org/10.1177/0093650219900632.
28. Bond BJ. Parasocial relationships as functional social alternatives during pandemic-induced social distancing. Psychol Pop Media. 2022;11(3):250–7. https://doi.org/10.1037/ppm0000364.
29. Chia SC, Poo YL. Media, celebrities, and fans: an examination of adolescents' media usage and involvement with entertainment celebrities. J Mass Comm. 2009;86(1):23–44. https://doi.org/10.1177/107769900908600103.
30. Theran SA, Newberg EM, Gleason TR. Adolescent girls' parasocial interactions with media figures. J Genet Psychol. 2010;171(3):270–7. https://doi.org/10.1080/00221325.2010.483700.
31. Gleason TR, Theran SA, Newberg EM. Connections between adolescents' parasocial interactions and recollections of childhood imaginative activities. Imagin Cogn Pers. 2020;39(3):241–60. https://doi.org/10.1177/0276236619825810.

# Online Self-Presentation and Identity: Insights from Diverse and Marginalized Youth

Chia-chen Yang, Angela Calvin, Sophia Choukas-Bradley, Koen Leurs, Adriana Manago, and Kaveri Subrahmanyam

## 1 Background

In the digital age, strategic self-presentation on social media has become commonplace among youth. By selectively posting texts, photos, and videos, young people present and communicate aspects of who they are and/or how they want to be seen [1]. Online self-presentation, also referred to as digital self-presentation, has important implications for identity development, such as identity clarity (in general and in specific areas, such as gender, sexual, and/or cultural identities), self-esteem, and body image [2–4]. In this chapter, we review recent studies about (1) different types of online self-presentation and their identity implications, (2) online self-presentation and body image, and (3) online self-presentation among marginalized youth. The first two topics are predominantly drawn from the research done with cisgender White youth in the Global North, whereas the last one focuses on youth who are usually underrepresented in research. In this review, "youth" refers to adolescents (13- to 17-year-olds) and emerging adults (18- to 29-year-olds).

## 2 Current State

### 2.1 Types of Online Self-Presentation

Whether online self-presentation facilitates or hinders identity development is contingent upon how youth present themselves. Research has examined self-presentation along different dimensions, including intimacy/depth, positivity, and authenticity.

*The second through fifth listed authors (AC, SCB, KL, AM,) made equal intellectual contributions to this chapter and share second authorship; these names are listed alphabetically.

C. Yang (✉)
School of Educational Foundations, Leadership and Aviation, Oklahoma State University, Stillwater, OK, USA
e-mail: chia-chen.yang@okstate.edu

A. Calvin
Common Sense Media, San Francisco, CA, USA
e-mail: acalvin@commonsense.org

S. Choukas-Bradley
Department of Psychology, University of Pittsburgh, Pittsburgh, PA, USA

K. Leurs
Department of Media and Culture Studies, Utrecht University, Utrecht, Netherlands

A. Manago
Department of Psychology, University of California, Santa Cruz, CA, USA

K. Subrahmanyam
Department of Psychology, University of North Florida, Jacksonville, FL, USA


D. A. Christakis, L. Hale (eds.), *Handbook of Children and Screens*,
https://doi.org/10.1007/978-3-031-69362-5_34

Intimate/deep self-presentation refers to revealing personal and private information on public or semi-public digital platforms [5]. Although it contributes to greater self-esteem by eliciting social support from the audience [5], it also has a direct relationship with lower self-esteem and identity clarity [2]. Furthermore, this self-presentation can reduce social attraction when perceived as oversharing [1], which may hurt youth's peer relations and thus self-esteem.

When youth engage in positive self-presentation, they aim to present a socially desirable image. Youth often consider the evaluation criteria held by peers and define positive self-presentation as presenting an interesting, likable, and attractive image [6]. Meanwhile, when youth take into account adult audiences, such as parents, relatives, teachers, and future employers, they understand the definition of "positive" may vary, and thus, they would need to tailor the image toward the audience's standards or adjust privacy settings to avoid tension [7, 8]. Scholars have proposed that positive self-presentation often directs presenters' attention to their positive traits and experiences, which affirms their identity and self-esteem [1].

Authentic self-presentation refers to presenting an image that is accurate (characterized by consistency between the online and offline images) and faithfully reflects one's inner, true self [1, 9]. For adolescents, it means the process of self-presentation should be spontaneous and unplanned, and the content should be raw and unedited [8]. For emerging adults, authenticity can be achieved by expressing angst through irony and humor and integrating various self-components into their online personas, such as family ties, cultural practices, and even political values that could potentially fuel tension or spark conflict [10]. Youth are able to present an authentic image when they feel safe and welcome [11]. In turn, presenting an authentic self, when validated by peers, makes youth feel that the true and unpolished self is accepted [8]. Unsurprisingly, authentic self-presentation has been found to be related to higher self-esteem by eliciting more supportive feedback from the audience [5].

Are positive and authentic self-presentations incompatible? The answer is unclear. In Yang and colleagues' studies of emerging adults, positive and authentic self-presentations had either a positive or null correlation [2, 5]. The authors argued that emerging adults did not think selective (and thus positive) self-presentation compromises their authenticity. Results from adolescents are less consistent. While some studies also reveal a positive correlation between positive and authentic self-presentations among adolescents [12], others indicate that teens associate authenticity with negative emotional expression, demoting oneself, and irreverence [8]. Perhaps there is a developmental difference: As youth get older and become more accepting of "adult" norms, it becomes easier to be positive and authentic simultaneously. Given the limited number of studies on this topic involving different age groups, further research is required to clarify how young people at various developmental stages negotiate different types of self-presentation.

Although positive and authentic self-presentations are generally associated with positive identity outcomes, there are caveats. Overemphasis on presenting a perfect image, especially in terms of appearance, can have negative implications for body image [3]. Presenting an authentic image or sharing authentic self-information online can have unintended consequences, especially for marginalized youth [13, 14]. We discuss these issues more carefully in the following sections.

## 2.2 Online Self-Presentation and Body Image

Youth are highly motivated to present a favorable self-image related to physical appearance. Body image concerns spike during adolescence, especially among girls, due to a complex coalescence of biological, cognitive, and social developmental processes [15]. For example, adolescents often experience the "imaginary audience," a social–cognitive phenomenon in which they feel acutely self-conscious and hyper-attuned to peers' reactions, during the same developmental period when puberty leads to rapid physical changes [3].

According to the "perfect storm" developmental–sociocultural framework, social media may intersect with these developmental processes to increase the risk for body image concerns among adolescent girls [3]. Social media presents the ideal opportunity for youth to engage in carefully curated self-presentations via photos and videos that showcase one's physical appearance with the goal of maximizing views and likes [16]. The online audience can feel ever-present; adolescents may be highly conscious of their online self-presentation even when not actively online. Higher levels of *appearance-related social media consciousness* (ASMC) have been linked to lower body esteem and greater mental health concerns among both girls and boys [17, 18]. Overall, research indicates that girls are on average more preoccupied with their online appearance than boys, but that among both boys and girls, higher levels of ASMC and other social media-related appearance concerns are associated with higher risk for body dissatisfaction and mental health concerns [3].

## 2.3 Online Self-Presentation Among Marginalized Youth

### 2.3.1 Sexual and Gender Minority Youth

Exploring, defining, and unveiling one's authentic identity online is a challenging but meaningful process for sexual and gender minority (SGM) youth. We use "SGM" to refer to individuals who identify with a gender that is not cisgender or a sexual orientation that is not heterosexual; examples include gay, lesbian, bisexual, transgender, and queer identities.

For SGM youth, sharing their authentic self includes disclosing their gender and sexual identity [19]. SGM youth often describe social media as a place to enact their authentic self without stigma because they offer safe, sometimes anonymous, communities [11], and youth have more control over whom, what, where, and when they share their true self [4]. Specifically, SGM youth report using multiple accounts, curating their network, and utilizing privacy controls to manage their public image [19]. Expressing their true self online facilitates gender and sexual identity development. By sharing honest self-expressions, SGM youth learn from each other's narratives of identity development and experience validation through shared experiences; this is especially meaningful for SGM youth who cannot find others with similar identities offline [4].

However, managing multiple accounts and identities across social media can be taxing over time [20]. Furthermore, sharing their true identity puts SGM youth at risk for cyberbullying and discrimination; even if they have not faced discrimination themselves, they have likely observed others with similar identities being harassed online [13]. Despite social media providers' efforts to manage discrimination through content moderation policies, many SGM content creators on social media are disproportionately censored [21]. Silencing these creators diminishes sexual health and gender-affirming care information that SGM youth often access for support.

### 2.3.2 Cultural and Racial/Ethnic Minority Youth

A burgeoning body of research on cultural differences in digital self-presentation demonstrates how uses of social media are culturally constructed [22]. Youth learn to present themselves on digital platforms within the context of cultural beliefs, values, and norms that shape purposes of self-presentation and what is considered authentic and ideal. The individualistic–collectivistic value dimension has been the most common framework for examining these cultural variations. For example, one study found that whereas self-promotion and self-documentation motivated (individualistic) White American college students' use of Instagram, social interaction primarily motivated (collectivistic) Croatian college students [23]. A recent content analysis using facial recognition software of over 3000 Instagram selfies from locations around the world found that selfies of Asian and Hispanic[1] users

[1] Bij de Vaate et al., (2022) used Hispanic rather than Latine because the participants were not necessarily people from Latin America (e.g., they could be people from Spain, Cuba, etc.).

were more likely to reflect interdependence values (more people in photos, less focus on the face, and more on context) compared to selfies of Black and White users [24]. Gender has also been an important focus of research on cultural variations in self-presentation. In cultural contexts undergoing changes in traditional gender roles such as the United Arab Emirates (UAE), social media have had emancipatory implications for emerging adult women's development by enabling greater exploration and control over their gender identity expression [25]. This study also reported that young men in UAE spent more time than women curating and editing their photos and posts, a reversal of common research findings in Western samples.

Research within the United States has demonstrated how social media have become critical tools for ethnically/racially marginalized youth to explore, express, and transform cultural identities. A study with Hmong-American emerging adults illustrated that they portrayed their cultural identities online through clothing, language, music, and association with famous figures to take pride in their heritage [26]. Social media also made them more aware of tensions in their bicultural identities, which they sought to manage through their digital self-presentations. Another example is a study with Black high school students in Detroit. Researchers found social media were tools for adolescents to resist and challenge racial stereotypes by showcasing their college ambitions, community commitments, and pride [27]. These studies suggest that self-presentations on social media are important avenues for exploring facets of one's identity and can generate feedback that strengthen the presented images and qualities in one's sense of self; however, there is lack of research examining this process longitudinally. Overall, research suggests that social media afford new opportunities for diverse cultural representations to flourish through adolescents' and emerging adults' identity development.

### 2.3.3 Migrant Youth

Similar to SGM and cultural/racial/ethnic minority youth, practices of migrant youth illustrate how marginalization amplifies the opportunities and challenges of online self-presentation. We use the term "migrant youth" to address the concerns and needs of a broad variety of young people. Its focus ranges from privileged migrants, including children of expatriates and young digital nomads who are predominantly White and/or hold "strong passports" issued in the Global North, to asylum seekers and refugees who have been forcibly displaced within their countries or across borders.

For migrant youth, self-presentation is a double-edged sword. On the positive side, youth are in charge of their appearance through text, visuals, moving images, hashtags, and sound; self-presentation practices thus provide opportunities to create a positive and empowering digital identity and for civic engagement and activism [14]. They can also use social media to bond with members of their communities by showcasing cultural traditions and achievements, as well as connecting with people outside of their communities who share similar interests, talents, and goals [28]. Migrant youth have to negotiate multi-layered, hybrid identities, with some highlighting the connection to their roots and others accentuating the changes they experience. In these negotiations, their digital self-presentation reveals how they satisfy, challenge, or balance the various expectations and demands related to gender, sexuality, diaspora, nationalism, generation, and youth culture, among others [29].

On the negative side, online self-presentation can have unintended consequences. In visa and asylum procedures across the world, social media and smartphone data are now used by immigration authorities as new vetting opportunities [30]. Migrant youth therefore are cautious about digital practices, as they are increasingly aware that self-presentations may inadvertently reveal personal information that could be used against them, or be taken as evidence of activities that could jeopardize their safety or legal status [31]. As a result, migrant youth are commonly sensitized into performing self-presentation practices in a mindful way [14]. Similarly, we see how migrant youth seek to negotiate context-collapse, meaning they have to face distinctive audiences (e.g., those in their home country versus host country) and curate their online self-presentations strategically towards them [14]. For these reasons, the digital practices of marginalized youth may also offer a corrective to dominant views of digital media literacy, showing how media literacy is situational, context-specific, and may be pioneered by non-mainstream youth [32].

## 3 Future Research

Below are some critical questions for future research:

- In what ways do youth's curation and self-presentation management strategies (e.g., using privacy settings and presenting on multiple accounts and platforms) relate to their well-being? Is curation perceived as less authentic, and does it therefore compromise well-being or does the control aspect of curation improve well-being?
- Does the flexibility in self-presentation afforded by social media help improve body esteem for some youth (e.g., SGM youth)?
- How do cultural beliefs, values, and norms shape what is considered ideal and authentic in digital self-presentation around the world? How does it impact youth's commitment to racial/ethnic or cultural identities when they face conflicting norms?
- How do youth manipulate their self-presentation in light of corporate financial interests (that seek to monetize niche trends), governmental monitoring (such as during asylum procedures), or intra-community policing (to conform to norms of gender, sexuality, and/or religion, for example)? Does the manipulation reflect or contribute to positive developmental outcomes (e.g., sensitivity to norms and ability to self-regulate and conform to norms) or negative ones (e.g., suppression of full-fledged identity development)?

## 4 Recommendations

### 4.1 For Researchers

- Future scholarship should explore how online self-presentation provides a means for youth to articulate their understanding of the intersections of various axes of difference, including gender, sexuality, ethnicity, race, age, generation, and ability, among others. This direction can be especially important for youth with multiple intersecting marginalized identities (e.g., a Black male in a same-sex relationship) that may conflict. Research should examine whether such youth view social media as a safe space to self-explore and self-present, and investigate the implications of their digital self-presentation for social support, cyberbullying, and well-being.

### 4.2 For Policymakers

- Policymakers should hold social media companies accountable for design tactics that encourage maladaptive social media use. They should also require social media companies to share data so that independent researchers can examine the long-term implications of different ways of social media use.

### 4.3 For Clinicians

- Instead of focusing on the overall amount of screen time, clinicians should ask young people what they do online, and encourage youth to examine the functions and outcomes of their specific digital behaviors.
- Clinicians should consider self-presentation practices when discussing social media use with adolescents and parents. Discussions could revolve around adolescents' goals of self-presentation. Based on the research discussed above, digital self-presentation has the potential to facilitate identity development when young people use it to explore, better understand, and communicate their identities.

It is also common that they seek validation and social connections with others who have similar identities and experiences. However, it can be concerning if youth are preoccupied with their appearance on social media. To assess whether youth engage in digital self-presentation in an adaptive manner, it is important to confer with them about their appraisal of the views, likes, and comments on their self-presentation.

## 4.4 For Educators

- Educators are encouraged to invite youth to reflect upon and discuss the benefits and risks of different forms of online self-presentation. The goal of these conversations is to help youth engage in adaptive and avoid detrimental forms of online self-presentation. For example, using social media to showcase positive experiences and express an authentic self is beneficial, but revealing more personal information than necessary and being preoccupied with having a perfect online image can be a red flag.
- Educators should advise youth to consider unforeseen consequences of their digital self-presentation (e.g., information being accessed and misused by unintended audiences).
- It is recommended that educators use or develop curricula aimed at helping young people to effectively use social media for self-presentation. For example, given the positive association between authentic self-presentation and identity development, youth are advised to present digital personas aligned with their true self rather than a false or embellished self. Exaggerating achievements to impress an audience, or pretending to share interests or experiences to gain peer approval, can negatively impact social relationships and self-esteem.
- For all young people, but especially those with marginalized identities, educators can teach them to carefully consider *where* they are disclosing information about their true selves. We encourage educators to discuss appropriate, safe, and supportive online spaces where youth can enact authentic and empowering self-presentation without fear of stigmatization.

**Conflict of Interest and Funding Disclosures** None.

## References

1. Yang CC, Holden SM, Ariati J. Social media and psychological well-being among youth: the multidimensional model of social media use. Clin Child Fam Psychol Rev. 2021;24(3):631–50. https://doi.org/10.1007/s10567-021-00359-z.
2. Yang CC, Holden SM, Carter MDK. Emerging adults' social media self-presentation and identity development at college transition: mindfulness as a moderator. J Appl Dev Psychol. 2017;52:212–21. https://doi.org/10.1016/j.appdev.2017.08.006.
3. Choukas-Bradley S, Roberts SR, Maheux AJ, Nesi J. The perfect storm: a developmental–sociocultural framework for the role of social media in adolescent girls' body image concerns and mental health. Clin Child Fam Psychol Rev. 2022;25(4):681–701. https://doi.org/10.1007/s10567-022-00404-5.
4. Bates A, Hobman T, Bell BT. "Let me do what I please with it... Don't decide my identity for me": LGBTQ+ youth experiences of social media in narrative identity development. J Adolesc Res. 2020;35(1):51–83. https://doi.org/10.1177/0743558419884700.
5. Yang CC, Brown BB. Online self-presentation on Facebook and self-development during the college transition. J Youth Adolescence. 2016;45(2):402–16. https://doi.org/10.1007/s10964-015-0385-y.
6. Yau JC, Reich SM. "It's just a lot of work": adolescents' self-presentation norms and practices on Facebook and Instagram. J Res Adolesc. 2019;29(1):196–209. https://doi.org/10.1111/jora.12376.
7. Charmaraman L, Chan HB, Chen S, Richer A, Ramanudom B. Asian American social media use: from cyber dependence and cyber harassment to saving face. Asian Am J Psychol. 2018;9(1):72–86. https://doi.org/10.1037/aap0000109.
8. Darr CR, Doss EF. The fake one is the real one: Finstas, authenticity, and context collapse in teen friend groups. Humphreys L, ed. J Comput-Mediat Commun. 2022;27(4):zmac009. https://doi.org/10.1093/jcmc/zmac009.
9. Sedikides C, Lenton AP, Slabu L, Thomaes S. Sketching the contours of state authenticity. Rev Gen Psychol. 2019;23(1):73–88. https://doi.org/10.1037/gpr0000156.
10. Santer N, Manago A, Bleisch R. Narratives of the self in polymedia contexts: authenticity and branding in generation Z. Qual Psychol. 2023;10(1):79–106. https://doi.org/10.1037/qup0000232.

11. McInroy LB, Craig SL. "It's like a safe haven fantasy world": online fandom communities and the identity development activities of sexual and gender minority youth. Psychol Popular Med. 2020;9(2):236–46. https://doi.org/10.1037/ppm0000234.
12. Tian L, Zhai R, Wang Y, Zhang H, Chen J. How different online self-presentations relate to different online feedback among adolescents: peer relationship as a mediator. Curr Psychol. 2024;43(12):10693–702. https://doi.org/10.1007/s12144-023-05190-z.
13. Berger MN, Taba M, Marino JL, et al. Social media's role in support networks among LGBTQ adolescents: a qualitative study. Newman C, ed. Sex Health. 2021;18(5):421–31. https://doi.org/10.1071/SH21110.
14. Leurs K. Communication rights from the margins: politicising young refugees' smartphone pocket archives. Int Commun Gaz. 2017;79(6–7):674–98. https://doi.org/10.1177/1748048517727182.
15. Markey CN. Invited commentary: why body image is important to adolescent development. J Youth Adolescence. 2010;39(12):1387–91. https://doi.org/10.1007/s10964-010-9510-0.
16. Chua THH, Chang L. Follow me and like my beautiful selfies: Singapore teenage girls' engagement in self-presentation and peer comparison on social media. Comput Hum Behav. 2016;55:190–7. https://doi.org/10.1016/j.chb.2015.09.011.
17. Choukas-Bradley S, Nesi J, Widman L, Galla BM. The appearance-related social media consciousness scale: development and validation with adolescents. Body Image. 2020;33:164–74. https://doi.org/10.1016/j.bodyim.2020.02.017.
18. Maheux AJ, Roberts SR, Nesi J, Widman L, Choukas-Bradley S. Longitudinal associations between appearance-related social media consciousness and adolescents' depressive symptoms. J Adolesc. 2022;94(2):264–9. https://doi.org/10.1002/jad.12009.
19. McConnell EA, Clifford A, Korpak AK, Phillips G, Birkett M. Identity, victimization, and support: Facebook experiences and mental health among LGBTQ youth. Comput Hum Behav. 2017;76:237–44. https://doi.org/10.1016/j.chb.2017.07.026.
20. Buss J, Le H, Haimson OL. Transgender identity management across social media platforms. Med Cult Soc. 2022;44(1):22–38. https://doi.org/10.1177/01634437211027106.
21. Haimson OL, Delmonaco D, Nie P, Wegner A. Disproportionate removals and differing content moderation experiences for conservative, transgender, and black social media users: marginalization and moderation gray areas. Proc ACM Hum-Comput Interact. 2021;5(CSCW2):1–35. https://doi.org/10.1145/3479610.
22. Manago AM, McKenzie J. Culture and digital media in adolescent development. In: Nesi J, Telzer EH, Prinstein MJ, editors. Handbook of adolescent digital media use and mental health. 1st ed. Cambridge University Press; 2022. p. 162–87. https://doi.org/10.1017/9781108976237.010.
23. Sheldon P, Rauschnabel PA, Antony MG, Car S. A cross-cultural comparison of Croatian and American social network sites: exploring cultural differences in motives for Instagram use. Comput Hum Behav. 2017;75:643–51. https://doi.org/10.1016/j.chb.2017.06.009.
24. de Bij Vaate NAJD, Veldhuis J, Konijn EA. Ethno-racial identity and digitalisation in self-presentation: a large-scale Instagram content analysis. Behav Inform Technol. Published online August 20, 2022:1–16. https://doi.org/10.1080/0144929X.2022.2112613.
25. Zaid B, Shin DD, Kteish SW, Fedtke J, Ibahrine M. Gendered self-representation and empowerment on social media in The United Arab Emirates. Commun Rev. 2021;24(3):199–217. https://doi.org/10.1080/10714421.2021.1957382.
26. McKenzie J. Digital media as sites for cultural identity development: the case of Hmong American emerging adults. J Adolesc Res. Published online August 23. 2022:074355842211163. https://doi.org/10.1177/07435584221116312.
27. Brown M, Pyle C, Ellison NB. "On my head about it": college aspirations, social media participation, and community cultural wealth. Soc Med Soc. 2022;8(2):205630512210915. https://doi.org/10.1177/20563051221091545.
28. Kutscher N, Kreß LM. The ambivalent potentials of social media use by unaccompanied minor refugees. Social Med Soc. 2018;4(1):205630511876443. https://doi.org/10.1177/2056305118764438.
29. Volpe CR. "What kind of girl is she?": good and bad diasporic daughters on social media. J Cult Geogr. 2021;38(2):177–205. https://doi.org/10.1080/08873631.2020.1864085.
30. Bolhuis MP, van Wijk J. Seeking Asylum in the digital era: social-media and mobile-device vetting in Asylum procedures in five European countries. J Refug Stud. 2021;34(2):1595–617. https://doi.org/10.1093/jrs/feaa029.
31. Literat I. Refugee Selfies and the (Self-)Representation of Disenfranchised Social Groups.
32. Bruinenberg H, Sprenger S, Omerović E, Leurs K. Practicing critical media literacy education with/for young migrants: lessons learned from a participatory action research project. Int Commun Gaz. 2021;83(1):26–47. https://doi.org/10.1177/1748048519883511.

# Youth Participatory Politics: Understanding and Supporting Civic Engagement in the Social Media Era

Ellen Middaugh, Mariah Kornbluh, Ashley Lee, Neta Kligler-Vilenchik, Srividya Ramasubramanian, Lynn Schofield Clark, and Tanner Vea

## 1 Background

### 1.1 Why Is Youth Civic Engagement Important to Foster?

Many arguments for the importance of youth civic engagement focus on the well-being of democracy and the need for an educated and engaged citizenry [1]. Taking a youth-centered perspective, there is ample evidence that the quality of our institutions (e.g., education, healthcare, juvenile justice/criminal punishment, immigration, child welfare/family policing, and media), and the policies that regulate directly impact youth well-being and potential to thrive, and that understanding these impacts require attention to youths' intersecting identities [2]. For example, Black American youth are impacted by multiple policy failures including—but not limited to—higher rates of exposure to police violence, health inequities, and unequal investment in education [3]. Globally, youth have reported high levels of climate anxiety about the impact of climate change on their opportunities and well-being [4]. Growing trends toward ideological hate, extreme partisanship, and belief polarization have significant implications for the well-being of minoritized youth. Research has documented the negative impact of political rhetoric and policies targeting LGBTQ+ and especially trans or gender nonconforming youth [3], Latine [3], Muslim [5], and Asian American youth [3] on their well-being. These trends point to the importance of supporting youth to advocate for their needs and participate in shaping the political rhetoric and policies that impact them.

The original version of the chapter has been revised. A correction to this chapter can be found at https://doi.org/10.1007/978-3-031-69362-5_88

E. Middaugh (✉)
San José State University, San José, CA, USA
e-mail: ellen.middaugh@sjsu.edu

M. Kornbluh
University of Oregon, Eugene, OR, USA

A. Lee
Harvard University, Cambridge, MA, USA

N. Kligler-Vilenchik
Hebrew University of Jerusalem, Jerusalem, Israel

S. Ramasubramanian
Syracuse University, Syracuse, NY, USA

L. S. Clark
University of Denver, Denver, CO, USA

T. Vea
University of Washington, Seattle, WA, USA


D. A. Christakis, L. Hale (eds.), *Handbook of Children and Screens*,
https://doi.org/10.1007/978-3-031-69362-5_35

### 1.2 Limitations of a Risk-Prevention-Only Approach

One common tension in research as it relates to children, youth, and screens is between a risk-prevention (or safety-and-privacy) approach and the participation and empowerment approach. The risk-prevention approach focuses on possible harms of technology (e.g., internet addiction, self-esteem, body image, etc.) and strategies to limit or avoid harm and encourage responsible use. The participation and empowerment approach emphasizes the affordances of technology (e.g. opportunities for creative expression and agency, social connection, and building social capital) and strategies for youth to take advantage of such affordances [6]. As digital technologies are now fully integrated into youths' lives, research has found the online/offline dichotomy to be obsolete, and current theory and practice focuses on taking a balanced approach to supporting children and youth to use media in healthy and responsible ways [7].

Furthermore, a risk-prevention-only approach is developmentally inappropriate. Decades of research from developmental sciences point to adolescents' expanding need for autonomy and the importance of opportunities during this period to learn to navigate risk with adult support [8]. As adolescents experience an expanded cognitive capacity to critically analyze social issues, they are frequently drawn to civic engagement opportunities that allow them to express their critiques of current systems. Accordingly, studies of youth–adult partnerships underscore the importance of giving youth the freedom to make decisions and power-sharing by adults in determining positive developmental outcomes [9]. This highlights the importance of working with adolescents and young adults to manage stressors associated with political action.

## 2 Current State

### 2.1 Benefits of Hybrid Civic and Political Participation

Online civic and political participation provides youth opportunities to exercise their voice, access and offer support, and organize around issues of injustice. Social media can enable youth to access sociopolitical education [10]. It also provides quick access to emerging news that influences social movement participation after events such as the murder of George Floyd [11]. Scholarship also suggests that social networking platforms can offer opportunities for exposure to de-radicalization processes [12]. Exposure to new information and perspectives has been found to enhance youths' critical consciousness, conceptualized as an understanding of structural inequities and one's positionality within such systems which provides them with the motivation and agency to engage in collective action [13].

Social networking sites also create opportunities for youth to engage in civic identity exploration with like-minded peers [14]. Youths have been found to demonstrate creativity in their political expression to initiate agency within the political process and provide their online peers with needed social-emotional support and distraction from sociopolitical distress [15]. Youth are also adept at engaging in narrative-based civic expression with the aim of intensifying sentiments around morality [16]. Developing a positive narrative around one's identity is a critical step in youth development [8]. Youth with historically marginalized identities often face harmful societal stereotypes. Therefore, they often must challenge and create new narratives that affirm and recognize the complexity of their own (and others') identities [10]. Social media provides one avenue for developing counter-narratives. For example, DREAMer (Development, Relief, and Education for Alien Minors) youth disseminated stories online to elevate their lived experiences, counteract anti-immigrant xenophobic rhetoric, and mobilize for community activism [17]. Artivism, a combination of art and activism, has also been used by LGBTQ+ youth as a tool for storytelling to inspire political change [18].

Online civic participation can also promote the development of communities that empower youth, especially marginalized and minoritized youth, by creating opportunities to foster civic identity formation [7]. These relationships may be particularly important for youth as this is a critical time period in social identity development [8]. For instance, the online engagement of Black women activists on college campuses provided critically affirming digital counterspace and helped them build a Black collegial community online. These youth tapped into the online community to both navigate and survive a hostile campus climate [19]. Such community-based connections can also offer vital information networks to seek support groups, and access advice and pertinent information [7]. Scholarship has found that such relational capital may be further bolstered by organizational and ad hoc locally based structures [20]. Such engagement has also been found to foster competencies in perspective taking [21], persuasive communication, and civic dissemination [22].

## 2.2 Risks and Challenges Associated with Youth Political Participation in a Hybrid World

As youth take on expanded rights and responsibilities to express their voices on societal issues, they grapple with some risks. Exposure to online hate speech is increasingly common, with the most frequent forms of hate speech focusing on race, sexuality and gender expression, religion, and immigration status, thus putting minoritized youth at greater risk [23]. Youth activists also report concerns about surveillance of online speech by adults, criminalization of dissent, and government use of digital tools (such as social media monitoring, data analytics, and facial recognition technology) to surveil protest activity [24]. While there is considerable attention to this type of risk in authoritarian regimes, studies of Black, LGBTQ+, Latine, and Muslim youth in the US also note they face similar concerns [24]. The risks of collective action are particularly pronounced for Muslim youth who are subject to religious discrimination and terrorism-related surveillance, which can lead to avoiding confrontation [5]. US-based studies of radicalization focus on how youth encounter and share hate speech, facilitated by the development of niche social network channels and the ease of spreading extremist content [25].

Navigating conflict and differences of opinion through dialogue is a hallmark of democratic participation. Not surprisingly, the majority of youth have encountered conflict between online users discussing political issues, and many find such conflict to be unproblematic as long as it falls short of personal attacks [26]. However, when asked about strategies for engaging in cross-cutting political conversations online, many report a lack of confidence in their capacity to navigate potential backlash or differences of opinion [27]. Another related set of challenges includes censorship (by government or school authorities) and self-censorship out of concern for how political speech might be perceived by future employers or cultural or academic gatekeepers [7, 24].

On the informational side, the challenges of misinformation and disinformation about political issues on social media are well-documented [28]. With the heightened awareness of the challenges in the information ecosystem, youth report fact-checking behaviors and preferences for social media posts that include evidence [29]. At the same time, many youths find it challenging to apply media literacy strategies to assess the credibility of information when consuming news through social media, especially news that is presented out of context or without clear indicators of the original source or credibility [28, 29]. The rapid advancement of generative artificial intelligence (AI) and deepfake technology presents additional challenges to information literacy practices [30].

## 2.3 Supportive Learning Environments for Hybrid Civic and Political Engagement

An emerging body of research has begun to focus on how to support the development of "civic media literacy" or the capacity to access, analyze, and communicate information for civic goals [29]. Several promising new strategies have emerged that build on adaptations of youth themselves—particularly young activists—and from media professionals. These strategies include:

- *Evaluating decontextualized news and information.* The decontextualized sharing of news in a social media feed alongside opinions and entertainment places additional burden on the user to analyze media for factual accuracy and political bias without the presence of pre-internet cues (author information, section of news as opinion/reporting, etc.) [28] Studies of youth strategies suggest a tendency to coordinate social information cues (likes, shares, comments) and identity cues (what they know about the political biases of the poster) from social media as part of an emerging approach to evaluating information [6]. A series of interventions under the umbrella of online civic reasoning have been developed to teach habits of questioning who is behind claims, lateral reading (checking additional sources) to determine whether claims are verified, and click restraint (developing a habit of waiting before clicking on salacious headlines) [28].
- *Teaching for curation.* As the majority of youth get at least some of their news through social media, the way they access news is through passive consumption (vs. effortful search) of frequently decontextualized posts shared by nonnews sources (friends, family, celebrities, or activist accounts) [29]. To manage such information, youth adaptations have included following reputable accounts and using endorsements (liking/hearting/sharing) to influence the algorithm to present certain types of news in the feed. Educators have begun to integrate attention to this strategy in civic media literacy interventions.
- *Practicing productive dialogue.* A common form of civic discourse on social media is topic-driven discourse, where users respond to emerging news stories without establishing an ongoing relationship between users. Such dialogue provides users with minimal opportunity to engage in productive exchanges of competing ideas and perspectives [31]. Youth who participate in sustained nonpolitical online communities to pursue hobbies or interests have demonstrated a more promising capacity to discuss political events productively [15]. Most recent educational interventions have focused on creating moderated online spaces where youth can engage with each other in a sustained fashion over time and providing tips on strategies to show active listening, encourage elaboration, and express disagreement in such settings [22, 26].
- *Civic storytelling and engaging an audience.* Using digital media to provide counter-narratives and tell their own stories is an area where young activists have innovated and excelled. Research has demonstrated the importance of media literacy interventions that explicitly teach online civic expression [32]. Thus, civic media interventions have learned from youth activist practices and are teaching youth to strategically identify audiences, craft narratives, and use internet-savvy strategies such as humor, design, and social engagement features on platforms (hashtags, stitches, duets, @ing) to engage audiences.

For such environments to be effective, it is important to tie the above elements together within a context of purposeful and socially rich learning environments where youth are using these strategies to accomplish civic goals. It is also important to recognize that youth are learning these practices in a context where political figures use dehumanizing rhetoric and propose policies that are harmful to minoritized youth. Engagement with political media (online or through broadcast) of this nature is inherently stressful. As such, it is important to craft trauma-informed, equity-minded approaches to teaching digital literacies within civic education [33].

## 3 Future Research

As technology and our understanding of *how* youth use hybrid tools and practices for civic and political engagement evolve, we see a few areas where future research can pick up from our current understanding to address pressing problems. Building the current knowledge base, a more systematic study of the impact of such engagement on youth well-being across intersectional identities. Within media literacy education, there is a need to build on the significant progress in identifying, testing, and evaluating educational strategies for evaluating and producing media, and to extend to additional work to teach habits of curation, circulation, and engaging in productive dialogue, particularly productive forms of disagreement and conflict. Finally, the rapid expansion of AI introduces new challenges in terms of evaluating information, and research on how such technology is being used for misinformation and radicalization as well as how youth themselves might be engaged in adaptive uses of AI is crucial.

## 4 Recommendations

### 4.1 For Parents

- One of the most consistent influences on youth civic engagement in the research is through parent modeling and socialization. Parents wishing to positively influence their children's capacity for informed, effective, and ethical civic engagement can and should engage their children in conversation about current issues, and importantly, as they relate to youth intersectional communities and identities [34–36].
- Talk to your children about what they are seeing online and the risks and benefits of online political expression. Resources like *Common Sense Media* translate research into Parent Tips and FAQs on a range of topics, including engagement with news, identity, and community [37].

### 4.2 For Educators

- Resist the urge to shy away from controversial issues in the classroom. This is easier said than done as legislators and parent activists seek to constrain content in K-12 classrooms. Furthermore, controversial conversations can feel risky. At the same time, young people *are* seeing controversial content and heated rhetoric through all media outlets, and they need opportunities to make sense of and discuss these things. Resources like *Facing History and Ourselves* provide practical, research-based curricular, and professional development resources for teachers to develop constructive approaches to controversy in the classroom [38].
- Integrate civic media literacy activities in the classroom with the social media practices that students will need outside of the classroom. Resources like the UC Irvine Civic Engagement Research Group's *Digital Civics Toolkit* provide example lessons and a professional community to innovate [39].
- Serve as allies to youth organizations that work outside of schools to address structural barriers to participation. Organizations like the *Philadelphia Student Union* provide effective models of youth leadership development and civic empowerment [40].

### 4.3 For Policymakers

- Recent efforts to regulate social media are necessary and important, particularly as they focus on transparency and accountability. Age restrictions and bans may be warranted at times, but in a context where social media and emerging technologies (most recently Generative AI) are in demand and integrated into our public life, more nuanced approaches to regulation are needed beyond bans. Regulations to encourage transparency around data use, algorithms, privacy, and content controls are necessary for parents, youth, and educators to understand the risks of online information-seeking, dialogue, and expression.
- One of the most challenging aspects of political life in the current climate is the tendency of political elites to use media to escalate tensions with extreme political rhetoric that dehumanizes people who disagree. As campuses grapple with issues of free speech and hate speech as well as concerns about escalations of protests into physical conflicts, they can play a critical role in fostering the capacity to engage in ways that encourage recognition of common humanity, for example via intergroup dialogue programs [41]. US Policymakers can also learn important lessons from the global community, where

organizations like UNESCO have long grappled with how to create educational opportunities that respond to a diversity of national, cultural, and political contexts, including areas impacted by political violence [42].

Across all areas of recommendation—parents, educators, and policymakers—it is critical to engage youth, listen to their experiences, consult with them, and give them opportunities to influence our public discussions around young people and social media.

**Conflict of Interest and Funding Disclosures** None.

## References


1. Cohen CJ, Kahne J. Participatory Politics. New Media and youth political action. Published online 2011. Accessed April 30, 2023. https://ictlogy.net/bibliography/reports/projects.php?idp=2180&lang=en
2. Crenshaw K. Demarginalizing the intersection of race and sex; a Black feminist critique of discrimination doctrine, feminist theory, and antiracist politics. Univ Chic Leg Forum. 1989;1:139–67.
3. Social policy for children and families. Sage Publications Inc. Published March 2, 2023. Accessed April 30, 2023. https://us.sagepub.com/en-us/nam/social-policy-for-children-and-families/book259364.
4. Vamvalis M. "We're fighting for our lives": centering affective, collective and systemic approaches to climate justice education as a youth mental health imperative. Res Educat. 2023:00345237231160090. https://doi.org/10.1177/00345237231160090. Published online March 3
5. Saleem M, Ramasubramanian S. Muslim Americans' responses to social identity threats: effects of Media representations and experiences of discrimination. Media Psychol. 2019;22(3):373–93. https://doi.org/10.1080/15213269.2017.1302345.
6. Yue A, Nekmat E, Beta AR. Digital literacy through digital citizenship: online civic participation and public opinion evaluation of youth minorities in Southeast Asia. MaC. 2019;7(2):100–14. https://doi.org/10.17645/mac.v7i2.1899.
7. Weinstein E, James C. Behind their screens: what teens are facing (and adults are missing). MIT Press; 2022.
8. Steinberg L. Adolescence. McGraw Hill; 2020.
9. Tivaringe T, Kirshner B. Learning to claim power in a contentious public sphere: a study of youth movement formation in South Africa. J Learn Sci. 2021;30(1):125–50. https://doi.org/10.1080/10508406.2020.1844713.
10. Sousa A, Ramasubramanian S. Challenging gender and racial stereotypes in online spaces. Alternative storytelling among Latino/a youth in the U.S. In: Nordicom Press; 2017. Accessed April 30, 2023. https://oaktrust.library.tamu.edu/handle/1969.1/188015.
11. Setter D, Nepstad SE. How social movements influence public opinion on political violence: attitude shifts in the wake of the George Floyd protests*. Mobilizat Int Quart. 2023;27(4):429–44. https://doi.org/10.17813/1086-671X-27-4-429.
12. Thorburn J. The (de-) radical (-ising) potential of r/IncelExit and r/ExRedPill. Eur J Cult Stud. 2023;26 https://doi.org/10.1177/13675494231153900.
13. Diemer MA, Pinedo A, Bañales J, et al. Recentering action in critical consciousness. Child Dev Perspect. 2021;15(1):12–7. https://doi.org/10.1111/cdep.12393.
14. Literat I, Kligler-Vilenchik N. Youth collective political expression on social media: the role of affordances and memetic dimensions for voicing political views. New Media Soc. 2019;21(9):1988–2009. https://doi.org/10.1177/1461444819837571.
15. Kligler-Vilenchik N, Literat I. Distributed creativity as political expression: youth responses to the 2016 U.S. presidential election in online affinity networks. J Commun. 2018;68(1):75–97. https://doi.org/10.1093/joc/jqx005.
16. Vea T. The ethical sensations of im-mediacy: embodiment and multiple literacies in animal rights activists' learning with media technologies. Br J Educ Technol. 2019;50(4):1589–602. https://doi.org/10.1111/bjet.12809.
17. Seif H. "We define ourselves": 1.5-generation undocumented immigrant activist identities and insurgent discourse. N Am Dialog. 2016;19(1):23–35. https://doi.org/10.1111/nad.12039.
18. Rhoades M. LGBTQ youth + video Artivism: arts-based critical civic praxis. Stud Art Educ. 2012;53(4):317–29. https://doi.org/10.1080/00393541.2012.11518872.
19. Race, Education and #BlackLivesMatter: how online transformational resistance shapes the offline experiences of Black College-age women – Tiera Tanksley, 2022. Accessed April 30, 2023. https://journals.sagepub.com/doi/full/10.1177/00420859221092970?casa_token=Rn7ugFbVRJ8AAAAA%3AItqr3VvnV1hIUdmgyYrU6uzIq_WZYptfTzeA2PxXZHo95-DeAJFmEjaBJ9V3r7bHy8kPDrSNdoE.
20. Yuen S, Tang G. Instagram and social capital: youth activism in a networked movement. Soc Mov Stud. 2021;22(5–6):706–827. https://doi.org/10.1080/14742837.2021.2011189.
21. Kornbluh ME. Building bridges: exploring the communication trends and perceived sociopolitical benefits of adolescents engaging in online social justice efforts. Youth Soc. 2019;51(8):1104–26. https://doi.org/10.1177/0044118X17723656.
22. Bell S, Kornbluh M. Networking in the digital age: identifying factors that influence adolescents' online

communication and relationship building. Appl Dev Sci. 2022;26(1):109–26. https://doi.org/10.1080/10888691.2019.1702042.
23. Costello M, Hawdon J. Hate speech in online spaces. In: The Palgrave handbook of international cybercrime and cyberdeviance. Springer; 2020. p. 1397–416.
24. Lee A. Hybrid activism under the radar: surveillance and resistance among marginalized youth activists in the United States and Canada. New Media Soc. 2022:14614448221105848. https://doi.org/10.1177/14614448221105847. Published online July 5
25. Turner N, Holt TJ, Brewer R, Cale J, Goldsmith A. Exploring the relationship between opportunity and self-control in youth exposure to and sharing of online hate content. Terror Polit Viol. 2022;35(7):1604–19. https://doi.org/10.1080/09546553.2022.2066526.
26. Middaugh E. More than just facts: promoting civic Media literacy in the era of outrage. Peabody J Educ. 2019;94(1):17–31. https://doi.org/10.1080/0161956X.2019.1553582.
27. Lee A. Breakdowns in mediated conversations: how and why youth exit cross-cutting political talk on social media. 2022. Accessed April 1, 2023. http://hdl.handle.net/10125/79728.
28. McGrew S, Breakstone J, Ortega T, Smith M, Wineburg S. Can students evaluate online sources? Learning from assessments of civic online reasoning. Theory Res Soc Educ. 2018;46(2):165–93. https://doi.org/10.1080/00933104.2017.1416320.
29. Middaugh E, Bell S, Kornbluh M. Think before you share: building a civic media literacy framework for everyday contexts. Information and Learning Sciences. 2022;123(7/8):421–44. https://doi.org/10.1108/ILS-03-2022-0030.
30. Shin SY, Lee J. The effect of Deepfake video on news credibility and corrective influence of cost-based knowledge about Deepfakes. Digit Journal. 2022;10(3):412–32. https://doi.org/10.1080/21670811.2022.2026797.
31. Kligler-Vilenchik N. Collective social correction: addressing misinformation through group practices of information verification on WhatsApp. Digit Journal. 2022;10(2):300–18. https://doi.org/10.1080/21670811.2021.1972020.
32. Jimenez C, Clark LS. BIPOC youth's TikTok and Instagram usage to create productive disruptions in the US. The Routledge handbook of Media education futures post-pandemic (pp. 488-498). Routledge.
33. Ramasubramanian S, Riewestahl E, Landmark S. The trauma-informed equity-minded asset-based model (TEAM): the six R's for social justice-oriented educators. Published online July 11, 2021. Accessed April 30, 2023. https://oaktrust.library.tamu.edu/handle/1969.1/194130.
34. Pinetta BJ, Blanco Martinez S, Cross FL, Rivas-Drake D. Inherently political? associations of parent ethnic–racial socialization and sociopolitical discussions with latinx youths' emergent civic engagement. Am J Community Psychol. 2020;66(1–2):94–105. https://doi.org/10.1002/ajcp.12435.
35. White ES. Parent values, civic participation, and children's volunteering. Child Youth Serv Rev. 2021;127:106115. https://doi.org/10.1016/j.childyouth.2021.106115.
36. Karras-Jean Gilles J, Astuto J, Niwa E, Ruck MD. Trajectories of civic socialization in context: examining variation among children in African American and Black immigrant families. Dev Psychol. 2020;56(12):2293–308. https://doi.org/10.1037/dev0001116.
37. Commonsense Media. Parenting, media, and everything in between. 2024. Accessed from https://www.commonsensemedia.org/articles.
38. Facing history and ourselves. Teaching Resources. 2024. Accessed from https://www.facinghistory.org/how-it-works/teaching-resources.
39. UC Irvine Civic Engagement Research Group. Digital Civics Toolkit (n.d.) Accessed from https://www.commonsensemedia.org/articles.
40. Philadelphia Student Union. (n.d.) About. Accessed from https://www.phillystudentunion.org/.
41. Nagda BA, Gurin P. Sorensen N & Zúñiga X Evaluating intergroup dialogue: engaging diversity for personal and social responsibility. Diver Democr. 2009;12(1):4–6.
42. UNESCO. Global citizenship and peace education. 2024. Accessed from: https://www.unesco.org/en/global-citizenship-peace-education.

# Part II

# Research on How Media Influence Relationships, Family, Culture, and Society

# Introduction to the Section on Race, Racism, and Digital Media

Rob Eschmann and Desmond Upton Patton

How does technology shape the lives of young people of color? This handbook provides a comprehensive set of answers to this question, with a critically reflexive focus on race, health, policy, cognition, education, gender, and more. Digital media and online technologies have a continuous effect on our daily lives, one that cannot simply be delineated between the digital and the physical. Jurgenson uses the term augmented reality to describe the ways our online and face-to-face realities overlap and coalesce [1].

The chapters in this section, *Race, Racism, and Digital Media*, investigate "the augmented reality of race and racism" [2] (p. 8) and its impact on youth. How does racism manifest online, and what effects does this have on young people, especially young people of color? Does technology contribute to, or challenge, racist structures or racial power dynamics? What types of technologies shape the ways youth experience and respond to race and racism?

People of color, young people, and youth of color are overrepresented in their use of nearly all social media platforms. While 97% of teens in the United States use the internet every day, around 55% of Black and Latinx teens use the internet "almost constantly," compared to just 37% of White teens [3]. Teens are more likely to use TikTok, Instagram, and Snapchat than are adults, and young adults (18–30) are more likely to use social media than are adults over 30 [3, 4]. As young people spend increasingly more time online, it is imperative that we understand the risks and rewards that are associated with different online behaviors and contexts.

For example, racism online—which is often more explicit and open than racism in most face-to-face settings—has forced many scholars and people of color to rethink how we understand racism [5–7]. Subtle forms of racism, like microaggressions, are more common than overt racism in most in-person, mainstream settings [8, 9]. Yet openly hateful rhetoric is much more prevalent in a variety of online contexts, from video games to anonymous comments on YouTube and other web pages [10]. The ubiquity of online racism is a fact of life, one that contrasts sharply with the friendly racial performances and subtle expressions of racism that characterize most mainstream spaces. What impact might this more explicit online racism have on youth wellbeing?

At the same time, social media has hosted some of the most noteworthy organizing efforts around issues of racial justice in past years, including the most used hashtag ever — #BlackLivesMatter — which is the name of a

R. Eschmann (✉)
Columbia University, School of Social Work, New York, NY, USA
e-mail: r.eschmann@columbia.edu

D. U. Patton
University of Pennsylvania, School of Social Policy and Practice, Annenberg School for Communication, Philadelphia, PA, USA


D. A. Christakis, L. Hale (eds.), *Handbook of Children and Screens*,
https://doi.org/10.1007/978-3-031-69362-5_36

singular organization, but has been used to demonstrate support of the broader Movement for Black Lives and the fight against anti-Black police violence [11]. Black Twitter is emblematic of biting social critiques of systems of oppression, including racism, sexism, homophobia, and the application of intersectional theory to everyday life [12]. Black feminists and Black women have been central to the development of counterpublics on social media that enable the dissemination of critical ideas around race [13]. Through social media and online technologies, resistance has taken new forms, and counter-narratives have been shared with viral effectiveness [14].

Technology is central to our understanding of the realities of race and racism in the twenty-first century. Concurrently, as the chapters in this section demonstrate, race and racism are central to the development of new digital technologies, online cultures, and online interactions.

## 1 In This Section

The section begins with an exploration of big-picture issues, including data and privacy, decisions being made by big tech that privilege capitalist interests over child wellbeing, and how the design and implementation of online technology shape the ways youth of color experience race and racism online. In their chapter entitled, "Structural Racism in Tech: Social Media Platforms, Algorithmic Bias, and Racist Tech," authors Safiya Noble, Sarah T. Roberts, Matt Bui, André Brock, and Olivia Snow (see chapter "Structural Racism in Tech: Social Media Platforms, Algorithmic Bias, and Racist Tech") discuss the ways racism is inherent in the structure of the internet. They insist we change the ways we regulate big tech and reevaluate the ways we build new technologies, including artificial intelligence (AI). The issues highlighted in this chapter provide context for all other chapters in this section.

The second chapter in the section is entitled "Is Social Media Increasing Risk for Mental Health Problems among Youth? It's Complicated." In this chapter, authors Ran Barzilay, David Pagliaccio, Carter J. Funkhouser, and Randy P. Auerbach (see chapter "Is Social Media Increasing Risk for Mental Health Problems Among Youth?: It's Complicated") discuss and evaluate the popular notion that increased time on the internet is associated with worse mental health outcomes for youth. In this very important investigation, the authors find that there is no causal link between time on social media and adolescent mental health. They suggest the literature is currently overly reliant on cross-sectional data and doesn't account for offline factors (including lack of access to health care and mental health care professionals) that can shape health outcomes. While there are risk factors associated with increased time online, including increased exposure to racism or discrimination (which is negatively associated with mental health for youth of color and LGBTQ+ youth, something that is explored more in the next chapter by Tynes and colleagues), there may also be increased access to community and support online. This should add complexity to the narrative that social media increases risk, as social media can be an important resource, especially for minoritized or marginalized youth.

The third chapter in this section comes from Brendesha M. Tynes, Henry A. Willis, Ashley Maxie-Moreman, Stephanie M. Ortiz, and Devin English (see chapter "Online Racism and Its Impact on Children, Adolescents, and Emerging Adults of Color"), as they present evidence detailing the ways exposure to online racism can have negative impacts on young adults. This chapter, "Online Racism and Its Impact on Children, Adolescents, and Emerging Adults of Color," reviews qualitative, quantitative, and big data research on the negative health effects of online experiences with discrimination. They note that Black and Latinx youth are more likely to be victims of cyberbullying than other racial groups. Since the pandemic, Black and Asian groups have seen increases in cyberbullying, with the highest increases among Asians, who were the least bullied before the pandemic. In one study they cite, Black people were found to experience racial discrimination more than five times each day, with most incidents taking place online

[15]. This important piece maps the dangers of online exposure to racism and details strategies for future research.

One example of an online setting that can expose youth to virulence and racism is online video game platforms. In "Racial Harms in Digital Gaming," Kishonna L. Gray, Tara McPherson, Gillian Russell, and Rachel Anderson (see chapter "Video Games and Race") write an engaging and informative discussion of racism in online gaming settings. Not only do the authors explore the ways communities of color are affected, but they also investigate the dangers for White youth online, as White supremacist groups have appropriated some online gaming spaces as recruiting and training grounds for racist ideologies. The authors suggest ways gaming platforms can be a part of the solution, creating real consequences for online racism, and "disrupting the alt-right pipeline." One such recommendation is that marginalized voices be included in video game design, something that overlaps with the next chapter.

A critical analysis of the child welfare system suggests it has been "designed to detect and punish the neglect on the part of poor parents and to ignore most middle-class failings (page 33)," something that has led many social workers, activists, and scholars to pursue child welfare abolition or a reframing: from mandated reporters to mandated supporters [16] (p. 33).

In their chapter, "Participation of Marginalized Youth in Designing a Machine Learning-based Model to Identify Child Abuse and Neglect," authors Aviv Y. Landau, Hannah Espeleta, Siva Mathiyazhagan, Ashley Blanchard, Paul Heider, Kenrick Cato, Rochelle F. Hanson, Desmond U. Patton, Leslie Lenient, and Maximum Tops (see chapter "Participation of Marginalized Youth in Designing a Machine Learning–Based Model to Identify Child Abuse and Neglect") discuss the racist and classist nature of child welfare policies, and the possible ways utilizing technology could reduce the bias inherent in child welfare policies that determine whether children should be removed from their homes.

The authors discuss trends in researchers taking advantage of the widespread use of electronic health records to develop machine learning models that can identify disorders, sicknesses, or risk factors faster and more effectively than more traditional methods. While one application of this technology is to identify potential child abuse and neglect, it is inevitable that those machine learning models reflect the same racist and classist biases inherent in child welfare policies and procedures. As a remedy, this chapter explores the participation of marginalized youth in the training of machine learning models, in order to limit the reproduction of dominant and biased understandings of child welfare and to introduce community-based and stakeholder understandings of child welfare into these new ways of using technology to identify risk. This process is reminiscent of Noble and colleagues' call in the first chapter of the section to include marginalized groups in decision-making in order to challenge and change racist structures.

In their chapter, "Radical and Untethered: Exploring the Health Benefits of Imagination in Virtual Reality for Black Youth," authors Courtney Cogburn, Valerie Taylor, Prema Fillipone, and Oyewole Oyekoya (see chapter "Radical and Untethered: The Health Benefits of Imagination in Virtual Reality for Black Youth") discuss emerging virtual reality (VR) technology and its affordances to doing antiracist work. They discuss the potential utility of embodiment in VR for social change, as users put on a headset and physically become someone else in immersive experiences. Then, they explore the power of imagination work, as Black youth use VR technologies to envision and explore new realities. This chapter expands our understanding of how innovative technologies can change the fundamental ways young people experience and understand the world.

The final chapter in the section is entitled "Online Resistance: The Past, Present, and Future of Challenging Racism with Digital Tools." Authors Rob Eschmann, Nkemka Anyiwo, Noor Toraif, and Stephanie M. Ortiz (see chapter "Online Resistance: The Past, Present, and Future of Challenging Racism with Digital Tools") explore the ways young people and activists use technology to challenge and resist racism at multiple levels, from structural to interpersonal, from clapping back to radical self-care. This chapter investigates organizing, activism, and the ways young people use online tools to get engaged in collective action. They also explore online support spaces where young people of color create affirming communities that challenge dominant narratives and provide a respite from oppressive racist norms. Lastly, they highlight research that documents the ways young people of color use technology to critique everyday racism, a practice that is less common offline.

## 2 Future Research and Recommendations

We began our journey of studying race, digital media, and youth wellbeing together in 2013 when we wrote our first conceptual chapter on the connection between social media use, youth, and violence in Chicago [17]. We followed this chapter up with an empirical study in 2014, investigating how Black and Latinx youth used social media to navigate high-violence neighborhoods, and the ways violence prevention workers used technology to bolster their interventions [18, 19]. Since these initial studies, we have both been concerned with understanding how technology shapes the risks faced by youth and their strategies for resilience in various contexts.

More than a decade later, we are grateful to be able to work with this esteemed group of scholars, many of whom have shaped our own understanding of the linkages between digital technologies, youth, and wellbeing and have pushed the field forward, innovating and creating a body of research that informs the ways we understand youth wellbeing online.

The work in this section provides a roadmap for the future of this work, highlighting the issues that plague research and practice, and outlining strategies for navigating the rapidly changing online landscape, where capitalist concerns are so often elevated over the needs of the most vulnerable in society, including children, and especially marginalized youth, including children of color, poor children, queer children, or children with disabilities. With these chapters as a guide, we have established a justice-oriented agenda that should drive future research, organizing, and educational efforts.

**Conflict of Interest and Funding Disclosures** None.

## References


1. Jurgensen N. Digital dualism versus augmented reality. Cyborgology, Published February 24, 2011. Accessed January 11, 2022. https://thesocietypages.org/cyborgology/2011/02/24/digital-dualism-versus-augmented-reality/.
2. Eschmann R. When the Hood comes off: racism and resistance in the digital age. University of California Press; 2023.
3. Vogels EA, Gelles-Watnick R, Massarat N. Teens, Social media and technology 2022. Pew Research Center: Internet, Science & Tech. Published August 10, 2022. Accessed May 1, 2023. https://www.pewresearch.org/internet/2022/08/10/teens-social-media-and-technology-2022/.
4. Auxier B, Anderson M. Social Media Use in 2021. Pew Research Center: Internet, Science & Tech. Published April 7, 2021. Accessed June 5, 2022. https://www.pewresearch.org/internet/2021/04/07/social-media-use-in-2021/.
5. Daniels J. Race and racism in internet studies: a review and critique. New Media Soc. 2013;15(5):695–719.
6. Daniels J. Cloaked websites: propaganda, cyber-racism and epistemology in the digital era. New Media Soc. 2009;11(5):659–83. https://doi.org/10.1177/1461444809105345.
7. Eschmann R. Unmasking racism: students of color and expressions of racism in online spaces. Soc Probl. 2020;67:418–36. https://doi.org/10.1093/socpro/spz026.
8. Bonilla-Silva E. Racism without racists: color-blind racism and the persistence of racial inequality in America. 6th ed. Rowman & Littlefield Publishers; 2021.
9. Sue DW. Microaggressions in everyday life: race, gender, and sexual orientation. Wiley; 2010.
10. Hughey MW, Daniels J. Racist comments at online news sites: a methodological dilemma for discourse analysis. Media Cult Soc. 2013;35(3):332–47. https://doi.org/10.1177/0163443712472089.
11. Anderson M. History of the hashtag #BlackLivesMatter: social activism on twitter. Pew Research Center: Internet, Science & Tech. Published August 15, 2016. Accessed April 8, 2021. https://www.pewresearch.org/internet/2016/08/15/the-hashtag-blacklivesmatter-emerges-social-activism-on-twitter/.

12. Hill ML. "Thank you, black twitter": state violence, digital Counterpublics, and pedagogies of resistance. Urban Educ. 2018;53(2):286–302. https://doi.org/10.1177/0042085917747124.
13. Jackson SJ, Bailey M, Welles BF. #Hashtag Activism: networks of race and gender justice. MIT Press; 2020.
14. Williams A. Black memes matter: #LivingWhileBlack with Becky and Karen. Soc Media Soc. 2020; 6(4):2056305120981047. https://doi.org/10.1177/2056305120981047.
15. English D, Lambert SF, Tynes BM, Bowleg L, Zea MC, Howard LC Daily multidimensional racial discrimination among Black US American adolescents. J Appl Dev Psychol. 2020;66:101068.
16. Roberts D. Shattered bonds: the color of child welfare. New York: Civitas Books.
17. Patton DU, Eschmann RD, Butler DA. Internet banging: new trends in social media, gang violence, masculinity and hip hop. Comput Hum Behav. 2013;29(5):A54–9. https://doi.org/10.1016/j.chb.2012.12.035.
18. Patton DU, Leonard P, Elaesser C, Eschmann RD, Patel S, Crosby S. What's a threat on social media? How Black and Latino Chicago young men define and navigate threats online. Youth Soc. 2019;51(6):756–72. https://doi.org/10.1177/0044118X17720325.
19. Patton DU, Eschmann RD, Elsaesser C, Bocanegra E. Sticks, stones and Facebook accounts: what violence outreach workers know about social media and urban-based gang violence in Chicago. Comput Hum Behav. 2016;65:591–600. https://doi.org/10.1016/j.chb.2016.05.052.

# Structural Racism in Tech: Social Media Platforms, Algorithmic Bias, and Racist Tech

Safiya U. Noble, Sarah T. Roberts, Matthew Bui, André Brock, and Olivia Snow

## 1 Background

A number of key research studies have been published over the last decade documenting the harmful effects of racist technologies, which include ways that algorithms are racially biased and produce harmful effects [1–4]. Scholars have also written critically about the broad landscape of algorithmic fairness and its limitations, which does not sufficiently account for structural racism and harm [5], and the ways in which racially discriminatory algorithms are used by the tech industry writ large without regulation or oversight. Beyond social media and advertising-led search companies, there are a number of scholars, journalists, and activists who have well documented the use of racist technologies that are often pointed at or exploitative of vulnerable and racialized communities, including children: predictive policing, facial recognition software [6], and racism embedded in emergent large language models and generative AI [7].

S. U. Noble (✉) · S. T. Roberts · O. Snow
University of California, Los Angeles, CA, USA
e-mail: snoble@ucla.edu

M. Bui
University of Michigan, Ann Arbor, MI, USA

A. Brock
Georgia Tech, Atlanta, GA, USA

## 2 Current State

### 2.1 Algorithmic Bias and Racist Tech

For more than 30 years, scholars have raised questions and documented concerns about the harms of digital tech, particularly with respect to racism, beginning in the early 1990s. Key scholars include Oscar Gandy Jr.'s [8] work on the racist, panoptic sorting of people online, Alondra Nelson, et al.'s [9] engagements with race, tech, and everyday life, Lisa Nakamura's Cybertypes [10], which signaled the perils of racial and ethnic profiling online, Wendy H.K. Chun's [11] argument that networked contact is experienced and negotiated through both sexuality and race, Anna Everrett's [12] counter-narrative of the contributions of African Americans to tech and what was lost by their erasures, Jessie Daniels' [13] chilling reminders of the origins of the web for organized racism, André Brock's [14, 15], research on resistance to racist tech, Safiya Umoja Noble's work on racism in search engines [16], the racial politics of technology as written by Rayvon Fouche [17], Simone Browne's [18] well-documented history of racist surveillance tech, Ruha Benjamin's [3] accounting of racist technologies, and Kishonna Gray and David Leonard's [19] volume on challenging racial oppression and video gaming, including its effects on children.


D. A. Christakis, L. Hale (eds.), *Handbook of Children and Screens*,
https://doi.org/10.1007/978-3-031-69362-5_37

Internet and digital media scholars have produced significant scholarship about the effects of social media on society, too, including the ways in which technologies can undermine the health and safety of vulnerable communities [20], how algorithms can reinforce harmful stereotypes and oppress people through racist search results that misrepresent Black girls and girls of color more broadly [2], how content moderation practices reproduce racism at a structural level across social media platforms, to which children are expressly exposed and harmed [20, 21], how social media practices are a threat to democracy and social welfare with no oversight or protections for the public and vulnerable people [22], and for 20 years, research has addressed racist narratives embedded in video games targeting young people, which reproduce dangerous and violent ideas about Black communities [23].

## 2.2 A History of Harmful Tech

Since the advent of the internet, there have been long-standing concerns about children's access to harmful content online, in addition to the myriad racist narratives they are exposed to in video games like Grand Theft Auto, on websites and on bulletin board systems, in early social networking sites like MySpace and more recently in web 2.0 social media sites like Facebook and Twitter, in web directories and search engines like Google, and in recommendation systems like YouTube. In the 1990s, debates ensued about whether libraries and schools should have filters on computers to ensure children's protection from harmful content, often to the exclusion of important health, medical, or educational materials [24]. In the more recent debates, the United States—the epicenter of global social media companies—has lagged behind the European Union and the United Kingdom in legislating around known harmful material that includes cyberbullying. Black youth are over-exposed to traumatic events online and persistent racial discrimination on the internet [25]. Black young people are also more likely to self-report post-traumatic stress disorder associated with their experiences of witnessing racism and the racial battle fatigue they experience due to algorithmic sorting mechanisms that expose them to harmful content [26]. Tynes, to date, has done the most extensive and systematic study of youth of color online and their experiences with racism. Meanwhile, Black people, and Black youth, in particular, are consistently saddled by myths predicated on discourses of technological deficiency, lack of access to tech, and invisibility as potential audiences for tech [27, 28], none of which bears resemblance to reality or lived experiences of Black people.

## 2.3 Regulating Children's Safety Online

Recent policy discussions illustrate the persistent and growing concern for children's safety and calls for digital media and internet regulation. For example, in 2021, Facebook came under fire again for its predatory targeted advertising model: mainly, internal research documents showed plans for expanding its user base by building products for children as young as six years old [29]. Coupled with general concerns about online marketing and design features, and exposure to harmful or "unhealthy" content, online business practices have come under greater scrutiny in bill proposals such as The Kids Internet Design and Safety (KIDS) Act (2021)—an attempt to reintroduce protections for children online, and to curb the reach and expansion of predatory targeted ad tactics, among other online issues. Similarly, the bipartisan but more controversial Kids Online Safety Act (KOSA, 2023) and Filter Bubble Transparency Act (2021) seek to address Congressional agreement around the need for tech regulation by pushing for increased privacy protections for children under 16 and greater algorithmic transparency about recommendation systems, including stronger content moderation practices and enforcement, respectively.

Although both the Democratic and Republican parties have signaled interest in Big Tech regulation in the United States, particularly over concerns about child safety, their bipartisan efforts have been hampered by their lack of agreement regarding appropriate strategies and tactics for such regulation. For one, there were concerns that the KIDS Act (2021) would enable greater data collection and impose additional surveillance on youth, especially LGBTQ+ youth.

Coupled with extant pushes for banning educational materials pertaining to issues of race, gender, and sexuality in Republican-led states such as Florida's Stop WOKE (Stop Wrongs to Our Kids and Employees) Act (2022), the chasm between the two major political parties in the United States seems to be even farther apart, making it much more difficult for bipartisan cooperation on regulating harmful content without immense compromises by either party. Anti-pornography laws and policies have blocked access to sex education and reproductive health information on social media [30]. Explicit legislation banning the ability to teach or discuss contemporary and historical structural racism (e.g. anti-critical race theory bills) in the U.S. further undermines the ability to keep Black, Indigenous, and other children of color at the forefront of conversations about racist or harmful technology. Nonetheless, in early 2023, Senate Majority Leader Chuck Schumer and President Joe Biden signaled that online protections for children are a high priority and supported the introduction of several regulatory bills on the topic that attest to this. While children have been at the heart of many of the important debates over online content moderation and algorithmic safety, civil, human, and privacy organizations have argued that these protections need to be extended to the public, regardless of age. This lack of protections presents general harms and risks to all children but is particularly harmful to Black, Indigenous, and other children of color.

## 2.4 Social Media Platforms

Meanwhile, even if social media platforms have lacked trust and safety measures from their inception [31], the industry continues to abdicate its responsibility to the public, in general, and to its most vulnerable members; among them, children. In a recent alarming trend, many of the major tech companies whose platforms and products lead the market worldwide have slashed positions, rolled back policies, and abandoned internal company business practices that addressed product trust and safety to protect users, due to a lack of pressure or accountability. This trend can be most dramatically traced to Elon Musk's takeover of Twitter and his subsequent dismantling of key groups and initiatives dedicated to ensuring user protections, such as the Twitter Trust & Safety, Health, Human Rights, Election Integrity, Equity Diversity and Inclusion (EDI), Machine Learning Ethics, Responsibility and Accountability (META) teams, all of which were concerned with eradicating racial bias in Twitter's products [32] and creating and enforcing policies that protected users based on their racial and/or ethnic identity. Under his direction, the company also slashed significant numbers of frontline content moderators already struggling under the Sisyphean burden of its mandate to remove racially abusive, violent, and threatening material, and a study in the immediate aftermath of the takeover found a massive increase in racist and antisemitic abuse [33].

Rather than decry these moves, other firms decided that the fallout Musk received was still less than the potential financial incentive for doing away with its own similar internal watchdogs. Soon, Meta, Microsoft, and Google began slashing their own personnel concerned with user welfare and social impact, including many of its own teams concerned with racial equity in products and policies. These firings and layoffs were largely dressed in cost-saving measures. Taken together, these moves demonstrate that whatever social contract the public may imagine it holds with social media platforms and the companies behind them, any implied commitment can vanish in the blink of an eye whenever the profit motive rears its head. Rather than improve upon their products and social media environments to safeguard them for the most vulnerable users, the companies have gone the other way entirely. We do not rely on the goodwill of other industry titans to ensure the safety of our children when consuming their products or making use of their services, and yet social media, specifically, and Big Tech, across the board, has been left to its own devices as far as whether or not it has any antiracist commitments and whether or not they have the means or the will to enforce them. Their products and practices, in fact, are part of the structural racism we experience online and off.

## 3 Future Research

We believe the most pressing research questions about internet regulation and children should focus on issues at the intersection of structural racism and exploitation of Black, Indigenous, and communities of color in the U.S. and Europe, and in countries of the global majority, given that these countries face persistent long-term harm from histories of occupation and colonization, and are the new frontiers for racist technology experimentation. Recent reports on the use of Kenyan workers labeling datasets used for generative [34], for example, demonstrate concerns about the escalation of ungovernable technologies around the world. Children are a difficult population to study, and privacy-focused legislation in the United States and Europe will either help or hinder the ability to effectively study the harms of digital technologies on children and intervene as advocates on behalf of them, and the public more broadly.

## 4 Recommendations

Based on the aforementioned analyses, we offer the following recommendations, separated by four distinct groups whom we identified as keenly interested and poised to act on these issues:

- First, *researchers* must elevate and make visible specific harms to children and young people from major, well-known technology firms, as well as how less well-understood technologies are deployed across education, housing, immigration, employment, health, and all aspects of decision-making that affect children's quality of life, including the lives of their parents, guardians, and caretakers. As the footprint of digital technologies expands into almost every aspect of young people's lives, its presence becomes all the more commonplace and, thus, unquestioned. These issues include cyberbullying and harassment as youth engage online—which open up questions about the role of educational institutions—but also issues pertaining to other spheres of children's lives, such as surveillance, invasive data collection practices, and children's rights (e.g., to be forgotten or deleted, mentioned later).
- Relatedly, we call on all *youth advocates* to continue to demand whether technologies of surveillance and control are in the service of youth, or at odds with their best interests, based on this research. Such advocates include parents and guardians but also educators and other individuals and groups that interface with children.
- Considering this, *policymakers* must legislate to protect the data that is collected on children, particularly as it's used to analyze and predict the possibilities for their futures. The European Union provides its citizens with the "right to be forgotten" or "right to deletion" to have their data and information removed from the internet and other digital services. This is an especially important right for those who have grown up digital and may wish, later in life, to redact their own online traces. No such law exists in the United States. Educators using data surveillance-based educational technologies that collect and analyze information about children are sorely under-studied and can have a profound impact on the futures of children and their perceived capabilities for success.
- Importantly, *technology providers* in medical and clinical settings, and *mental health and other professionals* are increasingly adopting technologies that collect troves of data on children, and that use predictive algorithms to

forecast all sorts of medical coverage, health diagnoses, treatment plans, and wellness opportunities that can affect children's quality of life and have long-term negative impacts.

In summary, we are at the beginning of understanding the consequences of technology as a facilitator and tool of structural racism, such as when it predicts success or failure in a variety of contexts that affect children and young people around the world. We believe that racist technologies, writ large, will be among the most pressing human, civil, environmental, and sovereign rights issues of the twenty-first century.

**Conflict of Interest and Funding Disclosures** None.

## References


1. Broussard M. Artificial unintelligence: how computers misunderstand the world. MIT Press; 2018.
2. Noble SU. Algorithms of oppression: how search engines reinforce racism. New York University Press; 2018.
3. Benjamin R. Race after technology: abolitionist tools for the new Jim code. Polity; 2019.
4. Eubanks V. Automating inequality: how high-tech tools profile police and punish the poor (First Picador edition. Paperback). Picador St. Martin's Press; 2019.
5. Bui M, Noble S. In: Dubber MD, et al., editors. Oxford handbook of ethics of AI. Oxford University Press, Incorporated, ProQuest Ebook Central; 2020.
6. Buolamwini J, Gebru T. Gender shades: Intersectional accuracy disparities in commercial gender classification. In Conference on fairness, accountability, and transparency; January 2018: 77–91. PMLR.
7. Bender EM, Gebru T, McMillan-Major A, Mitchell S. On the dangers of stochastic parrots: Can language models be too big? In Proceedings of the 2021 ACM conference on fairness, accountability, and transparency; March 2021:610–623.
8. Gandy OH Jr. Chapter 7: coming to terms with the panoptic sort. In: Lyon D, Zureik E, editors. Computers, surveillance, and privacy. University of Minnesota Press; 1996. p. 132.
9. Nelson A, Tu TLN, Hines AH. Technicolor: race technology and everyday life. New York University Press; 2001.
10. Nakamura L. Cybertypes: race, Ethnicity and Identity on the Internet. Routledge; 2002.
11. Chun WHK. Control and freedom: power and paranoia in the age of fiber optics. MIT Press; 2008.
12. Everett A. Digital diaspora: a race for cyberspace. SUNY Press; 2009.
13. Daniels J. Cyber racism: white supremacy online and the new attack on civil rights. Rowman & Littlefield Publishers; 2009.
14. Brock A. From the blackhand side: twitter as a cultural conversation. J Broadcast Electron Media. 2012;56(4):529–49.
15. Brock A Jr. Distributed blackness: African American Cybercultures. New York University Press; 2020.
16. Noble S. Searching for black girls: old traditions in new media (dissertation). University of Illinois at Urbana-Champaign; 2012.
17. Fouché R. From black inventors to one laptop per child: exporting a racial politics of technology. In: Nakamura L, Chow-White P, editors. Race after the internet. Routledge; 2013. p. 61–83.
18. Browne S. Dark matters: On the surveillance of blackness. Duke University Press; 2015.
19. Gray KL, Leonard DJ. Woke gaming: digital challenges to social injustice. University of Washington Press; 2018.
20. Roberts ST. Commercial content moderation: digital laborers' dirty work. In: Noble SU, Tynes B, editors. The intersectional internet: race, sex, class and culture online. Peter Lang Publishing; 2016.
21. Roberts ST. Behind the screen: content moderation in the shadows of social media. Yale University Press; 2019.
22. Vaidhyanathan S. Antisocial media: how Facebook disconnects us and undermines democracy. Oxford University Press; 2018.
23. Leonard D. Live in your world, play in ours: race, video games, and consuming the other. Stud Media Inf Lit Educ. 2003;3(4):1–9.
24. Kranich N. Why filters won't protect children or adults. Libr Adm Manag. 2004;18(1):14–8.
25. Maxie-Morema AD, Tynes BM. Exposure to online racial discrimination and traumatic events online in black adolescents and emerging adults. J Res Adolesc. 2022;32:254–69.
26. Tanksley TC. Race, education and# BlackLivesMatter: how social media activism shapes the educational experiences of black college-age women. Los Angeles: University of California; 2019.
27. Brock A. Critical technocultural discourse analysis. New Media Soc. 2018;20(3):1012–30.
28. Evans-Winters VE. Black feminism in qualitative inquiry: a mosaic for writing our daughter's body. 1st ed. Routledge; 2019.
29. Kaplan K. Documents reveal Facebook targeted children as young as 6 for consumer base. NBCnewscom 2021. URL last accessed on 4/26/2023: https://www.nbcnews.com/tech/social-media/facebook-documents-reveal-company-targeted-children-young-6-rcna4021.
30. Tildenberg E, van der Nagel K. Sex and social media. 1st ed. Emerald Group Publishing; 2020.
31. Knittel M, Menking A. Bridging theory & practice: examining the state of scholarship using the history of

trust and safety archive. J Online Trust Saf. 2024;2(2) https://doi.org/10.54501/jots.v2i2.173.
32. Chowdhury R. Sharing learnings about our image cropping algorithm. Twitter Engineering; 2021. URL last accessed on 4/26/2023 at https://blog.twitter.com/engineering/en_us/topics/insights/2021/sharing-learnings-about-our-image-cropping-algorithm.
33. Study finds hate speech on Twitter increased quickly after Elon Musk takeover. Press Room – Montclair State University; October 31, 2022. https://www.montclair.edu/newscenter/2022/10/31/study-finds-hate-speech-on-twitter-increased-following-elon-musk-takeover/.
34. Perrigo B. OpenAI used Kenyan workers on less than $2 per hour: exclusive. Time, January 18, 2023. https://time.com/6247678/openai-chatgpt-kenya-workers/.

# Is Social Media Increasing Risk for Mental Health Problems Among Youth?: It's Complicated

Ran Barzilay, David Pagliaccio,
Carter J. Funkhouser, and Randy P. Auerbach

## 1 Background

In recent decades, social media platforms have been proliferating [1], and they are nearly ubiquitous in adolescents' lives. Broadly, social media encapsulates digital platforms that facilitate social interaction. Typically, this involves generating user-developed profiles, posting text, photos, and videos, and interacting with other users [2]. Recent reports imply a *causal* association between social media use and the rise in mental health problems among adolescents in the United States [3]. Yet, causal interpretations are premature at best and dangerous at worst. Although social media can be a haven for misinformation, online victimization, and toxic portrayals of body image, it is reckless to lay blame at the hands of social media writ large without accounting for the potential benefits of social media as well as the broader societal failures to support adolescent mental health, particularly among marginalized youth (e.g., based on race, ethnicity, sexual preference, gender identity).

One challenge in attributing blame to social media is that the boundaries that define social media are constantly changing. Concerns about social media overlap with more general worries about the negative effects of *screen time*—the broader cumulative time spent in front of screens (e.g., smartphone, computer, TV, video games) [3, 4]. Complicating matters, many people use social media platforms for a variety of purposes, including direct one-on-one communication (e.g., Facebook Messenger), often in place of text messaging or email. Social media use also encompasses both passive (e.g., scrolling through online content) and active approaches (e.g., messaging, commenting, or postings), which may relate to different mental health trajectories [5]. There also are potentially varying associations with mental health based on interactions within public versus private spaces (e.g., posting on one's public Instagram account versus direct messaging on Instagram) as well as interacting with friends versus strangers. Taken together, social media use does not reflect monolithic behavior, and thus, directly testing impacts on adolescent mental health requires a more thorough understanding of *who* is engaging and how youth are engaging with these platforms.

R. Barzilay (✉)
Department of Psychiatry, University of Pennsylvania, Philadelphia, PA, USA

Department of Child and Adolescent Psychiatry and Behavioral Science, Children's Hospital of Philadelphia, Philadelphia, PA, USA

Lifespan Brain Institute of CHOP and Penn Medicine, Philadelphia, PA, USA
e-mail: ran.barzilay@pennmedicine.upenn.edu

D. Pagliaccio · C. J. Funkhouser · R. P. Auerbach
Department of Psychiatry, Columbia University, New York, NY, USA

Division of Child and Adolescent Psychiatry, New York State Psychiatric Institute, New York, NY, USA


D. A. Christakis, L. Hale (eds.), *Handbook of Children and Screens*,
https://doi.org/10.1007/978-3-031-69362-5_38

# 2 Current State

## 2.1 Social Media and Adolescent Mental Health

Despite widespread concerns about the potential harms of social media, research examining its impact on mental health is inconclusive. Meta-analyses and large-scale studies suggest social media use and screen time are cross-sectionally associated with worse mental health problems (e.g., depressive symptoms) [6, 7]. These associations are generally weak but are stronger for those who make more social comparisons [8] or use social media excessively [9]. Longitudinal studies examining the directionality of this effect have provided mixed findings. Social media use is associated with increased risk for future mental health problems in some studies [10], but unrelated to future mental health problems in others [11]. Research examining within-person associations at shorter time scales (e.g., hours) suggests that social media use is typically unrelated to momentary or daily mental health [12, 13]. Short-term effects of social media use may vary across individuals [13], however, this highlights the need for a more nuanced understanding of social media use in relation to mental health.

At the same time, it is well understood that greater social media use increases the risk of harassment as well as exposure to hate speech and misinformation, which negatively affects youth mental health [14]. Conversely, social media also can help youth build meaningful connections and can be empowering to share their voices and ideas with a wider audience. Particularly for marginalized youth, social media offers opportunities for emotional support, community building, and self-expression beyond their in-person communities [15]. Taken together, it is essential to better understand *how* adolescents engage with social media, especially disentangling positive from negative exposures, to identify those with increased susceptibility to negative social media exposure and inform the development of targeted strategies that promote well-being and reduce adverse mental health outcomes.

## 2.2 Social Media and Marginalized Youth

Societal marginalization can contribute to a disproportionate mental health burden (e.g., via discrimination, exclusion, and difficulty accessing services). This can include a wide range of experiences faced by youth of color, LGBTQIA+ youth, those of lower socioeconomic status, youth with disabilities, immigrants, and other populations. For example, compared to White and heterosexual youth, youth of color and sexual and gender minority adolescents exhibit higher suicide attempt rates, respectively [16]. This again may implicate many diverse experiences, including overt racism and homophobia. There are also sociodemographic differences in social media engagement, as nearly half of Black and Hispanic adolescents report being online "almost constantly" compared to about one-third of White youth [1]. Notwithstanding, the *direction* of the association between increased social media use and mental health burden among different marginalized youth remains unclear. Further, it is critical to consider social determinants influencing both social media use and adverse mental health outcomes among marginalized youth (e.g., unequal access to digital technology [17], discrimination) [18].

Research focused on social media use among different marginalized populations is in a nascent phase. Although untoward exposures on social media (e.g., cyberbullying) may be more prevalent among some marginalized youth [16], social media also has played a key role in facilitating connectedness [15]. There is ample evidence of strong community building among Black youth, connecting across geographic boundaries [19]. For sexual and gender minority youth, research has demonstrated clear benefits from online platforms supporting information-seeking regarding identity formation, finding peer support or role models, and navigating the coming out process [20]. These early findings underscore the need for research to clarify *when* and *which* aspects of social media use have protective effects that will foster resilience among marginalized youth as well as utilizing an intersectional approach to this work. Though we raise the potential issues facing marginalized populations broadly, there are numerous marginalized identities and populations that experience unique, nuanced risk and protective factors. More research is warranted to understand which aspects of social media use are common across marginalized populations and which may differentially impact certain marginalized groups.

## 2.3 Adolescent Mental Health: A Broader Landscape of Challenges

There are deeply entrenched systemic problems that, at the very least, are contributing to alarming rates of mental health problems among youth in the United States. Chief among them is a clinician shortage and lack of access to mental healthcare. Presently, there are 14 child and adolescent psychiatrists per 100,000 youth, and more broadly, ~45% of the US population resides in a community with a shortage of mental health professionals. These shortages are particularly acute in rural and marginalized communities [21] and were further exacerbated following the COVID-19 pandemic [22]. The scarce availability of clinicians has led many families to delay clinical services, often requiring 6 to 12 months for an initial appointment. Unsurprisingly, this delay has led to increased rates of emergency department services for suicide-related concerns [23]. Importantly, increases in the rate and severity of youth mental health problems coincide with alarming rates of psychiatric challenges for adults, with nearly 42% reporting symptoms of anxiety or depression [24], which increases intergenerational transmission of mental health concerns. Taken together, the lack of clinical services coupled with increased parental rates of mood and affective disorders may be playing an outsized role in increasing the risk for youth mental health problems.

A related challenge is that insurance-based coverage for mental health privileges treatment over prevention, which, again, delays access to care. Based on decades of research, there is a clear understanding of peak risk periods throughout childhood and adolescence regarding the emergence of internalizing and externalizing disorders. Leveraging these data, there are opportunities to offer prevention for youth when symptoms are subthreshold, and, perhaps, more responsive to our gold-standard psychotherapeutic interventions. Conversely, the US insurance-based care for mental health largely relies on a reactive versus a preventative model. Meaning, reimbursements are provided when there is a clear diagnosis as opposed to a risk for the disorder (e.g., elevated symptoms), which is unfortunate, given that our interventions are more effective for mild and moderate presentations, and at the more severe continuum, there is a greater impairment in everyday functioning and protracted recovery periods. Together, the clinician shortage and limited access to care based on current insurance-based approaches highlight key gaps in addressing adolescent mental health problems that may be more paramount relative to social media use.

# 3 Future Research

Additional research is needed to address current gaps in the literature linking social media to mental health outcomes, particularly: (a) to utilize objective measurement of social media behavior beyond self-reported measures of users' experience and patterns of behavior, (b) to leverage longitudinal data to examine potential causal and developmental effects, and (c) to take deeper account of prior vulnerabilities that may increase adolescent susceptibility to negative social media exposures [11, 25, 26]. Although self-report instruments offer insight into adolescent behavioral patterns (e.g., *what platforms are used, when social media is used, why and how long social media is used*), there are challenges with extracting more complex risk indicators that may be particularly important for understanding mental health among adolescents. To draw definitive links between social media and adolescent mental health, there are several core conceptual and methodological advances that can be made.

Research focused on social media and mental health requires rigorous and reliable methodological approaches. Presently, there is a reliance on self-report measures of social media use, which, at times, may not be accurate [27]. This is coupled with limited operationalizations of social media use (e.g., total screen time) that do not capture *how* social media is used [7], particularly in the context of cross-sectional designs which preclude inferences about directionality [6, 7]. Intensive longitudinal designs relying on user-derived content, as opposed to self-reported retrospective experiences, focusing on *how* (e.g., passively versus actively), *when* and *for how long* (e.g., time of day), *why* (e.g., seeking connectedness), and *with whom* (e.g., friends, strangers) youth use social media may provide key insights into potential risk and protective features of social media. Moreover, establishing a connection between social media and adolescent mental health requires carefully characterizing exposures present in their *digital lives* through a deep interrogation of real-time interactions. For example, research leveraging computational analysis of user-generated social media content across different social media platforms (e.g., Twitter, Instagram, TikTok) has the ability to capture dynamic interpersonal and associated affective changes with exceptional temporal resolution [28, 29].

Another key challenge is addressing the specificity of social media factors from non-digital risk exposures. This issue is nontrivial as one's interactions in digital space can, at times, spill into everyday life. For example, youth experiencing cyberbullying are more likely to report in-person bullying [30], and many marginalized youth are more likely than non-marginalized youth to experience adverse experiences (e.g., discrimination, trauma) both offline and online [18]. There is growing recognition that online and offline experiences may not be easily separable [31], and social media exposures and behaviors may be an extension of offline exposures and behaviors.

Critically, social media use is not likely to have a singular effect on mental health equally across all populations. It will be critical to examine differences in the quantity and quality of social media use that may help to explain mental health disparities and to understand that certain experiences may be risk factors in one population but promote resilience in another. With this in mind, future research can also seek to understand individual-level associations between social media and mental health to help bolster future intervention development.

### 3.1 Summary

The association between social media use and adolescent mental health is complex. Social media use does not reflect monolithic behavior, and current methods employed do not sufficiently disentangle digital from offline exposures. Given the increased use of social media, which is occurring at earlier ages in the developmental course, further research is warranted, particularly approaches that probe user-generated content while accounting for established social determinants that directly influence mental health and well-being among marginalized youth.

## 4 Recommendations

As social media use continues to increase and change over time among adolescents, it is essential to develop common-sense strategies that foster safer practices.

- There may be benefits to developing curricula to educate guardians about their children's social media use. At a minimum, it is advisable for guardians to have a clear understanding of *what* platforms their children are engaging with, *how* they are being utilized, and with whom they are interacting within these forums.

- There are important age-related differences with regard to parental monitoring practices. For younger and newer users, it may be advisable to have experiences with the youth and guardians together, wherein content is reviewed together, which will support ongoing conversations. In some families, this may include guardians having access to social media platform passwords, which would provide opportunities to review similar content.
- For older adolescents, guardians may opt to follow their teens and view their posted content and online interactions. Although these measures of oversight may be time-consuming, they will provide critical information about the different exposures—including positive and negative content—within youth digital lives, which may lead to safer online practices.
- Within schools there are often courses about physical health, sexual health, and for some, driver's education. At this critical crossroad, there may be a timely opportunity to develop directed education about social media engagement. Curricula within schools can explore common malicious exposures (e.g., online victimization, catfishing), practices to navigate safely (e.g., sexting, sharing revealing photos), and discuss potential dangers or worries. As social media platforms also may offer key support, particularly for marginalized youth, curricula can discuss safe havens, opportunities to remain protected, and protections as social media users.
- Treatment of adolescent mental health must consider the potential impact of social media use among adolescents. Accordingly, it is critical for mental health practitioners to obtain core competencies about if and how their patients are engaging with social media. Importantly, there may be opportunities for patients to benefit from social media engagement through connections made within specific fora, which facilitate youth being seen, heard, and connected. This may be particularly true among marginalized youth, and accordingly, practitioners may benefit from seeking guidance on how to best direct patients to engage in social media safely.

**Conflict of Interest and Funding Disclosures** This work was supported by the National Institute of Mental Health grants P50 MH115838 (RB, RPA), K23 MH120437 (RB), R01 MH119771 (RPA), U01 MH116923 (RPA), R01 MH126181 (DP), R21 MH125044 (DP); the American Foundation for Suicide Prevention [AFSP, grant number SRG-006-22 (RB)]; and the Morgan Stanley Foundation also supported this research project (RPA, DP). CJF was supported through a training fellowship awarded to the Division of Child and Adolescent Psychiatry at Columbia University (T32 MH016434–42). The content is solely the responsibility of the authors and does not necessarily represent the official views of the National Institutes of Health. RB serves on the scientific board and reports stock ownership in "Taliaz Health," with no conflict of interest relevant to this work. RPA is an unpaid scientific advisor for Ksana Health and a paid scientific advisor for Get Sonar, Inc. No other authors have conflicts of interest relevant to this chapter to disclose.

## References

1. Vogels EA, Gelles-Watnick R, Massarat N. Teens, social media and technology 2022. Published online August 10, 2022. Accessed January 4, 2023. https://policycommons.net/artifacts/2644169/teens-social-media-and-technology-2022/3667002/.
2. van Dijck J. The culture of connectivity: a critical history of social media. Oxford University Press; 2013.
3. Haidt J, Twenge JM. This is our chance to pull teenagers out of the smartphone trap. NY Times. Published online 2021. https://www.columbusschoolforgirls.org/uploaded/Upper_School/Opinion_This_Is_Our_Chance_to_Pull_Teenagers_Out_of_the_Smartphone_Trap_-_The_New_York_Times.pdf.
4. Leonhardt D. On the phone, alone. NY Times. Published online 2022. https://livelikesam.org/wp-content/uploads/2022/08/The-Morning_-Less-sleep-less-happiness.pdf.
5. Frison E, Eggermont S. Exploring the relationships between different types of Facebook use, perceived online social support, and adolescents' depressed mood. Soc Sci Comput Rev. 2016;34(2):153–71.
6. Odgers CL, Jensen MR. Annual research review: adolescent mental health in the digital age: facts, fears,

and future directions. J Child Psychol Psychiatry. 2020;61(3):336–48.
7. Valkenburg PM, Meier A, Beyens I. Social media use and its impact on adolescent mental health: an umbrella review of the evidence. Curr Opin Psychol. 2022;44:58–68.
8. Yoon S, Kleinman M, Mertz J, Brannick M. Is social network site usage related to depression? A meta-analysis of Facebook–depression relations. J Affect Disord. 2019;248:65–72.
9. Przybylski AK, Weinstein N. A large-scale test of the goldilocks hypothesis. Psychol Sci. 2017;28(2):204–15.
10. Boers E, Afzali MH, Newton N, Conrod P. Association of screen time and depression in adolescence. JAMA Pediatr. 2019;173(9):853–9.
11. Coyne SM, Rogers AA, Zurcher JD, Stockdale L, Booth M. Does time spent using social media impact mental health?: an eight year longitudinal study. Comput Hum Behav. 2020;104:106160. https://doi.org/10.1016/j.chb.2019.106160.
12. Jensen M, George M, Russell M, Odgers C. Young adolescents' digital technology use and mental health symptoms: little evidence of longitudinal or daily linkages. Clin Psychol Sci. 2019;7(6):1416–33.
13. Beyens I, Pouwels JL, van Driel II, Keijsers L, Valkenburg PM. The effect of social media on well-being differs from adolescent to adolescent. Sci Rep. 2020;10(1):10763.
14. Abi-Jaoude E, Naylor KT, Pignatiello A. Smartphones, social media use and youth mental health. CMAJ. 2020;192(6):E136–41.
15. Sadagheyani HE, Tatari F. Investigating the role of social media on mental health. Ment Health Soc Incl. 2021;25(1):41–51. https://doi.org/10.1108/mhsi-06-2020-0039.
16. CDC. Youth risk behavior surveillance data summary & trends report: 2011-2021. Published online 2023. https://www.cdc.gov/healthyyouth/data/yrbs/pdf/YRBS_Data-Summary-Trends_Report2023_508.pdf.
17. Cheshmehzangi A, Zou T, Su Z. The digital divide impacts on mental health during the COVID-19 pandemic. Brain Behav Immun. 2022;101:211–3.
18. Tao X, Fisher CB. Exposure to social media racial discrimination and mental health among adolescents of color. J Youth Adolesc. 2022;51(1):30–44.
19. Klassen S. Black twitter is gold: why this online community is worthy of study and how to do so respectfully. Interactions. 2022;29(1):96–8.
20. Craig SL, Eaton AD, McInroy LB, Leung VWY, Krishnan S. Can social media participation enhance LGBTQ+ youth well-being? Development of the social media benefits scale. Soc Media Society. 2021;7(1):2056305121988931.
21. Kuehn BM. Clinician shortage exacerbates pandemic-fueled "mental health crisis". JAMA. 2022;327(22):2179–81.
22. Chavira DA, Ponting C, Ramos G. The impact of COVID-19 on child and adolescent mental health and treatment considerations. Behav Res Ther. 2022;157:104169.
23. Madigan S, Korczak DJ, Vaillancourt T, et al. Comparison of paediatric emergency department visits for attempted suicide, self-harm, and suicidal ideation before and during the COVID-19 pandemic: a systematic review and meta-analysis. Lancet Psychiatry. Published online March 9, 2023. https://doi.org/10.1016/S2215-0366(23)00036-6.
24. Vahratian A, Blumberg SJ, Terlizzi EP, Schiller JS. Symptoms of anxiety or depressive disorder and use of mental health care among adults during the COVID-19 pandemic – United States, august 2020-February 2021. MMWR Morb Mortal Wkly Rep. 2021;70(13):490–4.
25. Bagot KS, Tomko RL, Marshall AT, et al. Youth screen use in the ABCD® study. Dev Cogn Neurosci. 2022;57:101150. https://doi.org/10.1016/j.dcn.2022.101150.
26. Nagata JM, Singh G, Sajjad OM, et al. Social epidemiology of early adolescent problematic screen use in the United States. Pediatr Res. 2022;92(5):1443–9. https://doi.org/10.1038/s41390-022-02176-8.
27. Verbeij T, Pouwels JL, Beyens I, Valkenburg PM. The accuracy and validity of self-reported social media use measures among adolescents. Comput Human Behav Rep. 2021;3:100090.
28. De Choudhury M, Kiciman E, Dredze M, Coppersmith G, Kumar M. Discovering shifts to suicidal ideation from mental health content in social media. Proc SIGCHI Conf Hum Factor Comput Syst. 2016;2016:2098–110.
29. Chancellor S, De Choudhury M. Methods in predictive techniques for mental health status on social media: a critical review. NPJ Digit Med. 2020;3(1) https://doi.org/10.1038/s41746-020-0233-7.
30. Waasdorp TE, Bradshaw CP. The overlap between cyberbullying and traditional bullying. J Adolesc Health. 2015;56(5):483–8.
31. Jurgenson N. When atoms meet bits: social media, the mobile web and augmented revolution. Future Internet. 2012;4(1):83–91.

# Online Racism and Its Impact on Children, Adolescents, and Emerging Adults of Color

Brendesha M. Tynes, Henry A. Willis,
Ashley Maxie-Moreman, Stephanie M. Ortiz,
and Devin English

## 1 Background

Despite early claims that the Internet would erase race and concomitant social problems, two decades of research suggest online racism, similar to its offline counterpart [1], is a major threat to public health. Scholars have argued that we are currently living through a second nadir of race relations [2], where racism and white supremacy are algorithmically amplified —the first occurred beginning in the 1870s as a white backlash to Black people's progress and included the highest number of lynchings to date as well as the passing of Jim Crow laws. As the bedrock of this twenty-first-century nadir, scholars have outlined online racism's nature, prevalence, and measurement, along with associations with a range of poor academic and health outcomes for young people of color. This chapter outlines the current state of online racism research, points out gaps, and makes recommendations for future directions.

B. M. Tynes (✉)
University of Southern California,
Los Angeles, CA, USA
e-mail: btynes@usc.edu

H. A. Willis
University of Pennsylvania, Philadelphia, PA, USA

A. Maxie-Moreman
Children's National Hospital, Washington, DC, USA

S. M. Ortiz
University of Massachusetts Lowell,
Lowell, MA, USA

D. English
Rutgers University, Newark, NJ, USA

## 2 Current State

### 2.1 Models of Online Racism

Online racism is defined as the virtual denigration, exclusion, terror, abuse, and dehumanization of groups or individuals due to race. It may be subtle or explicit, interpersonal or structural, direct or vicarious, and a single event or repeated (as in cyberbullying victimization) digital harms that place white individuals at an advantage and people of color at a compounded disadvantage. Several models of online racism conceptualize its nature, why it occurs, and how it adversely impacts communities of color. Although a full evaluation of each model is outside of the scope of this chapter, we will briefly highlight how these models have advanced our understanding of online racism. Tynes and colleagues' model [3] characterizes online racism as both ideological and structural, with factors such as algorithms and features of the interface influencing the likelihood of users having racist experiences. This model includes miseducation, microinvalidation, microinsult, misinformation/disinformation, online racial discrimination (individual and vicarious experiences), and online hate crimes


D. A. Christakis, L. Hale (eds.), *Handbook of Children and Screens*,
https://doi.org/10.1007/978-3-031-69362-5_39

(abuse, stalking, hacking, and certain privacy violations). Others have sought to explain why individuals engage in forms of online racism, explaining how online anonymity may facilitate disinhibition and deindividuation, in turn increasing prejudicial attitudes and expressions of racism [4]. Importantly, scholars have noted that games, and arguably a wide range of online contexts, are "racialized pedagogical zones" that train people in ways of doing race online [5].

Finally, scholars have also begun to conceptualize how online racism adversely affects the health and well-being of communities of color. Patton and colleagues proposed the framework of everyday racism in social media policing to explain how big data is used in criminal justice practices, and its adverse consequences for communities of color [6]. For instance, online public discourse between broader public society (which is influenced by racial prejudices and attitudes), and law enforcement leads to the decoding of social media posts by people of color as criminal. This leads to punitive actions being taken against communities of color, further exacerbating the negative effects of online racism. Volpe and colleagues [7] revised and extended Tynes and colleagues' model [3] to outline an additional framework to describe how online structural racism, such as racist healthcare algorithms, surveillance, traumatic events online, and mis- and disinformation (e.g., in the case of COVID-19) are a driving force behind ongoing health inequities in the country.

## 2.2 Measurement

Although numerous measures that assess in-person or offline experiences of racism exist [8, 9], to date, there are very few empirically validated measures of online racism, and very few researchers have investigated the negative impacts of online racism [10]. Furthermore, despite the frequency of direct and vicarious experiences, 29% vs 71%, respectively, for African Americans nearly two decades ago [11], early studies only used 1–2 items to measure online racism. To better assess the variety of ways youth may be exposed to online racism (e.g., racist images, cloaked websites, and jokes), individual and vicarious subscales of the Online Victimization Scale [12] were developed using a sample of adolescents. Both subscales show good reliability based on recently published peer-reviewed empirical papers utilizing the scales, with Cronbach's alphas ranging from 0.64 to 0.78 for the individual subscale, and from 0.79 to 0.84 for the vicarious subscale [13, 14]. Later, Keum and Miller created the Perceived Online Racism Scale [15] for adults, which consists of three subscales: personal and vicarious exposure to racial cyber aggression and online mediated exposure to racist reality. More recently, short and very brief versions of the Perceived Online Racism Scale were created to further optimize usability.

In response to the increased use of viral/trending videos and other images or recordings to call out "racial terror in the form of police violence, arrests, or state-sanctioned cruelty and deprivation via the Internet" [16] Tynes and colleagues developed the Traumatic Events Online Scale [17]. Questions in this scale ask the respondent about their exposure to images or videos of people of color being beaten, arrested, detained, killed as well as additional forms of violence against Black and Brown people that are propagated offline, but recorded and posted online. These existing online racism measures are the most used. They have been updated and will be included in a new measure that also includes more emergent forms of online racism such as algorithmic bias, also known as algorithmic oppression [18]—a set of often racist and sexist mathematical instructions that shape users' experiences (e.g., social media timelines and search results) and outcomes.

## 2.3 Qualitative Studies

Against a backdrop of white supremacist organizing and the empowerment of white youth to engage in racism and terror [19], online racism is an anticipated aspect of social life for adolescents and emerging adults of color [20]. Qualitative studies of online racism have utilized content analyses, virtual ethnography, and interviews to investigate the discourses, interactions, and meaning-making processes that inform the reproduction of racism online. For example, interview data suggests Black and Latinx adolescents experienced people framing them as criminals, unintelligent, lazy, dirty, and as people who should not have certain rights, such as voting [21]. They also experienced threats of violence and people justifying killings of Black people like Trayvon Martin. Black participants reported white people calling for their genocide. Additionally, a virtual ethnography provided unique insight into the ways that Black gamers are targeted for racism through linguistic profiling, questioning, provoking, and instigating [22].

Qualitative work has uncovered the strategies used to navigate, resist, and cope with mistreatment across online spaces [23, 24], as well as the broader narratives emerging adults of color draw upon to minimize and justify their racist experiences [20]. Respondents across studies have described the perceived negative impact of this racism on a host of social, academic, and health outcomes, noting anger, trouble focusing, and a sense of unease about their school racial climate [20, 25]. Further, intersectional studies have illuminated how gender is an important variable to consider, as young women of color receive gender-specific racialized insults from strangers and encounter victim-blaming from friends and family when they are vocal about their experiences of racism online [24]. Peers and adults also pressure young men of color to be "emotionally strong" and unscathed by online racism [26]. Qualitative work on online racism is therefore important to consider when evaluating coping styles, subjective reports of stress and well-being, and the social contexts that contribute to disparate health outcomes.

## 2.4 Quantitative Studies

Quantitative studies that include surveys, content, sentiment, social network, and spatial analyses as well as experimental designs allow researchers to examine larger groups of participants or racist posts online. Cross-sectional designs tend to be more represented in the literature whereas longitudinal, intensive longitudinal, and experimental designs are less common. Scholars argue that experimental designs are more methodologically rigorous because they eliminate retrospective reporting common in surveys, but recent studies using virtual reality deliberately expose participants to racial discrimination and they respond as if it were real life [27]. This may potentially compound the detrimental impacts young people of color already experience.

Research suggests there was an increase in online racism over the past decade aligned with the election of the first Black president, a global pandemic, and a racial reckoning against centuries of systemic racism against Black Americans. For example, African American, Latinx, Asian, and bi-racial 6-12th graders experienced increased online racial discrimination across three time points from 2010–2013, with 32% reporting seeing a racist image in the past year at time 1 and 50% at time 3 [28]. Similarly, across three nationally representative studies researchers found Black and Latinx 13–17 year olds were cyberbullied because of their race in the past 30 days significantly more than other groups from 2016 to 2019 [29]. All groups except Latinx and individuals and participants who identified their race or ethnicity "Other" experienced *more* cyberbullying from 2019 to 2021. A major concern with these studies is that whites were included when they did not experience online racism—note early studies included whites, but this practice ended in 2010. Additionally, scholars only used a single item to measure race-related cyberbullying. Finally, they assess past year or past 30 day's experiences. More intensive longitudinal studies are needed as the first study to use daily diary methods to examine a range of experiences both offline and online, found Black young people have more than five discriminatory experiences per day and most of these occur online [13].

Quantitative studies consistently show online racism is associated with poor outcomes for

Black, Indigenous, Asian, and Latinx adolescents and emerging adults. This includes depressive symptoms, anxiety, suicide ideation, alcohol use disorder, drug problems, decreased academic motivation, posttraumatic stress disorder symptoms, trauma symptoms of discrimination, internalized computing stereotypes, and problem behavior [16, 17, 30–34]. Studies also suggest that young people of color have a range of individual and cultural resources, such as self-esteem and racial-ethnic identity, that can be protective or promotive with respect to negative outcomes typically associated with online racism [14, 35]. Given the alarming rise in suicide rates, with Black 10–24-year-olds experiencing the highest proportional increase from 2018 to 2021 [36], more research is needed on the unique impact of online experiences in suicide ideation and behaviors.

### 2.5 Mixed, Multi-, AI, and Other Automated Methods

Some studies have used mixed, multi-methods, artificial intelligence (AI), and other automated data collection and analysis methods to broaden our understanding of the impact of online racism. A multi-method study included the use of Twitter's Streaming Application Programming Interface to collect 532 million tweets [37]. Researchers showed that discrimination targeted in tweets is associated with the number of race-ethnicity related hate crimes (e.g., assault, murder, arson, vandalism), with the most widely used words "f*cking n*gger" appearing in tweets of the top 10 cities. Similarly, a study of the heightened amount of online racism against Asians during the pandemic showed that negative sentiment proliferated on Twitter in alignment with policies to restrict entrance of Chinese people into the US as well as when Trump labeled the coronavirus the "Chinese Virus" in March of 2020 [38].

Extant research suggests the current rush to transform all aspects of personal, academic, and professional life with AI will have a detrimental impact on people of color. A groundbreaking study of AI systems in US healthcare showed systematic scoring of Black and white patients with the same level of risk though Black patients had more serious illness and health needs [39]. This has potential life or death implications for people of color in the United States because over 200 million people could be impacted by the algorithmic service's biased decision-making. The discourse from the tech industry is that AI systems will be less biased than humans [40], but given the fact that they train from biased data it is likely these systems will exacerbate inequity if left unchecked. There are equally detrimental outcomes in education where researchers note that machine learning can disadvantage English Learners (and, we argue, those who speak other dialects such as African American Vernacular English) in science assessments that use whiteness as the default [41]. More research is needed on the impact of AI in education [42], on marginalized young people, from AI instructors and personalized learning systems to automated assessments.

## 3 Future Research

Based on the current state of knowledge and pressing sociocultural issues there are several areas of future research stakeholders should consider as they continue to explore the impact of online racism on the development and psychosocial outcomes of youth of color. They include:

- How do we both measure the impact of how online racism is perpetuated on emerging forms of technology, as well as create policies [43] to reduce the proliferation of online racism in existing, emerging, and forthcoming forms of technology? The existence of the Metaverse [44], an iteration of the Internet that includes endless, interconnected, virtual worlds, promised to open new ways of engaging social interaction (though interest has waned), but this also exacerbates the deleterious harm that online racism may present for youth of color if there are no safeguards in place for protecting youth of color while reducing the ability for "bad actors" to use the Metaverse in harmful ways.

- How do previously established, evidence-based protective factors for youth of color (e.g., racial socialization messages, racial identity beliefs, among others) [45] function in the context of online racism? How do youth of color use emerging technologies to create new behaviors and strategies that protect against online racism?
  - We lack sufficient evidence of how previously established protective and productive mechanisms buffer the effects of racism experienced *online*. Further, technological advancements have ushered in *new* protective mechanisms and highlighted the novel strategies youth use to protect against online racism. For instance, the ability to critique racism in media and technology, which can buffer post-traumatic stress disorder symptoms when adults of color experience online racism [46], may also function as a protective factor for youth of color. There are undoubtedly *online* factors that have yet to be measured and explored, but they must be understood for their potential to protect against the impact of online racism.
- Given that burgeoning research has highlighted structural online racism (e.g., biased healthcare algorithms, policing, etc.), how do we extend this work by developing measures of structural online racism? How does structural online racism impact youths of color's physical and mental health, as well as academic and psychosocial development?
- Finally, what mechanisms account for the relationship between online racism and youth of color's academic, physical, and psychosocial outcomes? Are there developmental differences in these mechanisms? Recent research has not only identified rumination as a key factor that links racial discrimination experiences to Black youth's psychological well-being but also that the negative effect of rumination increases as these youth age [47].

## 4 Recommendations

Based on current knowledge, we have the following recommendations for researchers, the tech industry, policymakers, and practitioners:

- *Researchers* should consider ethical concerns when determining whether a method is more methodologically rigorous than extant designs. For example, recent arguments that experimental designs using virtual reality are more methodologically sound are problematic. Particularly if these studies deliberately expose people of color to racism [27]. Given the heightened amount of online and offline racism young people experience, we find deliberate exposure unethical and potentially harmful. The American Psychological Association Code of Ethics Section 3.04 [48] states that psychologists should avoid harm. We see potential in these emerging technologies and use VR/AR in the research of our coauthors but do so without simulating the daily racist violence young people witness.
- *Tech industry professionals, researchers, policymakers, and practitioners* need to adopt a critical race lens that informs their efforts. The current rhetoric that frames AI technologies as neutral, less biased than humans, or a new panacea for a range of problems, is dangerous. The AI-gold rush will move forward with exacerbating current racial inequity. If all stakeholders begin with the understanding that racism is systemic and pervasive in American institutions [49] and emerging technologies [18], that it intersects with other oppressions (e.g., sexism, classism, heterosexism), then we might take steps to curb the proliferation of online racism. We might also engage in more sophisticated and rigorous research into how emerging technologies impact people of color.
- We recommend diversifying the research, design, tech, and educator workforces with people who have training in Black Studies, whiteness, the histories, cultures, and development of people of color. These individuals will help teams center race and the racism built into technologies.

**Conflict of Interest and Funding Disclosures** None.

## References


1. AMA: Racism is a threat to public health. American Medical Association. Published November 16, 2020. Accessed May 16, 2023. https://www.ama-assn.org/delivering-care/health-equity/ama-racism-threat-public-health.
2. Daniels J. The algorithmic rise of the "alt-right". Contexts. 2018;17(1):60–5. https://doi.org/10.1177/1536504218766547.
3. Tynes BM, Lozada FT, Smith NA, Stewart AM. From racial microaggressions to hate crimes: a model of online racism based on the lived experiences of adolescents of color. In: Microaggression theory. Wiley; 2018. p. 194–212. https://doi.org/10.1002/9781119466642.ch12.
4. Keum BT, Miller MJ. Racism on the internet: conceptualization and recommendations for research. Psychol Violence. 2018;8:782–91. https://doi.org/10.1037/vio0000201.
5. Everett A, Watkins SC. The power of play: The portrayal and performance of race in video games. In: *The ecology of games: Connecting youth, games, and learning*. The John D. and Catherine T. MacArthur Foundation Series on Digital Media and Learning; 2007. p. 141–64. https://doi.org/10.1162/dmal.9780262693646.141.
6. Patton DU, Brunton DW, Dixon A, Miller RJ, Leonard P, Hackman R. Stop and frisk online: theorizing everyday racism in digital policing in the use of social media for Identification of criminal conduct and associations. Soc Media Soc. 2017;3(3):2056305117733344. https://doi.org/10.1177/2056305117733344.
7. Volpe VV, Hoggard LS, Willis HA, Tynes BM. Anti-Black structural racism goes online: a conceptual model for racial health disparities research. Ethn Dis. 2021;31(Suppl 1):311–8. https://doi.org/10.18865/ed.31.S1.311.
8. Atkins R. Instruments measuring perceived racism/racial discrimination: review and critique of factor analytic techniques. Int J Health Serv. 2014;44(4):711–34.
9. McNeilly MD, Anderson NB, Armstead CA, Clark R, Corbett M, Robinson EL, et al. The perceived racism scale: a multidimensional assessment of the experience of white racism among African Americans. Ethn Dis. 1996;6(1/2):154–66.
10. Bliuc AM, Faulkner N, Jakubowicz A, McGarty C. Online networks of racial hate: a systematic review of 10 years of research on cyber-racism. Comput Hum Behav. 2018;87:75–86. https://doi.org/10.1016/j.chb.2018.05.026.
11. Tynes BM, Giang MT, Williams DR, Thompson GN. Online racial discrimination and psychological adjustment among adolescents. J Adolesc Health. 2008;43(6):565–9. https://doi.org/10.1016/j.jadohealth.2008.08.021.
12. Tynes BM, Rose CA, Williams DR. The development and validation of the online victimization scale for adolescents. Cyberpsychol J Psychosoc Res Cyberspace. 2010;4(2) Accessed April 26, 2023. https://cyberpsychology.eu/article/view/4237
13. English D, Lambert SF, Tynes BM, Bowleg L, Zea MC, Howard LC. Daily multidimensional racial discrimination among Black U.S. American adolescents. J Appl Dev Psychol. 2020;66:101068. https://doi.org/10.1016/j.appdev.2019.101068.
14. Umaña-Taylor AJ, Tynes BM, Toomey RB, Williams DR, Mitchell KJ. Latino adolescents' perceived discrimination in online and offline settings: an examination of cultural risk and protective factors. Dev Psychol. 2015;51(1):87–100. https://doi.org/10.1037/a0038432.
15. Keum BT, Miller MJ. Racism in digital era: development and initial validation of the perceived online racism scale (PORS v1.0). J Couns Psychol. 2017;64:310–24. https://doi.org/10.1037/cou0000205.
16. Maxie-Moreman AD, Tynes BM. Exposure to online racial discrimination and traumatic events online in black adolescents and emerging adults. J Res Adolesc. 2022;32(1):254–69. https://doi.org/10.1111/jora.12732.
17. Tynes BM, Willis HA, Stewart AM, Hamilton MW. Race-related traumatic events online and mental health among adolescents of color. J Adolesc Health. 2019;65(3):371–7. https://doi.org/10.1016/j.jadohealth.2019.03.006.
18. Noble SU. Algorithms of oppression: how search engines reinforce racism. In: Algorithms of oppression. New York University Press; 2018. https://doi.org/10.18574/nyu/9781479833641.001.0001.
19. Tynes B. Children, adolescents and the culture of online hate. Handbook of children, culture and violence. Published online 2005. p. 267–289.
20. Ortiz SM. Racists without racism? From colourblind to entitlement racism online. Ethn Racial Stud. 2021;44(14):2637–57. https://doi.org/10.1080/01419870.2020.1825758.
21. Garcia AG, McGrew S, Mirra N, Tynes B, Kahne J. Rethinking digital citizenship: learning about media, literacy, and race in Turbulent Times.
22. Gray KL. Deviant bodies, stigmatized identities, and racist acts: examining the experiences of African-American gamers in Xbox live. New Rev Hypermedia Multimedia. 2012;18(4):261–76. https://doi.org/10.1080/13614568.2012.746740.
23. Eschmann R. Digital resistance: how online communication facilitates responses to racial microaggressions. Sociol Race Ethnicity. 2021;7(2):264–77. https://doi.org/10.1177/2332649220933307.
24. Ortiz SM. Call-in, call-out, care, and cool rationality: how young adults respond to racism and sexism online. Soc Probl. Published online October

19, 2021:spab060. https://doi.org/10.1093/socpro/spab060.
25. Eschmann R. Unmasking racism: students of color and expressions of racism in online spaces. Soc Probl. 2020;67(3):418–36. https://doi.org/10.1093/socpro/spz026.
26. Ortiz SM. "You can say I got desensitized to it": how men of color cope with everyday racism in online gaming. Sociol Perspect. 2019;62(4):572–88. https://doi.org/10.1177/0731121419837588.
27. Lui PP, Stringer E, Jouriles EN. Advancing knowledge on the health consequences of discrimination: the potential of virtual reality. Cult Divers Ethn Minor Psychol. 2023;29:96–105. https://doi.org/10.1037/cdp0000460.
28. Tynes BM, Zuckerman A, Seaton E. Online racial discrimination: a growing problem for adolescents. Published December 2015. http://www.apa.org/science/about/psa/2015/12/online-racial-discrimination.aspx (http://www.apa.org/science/about/psa/2015/12/online-racial-discrimination.aspx).
29. Patchin JW, Hinduja S. Cyberbullying among tweens in the United States: prevalence, impact, and helping behaviors. J Early Adolesc. 2022;42(3):414–30. https://doi.org/10.1177/02724316211036740.
30. Keum BT, Ángel CM. Online racism, depressive and anxiety symptoms, coping-related drinking motives, and alcohol use severity among Black, Latina/o/x, and Asian emerging adults. Addict Behav. 2023;136:107468. https://doi.org/10.1016/j.addbeh.2022.107468.
31. Tao X, Fisher CB. Exposure to social media racial discrimination and mental health among adolescents of color. J Youth Adolescence. 2022;51(1):30–44. https://doi.org/10.1007/s10964-021-01514-z.
32. Tynes BM, Rose CA, Hiss S, Umaña-Taylor AJ, Mitchell K, Williams D. Virtual environments, online racial discrimination, and adjustment among a diverse, school-based sample of adolescents. Int J Gaming Comput Mediat Simul. 2014;6(3):1–16. https://doi.org/10.4018/ijgcms.2014070101.
33. Tynes BM, Del Toro J, Lozada FT. An unwelcomed digital visitor in the classroom: the longitudinal impact of online racial discrimination on academic motivation. Sch Psychol Rev. 2015;44:407–24. https://doi.org/10.17105/SPR-15-0095.1.
34. Tynes BM, Maxie-Moreman A, Hoang T-MH, Willis HA, English D. Online racial discrimination, suicidal ideation, and traumatic stress in a National Sample of black adolescents. JAMA Psychiatry. 2024;81(3):312–6. https://doi.org/10.1001/jamapsychiatry.2023.4961.
35. Tynes BM, Umaña-Taylor AJ, Rose CA, Lin J, Anderson CJ. Online racial discrimination and the protective function of ethnic identity and self-esteem for African American adolescents. Dev Psychol. 2012;48(2):343–55. https://doi.org/10.1037/a0027032.
36. Stone DM. Notes from the field: recent changes in suicide rates, by race and ethnicity and age group — United States, 2021. MMWR Morb Mortal Wkly Rep. 2023;72 https://doi.org/10.15585/mmwr.mm7206a4.
37. Relia K, Li Z, Cook SH, Chunara R. Race, ethnicity and national origin-based discrimination in social media and hate crimes across 100 U.S. cities. Proc Int AAAI Conf Web Soc Media. 2019;13:417–27. https://doi.org/10.1609/icwsm.v13i01.3354.
38. Pei X, Mehta D. #Coronavirus or #Chinesevirus?!: Understanding the negative sentiment reflected in Tweets with racist hashtags across the development of COVID-19. Published online May 17, 2020. https://doi.org/10.48550/arXiv.2005.08224.
39. Obermeyer Z, Powers B, Vogeli C, Mullainathan S. Dissecting racial bias in an algorithm used to manage the health of populations. Science. 2019;366(6464):447–53. https://doi.org/10.1126/science.aax2342.
40. Benjamin R. Assessing risk, automating racism. Science. 2019;366(6464):421–2. https://doi.org/10.1126/science.aaz3873.
41. Cheuk T. Can AI be racist? Color-evasiveness in the application of machine learning to science assessments. Sci Educ. 2021;105(5):825–36. https://doi.org/10.1002/sce.21671.
42. Akgun S, Greenhow C. Artificial intelligence in education: addressing ethical challenges in K-12 settings. AI Ethics. 2022;2(3):431–40. https://doi.org/10.1007/s43681-021-00096-7.
43. Mathiyazhagan S. Field practice, emerging technologies, and human rights: the emergence of tech social workers. J Hum Rights Soc Work. 2022;7(4):441–8. https://doi.org/10.1007/s41134-021-00190-0.
44. EXPLAINER: What is the metaverse and how will it work? | NEWS10 ABC. Accessed May 16, 2023. https://www.news10.com/news/explainer-what-the-metaverse-is-and-how-it-will-work/.
45. Neblett EW. Racial, ethnic, and cultural resilience factors in African American youth mental health. Annu Rev Clin Psychol. 2023;19:361–79. https://doi.org/10.1146/annurev-clinpsy-072720-015146.
46. Volpe VV, Willis HA, Joseph P, Tynes BM. Liberatory media literacy as protective against posttraumatic stress for emerging adults of color. J Trauma Stress. 2021;34(5):1045–55. https://doi.org/10.1002/jts.22640.
47. Bernard DL, López CM, Banks DE, Hahn AM, Danielson CK. Developmental differences in the impact of racial discrimination on depression and anxiety among black youth: examining rumination as a mechanism. Am J rthopsychiatry, Published online May 8, 2023. https://doi.org/10.1037/ort0000679.
48. American Psychological Association. Ethical principles of psychologists and code of conduct. Copyright 2017. Accessed May 16, 2023. https://www.apa.org/ethics/code.
49. Crenshaw K. Mapping the margins: intersectionality, identity politics, and violence against women of color. Stanford Law Rev. 1991;43(6):1241–99. https://doi.org/10.2307/1229039.

# Video Games and Race

Kishonna L Gray, Tara McPherson, Gillian Russell, and Rachel Anderson

## 1 Background

As video game usage continues to increase, so does scholarship and research on its impacts on youth. Scholars have explored issues related to addiction, physical health, mental health outcomes, and more in relation to gaming. The scholarship outlines both the benefits and harms to youth around gaming. And while it is important to continue discussing the physical harms that may befall them in these spaces, it's also necessary to discuss the social harms as well. Using race as an anchor, we explore its impact on gaming practices, gameplay, and gaming culture.

Historically, racialized populations have been excluded from conversations related to game usage, game creation, and gaming culture. Related to gameplay, African Americans play games at and around the same rate as other racial groups despite the myth that Black people don't play video games. According to the Pew Research Center [1], forty-four percent (44%) of Black Americans often or sometimes play video games compared to forty percent (40%) of Whites and forty-eight (48%) percent of Hispanics. Data analytics company Nielsen stated African Americans comprise fourteen percent (14%) of the US population, and within that "Seventy-three percent (73%) of African Americans 13 and older identify as gamers compared to [sixty-six] 66% of the total population." [2]

The COVID-19 pandemic only exacerbated these numbers [3]. Researchers found that, during quarantine, video games increased movement, eased isolation, and reduced stress during isolation. Games like *Animal Crossing: New Horizons* became America's new pastime during the pandemic when it was released during the same time as the shutdown in 2020 [4, 5].

While people of color continue to play games at high rates breaking barriers around access and opportunities, the impacts of being a person of color in these spaces must be explored. As TaeHyuk and Hearns [6] found, racism continues to permeate the gaming landscape increasing psychological distress for Black, Asian, and Latinx gamers. Sadly, gamers of color normalize their experiences and become desensitized to the racism they face [7]. Not only that, researchers have found that gaming chatrooms and communication platforms have provided avenues for extremist groups to influence and promote racist

K. L. Gray (✉)
University of Michigan, Ann Arbor, MI, USA
e-mail: kishonna@umich.edu

T. McPherson
University of Southern California, Los Angeles, CA, USA

G. Russell
Simon Fraser University, Burnaby, BC, Canada

R. Anderson
University of Michigan, Ann Arbor, MI, USA

College of Medicine, University of Kentucky, Lexington, KY, USA


D. A. Christakis, L. Hale (eds.), *Handbook of Children and Screens*,
https://doi.org/10.1007/978-3-031-69362-5_40

ideologies among younger gamers [8]. But what exactly is the nature of the distress people of color face in online gaming? How have gaming environments also been used to radicalize young users in these spaces? The next section discusses the racialized harms that often befall racialized populations in gaming contexts.

# 2 Current State

## 2.1 Racial Harms in Gaming Spaces

In the late 1990s and early 2000s, some proponents of emerging online video games and of broader internet communities argued that these virtual spaces would create a "convergence" culture that fostered greater civic participation and increased access and diversity [9–11]. Other scholars countered that online multiplayer games and communities did not erase existing cultural patterns of racism, and they noted familiar and recurring racist behaviors among video game players [12, 13]. During the past 20 years, research has consistently shown that racism is a serious problem in online gaming. This problem has multiple dimensions that impact youth, including two elements discussed here. First, there is ongoing harm done to young players of color who are often exposed to racist stereotypes in games and to overtly racist language and harassment in video game chats. Second, these environments are also used by far-right extremists to recruit young white men into radical hate groups. Such recruitment produces a continuum of outcomes, from normalizing racist behaviors to deadly violence in the world outside of games.

Scholars have documented the prevalence of racist stereotypes and images in a wide variety of video games [14, 15], illustrating the persistence of patterns of racism from earlier literary and media forms. As in industries such as film and television, there are very few Black or Latino executives at game companies, and video game lead characters are disproportionately white males. Youths' harmful exposure to games containing racist imagery is exacerbated by the online communities that surround games in online chat spaces such as Discord and in popular online environments like Twitch. Players of color experience racism at heightened levels in many action and role-playing games, where racist behavior is more normative than in the offline world [16]. Research into the mental and physical impacts of such exposure indicates the possibility of lowered self-esteem, increased occurrences of severe depression, negative worldviews, heightened feelings of rage and helplessness, and elevated blood pressure levels [17]. Further research into the consequences of such immersive racism is needed.

If youth of color are at risk of harm from heightened exposure to racism in online games, white youth are at risk of coming to view racist behaviors as normative forms of interaction. Furthermore, these young white men are increasingly the target of white supremacist messaging and recruitment. Scholars, the federal government, and nonprofit groups have been tracking the rise of white supremacist groups in online environments for over two decades and have observed the rapid expansion of these activities. The Anti-Defamation League (ADL) found that in 2022 15% of gamers aged 10–17 reported in-game exposure to extreme white supremacist ideas alongside 20% of adults, up from 8% in 2021 [8]. Extremist white supremacist groups use gamer-aligned spaces such as Discord and in-game chat to recruit disaffected boys and young men, normalizing racist ideas and offering a sense of belonging through whiteness and separatism [18]. These processes produce a continuum of impacts from increasing the spread of racist harassment in games to the spread of violence in the offline world. For instance, the mass shooters in New Zealand in 2019 and in Buffalo, NY in 2022 were exposed to racist ideologies through video games.

The rise of hate and racism in online environments has serious consequences for gamers. Research into these impacts should continue at both the theoretical and the empirical level, including the development of harm reduction techniques.

### 2.2 What Happens When Racialized, Gender, and LGBTQIA+ Identities Collide Within Gaming Spaces?

As we have previously covered, youths of color and white youths are subjected to racial harm and racial supremacist ideologies in gaming spaces respectively. But what happens to young gamers who are both people of color and have different gender identifications and sexual orientations from their counterparts? Do these extra labels increase or decrease the probability of discrimination and harm? Current research shows that about 41% of adults who identify as transgender and about 42% who are part of the LGBTQIA+ community are people of color [19, 20]. Therefore, the impact of these combined identities on instigating discrimination and harm in gaming spaces is important to study.

As Richard and Gray [21] explored, queer gamers and gamers with disabilities are almost entirely absent from conversations related to gaming cultures. And until recently, intersectional work has been largely absent in studies on digital gaming, beyond content analysis of what is missing in games.[21(p. 117)] Intersectional Tech was one such engagement that explored identities at the crossroads and in this text, Gray found that the compounding effect of race, gender, sexuality, disability, class, and others often increase the harms experienced inside and around gaming [22]. The largest emerging trend at the intersection beyond gender is on understanding queer experiences and queering games, while many questions about racial experiences still remain.

While conversations on queer gaming are increasing, fan communities have been the ones that have continuously elevated these narratives. Fandoms and fan cultures on Tumblr, Reddit, Serebii, and others have been spaces that engaged in conversations of queering characters, and developing queer "ships" or relationships among seemingly heterosexual characters.

Fan labor has long provided places for discussion and dissemination of gaming and gaming technology news and cultural production. For example, the popular fan site Serebii.net, which began in 1999, provides in-depth coverage of Pokémon video games, trading card games, anime, and other cultural artifacts in and around gaming. Therefore, we urge for more racialized engagement of fandom communities, given the lack of diversity on screen, as their direct involvement in engaging with the content provided by these gaming spaces will offer them a keen-eyed view to spot and advocate against any form of racial or gender-related discrimination and harm.

## 3 Future Research

To better understand how racism impacts youth in gaming, we identify several areas necessary for future research. We offer suggestions based on what platforms can offer as well as what cultural changes are necessary to effect change and provide safety for youth:

- Platform stakeholders must identify ways to disrupt the alt-right pipeline. White youth are often radicalized in small ways on social media and in gaming. A focus should be on how this happens and what processes could be put in place to protect users.
- There needs to be more interoperability between digital media and gaming platforms. Regulatory agencies often cite an inability to urge platforms to reduce harm in their spaces beyond what violates the terms of service. Third-party apps are also negatively impacting the ability of platforms to support their users.
- Digital platforms must have better reporting systems in place. Many of them have no idea about the extent of the racial harms on their platforms. And even more problematic, many don't even offer ways to report these kinds of harms.
- Gaming platforms must also offer real consequences for engaging in harmful racial and racist behavior. Too often, racist behaviors occur, and there are rarely consequences. There must be incentives built into the system to support prosocial behavior to reduce the attractiveness of harming these platforms.

## 4 Recommendations

There are many ways to confront and address the harms experienced by people of color in gaming. After our brief study into the harms experienced in gaming spaces above, we propose the following recommendations to address the issue:

- *Developing digital literacies around gaming technology and its influence on social structures and institutions*: Research in the field of design and decolonial studies emphasizes that enabling effective and ethical responses requires the development of critical digital literacies that go beyond the practicalities of how technologies work to include an understanding of the value systems, contexts, and consequences of their creation. This critical intention entails revealing how digital tools are inexorably intertwined with politics, social norms, and market forces, so much so that it is impossible to speak of one without the others. When this literacy is missing, design's transformative power is restricted to instrumental solutions, such as content moderation, rather than engaging in the possibility of resisting or reshaping our technologies through a more values-based imagination [23, 24].
- *Rethinking experience-based design*: Critical to any discussion on race and gaming is a need to rethink how we imagine, design, and implement our technologies in ways that challenge, rather than reproduce, structural inequalities. Along with companies needing to hire more diverse teams to broaden the perspectives being represented in games, design teams need to move away from designing *for* people to designing *with* people. In other words, acknowledging the expertise that comes from lived experience, while amplifying those who have been historically marginalized to play an active role in building their own socio-technical encounters. Instead of rushing to quick solutions, we must pause and ask ourselves "What values do we want our technologies to uphold?" "What cultures do we want to nurture?" And "Who needs to be included?"
- *Implementation of regulations against racism on gaming platforms*: We agree there needs to be better platform and network-level support to address racial concerns in digital spaces. We also suggest an essential shift toward more socio-technical solutions, including the addition of critical digital literacies for youth in education, and amplifying the voices of marginalized people in both mitigation efforts and in the design and development of online games. While we understand that techno-solutions only offer a portion of support to ease racial concerns in digital spaces, we also suggest that platforms have processes to address the harms that occur. Medical professionals/societies must call for stronger regulations and support educational efforts that teach youth to navigate digital spaces and tools. Such efforts would prevent harm to youth since racist harm is both a mental and physical health issue.

**Conflict of Interest and Funding Disclosures** None.

## References

1. Brown A. Who plays video games? Younger men, but many others too. Pew Research Center; 2017. Retrieved March 6, 2023, from https://www.pewresearch.org/fact-tank/2017/09/11/younger-men-play-video-games-but-so-do-a-diverse-group-of-other-americans/.
2. Nielsen. Nielsen Examines the Digital Habits and Impact of Black Consumers. September 2018. Nielsen. Accessed, March 6, 2023, from https://www.nielsen.com/news-center/2018/nielsen-examines-the-digital-habits-and-impact-of-black-consumers/.
3. Barr M, Copeland-Stewart A. Playing video games during the COVID-19 pandemic and effects on players' well-being. Games Cult. 2022;17(1):122–39.
4. Zhu L. The psychology behind video games during COVID-19 pandemic: a case study of animal crossing: new horizons. Hum Behav Emerg Technol. 2021;3(1):157–9.
5. Comerford C. Coconuts, custom-play, and COVID-19: social isolation, serious leisure, and personas in 'Animal crossing: new horizons'. Persona Studies. 2020;6(2):101–17.
6. TaeHyuk Keum B, Hearns M. Online gaming and racism: impact on psychological distress among Black, Asian, and Latinx emerging adults. Games Cult. 2022;17(3):445–60.

7. Ortiz SM. You can say I got desensitized to it': how men of color cope with everyday racism in online gaming. Sociol Perspect. 2019;62(4):572–88.
8. ADL Center for Technology and Society. Hate is no game: hate and harassment in online games. 2022.
9. Jenkins H. Convergence culture. New York: NYU Press; 2008.
10. Boyd D. Can social network sites enable political action? International Journal of Media and Cultural Politics. 2008;4(2):241–4.
11. Rheingold H. Smart mobs: the next social revolution. New York: Basic Books; 2002.
12. Everett A, Watkins C. The power of play: the portrayal and performance of race in video games. In: Salen K, editor. The ecology of games: connecting youth, games, and learning. Cambridge, MA: MIT Press; 2008. p. 141–66.
13. Nakamura L. Don't hate the player, hate the game: the racialization of labor in world of Warcraft. In: Brookey R, ed. Crit Stud Media Commun. Special issue on massively multiplayer online games. 2009;26(2):128–44.
14. Gray K. Race, gender, and deviance in Xbox live: theoretical perspectives from the virtual margins. London: Routledge; 2014.
15. Nakamura L. Watching white supremacy on digital video platforms: "screw your optics, I'm going in". Film Quart. 2019;72(3):19–22.
16. Cary LA, Chasteen AL. Prejudice norms in online gaming: game context and gamer identification as predictors of the acceptability of prejudice. Psychol Pop Media. 2022;11(4):367–81. https://doi.org/10.1037/ppm0000377.
17. Keum BT, Miller MJ. Racism on the internet: conceptualization and recommendations for research. Psychol Violence. 2018;8(6):782–91. https://doi.org/10.1037/vio0000201.
18. Speckhard A, Ellenberg A, Garret T. White supremacists speak: recruitment, radicalization, & experiences of engaging and disengaging from hate groups. International Center for the Study of Violent Extremism; 2022.
19. Dawson L. Trans people in the U.S.: identities, demographics, and wellbeing, 2023.
20. LGBT Data & Demographics – The Williams Institute – UCLA. The Williams Institute, https://williamsinstitute.law.ucla.edu/visualization/lgbt-stats/?topic=lgbt#demographic, n.d. Accessed 25 April 2024.
21. Richard GT, Gray KL. Gendered play, racialized reality: black Cyberfeminism, inclusive communities of practice, and the intersections of learning, socialization, and resilience in online gaming. Front J Women Stud. 2018;39(1):112–48. https://doi.org/10.5250/fronjwomestud.39.1.0112.
22. Gray KL, Sarkeesian A. Intersectional tech black users in digital gaming. Baton Rouge, Louisiana: Louisiana State University Press; 2020.
23. Friedman B, Hendry DG. *Value sensitive design: shaping technology with moral imagination*. Cambridge: MIT Press; 2019.
24. Escobar A. Designs for the Pluriverse: radical interdependence, autonomy, and the making of worlds. Durham: Duke University Press; 2017.

# Participation of Marginalized Youth in Designing a Machine Learning–Based Model to Identify Child Abuse and Neglect

Aviv Y. Landau, Hannah Espeleta, Siva Mathiyazhagan, Ashley Blanchard, Paul Heider, Kenrick Cato, Rochelle F. Hanson, Desmond Upton Patton, Leslie Lenert, and Maxim Topaz

## 1 Background

Child abuse and neglect is a worldwide public health concern [1]. In 2021, the United States Child Protective Services received nearly four million referrals [2]. These early traumatic experiences are defined as any action (physical, emotional, and/or sexual) taken or failure to act by a caregiver that results in harm, potential harm, or threat of harm to a child [3]. Child abuse and neglect is challenging to identify in clinical practice due to the lack of a "gold standard" objective assessment [4]. There is also agreement among health providers that existing biases may directly impact racial and social class differences seen across reporting, identification, and intervention practices for child abuse [5]. Compared to White children, Black children in the USA are twice as likely to be investigated by child protective services by the time they reach adulthood [6]. While millions of children are affected by abuse and neglect, there has been insufficient child participation in defining or measuring abuse and neglect, and efforts to gain their input in clinical assessments, decision-making, and prevention efforts have historically been low [7]. Obtaining

A. Y. Landau (✉) · S. Mathiyazhagan
School of Social Policy & Practice, University of Pennsylvania, Philadelphia, PA, USA
e-mail: landauay@upenn.edu

H. Espeleta · P. Heider · R. F. Hanson · L. Lenert
Medical University of South Carolina, Charleston, SC, USA

A. Blanchard
Department of Emergency Medicine, Columbia University Irving Medical Center, New York, NY, USA

K. Cato
University of Pennsylvania School of Nursing, University of Pennsylvania, Philadelphia, PA, USA

Children's Hospital of Philadelphia, University of Pennsylvania, Philadelphia, PA, USA

D. U. Patton
School of Social Policy & Practice, University of Pennsylvania, Philadelphia, PA, USA

Annenberg School for Communication, University of Pennsylvania, Philadelphia, PA, USA

Department of Child and Adolescent Psychiatry and Behavioral Sciences, University of Pennsylvania, Philadelphia, PA, USA

M. Topaz
Columbia University School of Nursing, Columbia University, New York, NY, USA

Columbia University Data Science Institute, Columbia University, New York, NY, USA


D. A. Christakis, L. Hale (eds.), *Handbook of Children and Screens*,
https://doi.org/10.1007/978-3-031-69362-5_41

information from youth in matters concerning child abuse and neglect can contribute to a better understanding of real-world problems affecting their lives [8].

The extensive implementation of electronic health records (EHRs) in clinical settings has presented new opportunities for developing machine learning (ML)-based models to identify potential child abuse and neglect [9]. Despite these innovative advancements, the development and implementation of ML-based models are complicated due to fragmented EHRs, such as scattered social, family, and medical histories within EHRs [10]. Furthermore, key ethical concerns arise, such as including EHR data with possible inherent racial biases and developing and evaluating ML-based models that predict nonstandardized definitions of child abuse and neglect. Additional ethical challenges include balancing model sensitivity and specificity when errors have high stakes and ensuring clinical providers, families, and children have the necessary resources following model determinations [11, 12].

To develop an ethical and inclusive ML-based model for identifying child abuse and neglect in healthcare settings, we recommend involving marginalized youth such as BIPOC communities, people with disabilities, LGBTQA+ communities, and other vulnerable communities as domain experts in the development and design. Promoting their lived experiences as expertise can aid ML developers in being reflexive and designing technological tools that apply a youth and social justice lens to ML-based model design. This can reduce the possibility that the same model designed to identify risk may expose youth to new or heightened risks. Thus, the focus of this chapter is to describe opportunities, challenges, and recommendations for engaging marginalized youth and their communities in developing ML-based models to detect child abuse and neglect.

## 2 Current State

The design of inclusive and ethical ML-based models in healthcare requires a design justice approach, which prioritizes working with domain experts, such as clinicians, caregivers, and marginalized youth. This section will describe the current state of developing ethical ML-based models to identify child abuse and neglect.

### 2.1 Applying a Design Justice Approach in ML

Recent research has identified inherent bias in the medical field related to treatment for people of color [13]. Similarly, ML implementation in medical systems is subject to potential biases present in EHR systems and thus requires (1) the development of ethical guidelines for ML developers and (2) a culture shift concerning the relationships between clinicians, patients, and ML-based tools [11]. To understand misconceptions and inherent biases that affect abuse and neglect identification, it is necessary not only to elicit professional perceptions of abuse and neglect but also to incorporate the voices of impacted communities [14].

Applying a design justice lens can help tackle current challenges. As Costanza-Chock defines in their book *Design Justice*: "Design justice rethinks design processes, centers people who are normally marginalized by design, and uses collaborative, creative practices to address the deepest challenges our communities face." [15] Specifically, integrating the voices of individuals from marginalized communities, key stakeholders, researchers, and designers can help to challenge inequality and include the perspectives of those most impacted by the design of these ML-based models [15]. Fostering collaboration between clinicians and community experts with lived experiences, such as Black and Latinx youth, can improve accountability and transparency in healthcare and is essential for producing high-quality healthcare advancements [16].

The following examples illustrate the implications and challenges of involving clinical, community, and marginalized youth expertise in identifying child abuse and neglect and reducing racial bias in the development of ML-based models.

## 2.2 Clinician Engagement

Emergency department clinicians, primary care pediatricians, and medical stakeholders have significantly contributed to developing and implementing ML-based child abuse and neglect models. With their guidance, researchers have developed an EHR lexicon of risk factors associated with child abuse and neglect [17], provided evidence-based recommendations for screening for child abuse and neglect [18], and considerations for developing a phenotype to identify child abuse and neglect with implications for reducing racial bias [19]. Furthermore, clinical provider insights can reveal racism in medical documentation and settings that do not explicitly concern child abuse and neglect by illustrating how marginalized communities are described in EHR and where there may be inequalities in the quality of care provided to marginalized communities [20]. To combat racism in healthcare, it is imperative that data science research addresses the social contexts that lead to inequalities [21, 22].

## 2.3 Primary Caregiver Engagement

Primary caregivers have participated in and contributed to developing and validating various medical technologies. Examples include the development of online screening tools to support their children's healthy lifestyle behaviors [23], evaluation of how a digital tool can be implemented to manage childhood asthma [24], and the development of a web-based resource to support parents who have children diagnosed with autism [25].

As discussed, there has been little involvement of primary caregivers in the development of an ML-based model to identify child abuse and neglect. However, in a recent study, Black and Latinx primary caregivers were interviewed to gain insights about child abuse and neglect and their experiences with health providers to enhance the development of an ML-based model to identify child abuse and neglect and reduce racial bias in emergency department settings [14]. Primary caregivers contributed valuable insights into the design of ML-based models for identifying child abuse and neglect. Their perspectives provided several challenges ML developers must consider when designing and developing child abuse and neglect identification tools, which include:

1. Defining child abuse and neglect from a primary caregiver lens.
2. Miscommunication between patient and health provider can potentially lead to misidentification of child abuse and neglect and impact medical documentation.
3. Potential harm to communities due to the outcome and implementation of the ML-based models to identify child abuse and neglect.

## 2.4 Youth Engagement in ML Design: A Way Forward

The United Nations has actively promoted children's rights, empowering them as citizens capable of making decisions for themselves [26]. Despite global commitments, past research has suggested that children's voices are yet to be heard in decision-making discussions with child protection systems concerning their life trajectories [27]. Furthermore, several challenges may arise when youth are involved in discussions concerning abuse and neglect, such as the tension between participation and protection and appropriate management of the power differential between a professional and a child's viewpoint [7].

Recently, there has been an increased interest in engaging youth in designing digital products, such as ML-based models [28]. However, an ML shift in designing medical technology that includes the perspective or voice of youth is still warranted [29]. Several challenges must be considered when engaging marginalized youth to participate in designing technological tools. For example, identifying safe and accessible locations for marginalized youth to participate, balancing the desired research outcomes and the relatively packed schedules of youth, shifting power dynamics between adult stakeholders and marginalized youth, and overseeing and implementing new participation models that ensure children's rights and best interests are addressed [30]. Furthermore, when engaging marginalized youth to participate in the development of ML-based models to identify child abuse and neglect with implications for reducing racial bias, ML designers must center lived experiences, consider how and from whom data are collected and analyzed, discuss how the algorithms are deployed, and clearly specify the main benefits of this technology [31].

## 3 Future Research

As research and clinical teams globally leverage EHR data to develop ML-based risk models that help identify children at risk, several key ML modeling, data, and implementation issues concerning marginalized youth participation must be addressed in future research.

- **What are the influential roles of youth participation in designing ML-based models for identifying abuse and neglect?** Future research should engage youth not only as research participants but also as domain experts in designing, developing, and deploying ML models. The design of ML-based models for identifying child abuse and neglect can benefit significantly from the lived experiences of marginalized youth in several ways. First, they can help codesign, evaluate, and validate the ML-based models, discuss the outcomes, and add insight regarding potentially biased identification of abuse and neglect cases. Second, youth can contextually annotate and label training data and help to explore racial bias within the EHRs. For example, a recent study showed that the EHR notes of Black patients had higher odds of containing "judgment words" implying doubt (e.g., "claims" or "insists") and language suggesting mistrust (e.g., had a "reaction" to the medication), compared to notes of White patients [32]. Third, marginalized youth can help researchers better understand how child abuse and neglect are defined and provide insights to guide identification. Fourth, marginalized youth can inform best practices for intervention when potential child abuse and neglect is identified. Finally, youth can assist ML developers in better ways to present ML outcomes to diverse audiences. To ensure that marginalized youth are supported in this process, ML developers must constantly communicate with the youth about how their work is incorporated and if they have additional feedback to provide. Furthermore, ML developers are responsible for the youth's safety (please see the section below) and compensation based on their work and expertise.
- **What are the best practices to assure the safety of youth participation?** Ensuring the safety of marginalized youth is critical in developing ML-based models with implications for real-world problems. Future research should explore the involvement of marginalized youth and how to share medical and potentially harmful EHR data with them. When developing an ML-based model to identify abuse and neglect, it is critical to examine ways to find balance when conflict arises between stakeholders regarding the outcome of potential abuse and neglect. In addition, researchers should consider including social workers, counselors, psychologists, and caregivers as support for youth who participate in sensitive technological projects.
- **How can youth participation in ML design aid research in reimagining ethics for understanding ML and child abuse and neglect?** ML ethics should not be limited to data-centric approaches and should consider child-centeredness. ML researchers and developers should work with youth, primary caregivers, and community stakeholders to develop and implement ML-based models to identify child abuse and neglect. This collaboration can reduce racial bias and provide a holistic understanding of a child and family's social and cultural context regarding family structures, marginalized communities, and relationships between families and child

protective services. Furthermore, youth insights can provide critical and innovative thoughts on how abuse and neglect are identified by ML-based models and ways for clinicians to intervene in a culturally sensitive manner.

## 4 Recommendations

We offer the following recommendations to key stakeholders as ways to promote meaningful youth participation in the ML design, development, and deployment process to identify child abuse and neglect.

### 4.1 For Researchers

- Engage both individually and as a collective marginalized youth, primary caregivers, and stakeholders as research collaborators, participants, data labelers, and domain experts in developing and implementing clinical decision support systems for identifying child abuse and neglect. By doing so, we can better understand the effects of child abuse and neglect and develop technology that is more responsible for children's well-being.
- Apply a reflexive approach to culturally contextualized data sets while working on ML-based models that deal with marginalized communities and real-world problems.
- ML-based risk models for child abuse and neglect must be designed with a high level of interpretability, accountability, and transparency to give clinicians and caregivers an understanding of how they work and why they should assess potential abuse and neglect to make more informed decisions.
- Promote interdisciplinary health research with youth as coleaders in the end-to-end research project development process, and allocate adequate funds to support their participation.
- Researchers should explore the implementation of ML-based models identifying child abuse and neglect in primary and emergency care settings to understand better how they impact care and the relationship between clinicians and patients.
- Researchers must inform and discuss potential risks and ethical concerns with domain experts when developing innovative technologies capable of enhancing surveillance and targeting marginalized communities.
- Researchers must provide financial compensation to domain experts who contribute their lived experience as experts in developing machine learning-based models to identify child abuse and neglect.

### 4.2 For Clinicians

- Clinicians should become familiar with how ML-based models work in order to address questions and concerns on ML classifications/recommendations from patients and their families.
- ML systems are not comprehensive decision-makers; clinicians are still responsible for asking follow-up questions, requiring knowledge, and making final decisions, such as reporting potential abuse and neglect to child protective services.
- Clinicians should be open to engaging marginalized youth in meaningful discussions concerning child abuse and neglect and how to prevent and intervene.
- Clinicians should be open to learning from marginalized youth's lived experiences and engage them as community experts/advisors in a reverse mentorship model.

### 4.3 For Educators

- Develop an innovative curriculum around ethical technology, and include youth participation to obtain feedback.
- Offer skill training to youth on coding, user research experiences, and design justice methods.
- Create accessible youth-centered fellowships across academic environments, which emphasize the importance of lived experiences in ML design.

### 4.4 For Policymakers

- Marginalized youth and their communities should be included as impacted groups in algorithmic accountability legislation to formalize their participation in ML research and model design.
- MedTech policies should be updated to include youth participation in developing ML-based models from beginning to end.
- Meaningfully engage youth in the policy development process to make child-friendly policies concerning child abuse and neglect intervention and prevention programs.

**Conflict of Interest and Funding Disclosure** This research was partially supported by the Seeds Grant Fund at the Data Science Institute at Columbia University. In addition, AYL was awarded the Haruv Institution post-doctoral fellowship for researching child abuse and neglect.

## References

1. Child maltreatment. Children's Bureau. 2019. https://www.acf.hhs.gov/cb/research-data-technology/statistics-research/child-maltreatment. Accessed 16 Mar 2023.
2. National Child Abuse Statistics from NCA. National Children's Alliance. 2021. https://www.acf.hhs.gov/cb/report/child-maltreatment-2021. Accessed 13 Mar 2023.
3. Child Welfare Information Gateway. 2022. https://www.childwelfare.gov/topics/can/defining. Accessed 31 Mar 2023.
4. Pandya NK, Baldwin KD, Wolfgruber H, Drummond DS, Hosalkar HS. Humerus fractures in the pediatric population: an algorithm to identify abuse. J Pediatr Orthop B. 2010;19(6):535–41. https://doi.org/10.1097/bpb.0b013e32833ce424.
5. Najdowski CJ, Bernstein KM. Race, social class, and child abuse: content and strength of medical professional's stereotypes. Child Abuse Negl. 2018;86:217–22. https://doi.org/10.1016/j.chiabu.2018.10.006.
6. Hymel KP, Laskey AL, Crowell KR, Wang M, Armijo-Garcia V, Frazier TN. Pediatric Brain Injury Research Network (PediBIRN) Investigators. Racial and ethnic disparities and bias in the evaluation and reporting of abusive head trauma. J Pediatr. 2018;198:137–143.e1. https://doi.org/10.1016/j.jpeds.2018.01.048.
7. Kosher H, Ben-Arieh A. Children's participation: a new role for children in the field of child maltreatment. Child Abuse Neglect. 2020;110(Pt 1):104429. https://doi.org/10.1016/j.chiabu.2020.104429.
8. Toros K. A systematic review of children's participation in child protection decision-making: tokenistic presence or not? Child Soc. 2021;35(3):395–411. https://doi.org/10.1111/chso.12418.
9. Office-based Physician Electronic Health Record Adoption. https://www.healthit.gov/data/quickstats/office-based-physician-electronic-health-record-adoption. Accessed 13 Mar 2023.
10. Jensen PB, Jensen LJ, Brunak S. Mining electronic health records: towards better research applications and clinical care. Nat Rev Genet. 2012;13(6):395–405.
11. Char DS, Shah NH, Magnus D. Implementing machine learning in health care – addressing ethical challenges. N Engl J Med. 2018;378(11):981–3. https://doi.org/10.1056/NEJMp1714229.
12. Landau AY, Ferrarello S, Blanchard A, et al. Developing machine learning-based models to help identify child abuse and neglect: key ethical challenges and recommended solutions. J Am Med Inf Assoc (JAMIA). 2022;29(3):576–80. https://www.ncbi.nlm.nih.gov/pubmed/35024859. https://doi.org/10.1093/jamia/ocab286.
13. Benjamin R. Assessing risk, automating racism. Science. 2019;366(6464):421–2. https://doi.org/10.1126/science.aaz3873.
14. Landau AY, Blanchard A, Atkins N, et al. Black and Latinx primary caregiver considerations for developing and implementing a machine learning-based model for detecting child abuse and neglect with implications for racial bias reduction: qualitative interview study with primary caregivers. JMIR Format Res. 2023;7:e40194. https://www.ncbi.nlm.nih.gov/pubmed/36719717. https://doi.org/10.2196/40194.
15. Costanza-Chock S. Design justice: community-led practices to build the worlds we need. Cambridge, MA: The MIT Press; 2020. https://openresearchlibrary.org/viewer/41b0401f-8601-4b5c-b434-6b4a32a44c8c. https://doi.org/10.7551/mitpress/12255.001.0001.
16. McLemore MR, Choo EK. The right decisions need the right voices. Lancet (Br Edition). 2019;394(10204):1133. https://doi.org/10.1016/S0140-6736(19)32167-1.
17. Hanson RF, Zhu V, Are F, Espeleta H, Wallis E, Heider P, Kautz M, Lenert L. Initial development of tools to identify child abuse and neglect in pediatric primary care. BMC Med Inform Decis Mak. 2023;23(1):266.
18. Berger RP, Saladino RA, Fromkin J, Heineman E, Suresh S, McGinn T. Development of an electronic medical record–based child physical abuse alert system. J Am Med Inform Assoc. 2018;25(2):142–9.
19. Landau AY, Blanchard A, Cato K, et al. Considerations for development of child abuse and neglect phenotype with implications for reduction of racial bias: A qualitative study. J Am Med Inform Assoc. 2022;29(3):512–9. https://www.ncbi.nlm.nih.gov/

pubmed/35024857. https://doi.org/10.1093/jamia/ocab275.
20. Johnson TJ. Intersection of bias, structural racism, and social determinants with health care inequities. Pediatrics (Evanston). 2020;146(2):1. https://search.proquest.com/docview/2434257069. https://doi.org/10.1542/peds.2020-003657.
21. Cogburn CD. Culture, race, and health: Implications for racial inequities and population health. Milbank Q. 2019;97(3):736–61. https://www.jstor.org/stable/45218864. https://doi.org/10.1111/1468-0009.12411.
22. Hardeman RR, Medina EM, Kozhimannil KB. Structural racism and supporting black lives – the role of health professionals. N Engl J Med. 2016;375(22):2113–5. https://doi.org/10.1056/NEJMp1609535.
23. Avis JL, Cave AL, Donaldson S, et al. Working with parents to prevent childhood obesity: protocol for a primary care-based eHealth study. JMIR Re Protoc. 2015;4(1):e35. https://www.ncbi.nlm.nih.gov/pubmed/25831265. https://doi.org/10.2196/resprot.4147.
24. Kan K, Shaunfield S, Kanaley M, et al. Parent experiences with electronic medication monitoring in pediatric asthma management: qualitative study. JMIR Pediatr Parent. 2021;4(2):e25811. https://www.ncbi.nlm.nih.gov/pubmed/33890861. https://doi.org/10.2196/25811.
25. Rabba AS, Dissanayake C, Barbaro J. Development of a web-based resource for parents of young children newly diagnosed with autism: participatory research design. JMIR Pediatr Parent. 2020;3(2):e15786. https://search.proquest.com/docview/2509656040. https://doi.org/10.2196/15786.
26. UNCRC – United Nations Committee on the Rights of the Child. General comment No. 12 (2009): The right of the child to be heard (CRC/C/GC/12); 2009. Refworld.org. https://www.refworld.org/docid/4ae562c52.html.
27. Toros K. A systematic review of children's participation in child protection decision-making: tokenistic presence or not? Child Soc. 2021;35(3):395–411. https://onlinelibrary-wiley-com.proxy.library.upenn.edu/doi/10.1111/chso.12418
28. Mathiyazhagan S, La Fors K. Children's right to participation in AI: exploring transnational co-creative approaches to foster child-inclusive AI policy and practice. Inform Polity. 2022:1–13. https://www.narcis.nl/publication/RecordID/oai:ris.utwente.nl:publications%2F707ea302-9af5-4d13-9cd5-73f36a36922a. https://doi.org/10.3233/IP-229014.
29. Psihogios AM, Lane-Fall MB, Graham AK. Adolescents are still waiting on a digital health revolution: Accelerating research-to-practice translation through design for implementation. Arch Pediatr Adolesc Med. 2022;176(6):545–6. https://doi.org/10.1001/jamapediatrics.2022.0500.
30. Cortesi S, Hasse A, Gasser U. Youth participation in a digital world: designing and implementing spaces, programs, and methodologies. SSRN Electr J. 2021;2021–5). http://www.econis.eu/PPNSET?PPN=1806337797 https://doi.org/10.2139/ssrn.3844115.
31. Patton D. Social work thinking for UX and AI design. Interactions. 2020;27(2):86–9. https://doi.org/10.1145/3380535.
32. Beach MC, Saha S, Park J, et al. Testimonial injustice: linguistic bias in the medical records of black patients and women. J Gen Intern Med. 2021;36(6):1708–14. https://doi.org/10.1007/s11606-021-06682-z.

# Radical and Untethered: The Health Benefits of Imagination in Virtual Reality for Black Youth

Courtney D. Cogburn, Valerie Jones Taylor, Prema Filippone, and Oyewole Oyekoya

## 1 Background

Imagination is a powerful social and revolutionary force [1]. In this chapter, we interrogate the role of immersive virtual technologies, such as virtual reality, in facilitating the health benefits of imagination for Black youth. The paramount focus on understanding and attenuating threats that digital media pose to health should be complemented by research examining ways digital media may enrich the lives of young people. Immersive technologies have the potential to fundamentally change the ways we observe, learn, think, interact, and engage [2]. Virtual reality (VR) has been described as the most psychologically powerful medium in history and one we still do not understand [3]. In this chapter, virtual reality is examined as an imaginative medium for Black youth that may promote health, healing, and well-being. The discussion of the current state of research provides a critical overview of seminal empirical and creative work using VR to examine race, racism, and Black life. This discussion also highlights the contributions and promise of racial embodiment in VR, critiques the limited scope of race-related content in VR and the need to extend beyond understanding the effects of VR on empathy and bias. The discussion of future research highlights associations between imaginations and health. Following an overview of a relatively sparse empirical literature linking health, medicine, and imagination, the concepts and health benefits of radical and untethered imagination are introduced as processes that may be supported through the use of VR. Three recommendations for racial embodiment and health equity research are also provided.

C. D. Cogburn (✉)
Columbia University, New York, NY, USA
e-mail: cc3803@columbia.edu

V. J. Taylor
Rutgers University, New Brunswick, NJ, USA

P. Filippone
New York University, New York, NY, USA

O. Oyekoya
City University of New York, New York, NY, USA

## 2 Current State

### 2.1 Racial Embodiment in VR

Embodied perspective taking has been used in VR to create the sensation of the self being located in a digital body [4]. Racial embodiment in immersive virtual reality (IVR) has commonly focused on White users embodying Black digital bodies in experiences ranging from observing one's digital form in a mirror, physically mimicking the movements, to more direct encounters with racial discrimination and racism [3]. White participants embodying Black avatars in VR have


D. A. Christakis, L. Hale (eds.), *Handbook of Children and Screens*,
https://doi.org/10.1007/978-3-031-69362-5_42

been associated with reductions in implicit racial bias toward Black people and increases in indicators of social rapport [4], but the findings are mixed. Banakou and colleagues [5] examined the effects of different contextual cues (neutral, positive, and negative) and found that negative social experiences are more likely to be associated with increases in implicit racial bias for White participants embodying Black avatars compared to neutral and positive social experiences. Broader debates raise more fundamental questions regarding whether and for whom empathetic growth is even possible [6–8]. Emotional empathy may be insufficient for promoting sustained behavioral changes or in the analysis and engagement of complex social issues [6]. Nakamura [7] extends this critique and describes the recreational engagement of various experiences of social oppressions in VR as "toxic empathy" that serves as an illusion of authentic empathy and engagement, particularly among White users. The benefits of perspective taking for empathy may also depend on context [5]. Some conditions of perspective taking in VR (competitive or negative experiences), for instance, have been associated with *increased* stereotyping and victim blaming.

A recent meta-analysis of VR and empathy research has also found that VR may be more effective at improving emotional (compassion) versus cognitive (understanding another perspective) empathy and may not be more effective than other, less expensive modes of inducing emotional empathy (e.g., reading about another's experience) [9]. The authors contend that while emotional empathy may be stirred by witnessing in VR, cognitive empathy is more likely moved by effortful engagement and imagination [9]. In the context of racial embodiment in VR, cognitive empathy may be best supported when observation is accompanied by efforts to construct meaning about the historical and contemporary context and one's own relationship to the suffering being observed [9]. In contrast, observation without engaging meaning making may be more likely to elicit emotional but not cognitive empathy [9]. While there is very little work examining issues related to race and health in VR, these findings suggest that embodiment, perspective taking, and other racialized experiences in VR may be leveraged to enhance structural competencies (i.e., how race and racism are understood, framed, and applied to the framing and responses to racial health inequities) among medical and health professionals and researchers.

## 3 Future Research

If a key aim of racial embodiment in VR is to understand and improve the social conditions that lead to racial prejudice, discrimination, and systemic inequities [5], how else might racial embodiment and other racialized experiences in VR be leveraged? One alternative would be to, in the design of VR experiences, conceptualize and engage the ways systems of racial oppression are misunderstood and misframed [10, 11]. Let us consider the case of health equity research and practice. Medical and health researchers are increasingly considering "upstream" social determinants of health and reckoning with the historical roots of racism in American medicine [12]. In spite of these shifts and an abundance of evidence documenting the importance of social factors for health, there remains resistance to accepting and meaningfully addressing these factors in research and practice [12, 13]. There is a need for medical and health researchers and practitioners to build competencies related to the role of institutions, systems, policies, and practices in the production of racial inequities in health [14–16]. The development of these competencies may be improved by experiences and education that (a) frame racism as structural rather than individual phenomenon and (b) place racial statistics into a broader social context, supporting the competencies related to diagnosing how racial and social inequities across multiple domains are created and sustained [14, 17, 18]. Immersive VR may not only be beneficial for racial embodiment and perspective taking but may also be used to contextually ground racial and other social inequities in a manner that promotes structural competency. There is an emerging body of academic research examining more complex themes of race and racism in VR. In *1000 Cut Journey* [10], researchers are beginning to examine the psychosocial benefits of experiencing racism from the perspective of a Black male in multiple contexts and moments across the life course. There are very few immersive VR experiences, to my knowledge, that directly engage historic and contemporary complexities of race and racism in relation to inequities in health. One exception is a project utilizing data visualization in VR to represent inequities in the effects of the COVID-19 virus in New York City [19].

### 3.1 Imagination and Health

As medical and health researchers are increasingly urged to consider "upstream" social determinants of health and to have a "more complete sense" of patient care [12, 15, 20], pediatric health research may also consider existential factors that underlie the health and well-being of children. What are the preventative factors that may help young people to maintain health [21], avoid sickness, motivate affirmative relationships with health earlier in life, and perhaps even support health in the face of chronic threats? Antonovsky [22] was a proponent of searching for the origins of health as a complement to understanding the origins of disease. How might imagination, for instance, help promote and sustain health origins? There is a long history of exploring associations between imagination and medicine [20, 23], including imagination being viewed as "essential to genius" and a catalyst for medical and scientific discovery. Imagination, in the form of visual imagery, hypnosis, or meditation, may also influence physiological and disease processes [23]. Imagination may contribute to changes in expectations, coping, or how one is relating to the experience of illness or pain. While empirical evidence linking imagination and health is sparse, there is compelling empirical work examining the effects of narrativization that suggest storytelling related to one's suffering or condition is a meaning-making process that can aggravate or alleviate health and well-being [23, 24]. Social psychological research, for instance, has demonstrated that telling stories about pain and trauma can lead to healing [24] and has been directly associated with decreased physical and emotional distress, use of health care services, and increased well-being over time [23]. Storytelling is distinct from memory with the former requiring imagination and the latter recollection. Memories reproduce facts, whereas storytelling, like imagination, is a more creative process that rearranges memory to contextualize, discover meaning, and produce new knowledge [20].

In addition to making meaning of and healing from painful pasts, imagining the future may also be particularly important for those who are navigating chronic and evolving crisis and uncertainty [25]. Psychological connectedness to one's future self is an important determinant of "intertemporal choice" [26] or the ability to elaborate on future outcomes and decision-making related to one's future. This may have implications for health in (1) being able to envision the possibility of longevity and health and (2) more firmly establishing a connection between health and health behaviors in the present to the future. Narrative futuring (e.g., imagining the future through storytelling) may build the capacity to anticipate and navigate crisis and change [25]. Individuals may be more likely to neglect their future selves when they lack imagination and empathy for the future self [26, 27]. Hershfield and colleagues [26] used immersive virtual reality and interactive decision aids to allow users to interact with realistic, age-progressed renderings of themselves. They found that participants who embodied future self-renderings were more likely to concretely identify with their future selves and in turn were more motivated to make investments toward their futures. The ability to imagine future possibilities has also been associated with mental flexibility, which is considered to be critical to psychological well-being [25]. For young people who sit at the margins of society and whose well-being is perpetually threatened as a result of their positionality, imagining and reclaiming the story of the future and their place in it is not only a revolutionary act but may also be healing and promotive of health. In the subsequent discussion, we consider the particular benefits of imaginative processes for Black children and youth. Immersive virtual reality and other immersive technologies may be particularly powerful media for narrative futuring and imagination.

## 3.2 Radical and Untethered Imaginations in VR

> Without an image of tomorrow, one is trapped by blind history, economics, and politics, beyond our control. One is tied up in a web, in a net, with no way to struggle free. Only by having clear and vital images of the many alternatives, good and bad, of where one can go, will we have any control over the way we may actually get there in a reality tomorrow will bring all too quickly [28].

In this chapter, we reflect on two forms of imagination: radical and untethered. This brief discussion explores how these different forms of imagining might be engaged using VR and speculates about the potential health and social benefits of such imaginings.

### 3.2.1 Radical Imagination

In *Freedom Dreams: The Black Radical Imagination*, Kelley [1] described imagination as a dimension of collective revolution and psychological resistance. Consistent with narrative futuring [25], Black radical imagination surmises that oppression and struggle may serve as a powerful catalyst for imagination. The benefit to imagination does not remove the responsibility for sociopolitical action to diminish social inequity but rather posits that those steeped in social oppression are uniquely positioned to offer the most radical visions of the future. Ruha Benjamin [29] contends that "most people are forced to live inside someone else's imagination" and that imagination is not a fanciful exercise but rather a battleground that must be reclaimed to "craft the worlds (we) cannot live without, just as we dismantle the worlds we cannot live within." The benefits of radical imagination for survival and the soul [1, 29] may extend to physical and mental health as well [25, 26].

### 3.2.2 Untethered Imagination

Radical imagination may be described as revolutionary—it responds to, exists in spite of, and is perhaps even birthed from oppression. But the idea of untethered imagination begins somewhere else or what Kevin Quashie [30] describes as Black aliveness. Untethered imagination occurs without obligation, productive purpose, promise, resolution, repair, or responsibility to anyone or anything—it is imagination for the sake of imagination, and it is free. But even the notion of freedom suggests a release from a source of control. In principle, aliveness does not require a release because it does not exist in relation to any source of control but rather simply is just being. Whereas radical imagination may be seen as a necessary burden rooted in reality, untethered imagination is unrealistic and impractical. In this form, imagination would not be tethered to or begin with reimagining alternatives to or revision systems of racial oppression but would begin from a place of those systems having never existed or being referenced in any way. What might be created if imaginaries began with aliveness or the feeling and circumstances of freedom or aliveness? What might be the benefits of imagining oneself in the future, not as someone who has survived oppression but simply as someone who is alive? The specific charge being made here is to consider the health benefits of such imaginings, particularly for Black youth. The politics, digital bias, and threats embedded in immersive and other emerging technologies cannot be ignored. It is paramount for digital studies and health research to understand and attenuate the seemingly boundless threats to child and adolescent health, but that approach is also incomplete. The lives and health of Black youth are, too often, framed exclusively through a lens of death, disparity, threat, and trauma. The concept of untethered imagination does not disregard the circumstances of reality but rather temporarily suspends belief in that reality in service of unencumbered discovery that very well may have benefits for health.

Achieving untethered imagination in practice, however, may be challenging. How does one separate thought from reality, particularly when one's reality is mired in various systems of oppression? Virtual reality and other immersive and integrated technologies may be a medium that may support both radical and untethered imagination. It is possible that immersive virtual environments may function, at least symbolically, as a digital *tabula rasa*—a blank slate for the imaginings of Black youth. As opposed to regulating harassment and threats online, what might Black youth imagine if tasked with designing a social space where they feel free, alive, or to build an environment where they can be anyone or do anything? Perhaps most importantly, how might the health of Black youth benefit from engaging in processes that align their present and future selves and assume agency and control in designing the future? In addition to the possible benefits to their own health, how might our social collective benefit from the radical and untethered imaginations of Black youth? To imagine oneself in the future when consumed by a present that seeks to erase you is a revolutionary act, but to imagine merely for the sake of imagining embodies aliveness.

What would it mean to consider Black aliveness? [30]

## 4 Recommendations

- Empirical evidence evaluating factors that protect and maintain the health of Black youth is just as important as research seeking to identify threats to their health.
- Racial embodiment and other racialized experiences in immersive virtual reality must move beyond its near-exclusive aim to build empathy and reduce bias among dominant social groups (e.g., White people).
- The act of "witnessing" racial pain and trauma in racial embodiment VR can falsely juxtapose the user as a neutral observer as opposed to a participant and beneficiary of the oppression being observed. In order to build capacity for anti-racist analysis, practice, and research, this work will need to move toward building empirical evidence related to the development of critical self-awareness, social consciousness, and structural competency.
- It is shortsighted to only use VR to represent the past and present, and these technologies should also be leveraged to imagine and design the future. Black youth may be particularly well positioned to leverage these technologies to radically imagine the alternatives to social injustice and the circumstances of aliveness.
- Black youth imaginations may not only prove valuable to maintaining and protecting their own health but may very well protect us all.

**Conflict of Interest and Funding Disclosure** None.

## References

1. Kelley DG. Freedom dreams: the black radical imagination. 20th Anniversary ed. Beacon Press: Boston; 2022.
2. Ball M. The Metaverse: and how it will revolutionize everything. New York: W.W. Norton and Company; 2022.
3. Bailenson J. Experience on demand: what virtual reality is, how it works and what it can do. W.W. Norton and Company; 2018.
4. Gall D, Roth D, Stauffert J-P, Zarges J, Latoschik ME. Embodiment in virtual reality intensifies emotional responses to virtual stimuli. Front Psychol. 2021;12:674179.
5. Banakou D, Beacco A, Neyret S, Blasco-Oliver M, Seinfeld S, Slater M. Virtual body ownership and its consequences for implicit racial bias are dependent on social context. R Soc Open Sci. 2020;7(12):201848.
6. Bloom P. Empathy and its discontents. Trends Cogn Sci. 2017;21(1):24–31.
7. Nakamura L. Feeling good about feeling bad: Virtuous virtual reality and the automation of racial empathy. J Vis Cult. 2020;19(1):47–64.
8. Sora-Domenjó C. Disrupting the "empathy machine": the power and perils of virtual reality in addressing social issues. Front Psychol. 2022;13:1–13.
9. Martingano AJ, Hererra F, Konrath S. Virtual reality improves emotional but not cognitive empathy: A meta-analysis. Technol Mind Behav. 2021;2:1–39.
10. Cogburn CD, Bailenson J, Ogle E, Asher T, Nichols T. 1000 cut journey. In: ACM SIGGRAPH; 2018. p. 1–1.
11. Roswell RO, Cogburn CD, Tocco J, Martinez J, Bangeranye C, Bailenson JN, Wright M, Mieres JH, Smith L. Cultivating empathy through virtual real-

ity: advancing conversations about racism, inequity, and climate in medicine. Acad Med. 2020;95(12): 1882–6.
12. Bailey Z, Feldman JM, Bassett MT. How structural racism works – racist policies as a root cause of U.S. racial health inequities. N Engl J Med. 2021;384(8):768–73.
13. Haslam SA, McMahon C, Cruwys T, et al. Social cure, what social cure? The propensity to underestimate the importance of social factors for health. Soc Sci Med. 2018;198:14–21.
14. Metzl JM, Hansen H. Structural competency: theorizing a new medial engagement with stigma and inequality. Soc Sci Med. 2014;103:126–33.
15. Ray R, Lantz PM, Williams D. Upstream policy changes to improve population health and health equity: a priority agenda. Milbank Q. 2023;101(S1):20–35.
16. Phelan JC, Link BG. Is racism a fundamental cause of inequalities in health? Annu Rev Sociol. 2015;41:311–30.
17. Salter PS, Adams G, Perez MJ. Racism in the structure of everyday worlds: a cultural-psychological perspective. Curr Dir Psychol Sci. 2018;27(3):150–5.
18. Rucker J, Duker A, Richeson J. Structurally unjust: how lay benefits about racism relate to perceptions of and responses to racial inequality in criminal justice. 2019. https://doi.org/10.31234/osf.io/sjkeq
19. Goetschel E, Sekaran J, Ren W, He M, Ogbonnaya N, Nkereuwem M, Mapfunde I, Martin C, Cogburn CD, Feiner S. COVIZ: visualization of effects of COVID-19 on New York City through socially impactful virtual reality. In: IEEE conference on virtual reality and 3D user interfaces; 2021. https://doi.org/10.1109/VRW52623.2021.00234.
20. Altschuler S. The medical imagination: literature and health in the early United States. University of Pennsylvania Press; 2018.
21. Rush B. Lectures on the mind. JAMA J Am Med Assoc. 1981;246(16):1839–40.
22. Antonovsky A. Unraveling the mystery of health: how people manage stress and stay well. Josey-Bass; 1987.
23. Kirmayer LJ. Toward a medicine of imagination. New Lit Hist. 2006;37(3):583–601.
24. Pennbaker J, editor. Emotion, disclosure, and health. Washington, DC: American Psychological Association; 1995.
25. Sools A, Hein MJ. Towards narrative futuring in psychology: becoming resilient by imagining the future. Grad J Soc Sci. 2012;9(2):203–26.
26. Hershfield HE, Goldstein DG, Sharpe WF, et al. Increasing saving behavior through age-progressed renderings of the future self. J Mark Res. 2011;48:S23–37.
27. Parfit D. Personal identity. Philos Rev. 1971; 80(1):3–27.
28. Delany SR. Starboard wine. Revised ed. Middletown: Wesleyan University Press; 1984.
29. Benjamin R. Virtual commencement speech at the Columbia University School of Social Work, May 20, 2020. https://socialwork.columbia.edu/news/prof-ruha-benjamin-calls-on-class-of-2020-to-become-champions-of-the-social-contract/. Accessed 12 May 2023.
30. Quashie K. Black aliveness, or a poetics of being. Durham: Duke University Press; 2021.

# Online Resistance: The Past, Present, and Future of Challenging Racism with Digital Tools

Rob Eschmann, Nkemka Anyiwo, Noor Toraif, and Stephanie M. Ortiz

## 1 Background

What does it mean to resist racism? The most robust sociological definitions of racism suggest that racism is both attitudinal and structural: A racist ideology is a way of viewing race that supports and legitimates systems of racial inequality [3]. Resistance to racism, therefore, can take different forms, as people resist different manifestations of racism, from the macro—oppressive laws, policies, and institutions—to the micro—interpersonal experiences with racism, both overt and covert.

At a structural level, resistance can be direct action, protest, voting, and lobbying for change against unjust policies and programs. Interpersonal resistance can include direct challenges to microaggressions or racism, or building community among marginalized groups, providing space for healing, growth, or survival [4]. On an individual level, resistance might be self-care—choosing to devote time or energy to rest, in the midst of hostile racial environments [5].

Digital tools can amplify resistance efforts at all levels, as online users and activists create space for community growth and support across geographic boundaries, organize users to engage in collective or direct action, and facilitate the widespread sharing of anti-racist and anti-oppressive ideas, actions, and imaginaries. Digital resistance can change racial power dynamics as users challenge racism embedded in behaviors and attitudes that are often seen as being normal in a racial capitalist society [1].

In one of the earliest studies of online resistance against racism, André Brock wrote about Black bloggers during Hurricane Katrina [6]. As legacy media sources vilified Black people suffering at the hands of civic neglect during the natural disaster and its aftermath, Black bloggers disseminated counternarratives that challenged the racialized and racist framing of Hurricane survivors. These bloggers brought attention to the wide gulf separating the biased framing of Black communities by traditional, mainstream media, and critical narratives coming from marginalized groups.

While media bias is regretfully still an issue, digital tools provide activists and online users with access to ways to challenge dominant narratives and share critical and diverse narratives. For example, in a study mapping the influence of Twitter users, Groshek and Tandoc [7] found that

R. Eschmann (✉) · N. Anyiwo
Columbia University, School of Social Work, New York, NY, USA
e-mail: r.eschmann@columbia.edu

N. Toraif
University of Pennsylvania, School of Social Policy and Practice, Philadelphia, PA, USA

S. M. Ortiz
University of Massachusetts, Sociology Department, Lowell, MA, USA


D. A. Christakis, L. Hale (eds.), *Handbook of Children and Screens*,
https://doi.org/10.1007/978-3-031-69362-5_43

Black activists were the biggest hubs for information sharing during the Protests in Ferguson—even bigger than mainstream and traditional media accounts. Black Twitter (and Black women on Twitter, more specifically) has been central to bringing intersectional analyses of racism and anti-Black police violence to the mainstream, highlighting not just racism but also the ways racism intersects with other forms of oppression, including sexism, homophobia, ableism, or classism [8]. Activism-based hashtags (like #SayHerName) that challenge dominant and oppressive narratives and actions bring attention to activist and organizing demands for change [8]. Online campaigns like these are powerful and give everyday people the power to contribute to collective resistance against mainstream narratives and policies that continue and normalize racist ideologies.

Social media and online communication have been central to large-scale resistance efforts over the past decade, including the Movement for Black Lives, the #MeToo Movement, and the Arab Spring. No hashtag has been used more than #BlackLivesMatter. Beyond these large-scale movements, research finds that many young people feel more comfortable challenging racism online than they do in-person. In this chapter, we explore the current state of research on online resistance, discuss how future research can build on this body of knowledge, and make recommendations for scholars, activists, and educators who are invested in understanding and utilizing digital tools to empower online resistance to racism and oppression.

We situate our analysis of online resistance in adolescence and emerging adulthood—developmental periods where youth grapple with their identity, develop their ideologies about the world, and contend with dynamic, increasingly complex forms of racism that can threaten their safety, health, and life trajectory [9]. For youth who came of age as digital natives, the online context provides a unique, accessible space to explore their identity, assert their voice, build community, and challenge hegemonic racial structures that threaten their wellbeing [2, 10]. Online resistance may be a particularly salient tool for youth who are politically disenfranchised as it allows them to reclaim their power and have access to novel forms of political participation [11, 12]. While we emphasize empirical investigations of youth engaging in resistance work, we may also explore broader resistance activities that shape the styles, tools, and resistance possibilities for youth in online spaces.

## 2 Current State

### 2.1 Collective Action for Consciousness Raising and Racial Justice

The online space has been a quintessential context for today's youth to engage in organizing for consciousness raising and collective action. Mainstream media can reproduce racial hierarchies that can inform youth's self-concepts and perpetuate victim blaming [13, 14]. However, youth have used social media as a tool for storytelling that allows them to bear witness to harm inflicted on racially marginalized communities and present counternarratives of stereotypes [15–17]. For example, in response to the media coverage of Michael Brown, a 17-year-old Black boy killed in Ferguson, Missouri by police officer Darren Wilson, Black youth used the hashtag #IfTheyGunnedMeDown coupled with images of themselves to engage in "visual resistance" to challenge the villainization of Black victims of violence in the media [18]. In addition to racial justice hashtags, youth use a multitude of tools online to facilitate their resistance. For example, in their analysis of the Philadelphia Student Union—a longstanding student-led advocacy—Conner and Slatter found that youth created media (e.g., music, videos, and podcasts) and utilized online communication and documentation tools such as Facetime and Dropbox as strategies to organize around educational inequities [19]. Youth's multifaceted strategies for online resistance serve to galvanize racial justice actions offline and online around issues like educational inequities [12, 20, 21], immigration [22], and policing [23].

Youth's engagement in online action may be catapulted by their belief in media as a transformative tool. For example, in a qualitative study, examining the effects of online vicarious racism on adolescents of diverse backgrounds, youth identified online activism (e.g., sharing stories, challenging racist comments) as a tool to heal from media-based racism [24]. However, online action may also come at a cost. Youth described being targeted with racial epithets and threatened, experiencing surveillance for speaking up online and experiencing marginalization from adults who devalue the significance of their online activism [15, 25]. Thus, examining youth's online collective action must also include an examination of the psychological and emotional implications of their work and how they navigate complex stressors.

## 2.2 Cultivating Spaces of Care and Joy

Although less commonly examined, emerging scholarship has considered the ways that racially marginalized youth utilize the online sector to cultivate spaces of healing, care, and joy. Scholars argue that digital spaces can provide context for community building, identity exploration, and engagement in radical imagination that create liberated realities [10, 26]. Youth organizers described using digital space to build community, envision futures, engage in self-love, and receive emotional support as they navigated the stresses of organizing against oppression [17]. Indeed, youth have identified organizing as a tool for collective self-care to heal from historical trauma [27]. As they heal, racially marginalized communities use social media as a tool to build narratives of Black youth joy and thriving irrespective of and despite racial oppression (e.g., #BlackBoyJoy and #BlackgirlMagic) [28, 29]. Recent research suggests that Black youth draw on such presentations in social media to construct affirming intersectional identities [28]. Using social media, online users can leverage and sidestep algorithmic oppression in order to circulate anti-racist content [30].

Wilf and Wray-Lake show how youth involved with Black Lives Matter ascribe a variety of meanings and purposes to their civic engagement online, such as envisioning new futures, allyship and emotional support of a community, and holding others accountable [17]. Taken together, the online sector may be a unique space for youth to engage in collective community spaces where they can safely explore their identity and engage in care for each other and ground themselves in uplifting narratives as they navigate multisystemic forms of oppression.

## 2.3 Interpersonal Resistance

Apart from broader organizing and activist efforts, research has found that online tools also enable new forms of resistance on an interpersonal level. For example, Ortiz [31] found that while women of color college students do not necessarily consider themselves activists for their efforts, they nevertheless care for each other and call out racist and sexist students online as forms of resistance, particularly in the absence of institutional mechanisms of protection and accountability. This is unique, especially given the large literature on racism and microaggressions on college campuses, which suggests that students of color rarely challenge microaggressions directly; students of color discuss witnessing and participating in more responses to racism online than in person, a practice that can upend the racial power dynamics that privilege silence in response to racism or microaggressions in mainstream, face-to-face settings [1].

In one of the only quantitative studies of the effectiveness of online resistance to racism, Eschmann et al. [32] found that among users who were anti-Colin Kaepernick (the NFL quarterback who knelt during the national anthem to protest anti-Black police violence), those who received more messages in response to their posts on on Twitter were more likely to make concessions (i.e. admit that Kaepernick had the right to protest or was protesting for a valid reason). Challenging racist narratives online, it seems, can lead to attitude change.

## 3 Future Research

As online spaces increasingly serve as platforms for youth to build community and organize, digital resistance to racism has continued to evolve as a crucial area of research. As such, understanding the contours of digital resistance—including the strategic utilization of digital tools for mobilizing direct action and fostering solidarity—is necessary for building a digital landscape that is more inclusive, equitable, and just. To advance knowledge in this area, future research directions on digital resistance should explore both the forms of this resistance and their efficacy. This includes investigating how digital activism translates into real-world activism, examining the mechanisms through which online movements gain momentum, and identifying the factors that contribute to successful online–offline mobilization.

Second, researchers should investigate the role and scope of AI as a tool for organizing digital resistance. AI technologies may enhance the efficiency and reach of organizing initiatives, automate logistics and tasks, and provide data-driven insights to organizers on the reach of their efforts. Investigating the use of AI in organizing can shed light on how it may diminish or amplify the voices of marginalized communities and its potential for expanding the political power of historically silenced populations.

Another significant research direction involves the development, implementation, and evaluation of democratic and participatory coding interventions aimed at reducing algorithmic bias. As scholars have demonstrated in prior research, algorithms have perpetuated various forms of discrimination and particularly racial discrimination. Research should investigate the outcomes of incorporating democratic principles and involving diverse stakeholders in the coding process as a mechanism for mitigating biases and ensuring the accountability of new technological developments to the people and communities they impact.

Finally, advocates and organizers in both offline and online spaces draw attention to the importance of intersectional frameworks in responding to and resisting oppression. These frameworks recognize that people with different identities have unique experiences of both privilege and oppression. Researchers should investigate the types of intersectional analyses present in the digital landscape, including how they are negotiated, contested, and affirmed, as well as the extent to which these intersectional approaches permeate digital resistance initiatives and platforms.

## 4 Recommendations

- Resistance to racism online intersects with other systemic inequities. Practitioners, researchers, and educators will be much better positioned to intervene in online racism and support resistance efforts if we understand that people of color are not only resisting racism online but are also resisting homophobia, colorism, transphobia, fatphobia, misogyny, colonization, ableism, and other forms of structural violence which rely on and reproduce racism. Honoring intersectionality should involve taking cues from activists and everyday people who create and deploy strategies to resist racism across space and across issues.
- While online resistance is often conceptualized as a safer form of organizing in that there are no *physical* confrontations involved, these forms of resistance are not without real costs to the people who do the work. There is immense stress involved in online resistance which practitioners should be attuned to in order to address mental health consequences. Furthermore, those who resist racism may be at risk for doxxing, hacking, and stalking and need financial support to protect themselves and recover from cyberattacks.
- In order to support resistance efforts, educators must take online racism itself seriously. We recommend redesigning curricula to include and validate the online experiences of people of color, who are often told those interactions are not "real."
- Conversations around forms of resistance are also crucial, especially during this

sociopolitical moment when such discussions are the target of a white backlash. Learning activities can be designed to empower students to collectively organize and resist the silences they might otherwise adopt.

- We also recommend connecting students to community resources and activists who will foster sustained resistance efforts and incorporate youth into a community. Resistance efforts can also be bolstered through algorithmic reparations [33]. Practitioners, politicians, educators, and scholars should hold tech accountable and demand changes around how AI is designed and deployed, especially considering such tools are used for surveillance and to criminalize people of color who do resist online and offline. In service of this, efforts to assess and audit algorithms must recognize people of color and other marginalized communities as domain experts in their own right.

**Conflict of Interest and Funding Disclosures** None.

## References


1. Eschmann R. Digital resistance: how online communication facilitates responses to racial microaggressions. Sociol Race Ethn. 2021;7(2):264–77. https://doi.org/10.1177/2332649220933307.
2. Anyiwo N, Palmer GJ, Garrett JM, Starck JG, Hope EC. Racial and political resistance: an examination of the sociopolitical action of racially marginalized youth. Curr Opin Psychol. 2020;35:86–91.
3. Bobo L. Racism in Trump's America: reflections on culture, sociology, and the 2016 US presidential election. Br J Sociol. 2017;68:S85–S104. https://doi.org/10.1111/1468-4446.12324.
4. Eschmann R. When the Hood comes off: racism and resistance in the digital age. University of California Press; 2023.
5. Bell H. Yearning: race, gender, and cultural politics. South End Press; 1990.
6. Brock A. Race matters. African Americans on the web following Hurricane Katrina. In: Proceedings of cultural attitudes towards communication and technology; 2008. p. 91–105. http://sammelpunkt.philo.at:8080/2376/. Accessed 21 Sept 2016.
7. Groshek J, Tandoc E. The affordance effect: gatekeeping and (non)reciprocal journalism on Twitter. Comput Hum Behav. 2017;66:201–10. https://doi.org/10.1016/j.chb.2016.09.020.
8. Jackson SJ, Bailey M, Welles BF. #HashtagActivism: networks of race and gender justice. MIT Press; 2020.
9. Hope EC, Hoggard LS, Thomas A. Emerging into adulthood in the face of racial discrimination: physiological, psychological, and sociopolitical consequences for African American youth. Transl Issues Psychol Sci. 2015;1(4):342.
10. Tynes BM, Coopilton M, Schuschke J, Stewart A. Toward developmental science that meets the challenges of 2044: afrofuturist development theory, design, and praxis. In: Diversity and developmental science: bridging the gaps between research, practice, and policy. Springer; 2023. p. 245–70.
11. Cohen CJ, Kahne J. Participatory politics: new media and youth political action. Youth and Participatory Politics Research Network; 2012. https://ypp.dmlcentral.net/sites/default/files/publications/Participatory_Politics_New_Media_and_Youth_Political_Action.2012.pdf. Accessed 18 July 2016.
12. Stornaiuolo A, Thomas EE. Disrupting educational inequalities through youth digital activism. Rev Res Educ. 2017;41(1):337–57.
13. Anyiwo N, Richards-Schuster K, Jerald MC. Using critical media literacy and youth-led research to promote the sociopolitical development of Black youth: strategies from "Our Voices". Appl Dev Sci. 2021;25(3):201–16.
14. Dukes KN, Gaither SE. Black racial stereotypes and victim blaming: implications for media coverage and criminal proceedings in cases of police violence against racial and ethnic minorities. J Soc Issues. 2017;73(4):789–807.
15. Kelly LL. A snapchat story: how black girls develop strategies for critical resistance in school. Learn Media Technol. 2018;43(4):374–89.
16. George Mwangi CA, Bettencourt GM, Malaney VK. Collegians creating (counter)space online: a critical discourse analysis of the I, Too, Am social media movement. J Divers High Educ. 2018;11(2):146–63. https://doi.org/10.1037/dhe0000054.
17. Wilf S, Wray-Lake L. "That's how revolutions happen": psychopolitical resistance in Youth's online civic engagement. J Adolesc Res. 2021:07435584211062121.
18. Gross N. # IfTheyGunnedMeDown: the double consciousness of Black youth in response to oppressive media. Souls. 2017;19(4):416–37.
19. Conner J, Slattery A. New media and the power of youth organizing: minding the gaps. Equity Excell Educ. 2014;47(1):14–30.
20. George Mwangi CA, Bettencourt GM, Malaney VK. Collegians creating (counter) space online: a critical discourse analysis of the I, Too, Am social media movement. J Divers High Educ. 2018;11(2):146.
21. Reynolds R, Mayweather D. Recounting racism, resistance, and repression: examining the experiences and# hashtag activism of college students with critical race theory and counternarratives. J Negro Educ. 2017;86(3):283–304.
22. Clark R. "Hope in a hashtag": the discursive activism of #WhyIStayed. Fem Media Stud.

2016;16(5):788–804. https://doi.org/10.1080/14680777.2016.1138235.
23. Welton AD, Harris TO. Youth of color social movements for racial justice: the politics of interrogating the school-to-prison pipeline. Educ Policy. 2022;36(1):57–99.
24. Heard-Garris N, Ekwueme PO, Gilpin S, et al. Adolescents' experiences, emotions, and coping strategies associated with exposure to media-based vicarious racism. JAMA Netw Open. 2021;4(6):e2113522.
25. Fine M, Finesurrey S, Rodriguez A, Almonte J, Contreras A, Lam A. "People are demanding justice": pandemics, protests, and remote learning through the eyes of immigrant youth of color. J Adolesc Res. 2021;36(5):437–66.
26. Volpe VV. "Easier said than done": a qualitative investigation of Black emerging adults coping with multilevel racism. Cult Divers Ethn Minor Psychol. 2021;27(3):495. https://doi.org/10.1037/cdp0000446.
27. Ortega-Williams A. Organizing as "Collective-Self" care among African American youth in precarious times. J Afr Am Stud. 2021;25(1):3–21.
28. Rogers LO, Butler Barnes S, Sahaguian L, Padilla D, Minor I. # BlackGirlMagic: using multiple data sources to learn about Black adolescent girls' identities, intersectionality, and media socialization. J Soc Issues. 2021;77(4):1282–304.
29. Williams KD, Dougherty SA, Lattie EG, Guidry JP, Carlyle KE. Examining hashtag use of# blackboyjoy and# theblackmancan and related content on Instagram: descriptive content analysis. JMIR Form Res. 2022;6(8):e34044.
30. Peterson-Salahuddin C. "Pose": examining moments of "digital" dark sousveillance on TikTok. New Media Soc. 2022:14614448221080480. https://doi.org/10.1177/14614448221080480.
31. Ortiz SM. Call-in, call-out, care, and cool rationality: how young adults respond to racism and sexism online. Soc Probl. 2021;70:665.
32. Eschmann R, Groshek J, Li S, Turaif N, Thompson J. Bigger than sports: identity politics, Colin Kaepernick, and concession making in #BoycottNike. Comput Hum Behav. 2021;114:106583. https://doi.org/10.1016/j.chb.2020.106583.
33. Davis JL, Williams A, Yang MW. Algorithmic reparation. Big Data Soc. 2021;8(2):20539517211044808.

# Introduction to the Section on Gender, Sexuality, and Digital Media

Megan K. Maas

Adolescence is a developmental period of transition and experimentation, marked by significant physical, emotional, social, and cognitive changes. Sexual development is an integral part of this transition, and the use of media and technology to learn about and engage in sexual experiences has become increasingly prevalent among adolescents. The availability of pornography, social media, sexual health websites, and dating apps has revolutionized the way adolescents explore and express their sexuality. However, these technologies and other media pose the potential to influence adolescent behavior, both positively and negatively. This section provides an overview of the academic research on the role of media and technology use in the development of gender and sexuality among children and adolescents.

## 1 Representation of Gender and Sex in Entertainment Media and Pornography

For children, film and television shows offer a way to learn more about abstract concepts such as gender roles and stereotypes through the experiences of the characters they watch. This process is part of broader gender socialization, where children incorporate observations of commonalities within and differences between gender groups. Dr. Jennifer Stevens Aubrey (see Chap. 45) and colleagues discuss how entertainment media for youth represent gender in such a way that supports many commonly held gender stereotypes. For example, male characters still outnumber female characters in film and television programming made for youth [1, 2]. Male characters are also depicted as larger and more muscular [2, 3], whereas female characters are often sexualized and expected to be thin [1, 2, 4], occupying less space than male characters. This binary betrayal reinforces ideas that boys and men are more important and powerful than girls and women. Gender stereotypes are also reinforced by dividing interests, hobbies, and occupations by gender, where male characters are more likely to be interested in and/or performing in STEM activities and female characters are seen more in caretaking roles or interested in the arts and humanities [1–3]. In response to the very recent expansion of racially and ethnically diverse characters in entertainment media for youth, Dr. Aubrey and colleagues have called for more content analyses that address intersecting identities (e.g., race and gender) within characters to chart how representations of gender are changing over time.

As interest in sexuality and romantic relationships accelerates after puberty, adolescents

M. K. Maas (✉)
Michigan State University, East Lansing, MI, USA
e-mail: maasmeg1@msu.edu


D. A. Christakis, L. Hale (eds.), *Handbook of Children and Screens*,
https://doi.org/10.1007/978-3-031-69362-5_44

become more oriented toward media that contain sexual or romantic content. Although explicit sexual behavior is not seen in entertainment medium that is created for youth, sexual innuendos, discussions about sex, and sexual behaviors are frequently depicted. Heterosexual experiences showcasing the sexual double standard are central [5]. For example, boys are typically depicted as obsessed with sex, whereas girls are depicted as the ones who have to cope with the negative consequences for sexual experiences [5, 6]. Portrayals of LGBTQ+ sexual relationships are rare [5]. However, Dr. Lauren McInroy (see Chap. 46) and colleagues discuss how emerging new media, particularly shows on Netflix such as Sex Education and Heartstopper, have been found to be enjoyable and affirming for LGBTQ+ youth, which suggests a promising shift for future viewers. In addition to sexual content in traditional media, adolescents are viewing sexually explicit material on mainstream Internet pornography websites. The sexual behavior portrayed on "tube site" platforms similar to YouTube mimics the sexual double standard and often feature acts of aggression or even violence [7, 8]. Even while seemingly consensual, studies have shown that pornography often portrays women as submissive and passive, whereas men are depicted as dominant and in control [7–9]. Thus, a great deal of attention has been paid to investigating the role of pornography use in the sexual socialization of youth.

## 2 Seeking Sexual Norms and Sexual Health Information Online

As Drs. Megan Maas (see Chap. 47) and Eric Walsh-Buhi (see Chap. 48) and their colleagues discuss in their respective chapters, the absence or inconsistent implementation of comprehensive sex education (particularly, in the USA) has led many young people to turn to Internet pornography to learn about sex. Although heterosexual cisgender male adolescents are the largest group of underage consumers of pornography, LGBTQ+ youth have been shown to seek out pornography more often and at younger ages than their cisgender, heterosexual peers [10]. Pornography use appears to be a poor source of sex education for youth, as the use of pornography among adolescents has been found to be associated with various harmful sexual beliefs and perceptions. Studies have demonstrated that frequent consumption of pornography is linked to more recreational attitudes toward sex, particularly among cisgender boys [11, 12]. Adolescents who use pornography have also been found to hold more erroneous beliefs about sex, such as the belief that most people prefer rough to gentle sex [13]. The frequency of pornography use has also been shown to be associated with greater acceptance of rape myths, particularly for violent pornography.

In contrast to pornography, sexual health websites provide generally safe, non-embarrassing, and standardized ways for adolescents to learn about body parts, sexual processes, and other sensitive topics essential for promoting healthy sexual development [14, 15]. As Dr. Eric Walsh-Buhi and colleagues detail, a growing number of adolescents are turning to the Internet for sexual health information, mostly due to privacy reasons, particularly for LGBTQ+ youth [15–17]. As both Drs. McInroy and Walsh-Buhi and their colleagues report in their respective chapters, gender diverse youth seek out sexual health information online more often than their cisgender peers because they face many barriers while seeking affirming care within clinics [15, 17, 18].

Although seeking sexual health information online is becoming more common among adolescents, it is very difficult to determine the quality of the content they come across. For instance, Google searches are driven by individualized algorithms, making it difficult to know what adolescents are being exposed to when they search terms (e.g., condoms, birth control) on Google. Adolescents themselves also face barriers in their search for sexual health information online such as fatigue sifting through content that may not be relevant and not knowing which information source to trust [17, 18]. In contrast, sexual health content may be presented without searching at all on platforms such as TikTok. A recent content analysis showed that the majority of 100 sexual health–themed TikTok videos discussed female anatomy and orgasm as well as sexual pleasure and arousal [19]. Therefore, TikTok may provide alternative and additional information than what is typically offered in school-based sex education programming.

Studies with adolescent samples are rare; however, a scoping review with emerging adults in the UK showed that digitally implemented sexual health education can have a positive impact on sexual health knowledge, attitudes, and behaviors [14]. As Dr. Walsh-Buhi and colleagues discuss, studies should consider how sexual health websites can help adolescents to make more informed decisions about sexual activity and reduce their risk of negative sexual health outcomes (e.g., sexually transmitted infections, unintended pregnancy). They also call for future research efforts to unpack longer-term benefits of receiving sexual health information online and the consideration of social media to leverage adolescents' sexual health knowledge, attitudes, and behaviors.

## 3 Romantic Relationship and Interpersonal Development with Online Platforms

As adolescents use the Internet and digital technology to learn about sexuality and romantic relationships, they also use the same resources to communicate with current or potential romantic and sexual partners and engage in sexual expression in private and public ways. In their chapter, Dr. Kathryn Macapagal (see Chap. 49) and colleagues describe how using technology-facilitated communication can be a positive way for adolescents to flirt or discuss sexual health needs and practices with partners [20, 21]. For example, adolescents were found to be more likely to discuss contraception (including condoms) and set sexual consent boundaries ahead of time via texting than face-to-face communication. Moreover, adolescents who did communicate about sexual health through text were three times more likely to use condoms during sex [21].

Dating apps are primarily used by emerging adults (18–25 years old) but are sometimes used by adolescents who fake their date of birth to create a profile. As Drs. McInroy and Macapagal consider in their respective chapters, dating apps can offer a convenient way for more marginalized groups like LGBTQ+ adolescents [22], those with physical disabilities [23], or even those who are ashamed of their weight status [24] to find or communicate with existing romantic partners. For example, LGBTQ+ youth use dating apps and social media platforms to seek platonic friendships (in addition to romantic relationships) as a means of finding like-minded support [25]. It can be dangerous for LBGTQ+ adolescents and emerging adults to seek out sexual and romantic experiences in person; therefore, turning to dating apps or other online platforms that are curated by sexual identity can feel safer. However, gay and bisexual male adolescents have been shown to engage in more sexual risk-taking and substance use with partners met online [26].

Dr. Joris Van Ouytsel (see Chap. 50) and colleagues describe the current state of the literature on sexting or the practice of sending sexually explicit messages or images via mobile devices among adolescents. Although consistent prevalence rates (14.5–34.8%) are difficult to determine for youth under the age of 18 years [27], it is prevalent enough to warrant scientific attention that simultaneously considers positive aspects of adolescent sexual development and legal issues of sharing and receiving nude images of minors. This is particularly important as laws are changing rapidly across many countries to decriminalize consensual sexual image sharing among minors. Research with adolescent samples suggests that sexting is associated with several risks, such as sexual coercion, emotional distress, and legal consequences [28, 29]. However, these consequences appear to vary greatly by gender and sexual identity as discussed below.

## 4 Sexual Media Use as a Risk Factor for Sexual Violence Perpetration and Victimization

Engagement with various other or self-produced sexualized media (e.g., pornography, dating apps, and sexting) is consistently associated with or predictive of sexual and intimate partner violence when investigated in adolescent samples. Given that Internet pornography does depict various violent and aggressive sex acts, it may not be surprising that adolescents' use of pornography has been shown to be predictive of increases in sexual harassment [30], sexual aggression perpetration [30, 31], and sexual violence victimization [32]. Adolescents also use online technology to perpetrate intimate partner violence through digital stalking and harassment [33], often resulting in anxiety and depression for the victim [25].

Despite adult discomfort with it, when sexting occurs between two consenting adolescents and the images are not shared outside of that exchange, the negative mental health impacts are mitigated [28]. However, sexting can become coercive if one partner is repeatedly asking for nudes, in which case sexting is associated with anxiety and depression, particularly for girls. This kind of unwanted sexual solicitation can also occur from peers or strangers via social media and dating apps and is disproportionately experienced by girls as well as gay and bisexual male adolescents [34, 35]. In contrast, heterosexual boys are more likely to ask for nude images, send their own images without first asking for consent, and are more likely to nonconsensually disseminate those images to peers or online. When images are exchanged but are then disseminated throughout the school or online, victims can experience mental health issues including thoughts of suicide and a fear of going to school [36]. Indeed, youth often react to this kind of image-based sexual abuse as humorous and engage in slut-shaming, a form of sexual harassment. Thus, the victim experiences further trauma beyond the initial betrayal of the recipient forwarding the image. In their chapter, Dr. Joris Van Ouytsel and colleagues call for future research to consider how nonconsensual sexting experiences impact multiple areas of adolescents' lives (e.g., mental health, academic experiences, and self-esteem).

## 5 Recommendations for Policy, Programming, and Practices

### 5.1 Educational Settings

One of the most common recommendations across these review articles is for systemic, medically accurate, comprehensive sex education implemented in public schools. Specifically, such education should include information on healthy relationships, consent, diverse sexual identities, and the risks associated with engaging in sexual behaviors online. To alleviate the curriculum burden that comes with concentrating health education during selected years, comprehensive sex education should be provided in an age-appropriate manner across many years, scaffolding concepts that build upon anatomy, reproduction, healthy relationships, delaying sexual activity, and engagement in safer sexual behaviors. Such education should also be delivered in a culturally sensitive manner and should be inclusive of all genders, sexual orientations, and identities. Schools can also provide education on digital citizenship and responsible online behavior, including the responsible use of social media and dating apps that acknowledge sexual harassment under the umbrella of safety education and not sex education.

Developing student conduct policies that reflect the digital lives of students today is also suggested as an avenue for preventing problems that can arise from adolescents' use of pornography at school, sexting, and dating apps. Policies serve as guidelines for appropriate online behavior and can help prevent online violence such as cyberbullying, sexual harassment, and nonconsensual sexting and pornography. Schools should establish clear consequences for disseminating nude images of students throughout the school or online, which may include counseling, parental involvement, or disciplinary action. Schools should designate specific personnel responsible for implementing the policy and providing resources to students. Lastly, considering the intersecting identities of students' experiences when implementing would also be important for increasing equitable experiences for all students.

### 5.2 Therapeutic Settings

Whether situated within schools or larger healthcare systems, counseling and mental health services that are meant to address substance abuse, sexual violence, and other related issues among youth should also be equipped with how to respond to issues of problematic pornography use, nonconsensual sexting, online sexual harassment, and sexual health needs in general. Understanding the digital lives of youth and how those experiences vary greatly based upon gender and sexual identity is vital knowledge for providing trauma-informed, affirming, and holistic mental healthcare to adolescents. Clinicians could also consider running individual or group counseling sessions for victims of online sexual violence and may include a focus on issues such as self-esteem, healthy relationships, and communication skills.

### 5.3 Pediatric Healthcare Settings

Pediatricians are on the frontlines of adolescent health and provide a unique opportunity to systemically screen for or respond to emerging issues. Given this widespread access to youth, the authors throughout this section noted the need for pediatricians to have a better understanding of media's role in gender and sexuality development. For example, systematic professional development opportunities that build skills to respond to issues related to online sexual experiences could assist pediatricians in providing appropriate resources for their patients and families. For example, providers can deliver information on how to talk to children and adolescents about sexuality and how to identify and address risky behaviors related to pornography, sexting, and dating apps. In addition, pediatric providers can support parents of LGBTQ+ youth with apps and other resources that aim to improve mental health, particularly suicide prevention, among this at-risk population.

## 6 Conclusion

Media and digital technology have changed the way that children and adolescents communicate, socialize, and develop their identities. Adolescents have unprecedented access to a vast array of online content that provides fictional and factual implicit and explicit messages about gender and sexuality in the form of streaming services, pornography, sexting, sexual health websites, and dating apps. As these activities become more available, increasing statistics suggest that adolescents are having more sexual experiences online than they are offline. While these technologies offer new opportunities for gender and sexual exploration and expression, they also come with risks that must be addressed. In the chapters throughout this section, the authors have noted the need to further investigate marginalized youths (e.g., LGBTQ+, racially minoritized, maltreated) online sexual experiences in such a way that honors the unique contextual factors that interact with those experiences. Future research in this area should focus on identifying effective strategies for promoting healthy sexual development among adolescents while minimizing the potential risks associated with technology use.

**Conflict of Interest and Funding Disclosure** None.

## References

1. Shawcroft JE, Coyne SM, Zurcher JD, Brubaker PJ. Depictions of gender across eight decades of Disney animated film: the role of film producer, director, and writer gender. Sex Roles. 2022;86:346–65. https://doi.org/10.1007/s11199-022-01273-6.
2. Gerding A, Signorielli N. Gender roles in tween television programming: a content analysis of two genres. Sex Roles. 2014;70:43–56. https://doi.org/10.1007/s11199-013-0330-z.

3. Brubaker PJ, Zurcher JD, Parks M, King J, Coyne SM, Robinson T. The fairest of them all: representations of bodies across Disney animated films from 1937 to 2019. Psychol Pop Media. 2023;12:312–23. https://doi.org/10.1037/PPM0000411.
4. Lynch T, Tompkins JE, van Driel II, Fritz N. Sexy, strong, and secondary: a content analysis of female characters in video games across 31 years. J Commun. 2016;66(4):564–84. https://doi.org/10.1111/JCOM.12237.
5. Aubrey JS, Yan K, Terán L, Roberts L. The heterosexual script on tween, teen, and young-adult television programs: a content analytic update and extension. J Sex Res. 2019;57(9):1134–45. https://doi.org/10.1080/00224499.2019.1699895.
6. Van Damme E, Van Bauwel S, Van DE. Sex as spectacle. J Child Media. 2013;7(2):170–85. https://doi.org/10.1080/17482798.2012.673499.
7. Fritz N, Malic V, Paul B, Zhou Y. A descriptive analysis of the types, targets, and relative frequency of aggression in mainstream pornography. Arch Sex Behav. 2020;49(8):3041–53. https://doi.org/10.1007/s10508-020-01773-0.
8. Vera-Gray F, Mcglynn C, Kureshi I, Butterby K. Sexual violence as a sexual script in mainstream online pornography. Br J Criminol. 2021;61:1234–60. https://doi.org/10.1093/bjc/azab035.
9. Seida K, Shor E. Aggression and pleasure in opposite-sex and same-sex mainstream online pornography: a comparative content analysis of dyadic scenes. J Sex Res. 2019;58(3):292–304. https://doi.org/10.1080/00224499.2019.1696275.
10. Bőthe B, Vaillancourt-Morel MP, Girouard A, Štulhofer A, Dion J, Bergeron S. A large-scale comparison of Canadian sexual/gender minority and heterosexual, cisgender adolescents' pornography use characteristics. J Sex Med. 2020;17(6):1156–67. https://doi.org/10.1016/J.JSXM.2020.02.009.
11. Valkenburg PM. Adolescents and pornography: a review of 20 years of research. J Sex Res. 2016;53(4–5):509–31. https://doi.org/10.1080/00224499.2016.1143441.
12. Doornwaard SM, Bickham DS, Rich M, ter Bogt TFM, van den Eijnden RJJM. Adolescents' use of sexually explicit internet material and their sexual attitudes and behavior: parallel development and directional effects. Dev Psychol. 2015;51(10):1476–88. https://doi.org/10.1037/DEV0000040.
13. Wright PJ, Tokunaga RS, Herbenick D, Paul B. Pornography vs. sexual science: the role of pornography use and dependency in U.S. teenagers' sexual illiteracy. Commun Monograph. 2022;89:332–53. https://doi.org/10.1080/03637751.2021.1987486.
14. Bailey J, Mann S, Wayal S, et al. Sexual health promotion for young people delivered via digital media: a scoping review. Public Health Res. 2015;3(13):1–120. https://doi.org/10.3310/PHR03130.
15. Mitchell KJ, Ybarra ML, Korchmaros JD, Kosciw JG. Accessing sexual health information online: use, motivations and consequences for youth with different sexual orientations. Health Educ Res. 2014;29:147–57. https://doi.org/10.1093/her/cyt071.
16. Lindberg LD, Kantor LM. Adolescents' receipt of sex education in a nationally representative sample, 2011–2019. J Adolesc Health. 2022;70(2):290–7. https://doi.org/10.1016/J.JADOHEALTH.2021.08.027/ATTACHMENT/DF3BB52A-15FD-42A3-8F0A-25F767D0B806/MMC1.PDF.
17. Magee JC, Bigelow L, DeHaan S, Mustanski BS. Sexual health information seeking online: a mixed-methods study among lesbian, gay, bisexual, and transgender young people. Health Educ Behav. 2011;39:39. https://doi.org/10.1177/1090198111401384.
18. Patterson SP, Hilton S, Flowers P, Mcdaid LM. What are the barriers and challenges faced by adolescents when searching for sexual health information on the internet? Implications for policy and practice from a qualitative study. Sex Transm Infect. 2019;95(6):462–7. https://doi.org/10.1136/SEXTRANS-2018-053710.
19. Fowler LR, Schoen L, Stevens Smith H, Morain SR. Resources, frameworks, and perspectives sex education on TikTok: a content analysis of themes. Health Promot Pract. 2022;23(5):739–42. https://doi.org/10.1177/15248399211031536(19).
20. Lykens J, Pilloton M, Silva C, Schlamm E, Wilburn K, Pence E. Google for sexual relationships: mixed-methods study on digital flirting and online dating among adolescent youth and young adults. JMIR Public Health Surveill. 2019;5(2):e10695. https://doi.org/10.2196/10695.
21. Widman L, Nesi J, Choukas-Bradley S, Prinstein MJ. Safe sext: adolescents' use of technology to communicate about sexual health with dating partners. J Adolesc Health. 2014;54:612–4. https://doi.org/10.1016/j.jadohealth.2013.12.009.
22. Korchmaros JD, Ybarra ML, Mitchell KJ. Adolescent online romantic relationship initiation: differences by sexual and gender identification. J Adolesc. 2015;40:54–64. https://doi.org/10.1016/J.ADOLESCENCE.2015.01.004.
23. Mazur E. Diverse disabilities and dating online. In: Identity, sexuality, and relationships among emerging adults in the digital age. IGI Global; 2017. p. 150–67. https://doi.org/10.4018/978-1-5225-1856-3.CH010.
24. Walsh Ó, Dettmer E, Regina A, et al. 'Teenagers are into perfect-looking things': dating, sexual attitudes and experiences of adolescents with severe obesity. Child Care Health Dev. 2022;48(3):406–14. https://doi.org/10.1111/CCH.12940.
25. Ybarra ML, Mitchell KJ, Palmer NA, Reisner SL. Online social support as a buffer against online and offline peer and sexual victimization among U.S. LGBT and non-LGBT youth. Child Abuse Negl. 2015;39:123–36. https://doi.org/10.1016/J.CHIABU.2014.08.006.
26. Macapagal K, Moran K, Newcomb ME, Moskowitz DA, Owens C, Mustanski B. Patterns of online and offline partnering, partnership characteristics, and

Condomless sex among adolescent sexual minority males in the USA. AIDS Behav. 2021;25:2033–45. https://doi.org/10.1007/s10461-020-03133-4.
27. Mori C, Park J, Temple JR, Madigan S. Are youth sexting rates still on the rise? A meta-analytic update. J Adolesc Health. 2022;70(4):531–9. https://doi.org/10.1016/J.JADOHEALTH.2021.10.026.
28. Mori C, Temple JR, Browne D, Madigan S. Association of sexting with sexual behaviors and mental health among adolescents: a systematic review and meta-analysis. JAMA Pediatr. 2019;173(8):770–9. https://doi.org/10.1001/JAMAPEDIATRICS.2019.1658.
29. Mitchell KJ, Jones L, Finkelhor D, Wolak J. Youth involvement in sexting: findings from the youth internet safety studies. YISS. 2014;3:1–8.
30. Waterman EA, Wesche R, Morris G, Edwards KM, Banyard VL. Prospective associations between pornography viewing and sexual aggression among adolescents. J Res Adolesc. 2022;32(4):1612–25. https://doi.org/10.1111/JORA.12745.
31. Wright PJ, Paul B, Herbenick D. Preliminary insights from a U.S. probability sample on adolescents' pornography exposure, media psychology, and sexual aggression. J Health Commun. 2021;26:39–46. https://doi.org/10.1080/10810730.2021.1887980.
32. Maas MK, Bray BC, Noll JG. Online sexual experiences predict subsequent sexual health and victimization outcomes among female adolescents: a latent class analysis. J Youth Adolescence. 2019;48:837–49. https://doi.org/10.1111/jora.12364.
33. Muñoz-Fernández N, Sánchez-Jiménez V. Cyber-aggression and psychological aggression in adolescent couples: a short-term longitudinal study on prevalence and common and differential predictors. Comput Hum Behav. 2020;104 https://doi.org/10.1016/J.CHB.2019.106191.
34. Madigan S, Van Ouytsel J, Temple JR. Nonconsensual sexting and the role of sex differences—reply. JAMA Pediatr. 2018;172:890–1. https://doi.org/10.1001/jamapediatrics.2018.1951.
35. Van Ouytsel J, Walrave M, De Marez L, Vanhaelewyn B, Ponnet K. A first investigation into gender minority adolescents' sexting experiences. J Adolesc. 2020;84:213–8. https://doi.org/10.1016/j.adolescence.2020.09.007.
36. Gámez-Guadix M, Sorrel MA, Martínez-Bacaicoa J. Technology-facilitated sexual violence perpetration and victimization among adolescents: a network analysis. Sex Res Soc Policy. 2023;20:1000–12. https://doi.org/10.1007/S13178-022-00775-Y/FIGURES/3.

# Representations of Gender and Sexuality in Youth Media

Jennifer Stevens Aubrey, Megan K. Maas, Sophia Choukas-Bradley, Sarah M. Coyne, Meenakshi Gigi Durham, Tracy M. Scull, Johanna M. F. van Oosten, and L. Monique Ward

## 1 Background

In the first few years of life, children begin understanding their gender identity and the rules associated with gender (i.e., gender stereotypes), through a complex process known as gender socialization. Indeed, children are often called "gender detectives," as they have a strong motivation to learn how they should act according to their gender. Children pick up clues about gender from parents, peers/siblings, and teachers, but one consistent source of socialization is entertainment screen media. Media have traditionally relied on prescriptive gender stereotypes that could ultimately restrict youth's conception of what is possible or appropriate for their identity, relationships, and well-being.

In adolescence, this motivation to learn about gender roles expands to include sexual roles and sexuality, through the process of sexual socialization. The development of healthy sexual behaviors and self-concept is an important milestone in adolescence, and understanding the multiple aspects of sexuality is critical to that endeavor. In this context, too, youth will learn about sexual behaviors from parents, peers/siblings, and schools, but where those sources are deficient, the media will serve as de facto sex educators. Because entertainment media often depict behavioral scripts that provide procedural details about how sex will unfold, they can be quite effective in teaching adolescents how to think, feel, and behave in relation to their sexuality, a term we

Because the contributions of the third through eighth authors were equal, their names are listed alphabetically.

J. S. Aubrey (✉)
Department of Communication, University of Arizona, Tucson, AZ, USA
e-mail: jlsa@arizona.edu

M. K. Maas
Department of Human Development & Family Studies, Michigan State University, East Lansing, MI, USA

S. Choukas-Bradley
Department of Psychology, University of Pittsburgh, Pittsburgh, PA, USA

S. M. Coyne
School of Family Life, Brigham Young University, Provo, UT, USA

M. G. Durham
School of Journalism and Mass Communication and Department of Gender, Women's and Sexuality Studies, University of Iowa, Iowa City, IA, USA

T. M. Scull
Innovation Research & Training, Durham, NC, USA

J. M. F. van Oosten
University of Amsterdam, Amsterdam School of Communication Research, Amsterdam, The Netherlands

L. M. Ward
Department of Psychology, University of Michigan, Ann Arbor, MI, USA


D. A. Christakis, L. Hale (eds.), *Handbook of Children and Screens*,
https://doi.org/10.1007/978-3-031-69362-5_45

use to broadly refer to sexual expressions, behaviors, desires, and attitudes.

To understand how media affect children and adolescents (herein "youth") in terms of gender and sexuality, we must first understand the messages in their media. After all, the effects that media have on youth will be connected to the messages that they are consuming. In this vein, we review recent content analyses of portrayals of gender and sexuality in entertainment screen media that are created for or popular with youth (herein "entertainment media for youth"). Such studies lend important insight to the *system* of representation that exists in entertainment screen media, despite the existence of salient exceptions.

With an eye toward *current* representations of gender and sexuality, we limited our review to studies published in or after 2010 and did not include studies on media created for adults. Qualitative and quantitative studies were included, but each study had to use an empirical method that was described and systematically applied. Priority was given to studies that were published in peer-reviewed academic journals, but in some cases, we included professional reports. Practically speaking, our review covers studies on television, films, and video games, from a variety of cultures and countries, but not other well-studied media such as advertising, news, books, and pornography. We also excluded studies on media created *by* youth, such as social media posts. Television, films, and video games are still relevant to the media diets of adolescents. Among teens (ages 13–18), their most frequent type of media exposure is still television/videos at 3 h 16 min per day, followed by video games at 1 h 46 min [1]. In comparison, teens spend 1 h and 27 min on social media.

## 2 Current State

### 2.1 Representations of Gender in Entertainment Media for Youth

Based on the current content analytic literature, we make five conclusions about the representations of gender in entertainment media for youth. First, the most pervasive representation of gender in entertainment media for youth is the visibility of men and boys. Male characters outnumber female characters, typically at a rate of 1.5–2 to 1. This unequal distribution occurs in films [2–4] and television created for children [5–8], including television created for infants and toddlers [9]. It also occurs in television popular among children [10] and tweens/adolescents [11]. A recent content analysis demonstrated that television *created* for children ages 2–11 did conform to the disproportionate representation of male characters, but in the same study, television programs *popular* among children aged 2–11 had a more balanced gender representation: 48.8% of lead characters were women/girls [7]. Although too early for conclusions about a change on the horizon, this example of relative parity should be underscored.

Our second conclusion is that appearance is a multidimensional concern for female characters in entertainment media for youth. They care about their appearance more than male characters [6, 9, 11]; indeed, their value is based largely on how they appear to others. Moreover, female characters should and do want to be thin, and thinness is associated with "goodness" (i.e., positive personality characteristics and admiration from other characters) [3, 8, 12]. At the same time, media characters could express positive body image messages, such as body appreciation, self-care, and resilience against body image-threatening input [13]. In a content analysis of youth-oriented series on Netflix (e.g., *Riverdale*, *Big Mouth*, and *Sex Education*), these positive body image messages were rare (3.4% of scenes) but were disproportionately expressed by girl-identifying characters, supporting the stereotype that appearance concerns are the domain of girls and women. In video games, television, *and* films, female characters' bodies are often sexualized, variably defined by sexual clothing, nudity/body exposure, and occupying an overtly sexual role [3, 7, 10, 14]. Compared to female characters, the appearance stereotype for male characters is more uniform; they are expected to be muscular and to take up more space than female characters. Moreover, their muscularity/size is connected to power, strength, and athleticism [12, 15–17].

Although not as pervasive as gender differences in physical appearance foci, the other conclusions we draw are also supportive of gender stereotypes. Our third conclusion is that male characters are more likely to be physically aggressive than female characters [16, 18], whereas female characters are likely to use relational aggression (i.e., actions that degrade persons' self-esteem and/or social standing) more than male characters [18, 19]. The latter conforms to the "mean girls" trope often seen in entertainment media for youth. Fourth, interests, hobbies, and occupations are divided by gender. Science, technology, engineering, and mathematics (STEM) careers are still more likely to be held by male characters than female characters [5, 20, 21]. Meanwhile, the visual arts, the performing arts (including modeling), and humanities-related jobs and hobbies are associated with female characters more than male characters [5, 8, 21]. Finally, male characters are more likely to be leaders than female characters [2, 4, 12], and leadership is associated with other desirable characteristics, such as intellect, bravery, and heroism [15].

Although these conclusions support traditional gender stereotypes, we note that some gender stereotypes are less consistently supported, particularly when compared to older content analyses. For example, although boys/men are more likely to be leaders, the evidence does not consistently support the idea that girls are more likely to be followers [4] or in need of rescue [22]. Additionally, the stereotype that girls value romance is also contentious in the content analytic literature [4, 22]. For example, Disney princesses are less romantically attached in recent movies compared to older Disney princess movies [22]. Thus, progress in the representation of gender seems to apply to female characters more than male characters.

## 2.2 Representations of Sexuality in Entertainment Media for Youth

We make four conclusions about the representations of sexuality in entertainment media for youth. First, in terms of quantity, depictions of sexual talk and behaviors are quite frequent in entertainment media for youth [23–25]. For example, in "teen sex romps" (i.e., comedic films featuring adolescent and/or young adult characters in which a dominant theme is the pursuit of sexual gratification), sexual behaviors were portrayed an average of four times per hour, whereas talk about sex occurred five times per hour [23]. In television shows popular with tweens, there were an average of five sexual behaviors per episode, and in shows popular with teens, there were 15 sexual behaviors per episode, but most behaviors were mild (innuendo, physical flirting, affectionate touching, and kissing) [25].

Second, content analyses suggest that heterosexuality is still assumed and naturalized; portrayals of LGBTQ+ sexual relationships are rare [15, 24, 26, 27]. Although gender-diverse sexual relationships are emerging for youth on streaming services, these portrayals are not yet reflected in the content analytic literature. Furthermore, LGBTQ+ characters are sources of humor and derision in entertainment media for youth [26, 27].

Third, the pervasive theme about sexuality in entertainment media for youth conforms to a "heterosexual script," which broadly overlaps with the sexual double standard [28]. A major component of the heterosexual script is that sex is risky for girls, both physically and emotionally; thus, it is incumbent upon girls to be responsible for when and what sex will occur in relationships [24]. When female characters engage in sex, they will deal with mostly negative consequences more often than male characters (e.g., reputational damage, unplanned pregnancy) [29, 30]. A final component of the heterosexual script, and the most frequently portrayed, is that boys are obsessed with sex because an active heterosexual experience is a defining aspect of masculinity [28, 30].

Fourth, the overall portrayal of sex in entertainment media for youth reflects a recreational approach toward sex. This approach is evidenced in three ways: (1) Although sex most often occurs in the context of committed relationships, recent content analyses suggest that sex occurs quite often in casual sex relationships or "hookups," [23, 30, 31] (2) the percentage of sexually active teens in entertainment media for youth is significantly greater than the percentage of actual teens who have had sex, thereby overrepresenting teen sex [25], and (3) portrayals of sexual behaviors are largely unencumbered by discussions of risks (e.g., sexually transmitted infections) and responsibility (e.g., condom use) [23, 32].

Taken together, we conclude that the portrayal of sexuality in adolescent media is pervasive, heterosexual, the object of emotional turmoil for female adolescents, the object of obsession for male adolescents, and, overall, recreational in nature. We note that our review did not capture entertainment media produced for or popular among emerging adults (typically ages 18–25), even though adolescents will often consume these media in an aspirational way (i.e., they look up to older characters).

## 3 Future Research

The conclusions we have drawn are limited by the research questions that were asked. Thus, we make four recommendations for future research on the representation of gender and sexuality in entertainment media for youth.

First, to understand how portrayals are changing over time, we recommend more prospective longitudinal content analyses. Currently, we can only make limited comparisons across studies from different time points, especially in cases in which researchers operationalize constructs differently. Additionally, because sociocultural norms about gender and sexuality are changing rapidly, we need to track changes over time if we want to determine whether and/or how media are keeping pace. Certainly, high-quality content analyses are labor-intensive; thus, there will necessarily be a time lag between what is happening in entertainment media for youth and what the research can reflect.

Second, more content analyses that address intersectionality in representation are needed. Examining how gender stereotypes and depictions of sexuality intersect with other identity markers, such as sexual orientation, race, ethnicity, nations, and age, will provide important context to how these messages resonate with youth from differing backgrounds. For example, many gender stereotypes are also racialized (e.g., the Jezebel and Sapphire stereotypes) [33]. Examination of such stereotypes in entertainment media for youth will lay the foundation for culturally informed future research that can examine how portrayals of gender and sexuality impact attitudes and behavior among youth of color.

Third, although we did not review research on representations of gender and sexuality on social media due to space limitations, it will be important to examine how youth use social media to create spaces for resistance, critique, solidarity, and community concerning general issues related to sexuality, sexual orientation, gender identity, and sexual violence. Additionally, given that many youths are turning to short-form, user-generated video content, such as that found on YouTube and TikTok, to satisfy their entertainment needs, future research will need to examine representations of gender and sexuality on those platforms, as well. The content produced by social media personalities and influencers is highly consequential for youth, as social media provide more explicit avenues for audience engagement than traditional media. For example, Andrew Tate, a social media personality and influencer who expresses openly misogynistic viewpoints, has a largely young male audience; the long-term impacts of his views on his young male audience are unknown and potentially troubling.

Fourth, the emphasis on research on representation of sexuality is typically on risks, instead of approaching sexuality as a positive developmental milestone. Further research examining prosocial sexuality messages would expand our understanding of sexuality representation in entertainment media for youth [34]. For example, shows like Netflix's critically acclaimed *Sex Education,* which followed the lives of British teenagers of diverse sexual and gender identities, contained themes of positive sexuality, active sexual consent, and respectful treatment of diverse sexual expressions.

## 4 Recommendations

Our review of research on the portrayals of gender and sexuality motivates several recommendations that we make to stakeholders interested in youth's well-being, including media content producers and providers, policymakers/foundations/governmental organizations, and clinicians/educators.

- For media content producers and providers, parity in gender representation should be the goal. The disproportionate representation of male characters likely teaches child viewers that girls/women are not as important as boys/men. The media industry adage that boys will not have interest in girl-led narratives prevents the opportunity to normalize parity, and smart, creative girl-led narratives, such as *The Hunger Games* franchise, have proven to be globally successful [35].
- More diversity in gender identity (e.g., transgender and nonbinary characters) and sexual identity (e.g., lesbian and gay characters) in content produced for youth is sorely needed, in addition to diversity in representation of race, ethnicity, and nations. Youth who are exposed to positive portrayals of characters representing marginalized groups and with whom the viewers have a one-way relationship (i.e., "parasocial contact") will likely experience benefits in empathy and prejudice reduction [36].
- Media producers should also continue to expand portrayals of both boys and girls to be less gender-stereotyped. Although there are examples of counter-stereotyped female characters in children's media (e.g., *Doc McStuffins*, *Dora the Explorer*), there appear to be fewer counter-stereotypical representations of boys/men.
- Lastly, the reduction of messages that conform to the heterosexual script in entertainment media for youth is recommended. The heterosexual script, which pits women against men in sexual interactions and relationships, implies that girls should take on the emotional labor of sexual interactions, including sexual negotiations, the procuring of sexual consent, and the fallout from mostly negative consequences including sexual harassment and violence.
- We also recommend more funding from governmental agencies and/or foundations to conduct prospective longitudinal content analyses of not only traditional screen media but also social media and influencers, which would allow researchers to track changes over time. Prospective longitudinal survey research is also needed to examine the effects of these representations on youth. After all, the essential consideration of this research is whether media exposure to portrayals of gender and sexuality is limiting what youth grow up to be.
- Clinicians and educators have remarkable opportunities to augment positive portrayals of gender and sexuality and counteract negative ones. Some well-developed and evaluated media literacy programming that addresses issues concerning gender and sexuality already exists. For example, *Media Aware*, a comprehensive sexual health program that uses a media literacy education approach, was found to improve high school students' sexual health knowledge, correct inaccurate normative beliefs about the frequency of risky teen sex, improve critical thinking about media messages, and decrease the perceived realism of media messages [37]. Thus, more widespread deployment of such programming in schools, other educational settings, and clinical settings is recommended.

**Conflict of Interest and Funding Disclosure** None.

## References

1. Rideout V, Peebles A, Mann S, Robb MB. Common sense census: media use by tweens and teens, 2021. San Francisco: Common Sense; 2022. https://www.commonsensemedia.org/sites/default/files/research/report/8-18-census-integrated-report-final-web_0.pdf
2. Aley M, Hahn L. The powerful male hero: a content analysis of gender representation in posters for children's animated movies. Sex Roles.

2020;83(7–8):499–509. https://doi.org/10.1007/s11199-020-01127-z.
3. Shawcroft JE, Coyne SM, Zurcher JD, Brubaker PJ. Depictions of gender across eight decades of Disney animated film: the role of film producer, director, and writer gender. Sex Roles. 2022;86(5–6):346–65. https://doi.org/10.1007/s11199-022-01273-6.
4. Gonzalez MPL, Infantes-Paniagua A, Thornborrow T, Jordan OC. Associations between media representations of physical, personality, and social attributes by gender: a content analysis of children's animated film characters. Int J Commun. 2020;14:6026–48.
5. Hamlen KR, Imbesi KJ. Role models in the media: a content analysis of preschool television programs in the U.S. J Child Media. 2020;14(3):302–23. https://doi.org/10.1080/17482798.2019.1689369.
6. Hentges B, Case K. Gender representations on Disney channel, cartoon network, and nickelodeon broadcasts in the United States. J Child Media. 2013;7(3):319–33. https://doi.org/10.1080/17482798.2012.729150.
7. Meyer M, Conroy, M. What children are seeing on TV. Seejane.org. https://seejane.org/wp-content/uploads/GDI-See-It-Be-It-TV-2022-Report-v2.pdf. Accessed 3 Apr 2023.
8. Walsh A, Leaper C. A content analysis of gender representations in preschool children's television. Mass Commun Soc. 2020;23(3):331–55. https://doi.org/10.1080/15205436.2019.1664593.
9. Kang S, Hust SJT. Traditionally and narrowly defined: gender portrayals in television programming targeting babies and toddlers. Sex Roles. 2022;86(9–10):576–86. https://doi.org/10.1007/s11199-022-01286-1.
10. Rousseau A, Eggermont S, Bels A, Van den Bulck H. Separating the sex from the object: conceptualizing sexualization and (sexual) objectification in Flemish preteens' popular television programs. J Child Media. 2018;12(3):346–65. https://doi.org/10.1080/17482798.2018.1425888.
11. Gerding A, Signorielli N. Gender roles in tween television programming: a content analysis of two genres. Sex Roles. 2014;70(1–2):43–56. https://doi.org/10.1007/s11199-013-0330-z.
12. Brubaker PJ, Zurcher JD, Parks M, King J, Coyne SM, Robinson T. The fairest of them all: representations of bodies across Disney animated films from 1937 to 2019. Psychol Pop Media. 2022; https://doi.org/10.1037/ppm0000411.
13. Maes C, Vandenbosch L. "I love my body; I love it all": body positivity messages in youth-oriented television series. Mass Commun Soc. 2023;26(1):122–46. https://doi.org/10.1080/15205436.2022.2030756.
14. Lynch T, Tompkins JE, van Driel II, Fritz N. Sexy, strong, and secondary: a content analysis of female characters in video games across 31 years: female game characters across 31 years. J Commun. 2016;66(4):564–84. https://doi.org/10.1111/jcom.12237.
15. Birthisel J. How body, heterosexuality and patriarchal entanglements mark non-human characters as male in CGI-animated children's films. J Child Media. 2014;8(4):336–52. https://doi.org/10.1080/17482798.2014.960435.
16. Harriger JA, Wick MR, Trivedi H, Callahan KE. Strong hero or violent playboy? Portrayals of masculinity in children's animated movies. Sex Roles. 2021;85(11–12):677–87. https://doi.org/10.1007/s11199-021-01247-0.
17. Martins N, Williams DC, Ratan RA, Harrison K. Virtual muscularity: a content analysis of male video game characters. Body Image. 2011;8(1):43–51. https://doi.org/10.1016/j.bodyim.2010.10.002.
18. Coyne SM, Callister M, Robinson T. Yes, another teen movie: three decades of physical violence in films aimed at adolescents. J Child Media. 2010;4(4):387–401. https://doi.org/10.1080/17482798.2010.510006.
19. Martins N, Wilson BJ. Mean on the screen: social aggression in programs popular with children. J Commun. 2012;62(6):991–1009. https://doi.org/10.1111/j.1460-2466.2012.01599.x.
20. Aladé F, Lauricella A, Kumar Y, Wartella E. Who's modeling STEM for kids? A character analysis of children's STEM-focused television in the US. J Child Media. 2021;15(3):338–57. https://doi.org/10.1080/17482798.2020.1810087.
21. Hunting K, Grumbein A, Cahill M. Watch and learn: gendered discrepancies in educational messages on television channels targeted at boys versus girls. Mass Commun Soc. 2018;21(1):115–41. https://doi.org/10.1080/15205436.2017.1370114.
22. Hine B, England D, Lopreore K, Horgan ES, Hartwell L. The rise of the androgynous princess: examining representations of gender in prince and princess characters of Disney movies released 2009–2016. Soc Sci (Basel). 2018;7(12):245. https://doi.org/10.3390/socsci7120245.
23. Alexopoulos C, Taylor LD. Risky business: sexual risk and responsibility messages in teen sex romps. Sex Cult. 2020;24(6):2161–82. https://doi.org/10.1007/s12119-020-09742-4.
24. Kinsler JJ, Glik D, de Castro BS, et al. A content analysis of how sexual behavior and reproductive health are being portrayed on primetime television shows being watched by teens and young adults. Health Commun. 2019;34(6):644–51. https://doi.org/10.1080/10410236.2018.1431020.
25. Signorielli N, Bievenour A. Sex in adolescent programming: a content analysis. Commun Res Rep. 2015;32(4):304–13. https://doi.org/10.1080/08824096.2015.1089856.
26. Bond BJ. Sex and sexuality in entertainment media popular with lesbian, gay, and bisexual adolescents. Mass Commun Soc. 2014;17(1):98–120. https://doi.org/10.1080/15205436.2013.816739.
27. Thorfinnsdottir D, Jensen HS. Laugh away, he is gay! Heteronormativity and children's television

in Denmark. J Child Media. 2017;11(4):399–416. https://doi.org/10.1080/17482798.2017.1312470.
28. Aubrey JS, Yan K, Terán L, Roberts L. The heterosexual script on tween, teen, and young-adult television programs: a content analytic update and extension. J Sex Res. 2020;57(9):1134–45. https://doi.org/10.1080/00224499.2019.1699895.
29. Aubrey JS, Miller B, Bond BJ, Roberts L. The lessons will be televised: examining television portrayals of sexual consequences by gender. J Mass Commun Q. 2023;100(1):172–92. https://doi.org/10.1177/10776990211073953.
30. Van Damme E, Van Bauwel S. Sex as spectacle: an overview of gender and sexual scripts in teen series popular with Flemish teenagers. J Child Media. 2013;7(2):170–85. https://doi.org/10.1080/17482798.2012.673499.
31. Dajches L, Aubrey JS. Defining the relationship: an examination of sexual behaviors and relational contexts across tween, teen, and young adult U.S. television. Commun Rep. 2020;33(3):136–47. https://doi.org/10.1080/08934215.2020.1803389.
32. Masterson AM, Messina NM. Love and sexual scripts: a content analysis of 19 Netflix teen series. J Child Media. 2023;17(2):161–79. https://doi.org/10.1080/17482798.2023.2165517.
33. Jerald MC, Ward LM, Moss L, Thomas K, Fletcher KD. Subordinates, sex objects, or sapphires? Investigating contributions of media use to black students' femininity ideologies and stereotypes about black women. J Black Psychol. 2017;43(6):608–35. https://doi.org/10.1177/0095798416665967.
34. Maes C, Vandenbosch L. "Consent is sexy": exploring the portrayal of prosocial sexuality messages in youth-oriented series. J Child Media. 2022;16(3):332–51. https://doi.org/10.1080/17482798.2021.1982741.
35. Dockterman E. Despite success of Hunger Games, frozen, women still struggle in film. Time. 2014. https://time.com/3419411/women-led-blockbuster-successes-havent-killed-movie-gender-gap/. Accessed 11 Apr 2023.
36. Massey ZB, Wong NC, Barbati JL. Meeting the (trans) parent: test of Parasocial contact with transgender characters on reducing stigma toward transgender people. Commun Stud. 2021;72(2):232–50. https://doi.org/10.1080/10510974.2021.1876125.
37. Scull TM, Dodson CV, Geller JG, Reeder LC, Stump KN. A media literacy education approach to high school sexual health education: immediate effects of Media Aware on adolescents' media, sexual health, and communication outcomes. J Youth Adolesc. 2022;51(4):708–23. https://doi.org/10.1007/s10964-021-01567-0.

# Gender and Sexuality: LGBTQ+ Youth Experiences

Lauren B. McInroy, Kathryn Macapagal, Oliver W. J. Beer, and Claire Coyne

## 1 Background

Youth in the United States (US) and other countries around the world are prolific users of information and communication technologies (ICTs) [1, 2]. ICTs encompass Internet-enabled devices (e.g., mobile devices), as well as various other Internet-mediated platforms and contexts (e.g., social media). In 2022, half of US adolescents (46%; age 13–17) were online "almost constantly" and effectively all had access to mobile devices [1]. This use is comparable to other developed countries (e.g., Canada, United Kingdom) [3]. Youth who identify as lesbian, gay, bisexual, transgender, queer, intersex, asexual, or otherwise sexual and/or gender diverse (LGBTQ+) may be particularly active ICT users, although comparisons to non-LGBTQ+ (i.e., cisgender, heterosexual) youth are relatively scarce [4]. One recent study by Nagata et al. [38] found that "sexual minority (compared to heterosexual) identification was associated with 3.72… more hours of daily recreational screen time." [38] (p. 54) What has been established is that LGBTQ+ youth experience distinct identity-based risks *and* opportunities via ICTs [5, 6]. This chapter considers extant knowledge regarding LGBTQ+ youths' experiences with ICTs, followed by proposed areas of inquiry for future research and recommendations for stakeholders.

LGBTQ+ youth experience disproportionate mental (e.g., depression, suicidal ideation) and behavioral (e.g., suicidal behavior, substance misuse) health risks [7]. LGBTQ+ youth who are gender diverse (e.g., transgender, gender nonconforming) are at particular risk for poor health outcomes [7, 8]. Health disparities stem from the discrimination and violence LGBTQ+ youth experience in their homes, schools, and communities, including rejection and victimization from family and peers, bias-based bullying, and harassment [7, 9]. Again, gender minority youth may be particularly vulnerable to these challenges [7]. Interpersonal imparities are accompanied by a lack of institutional support [7]. For example, anti-LGBTQ+ bills being enacted across the USA focus on "restricting…the safety of transgender students, and access to [affirmative] health care." [10] LGBTQ+ youth report significant unmet health needs and barriers to supportive care. They frequently encounter discrimination and lack of competence from healthcare providers, leading to hesitancy to disclose LGBTQ+ status or access services [11]. Competent care

L. B. McInroy (✉)
The Ohio State University, Columbus, OH, USA
e-mail: mcinroy.1@osu.edu

K. Macapagal
Northwestern University, Evanston, IL, USA

O. W. J. Beer
The University of Plymouth, Plymouth, UK

C. Coyne
Ann & Robert H. Lurie Children's Hospital of Chicago, Chicago, IL, USA


D. A. Christakis, L. Hale (eds.), *Handbook of Children and Screens*,
https://doi.org/10.1007/978-3-031-69362-5_46

may be particularly limited for certain subpopulations [12], and COVID-19 has exacerbated extant issues [13].

## 2 Current State

### 2.1 Risks

A 2018 systematic review found that LGBTQ+ youth are at elevated risk for cyberbullying victimization compared to their non-LGBTQ+ peers. Rates of victimization across studies ranged from 10.5% to 71.3% [5]. Cyberbullying has adverse impacts, including negative mental (e.g., depression, suicidality), behavioral (e.g., isolation), and academic (e.g., lower grade point average) outcomes [5]. Other studies have demonstrated similar findings regarding the prevalence and outcomes of cyberbullying for LGBTQ+ youth [9, 14]. Research has indicated sexually diverse youth may also be more likely to perpetrate cyberbullying [9]. However, complexities of power and hierarchies in cyberbullying interactions require further consideration. A lack of research persists on the prevalence, roles (e.g., victim, perpetrator, and bystander), and specific experiences of LGBTQ+ youth regarding cyberbullying [5].

There are also indications of vulnerabilities for LGBTQ+ youth to other ICT-based issues—including online harassment, exploitation, overuse, and risk-taking behavior [14–16]. For example, a study of male LGBTQ+ adolescents (aged 14–19) found that "[c]ompulsive Internet use was positively and significantly associated with both loneliness and internalized homophobia." [15] Another study of adolescents (aged 13–18) found sexually diverse youth were more likely to experience both online peer victimization and sexual harassment than their heterosexual peers [14]. Importantly, some subpopulations (e.g., bisexual and pansexual youth) may experience more online harassment and exclusion than others (e.g., lesbian and gay youth) [17].

The unique potential risks of specific types of ICTs for LGBTQ+ youth should be more fully explored and nuanced. For example, research suggests that dating apps (e.g., Tinder) may pose risks to young gay males, such as escalating sexual and/or substance-related risk-taking [18]. Yet, studies on sexual risk behaviors comparing where partners are met (online vs. offline) suggest that it is not the modality, but the characteristics of the young person—such as a greater tendency to engage in risk-taking behavior—that are most important. Little research has focused on the online dating of gender diverse and cisgender female LGBTQ+ youth. Thus, more research is needed to understand the potential risks posed to these populations. Similarly, research suggests that while LGBTQ+ youth use more pornography at younger ages than their non-LGBTQ+ peers, they may not be more prone to developing problematic pornography use. LGBTQ+ youth may use pornography in multiple ways: to experience sexual pleasure, learn about sexuality, and engage in sexual identity development [19].

### 2.2 Opportunities

ICTs provide critical opportunities for LGBTQ+ youth to engage in important developmental and communal activities in comparatively safe and anonymous contexts that are frequently unavailable in their in-person environments [6, 12]. These opportunities may be particularly salient to subpopulations of LGBTQ+ youth with greater barriers to in-person socialization and service access. For example, gender diverse youth may be the most active online [4], likely due to increased identity-based hostility and difficulty accessing gender-affirming care. Similarly, rural LGBTQ+ youth can reduce geographic isolation by using ICTs to circumvent potentially unsupportive offline communities and access identity-specific services and social connections [12].

Among the resources available via ICTs is identity-specific health information, including on sexual health and safer sex practices. These types of resources are particularly consequential for LGBTQ+ youth given barriers to healthcare access and the lack of comprehensive sex education in US school curricula [20]. Information on gender and sexuality is also available. ICTs offer unique opportunities to explore, experiment with, and rehearse LGBTQ+ identities, "coming out" processes, and other identity-based developmental activities in relative safety before doing so offline [6].

An important resource is the breadth of LGBTQ+ representation found online. While legacy media (e.g., print, television) are slowly increasing the quantity and quality of LGBTQ+ characters and storylines, a lack of representation persists. In contrast, LGBTQ+ youth have articulated the value of ICTs (e.g., social media, streaming services) for providing authentic, identity-based, and community-oriented media narratives [6, 12, 21].

Of particular significance may be content produced by individuals perceived by LGBTQ+ youth as sharing their experiences. Such content is often perceived as having a greater degree of relevance and authenticity [6, 12, 21]. As an example of affirming, youth-led content, see the Netflix series Heartstopper, adapted from the webcomic and graphic novels of the same name by Alice Osman. Social media creators (i.e., "influencers") are easily accessible and may provide affirmational and informational support, as well as serve as diverse role models for LGBTQ+ youth [39]. Additionally, the same dating apps and pornography posing risks to LGBTQ+ youths' health may simultaneously build a sense of community, enhance perceptions of safety, and increase representation, while offering potential opportunities for education and intervention [18, 19]. Yet, it is important to recognize that the quality and accuracy of available ICT resources for LGBTQ+ youth vary wide, and the potential consequences of inaccurate, misleading, or unsafe information should be seriously considered [22].

LGBTQ+ youth employ ICTs for identity-specific socialization and community connectedness, which may otherwise be unavailable in person due to a variety of identity-based (e.g., unsupportive family) and practical (e.g., transportation) constraints [6]. LGBTQ+ youth use ICTs for acquiring social support from similar peers and increasing their sense of belonging [6]. LGBTQ+ youth may be more likely than their non-LGBTQ+ peers "to have online friends and to appraise these friends as better than their in-person friends at providing emotional support." [14] A systematic review found that social media promotes LGBTQ+ youths' mental health by leveraging benefits, though findings were limited [23]. As discussed elsewhere in this supplement, LGBTQ+ youth use ICTs to mediate developmentally beneficial opportunities for romantic, sexual, and other types of intimate relationships [24].

Finally, the independent and communal activities undertaken by LGBTQ+ youth include engagement in a variety of identity-based empowerment and social action activities (e.g., challenging discrimination, advocacy, building identity pride) [12, 25]. Many LGBTQ+ youth proactively navigate and cultivate their online spaces—including platform selection, use of platform-based safety features, and online profile and presence management—to cope with hostility, engage in developmentally important activities, and enhance their well-being [12, 25].

## 3 Future Research

Significant knowledge gaps persist, including LGBTQ+ youths' experiences of simultaneous risks *and* opportunities. Sustained attention is necessary to understand contemporary youths' experiences and the impact on their developmental processes as well as to identify opportunities for education and intervention. Among the most pressing research questions are the following:

- *What are the specific experiences of LGBTQ+ youth regarding ICTs?* Scarcity of research into the specific risks and opportunities LGBTQ+ youth experience may reflect a broader lack of attention to their Internet-mediated experiences. While research is increasingly addressing some forms of overt violence experienced by LGBTQ+ youth (e.g., cyberbullying, harassment), scant research has investigated their experiences with more covert forms of violence [26]. This includes digital microaggressions—commonplace instances of discrimination encountered by marginalized groups via ICTs. While the potentially deleterious psychophysiological consequences of in-person microaggressions have been identified for LGBTQ+ youth, the same attention has not been given to digital microaggressions despite indications of the potential for adverse impacts [26]. Altogether, the Internet-mediated experiences of LGBTQ+ youth is an area primed for further scholarship, including a detailed understanding of bidirectional relationships between experiences with specific ICTs and mental, physical, and behavioral health outcomes. For example, there is evidence of the particular importance of online friendships for LGBTQ+ youth, especially for those with scarce in-person supports [14]. Yet, limited information exists about how youth navigate online friendships and manage conflict in Internet-only relationships and the impact of ruptures in those relationships. The ways in which these relationships may be similar or different to in-person relationships necessitate examination.

- *What are the specific experiences of subpopulations of LGBTQ+ youth regarding ICTs?* Knowledge deficits persist regarding the experiences of LGBTQ+ youth subpopulations. While research has considered some subpopulations (e.g., gender diverse, rural) [4, 12], there is a continued lack of attention to intersectionality. Little is known about how LGBTQ+ youth who are ethnic and racial minorities use ICTs to access intersectional communities and supports, consistent with a general lack of scholarship on the subpopulation. Similarly, LGBTQ+ youth, overrepresented among those who are homeless and/or foster care involved [27], may be especially active ICT users. Technology may offer improved access to necessary resources (e.g., crisis services) [28], though little scholarship has been undertaken.
- *What are the opportunities for digital intervention with LGBTQ+ youth?* Rapid growth in digital interventions has increasingly reflected LGBTQ+ youths' needs and wants. A study recently found that 76% of LGBTQ+ youth prefer online chat or texting options when seeking crisis support [29]. Rigorously evaluated interventions designed specifically for LGBTQ+ youth are emerging for a variety of concerns. These include AFFIRM [30], Q Chat Space [13], SMART [31], Project RISE [32], and many others [33]. Importantly, these digital interventions somewhat address the acknowledged lack of competent LGBTQ+ mental and behavioral health providers. However, a paucity of interventions persists—particularly those having undergone rigorous evaluation or attending to particular health issues, such as suicide [33]. Specific interventions are also needed "tailored exclusively to a [gender diverse] user base, incorporate gender-affirming features, and… [optimized for] mobile technologies." [33]

## 4 Recommendations

Online activities and peer connections offer important benefits for LGBTQ+ youth, especially those otherwise without access to such developmentally important opportunities. Yet, the continued importance of in-person resources and support indicates that "one is not a replacement for the other." [14] Internet-mediated *and* in-person activities, resources, and connections are important for the development and well-being of contemporary LGBTQ+ youth. Scholarship regarding LGBTQ+ youths' experiences with both the risks and opportunities of ICTs is increasing, yet there remain many areas of inquiry for research and practice. American literature may be extrapolated to other developed countries with similar rates of ICT use by youth [3]. However, research is also needed in other regions to understand how cultural and sociopolitical contexts may influence LGBTQ+ youths' experiences and consider the need for context-specific protections. As ICTs constantly evolve, continued investigation into how ICTs impact LGBTQ+ youth's lives is critical: informing education, service provision, policy development, and creation of technologies that consider their unique needs.

### 4.1 For Researchers

- The ubiquity of ICTs in developed countries warrants the expansion of digital methodologies. While the use of online survey-based platforms is broadly accepted, other types of platforms with the potential for innovative data collection should be thoughtfully considered. For example, qualitative arts-based methods may be undertaken with LGBTQ+ youth using online design tools (e.g., digital whiteboards) [3, 13, 26], and novel online data may be used for secondary analyses.
- Importantly, digital methodologies facilitate opportunities to enhance ethical principles when engaging in research with youth, including augmenting informed consent processes and improving responses to participant distress [34].
- Robust and rigorous mixed-method and longitudinal studies can aid future research on the impact of ICTs.

### 4.2 For Policy Professionals and Technologists

- LGBTQ+ youth are at elevated risk for various forms of victimization via ICTs. However, they are *also* at higher risk of discrimination and physical violence (e.g., at home, with peers, at school). In a reality of ubiquitous online *and* offline risks, ICTs offer critical opportunities for safety, respite, social support, and service access not otherwise available to LGBTQ+ youth [14].
- LGBTQ+ youth actively cultivate online spaces and utilize platform safety features (when available) to effectively navigate and respond to the online hostility they experience [25, 26].
- Recommendations for enhancing the safety of youth when using ICTs often actually inhibit the safety of LGBTQ+ youth (e.g., increasing their risk of being "outed" to unsupportive families).
- Their access to wellness-enhancing resources may also be constrained. For example, content on LGBTQ+ populations is "singled out for censorship by many of the most prominent" filtering programs used in schools and libraries [35].
- Given the rapidly changing popularity and features of platforms, policy professionals, technologists, and others should consider how legislating, restricting, or otherwise regulating youths' Internet-mediated activities may adversely impact subpopulations experiencing disproportionate challenges.
- Experts should attend to developing and leveraging ICTs to address the critical health disparities of LGBTQ+ youth experience, particularly their elevated risk for negative outcomes such as self-harm, suicidal ideation, and suicide attempts. For example, technologists should more thoroughly explore web-based support services or algorithmic tools that can screen for suicidality and intervene in real time.
- Finally, professionals need to engage with LGBTQ+ youth directly to better understand their needs, wants, etc. regarding ICTs.

### 4.3 For Educators and Service Providers

- Arguably, the most effective mechanism for enhancing the safety of LGBTQ+ youth is improving their digital literacy and competence to safely navigate ICTs, including interpersonal interactions [36].
- For educators and direct service providers (e.g., social workers, clinical psychologists) digital competence and knowledge of youths' Internet-mediated activities are critical. A feasible first step is integration of comprehensive inquiries regarding ICT activities into intakes and other forms of assessment, rather than the typical handful of general questions on usage.
- Integrating ICTs into in-person services (e.g., using tablets in clinical sessions) could also aid in assessing and fostering youths' digital literacy and providers' knowledge of their clients' activities [37].

- A dearth of purposefully developed evidence-based resources and digital interventions to address LGBTQ+ youths' health disparities and risk behaviors persists. Efforts to develop such innovations must meaningfully involve educators, service providers, LGBTQ+ youth, and other stakeholders. Collaborative inquiry is an effective mechanism for engaging with youth and codesigning accurate, relevant, and accessible information and programming.

**Conflict of Interest and Funding Disclosure** KM was supported by R01MH129207. The content is solely the responsibility of the authors and does not necessarily represent the official views of the National Institutes of Health.

## References

1. Vogels EA, Gelles-Watnick R, Massarat N. Teens, social media and technology 2022. PEW Research Center; 2022. https://www.pewresearch.org/internet/2022/08/10/teens-social-media-and-technology-2022/. Accessed 24 Feb 2023.
2. Internet/broadband fact sheet. PEW Research Center. Published April 7, 2021. https://www.pewresearch.org/internet/fact-sheet/internet-broadband/. Accessed 24 Feb 2023.
3. McInroy LB, Beer OWJ. Adapting vignettes for internet-based research: eliciting realistic responses to the digital milieu. Int J Soc Res Methodol. 2022;25(3):335–47. https://doi.org/10.1080/13645579.2021.1901440.
4. Out online: The experiences of lesbian, gay, bisexual and transgender youth. GLSEN. Published July 10, 2013. https://www.glsen.org/news/out-online-experiences-lgbt-youth-internet. Accessed 1 Mar 2023.
5. Abreu RL, Kenny MC. Cyberbullying and LGBTQ Youth: a systematic literature review and recommendations for prevention and intervention. J Child Adolesc Trauma. 2017;24(11):81–97. https://doi.org/10.1007/s40653-017-0175-7.
6. Craig SL, McInroy LB, McCready LT, Di Cesare DM, Pettaway LD. Connecting without fear: clinical implications of the consumption of information and communication technologies by sexual minority youth and young adults. Clin Soc Work J. 2015;43(2):159–68. https://doi.org/10.1007/s10615-014-0505-2.
7. Russell ST, Fish JN. Mental health in lesbian, gay, bisexual, and transgender (LGBT) youth. Annu Rev Clin Psychol. 2016;12:465–87. https://doi.org/10.1146/annurev-clinpsy-021815-093153.
8. Connolly MD, Zervos MJ, Barone CJ II, Johnson CC, Joseph CL. The mental health of transgender youth: advances in understanding. J Adolesc Health. 2016;59(5):489–95. https://doi.org/10.1016/j.jadohealth.2016.06.012.
9. Hinduja S, Patchin JW. Bullying, cyberbullying, and LGBTQ students. Cyberbullying Research Center; 2020. https://www.humanitarianlibrary.org/sites/default/files/2020/07/Bullying%2C%20Cyberbullying%2C%20and%20LGBTQ%20Students.pdf. Accessed 1 Mar 2023.
10. Over 120 bills restricting LGBTQ rights introduced Nationwide in 2023 so far. American Civil Liberties Union. Published January 19, 2023. https://www.aclu.org/press-releases/over-120-bills-restricting-lgbtq-rights-introduced-nationwide-2023-so-far. Accessed 1 Mar 2023.
11. Rider GN, McMorris BJ, Gower AL, Coleman E, Eisenberg ME. Health and care utilization of transgender and gender nonconforming youth: a population-based study. Pediatrics. 2018;141(3):e20171683. https://doi.org/10.1542/peds.2017-1683.
12. Escobar-Viera CG, Choukas-Bradley S, Sidani J, Maheux AJ, Roberts SR, Rollman BL. Examining social media experiences and attitudes toward technology-based interventions for reducing social isolation among LGBTQ youth living in rural United States: an online qualitative study. Front Digital Health. 2022;4 https://doi.org/10.3389/fdgth.2022.900695.
13. Fish JN, McInroy LB, Paceley MS, Williams ND, Henderson S, Levine DS, Edsall RN. "I'm kinda stuck at home with unsupportive parents right now": LGBTQ youths' experiences with COVID-19 and the importance of online support. J Adolesc Health. 2020;67(3):450–2. https://doi.org/10.1016/j.jadohealth.2020.06.002.
14. Ybarra ML, Mitchell KJ, Palmer NA, Reisner SL. Online social support as a buffer against online and offline peer and sexual victimization among US LGBT and non-LGBT youth. Child Abuse Negl. 2015;39:123–36. https://doi.org/10.1016/j.chiabu.2014.08.006.
15. DeLonga K, Torres HL, Kamen C, Evans SN, Lee S, Koopman C, Gore-Felton C. Loneliness, internalized homophobia, and compulsive internet use: factors associated with sexual risk behavior among a sample of adolescent males seeking services at a community LGBT center. Sex Addict Compuls. 2011;18(2):61–74. https://doi.org/10.1080/10720162.2011.581897.
16. Hightow-Weidman LB, Muessig KE, Bauermeister J, Zhang C, LeGrand S. Youth, technology, and HIV: recent advances and future directions. Curr HIV/AIDS Rep. 2015;12:500–15. https://doi.org/10.1007/s11904-015-0280-x.
17. Nelson R, Robards B, Churchill B, Vivienne S, Byron P, Hanckel B. Social media use among bisexuals and pansexuals: connection, harassment and mental

health. Cult Health Sex. 2022;25:711. https://doi.org/10.1080/13691058.2022.2092213.
18. Gaudette M, Hesse CL, Kia H, Chanady T, Carson A, Knight R, Ferlatte O. "A Double-Edged Sword": health professionals' perspectives on the health and social impacts of gay dating apps on young gay, bisexual, trans and queer men. J Sex Res. 2022;60:656. https://doi.org/10.1080/00224499.2022.2153786.
19. Bőthe B, Vaillancourt-Morel MP, Bergeron S, Demetrovics Z. Problematic and non-problematic pornography use among LGBTQ adolescents: a systematic literature review. Curr Addict Rep. 2019;6:478–94. https://doi.org/10.1007/s40429-019-00289-5.
20. Delmonaco D, Marcu G, Haimson OL. Search engines and the sex education information practices of LGBTQ+ youth. Proc Assoc Inf Sci Technol. 2020;57(1):e364. https://doi.org/10.1002/pra2.364.
21. McInroy LB, Craig SL. Perspectives of LGBTQ emerging adults on the depiction and impact of LGBTQ media representation. J Youth Stud. 2017;20(1):32–45. https://doi.org/10.1080/13676261.2016.1184243.
22. McInroy LB, Hawkins BW, Zapcic I, Fregoli C. Using design thinking to address health disparities and interdisciplinary knowledge translation: an LGBTQ+ youth health literacy project. Health Soc Work. 2023;48(1):21–32. https://doi.org/10.1093/hsw/hlac035.
23. Berger MN, Taba M, Marino JL, Lim MS, Skinner SR. Social media use and health and Well-being of lesbian, gay, bisexual, transgender, and queer youth: systematic review. J Med Internet Res. 2022;24(9):e38449. https://doi.org/10.2196/38449.
24. Macapagal K, Wongsomboon V, Gordon JD, Widman LM. Online dating, sexual behavior, and sexual communication among adolescents. (Under review).
25. Craig SL, Eaton AD, McInroy LB, D'Souza SA, Krishnan S, Wells GA, Twum-Siaw L, Leung VW. Navigating negativity: a grounded theory and integrative mixed methods investigation of how sexual and gender minority youth cope with negative comments online. Psychol Sex. 2020;11(3):161–79. https://doi.org/10.1080/19419899.2019.1665575.
26. McInroy LB, Beer OWJ, Scheadler TR, Craig SL, Eaton AD. Exploring the psychological and physiological impacts of digital microaggressions and hostile online climates on LGBTQ+ youth. Curr Psychol. in press;
27. Gambon TB, Gewirtz O'Brien JR, Lavin A, Askew GL, Baum R, Berger-Jenkins E, Johnson T, Jutte D, Nasir A, Duffee J, Dilley KJ. Runaway youth: caring for the nation's largest segment of missing children. Pediatrics. 2020;145(2) https://doi.org/10.1542/peds.2019-3752.
28. Rhoades H, Rusow JA, Bond D, Lanteigne A, Fulginiti A, Goldbach JT. Homelessness, mental health and suicidality among LGBTQ youth accessing crisis services. Child Psychiatry Hum Dev. 2018;49:643–51. https://doi.org/10.1007/s10578-018-0780-1.
29. National survey on LGBTQ mental health. The Trevor Project. 2019. https://www.thetrevorproject.org/survey-2019/. Accessed 1 Mar 2023.
30. Craig SL, Leung VW, Pascoe R, Pang N, Iacono G, Austin A, Dillon F. AFFIRM online: utilising an affirmative cognitive–behavioural digital intervention to improve mental health, access, and engagement among LGBTQA+ youth and young adults. Int J Environ Res Public Health. 2021;18(4):1541. https://doi.org/10.3390/ijerph18041541.
31. Mustanski B, Saber R, Macapagal K, Matson M, Laber E, Rodrgiuez-Diaz C, Moran KO, Carrion A, Moskowitz DA, Newcomb ME. Effectiveness of the SMART sex Ed program among 13-18 year old English and Spanish speaking adolescent men who have sex with men. AIDS Behav. 2023;27(2):733–44. https://doi.org/10.1007/s10461-022-03806-2.
32. Shen J, Rubin A, Cohen K, Hart E, McDanal R, Sung J, Roulston CA, Sotomayor I, Fox K, Schleider JL. Randomized evaluation of an online single-session intervention for minority stress in LGBTQ+ adolescents. Internet Interv. 2023; https://doi.org/10.31234/osf.io/6yj9b.
33. Skeen SJ, Cain D, Gamarel KE, Hightow-Weidman L, Reback CJ. mHealth for transgender and gender-expansive youth: harnessing gender-affirmative cross-disciplinary innovations to advance HIV prevention and care interventions. Mhealth. 2021;7 https://doi.org/10.21037/mhealth-20-60.
34. McInroy LB. Innovative ethics: using animated videos when soliciting informed consent of young people for online surveys. Soc Work Res. 2017;41(2):121–8. https://doi.org/10.1093/swr/svx004.
35. Robinson T. Overcoming social exclusion in public library services to LGBTQ and gender variant youth. Public Libr Q. 2016;35(3):161–74. https://doi.org/10.1080/01616846.2016.1210439.
36. Hartikainen H, Iivari N, Kinnula M. Should we design for control, trust or involvement? A discourses survey about children's online safety. In: Proceedings of the 15th international conference on interaction design and children; 2016. p. 367–78. https://doi.org/10.1145/2930674.2930680.
37. Coyne CA, Wongsomboon V, Korpak AK, Macapagal K. "We have to figure it out ourselves": transfeminine adolescents' online sexual experiences and recommendations for supporting their sexual health and wellbeing. Front Reprod Health. 2023;4:1034747. https://doi.org/10.3389/frph.2022.1034747.
38. Nagata JM, Lee CM, Yang J, Al-Shoaibi AA, Ganson KT, Testa A, Jackson DB. Associations between sexual orientation and early adolescent screen use: findings from the Adolescent Brain Cognitive Development (ABCD) Study. Ann Epidemiol. 2023;82:54–8. https://doi.org/10.1016/j.annepidem.2023.03.004.
39. Bond BJ, Miller B. YouTube as my space: the relationships between YouTube, social connectedness, and (collective) self-esteem among LGBTQ individuals. New Media Soc. 2024;26(1):513–33.

# Pornography Use During Adolescence: The Current State of Knowledge and Recommendations

Megan K. Maas, Paul J. Wright, Emily F. Rothman, Kimberly M. Nelson, Paul Weigle, and Debby Herbenick

## 1 Background

As the Internet remains a ubiquitous presence in the lives of adolescents, it is not surprising that large-scale, representative studies show that many have seen pornography, whether intentionally or not (approximately 60–75% of boys and 40–52% of girls) [1, 2]. Although point estimates vary across studies, the median age at first exposure to pornography ranges from 12 to 15 years old [3], with a recent study reporting that 54% of adolescents first saw online pornography at age 13 years or younger [2]. More frequent pornography use has been seen in older adolescents, cisgender boys, those higher in sensation seeking, and sexual or gender diverse youth [2–4]. In this chapter, we review quantitative studies of pornography use (typically defined as videos or images of nudity and/or sexual activity intended to arouse the viewer) among adolescent samples only. To be included, priority was given to studies published in peer-reviewed academic journals published in or after 2010. The study also had to be empirical, using a method that was described and systematically applied. Of note, research studies examining the potential effects of pornography are becoming more prevalent, with annual PubMed Publications found with search terms "pornography" and "youth" doubling between 2010 and 2020.

Mainstream pornography that adolescents routinely access (as it is often free and easily accessible both on pornographic websites and some social media sites) depicts what would have been considered "extreme" content in former generations. At its most extreme, pornography on what are known as "tube-sites" that act as streaming platforms similar to YouTube frequently portrays sexual violence and coercion [5], rough or aggressive sex [6], BDSM without relational context, and step-sibling or parent incest [5, 6]. While seemingly consensual, pornography rarely

M. K. Maas (✉)
Department of Human Development & Family Studies, Michigan State University, East Lansing, MI, USA
e-mail: maasmeg1@msu.edu

P. J. Wright
Communication Science, The Media School, Indiana University, Bloomington, IN, USA

E. F. Rothman
Department of Occupational Therapy, Boston University, Boston, MA, USA

K. M. Nelson
Department of Community Health Sciences, Boston University School of Public Health, Boston, MA, USA

Department of Psychiatry, Boston University School of Medicine, Boston, MA, USA

P. Weigle
Department of Psychiatry, University of Connecticut School of Medicine, Farmington, CT, USA

D. Herbenick
Department of Applied Health Science, Indiana University, Bloomington, IN, USA


D. A. Christakis, L. Hale (eds.), *Handbook of Children and Screens*,
https://doi.org/10.1007/978-3-031-69362-5_47

portrays effective sexual communication, the use of condoms, or caring behaviors [5, 6]. Given the regular exposure to depictions of sexual violence and condomless sex while watching Internet pornography, it is vital to understand what role pornography plays in the sexual socialization of youth and how parents and professionals can prepare them to be more resilient to any subsequent harmful impacts from viewing it.

Adolescents generally do not have the life experience or comprehensive sex education to understand or contextualize what they see in pornography the way that more sexually experienced adults can. They are beginning their sexual lives with few in-person experiences to provide a frame of reference to judge what is likely to be realistic, mutually acceptable, or pleasurable with a partner. Indeed, data demonstrates that pornography is now the primary source of information for emerging adults on how to have sex, and many adolescents perceive pornography to be a realistic portrayal of sexual behaviors [7–9]. One longitudinal study showed that as adolescents' pornography use continued across 23 months, their perceptions of its realism decreased [7], indicating that the maturity and analytical skills gained rapidly during adolescence may make pornography's impact different for younger compared to older adolescents. Regardless of the variance in maturity and analytic skills, most adolescents (particularly in the US) do not have widespread access to comprehensive sex education [10], potentially rendering them more vulnerable to negative impacts from pornography use. Indeed, sex education rarely includes the topics of sexual communication or sexual pleasure, nor does it cover the diversity of sexual and gender identities [10], leaving teens to turn to the Internet to learn how to have sex in ways that appear pleasurable, particularly between same-gender partners [11].

Most research on adolescent pornography use was not designed to focus on pornography as a root cause of attitude or behavior change. However, some longitudinal studies provide evidence for changes in attitudes and behaviors that correspond to differences in pornography use over time, providing support for media socialization models. For example, much evidence has been generated supporting the sexual script acquisition, activation, and application model's ($_3$AM) hypotheses regarding the role of sexual scripts (symbolically imparted directives for sexual behavior) in sexual media socialization processes [12].

## 2 Current State

### 2.1 Pornography Use, Sexual Attitudes, Beliefs, and Satisfaction

Inquiries into adolescents' pornography use have revealed associations with sexual beliefs and perceptions. For example, more frequent use of pornography has consistently been found to be associated with more recreational attitudes toward sex [3], even across 1 year, and particularly among cisgender boys [13]. Adolescents who consume pornography were also found to hold more erroneous beliefs about sex (e.g., "most people prefer rough to gentle sex") than those who did not consume pornography. These beliefs were especially salient for those who viewed pornography more frequently or depended upon pornography as a primary source of sexual knowledge [14]. Similarly, when male adolescents perceived pornography to be less real, they experienced less rapid development of permissive sexual attitudes over time than boys who perceived it as more real; whereas changes in female adolescents' sexual attitudes over time were not as dependent upon their perceptions of pornography [8]. Pornography use has also been associated with more negative sexual self-perceptions [15] and lower sexual satisfaction with partners [16] among adolescents. However, some results indicate that there are differences (e.g., cultural, measurement, and social norms) that have yet to be accounted for, as pornography use was found to be longitudinally associated with lower sexual satisfaction among Dutch adolescents [3], but not among Croatian adolescents [17].

Studies involving adolescent samples have shown consistent associations between pornography use and harmful gendered perceptions. A meta-analysis demonstrated that adolescent pornography use—and particularly violent pornography use—was associated with greater acceptance of rape myths (e.g., the victim deserved it due to provocative clothing), regardless of gender identity [18]. In a longitudinal study of adolescents, pornography viewing and attitudes toward women as sexual objects had a reciprocal association, where more endorsement of the sexual objectification of women predicted more frequent pornography use, and more frequent pornography use predicted more endorsement of the sexual objectification of women [3]. Among Croatian female adolescents, higher baseline levels of pornography use predicted more endorsement of hyperfemininity (i.e., emphasis on sexiness and submissiveness), but also a greater feeling of sexual agency 2 years later [19]. An alternative study showed that the prospective association between earlier pornography use and later sexual objectification endorsement was weaker when adolescents indicated they had received more pornography education in school and stronger when they indicated they had received less pornography education in school.

## 2.2 Online Pornography Use and In-Person Sexual Experiences

Perhaps the most common question among scientists, practitioners, and parents is whether pornography causes adolescents (who might otherwise engage in healthier sexual activity) to engage in more risky or otherwise harmful sexual behavior. For example, a path analysis supported a conceptual model, where youth with more frequent exposure to pornography were more likely to engage in sexually dominant behaviors (e.g., choking/strangulation, name-calling, and spanking), emotionally distancing them from their partners, and reducing their sense of sexual satisfaction [16]. Of note for physically risky sexual behavior, there are consistent findings that have shown pornography use to be associated with younger age of onset of sexual activity [20] and condomless sex among adolescents [21] (particularly for heterosexual [22] and sexual minority [11] male adolescents). However, one study demonstrated that pornography use was not associated with condomless sex for adolescents with parents who engaged them in discussions of sexual health [23], again highlighting the protective power of sex education.

Sexual violence (e.g., sexual harassment, sexual coercion, and physical rape) victimization has been disproportionately experienced by female adolescents and sexual or gender minority youth (compared to cisgender, heterosexual male adolescents), particularly in the last 5 years [24]. Given the depiction of sexual objectification, coercion, and even violence in Internet pornography [5, 6], researchers have investigated if pornography use may be predictive of both sexual violence perpetration and victimization. A recent longitudinal study of US adolescents showed a positive reciprocal correlation between pornography use and sexual harassment perpetration when adolescents were surveyed five times in 3 years. For male adolescents in this study, pornography use longitudinally predicted sexual assault perpetration during two waves of data collection [25]. However, another study showed that not simply viewing but having viewed and perceived pornography to be realistic, was associated with an increased probability of sexual aggression for male (but not female) adolescents [9].

In terms of victimization, female adolescents who sought out pornography in addition to online chatting about sex were found to have had a higher likelihood of intimate partner violence (including sexual assault) victimization 1 year later compared to those who sought out pornography or engaged in sexual chatting alone [26]. This finding suggests that future measurement of pornography use needs to consider related online experiences when investigating outcomes such as violence victimization. For example, high rates of violent pornography exposure and intimate partner violence victimization were documented among female adolescents in another study, particularly for girls with diverse sexual identities

[27], but pornography use was not a predictor of victimization. More research on victimization should include sexually explicit fan fiction as part of pornography assessment. For example, in a qualitative study of female adolescent fanfiction writers, participants revealed their love of bad boys (who were sexually aggressive or emotionally manipulative) in fan fiction and reported tolerating similar behavior from real-life romantic partners [28].

## 2.3 Conclusion

In conclusion, adolescents will continue to have a variety of experiences in online spaces that are difficult to monitor as they engage with smartphones, laptops, and school-issued devices that may facilitate access to pornographic content. Overall, pornography use has been shown to play a role in the development of potentially harmful sexual attitudes and behaviors among adolescents, especially younger adolescents. Therefore, it is imperative for parents, educators, and clinicians to discuss pornography with youth and offer support and guidance on navigating healthy sexual experiences. We recommend interdisciplinary approaches to pornography research that can account for physiological impacts to accompany the psychological and social impacts that have already been investigated. We also strongly urge for the mobilization of resources to ensure that widespread, comprehensive, medically accurate sex education occurs in schools. Compared to parent-based sex education, school-based sex education has the ability to change individual-level behavior as well as the social norms within a school, resulting in a healthier environment for all adolescents [10]. Despite societal discomfort with pornography discourse, it is imperative that we include pornography in the discussion of sexuality across contexts as it will continue to be an immersive online activity deserving of the same scientific attention we give to understanding how gaming, social media, and traditional media shape adolescent development.

# 3 Future Research

First, there are several ways to improve the current state of measurement of pornography use that could help identify person-specific factors for risk and resilience in terms of exposure frequency. More nuanced, within-person (e.g., longitudinal panel or momentary assessment designs) and/or person-specific (e.g., latent class and profile) analyses would advance our understanding of the multidimensional processes of how adolescents use pornography (e.g., devices and contexts), better recall of what kinds of sex they see depicted, and resultant behavior changes after pornography use [20, 26]. For example, will most adolescents who view sexual violence in pornography then perpetrate or become victims of sexual violence? If not, what factors contribute to their resilience?

Second, we need more research that focuses on the specific health impacts of pornography use among marginalized youth (e.g., minoritized racial/ethnic backgrounds, sexual and gender minorities, maltreatment). Marginalized youth are at greater risk for a myriad of adverse sexual health outcomes, including HIV/STIs, unintended pregnancy, and experiences of sexual violence [11, 26, 27]. There are preliminary studies indicating that marginalized youth may be more likely to view pornography earlier and more often than their nonmarginalized peers [3, 4, 26]. It would be helpful to assess whether pornography use is meaningfully and differentially impacting their sexual health behaviors and outcomes. This information could lead to considerations for tailoring sex education efforts to address their specific sexual health needs, including the use of pornography.

Third, interdisciplinary approaches that simultaneously consider neurological, developmental, and sociological aspects of behavior need to be applied to pornography use among adolescents. Adolescence is a sensitive period of brain development, with physiological pubertal processes causing neuronal "branching" to occur at rates similar to infancy [29]. Thus, sexual experiences are likely just as formative for brain development as other psychosocial processes. Differing pornography use patterns may not only play a role in developing attitudes or ideas about sexuality but also in developing sexual arousal patterns that could be dependent upon rapidly changing visual stimuli, for example. Although scientific understanding of problematic pornography use among adolescents is nascent [30], one longitudinal study showed that more negative emotions and impulsivity predicted higher levels of problematic pornography use among Croatian male adolescents 3 years later [31]. Additional data could be beneficial for understanding if or when an individual adolescent's pornography use should receive clinical attention. For adolescents in general, understanding motivations and consequences for different patterns of pornography use could also be key in understanding when pornography should be targeted in the prevention of undesired outcomes (e.g., sexual violence).

## 4 Recommendations

- **For decision makers:** Policies that support school-based comprehensive sex education and violence prevention to address sexualized media, as vital supports for the health and well-being of youth. In the absence of medically accurate, factual information about sex and how to have sex, most adolescents will likely continue to turn to online, free, and mainstream pornography to learn about sex because it is readily available and designed to be visually engaging and arousing.
- **For educators:** As school-based sex education curricula and standards are typically decided at the district level [10], we urge sex education advisory boards to recommend programming that includes empirically supported, nonjudgmental information about pornography for students, school staff, and parents.
- **For parents:** Educational opportunities that describe the nature and impact of online pornography, explain the need to scaffold autonomous Internet use among older adolescents by first monitoring younger adolescents' online activities, and support skill building for discussing healthy sexuality with children. Many parents underestimate their children's exposure to pornography and may not be fully aware of what their children are potentially learning from it [1]. Therefore, parents would also benefit from.
- **For pediatricians:** Professional development opportunities to gain a deeper understanding of the online sexual experiences of teens (including pornography use). These training opportunities could help providers respond to any issues that may arise. It may be especially important to screen for pornography use in cases of suspected sexual abuse. As overt consent is often missing from pornography and some mainstream pornography sites portray behaviors that would be considered abusive (e.g., incest, rape) [6], it is possible that youth who see such content may minimize the seriousness of the abuse they are enduring.
- **For Mental Healthcare Providers**: It is important to note when pornography use has become a source of distress for an adolescent where they describe obsession or loneliness, as seen in samples of adolescents with mental health disorders, where problematic pornography use models may be helpful for guiding treatment [30]. That being said, sexual curiosity and masturbation are normal processes of adolescent development that should not be pathologized by healthcare providers [32]. It is important that parents, educators, and clinicians do not conflate sexual curiosity and masturbation with pornography use during discussions of sexuality with youth.

**Conflict of Interest and Funding Disclosures** DH has received grant funding and/or provided consultation to Pure Romance, Reckitt Benckiser, and Church & Dwight. KN and ER's contributions were supported by the National Institute of Child Health and Human Development [R21HD105482]. Any opinions, findings, conclusions, or recommendations expressed in this material are those of the authors and do not necessarily reflect the views of the National Institutes of Health.

## References


1. Wright PJ, Herbenick D, Paul B, Tokunaga RS. U.S. Parents underestimate their children's pornography use and learning, vol. 52. Springer; 2023. https://doi.org/10.1007/S10508-022-02449-7/METRICS.
2. Micheal, Robb B, Supreet M. Teens and pornography.; 2023. https://www.commonsensemedia.org/sites/default/files/research/report/2022-teens-and-pornography-final-web.pdf.
3. Peter J, Valkenburg PM. Adolescents and pornography: a review of 20 years of research. J Sex Res. 2016;53:509–31. https://doi.org/10.1080/00224499.2016.1143441.
4. Bőthe B, Vaillancourt-Morel MP, Girouard A, Štulhofer A, Dion J, Bergeron S. A large-scale comparison of Canadian sexual/gender minority and heterosexual, cisgender adolescents' pornography use characteristics. J Sex Med. 2020;17(6):1156–67. https://doi.org/10.1016/J.JSXM.2020.02.009.
5. Fritz N, Malic V, Paul B, Zhou Y. A descriptive analysis of the types, targets, and relative frequency of aggression in mainstream pornography. Arch Sex Behav. 2020;49(8):3041–53. https://doi.org/10.1007/s10508-020-01773-0.
6. Vera-Gray F, Mcglynn C, Kureshi I, Butterby K. Sexual violence as a sexual script in mainstream online pornography. Br J Criminol. 2021;61:1243. https://doi.org/10.1093/bjc/azab035.
7. Wright PJ, Štulhofer A. Adolescent pornography use and the dynamics of perceived pornography realism: does seeing more make it more realistic? Comput Hum Behav. 2019;95:37–47. https://doi.org/10.1016/J.CHB.2019.01.024.
8. Baams L, Overbeek G, Dubas JS, Doornwaard SM, Rommes E, van Aken MAG. Perceived realism moderates the relation between sexualized media consumption and permissive sexual attitudes in Dutch adolescents. Arch Sex Behav. 2015;44(3):743–54. https://doi.org/10.1007/S10508-014-0443-7/METRICS.
9. Wright PJ, Paul B, Herbenick D. Preliminary insights from a U.S. probability sample on adolescents' pornography exposure, media psychology, and sexual aggression. J Health Commun. 2021;26:39. https://doi.org/10.1080/10810730.2021.1887980.
10. Lindberg LD, Kantor LM. Adolescents' receipt of sex education in a nationally representative sample, 2011–2019. J Adolesc Health. 2022;70(2):290–7. https://doi.org/10.1016/J.JADOHEALTH.2021.08.027/ATTACHMENT/DF3BB52A-15FD-42A3-8F0A-25F767D0B806/MMC1.PDF.
11. Nelson KM, Perry NS, Carey MP. Sexually explicit media use among 14–17-year-old sexual minority males in the U.S. Arch Sex Behav. 2019;48(8):2345–55. https://doi.org/10.1007/S10508-019-01501-3/METRICS.
12. Wright PJ. Media and sexuality. In: Oliver MB, Raney AA, Bryant J, editors. Media effects: advances in theory and research. Routledge; 2020. p. 227–42.
13. Doornwaard SM, Bickham DS, Rich M, ter Bogt TFM, van den Eijnden RJJM. Adolescents' use of sexually explicit internet material and their sexual attitudes and behavior: parallel development and directional effects. Dev Psychol. 2015;51(10):1476–88. https://doi.org/10.1037/DEV0000040.
14. Wright PJ, Tokunaga RS, Herbenick D, Paul B. Pornography vs. sexual science: the role of pornography use and dependency in U.S. teenagers' sexual illiteracy. Commun Monogr. 2021;89:332. https://doi.org/10.1080/03637751.2021.1987486.
15. Doornwaard SM, Bickham DS, Rich M, Vanwesenbeeck I, Van Den Eijnden RJJM, Ter Bogt TFM. Sex-related online behaviors and adolescents' body and sexual self-perceptions. Pediatrics. 2014;134(6):1103–10. https://doi.org/10.1542/PEDS.2014-0592.
16. Wright PJ, Herbenick D, Paul B, Tokunaga RS. Exploratory findings on U.S. adolescents' pornography use, dominant behavior, and sexual satisfaction. Int J Sex Health. 2021;33(2):222–8. https://doi.org/10.1080/19317611.2021.1888170.
17. Milas G, Wright P, Štulhofer A. Longitudinal assessment of the association between pornography use and sexual satisfaction in adolescence. J Sex Res. 2019;57(1):16–28. https://doi.org/10.1080/00224499.2019.1607817.
18. Burnay J, Kepes S, Bushman BJ. Effects of violent and nonviolent sexualized media on aggression-related thoughts, feelings, attitudes, and behaviors: a meta-analytic review. Aggress Behav. 2022;48(1):111–36. https://doi.org/10.1002/AB.21998.
19. Klein V, Šević S, Kohut T, Štulhofer A. Longitudinal assessment of the association between the use of sexually explicit material, hyperfemininity, and sexual agency in adolescent women. Psychol Sex. 2020;13:213. https://doi.org/10.1080/19419899.2020.1757500.
20. Pirrone D, Zondervan-Zwijnenburg M, Reitz E, van den Eijnden RJJM, ter Bogt TFM. Pornography use profiles and the emergence of sexual behaviors in adolescence. Arch Sex Behav. 2022;51(2):1141–56. https://doi.org/10.1007/S10508-021-02140-3/TABLES/7.
21. Tokunaga RS, Wright PJ, Vangeel L. Is pornography consumption a risk factor for condomless sex? Hum Commun Res. 2020;46(2–3):273–99. https://doi.org/10.1093/hcr/hqaa005.
22. Luder M-T, Pittet I, Berchtold A, Akré C, Michaud P-A, Surís J-C. Associations between online pornography and sexual behavior among adolescents: myth or reality? Arch Sex Behav. 2011;40:1027–35. https://doi.org/10.1007/s10508-010-9714-0.
23. Wright PJ, Herbenick D, Paul B. Adolescent condom use, parent-adolescent sexual health communication, and pornography: findings from a U.S. probability

sample. 2019. https://doi.org/10.1080/10410236.2019.1652392
24. Centers for Disease Control and Prevention. Youth risk behavior survey data summary & trends report: 2011–2021.; 2023.
25. Waterman EA, Wesche R, Morris G, Edwards KM, Banyard VL. Prospective associations between pornography viewing and sexual aggression among adolescents. J Res Adolesc. 2022;32(4):1612–25. https://doi.org/10.1111/JORA.12745.
26. Maas MK, Bray BC, Noll JG. Online sexual experiences predict subsequent sexual health and victimization outcomes among female adolescents: a latent class analysis. J Youth Adolesc. 2019;48:837–49. https://doi.org/10.1111/jora.12364.
27. Herbitter C, Norris AL, Nelson KM, Orchowski LM. Understanding associations between exposure to violent pornography and teen dating violence among female sexual minority high school students. J Interpers Violence. 2021;37(17–18):NP17023-NP17035. https://doi.org/10.1177/08862605211028314.
28. Hedrick A. 'He's so bad but he does it so well': interviews with one direction fans about writing romantic and erotic fiction online. Sex Educ. 2021;21(6):693–707. https://doi.org/10.1080/14681811.2020.1852075.
29. Goddings A-L, Beltz A, Peper JS, Crone EA, Braams BR. Understanding the role of puberty in structural and functional development of the adolescent brain. J Res Adolesc. 2019; https://doi.org/10.1111/jora.12408.
30. Testa G, Mestre-Bach G, Chiclana Actis C, Potenza MN. Problematic pornography use in adolescents: from prevention to intervention. Curr Addict Rep. 2023;1:1–9. https://doi.org/10.1007/S40429-023-00469-4/TABLES/2.
31. Rousseau A, Bőthe B, Štulhofer A. Theoretical antecedents of male adolescents' problematic pornography use: a longitudinal assessment. J Sex Res. 2021;58(3):331–41. https://doi.org/10.1080/00224499.2020.1815637.
32. Fortenberry JD, Hensel DJ. Sexual pleasure in adolescence: a developmental sexual embodiment perspective. In: Gender and sexuality development: contemporary theory and research; 2022. p. 357–84. https://doi.org/10.1007/978-3-030-84273-4_13.

# Sexual Health Information Online

Eric R. Walsh-Buhi, Hannah Javidi,
and Kathryn Macapagal

## 1 Background

Digital access, including Internet usage among adolescents, is at its highest point in history. As of 2023, over 90% of US teens aged 13–17 years reported that they use the Internet daily, with nearly half of teens reporting that they use the Internet "almost constantly" (see previous chapter) [1]. Mobile Internet access is prevalent among adolescents and, in particular, older adolescents. Approximately 95% of teens own or have access to a smartphone; 90% also report owning or having access to a desktop/laptop computer [1]. Regarding social media, in 2023, roughly 9 in 10 US teens reported using YouTube—by far the most popular social media application (app)/platform [1]. TikTok, Snapchat, and Instagram are used by 63%, 60%, and 59% of teens ages 13–17, respectively, while this increases to about 70% for teens aged 15–17 [1]. Facebook and Twitter are less popular, but still used, social media platforms among adolescents [1].

E. R. Walsh-Buhi (✉) · H. Javidi
Department of Applied Health Science, Indiana University School of Public Health-Bloomington, Bloomington, IN, USA
e-mail: erwals@iu.edu

K. Macapagal
Institute for Sexual and Gender Minority Health and Wellbeing, Northwestern University, Chicago, IL, USA

Department of Medical Social Sciences, Feinberg School of Medicine, Northwestern University, Chicago, IL, USA

## 2 Current State

### 2.1 Online Sexual Health Information Seeking: Prevalence, Sources, and Topics

Adolescents consistently engage with online sexual health information (OSHI). In fact, sexual health is the *most widely-searched-for topic online* (e.g., compared to searches related to diet/nutrition, mental health, fitness, or specific diseases/conditions) [2]. Collectively, studies report that between 20% and 77% of young people use the Internet for sexual health and sex education purposes.

Search engines, specifically, are very common methods for retrieving OSHI, though barriers remain. In one observational study [2], researchers found that young people do not go straight to trusted websites or sources for OSHI. Instead, their first step is usually a search engine like Google. However, in a study querying sexually transmitted infection (STI) and human immunodeficiency virus (HIV) testing services on Google for six geographically unique locations in the United States [3], researchers found that searches


D. A. Christakis, L. Hale (eds.), *Handbook of Children and Screens*,
https://doi.org/10.1007/978-3-031-69362-5_48

for information in larger cities were more likely to yield relevant results compared with searches for information in smaller cities. Accordingly, OSHI searches do not always yield consistent results enabling adolescents' access to sexual and reproductive health (SRH) care services and information that can guide SRH-related behavioral decisions.

While social media use is very common among adolescents, it is not the preferred or most frequently used source for OSHI. In a study of African American and Latino adolescents, for example, social media was the fourth most commonly cited source of sexual risk reduction information behind television and movies, school, and parents, with just under half of participants reporting social media as a source of *recent* sexual risk reduction information [4]. Numerous mobile apps also have been created with the intention of enhancing sexual health knowledge and outcomes among adolescents (e.g., Tia: Female Health Advisor) [5]. While these apps exhibit some strengths, such as high functionality, user-friendliness, and navigability, the majority of them do not provide comprehensive, reliable, and evidence-based information on sexual health [6].

What sexual health-related topics are adolescents looking for? Simon and Daneback [7] reported that the most commonly cited OSHI topics of interest pertained to (1) HIV/acquired immunodeficiency syndrome (AIDS) and STIs, (2) pregnancy/childbirth, (3) sex acts/sexual behavior, (4) contraception, (5) information about the body (e.g., genitalia, anatomy, and physiology), (6) relationships/social issues, and (7) gender identity and sexual orientation [7]. In other research, however, clinicians/medical providers remain the most important sources of *contraception* information for young people [8].

## 2.2 Barriers to Engagement with Online Sexual Health Information

In their searches for sexual health information online, adolescents may face a number of barriers and challenges. Patterson et al. [9] reported that some of the more common barriers mentioned by young people included difficulty filtering an overabundance of content, limited awareness of specific, relevant, trusted online sources, difficulties with finding locally relevant information about sexual health services (as also noted above), and challenges in navigating large organizations' websites. In fact, in one observational study [2], researchers found that some young people gave up on their searches for OSHI due to frustration and difficulties navigating certain organizations' websites.

There are also sociocultural barriers to searching for and retrieving OSHI, including privacy issues (e.g., fear of being observed), uncertainty about engaging with visual and auditory content (heightening their risk of "being seen"), concerns regarding unintentionally accessing sexually explicit materials, and reticence to access sexual health information on social media platforms or through smartphone apps given the possibility of their peers coming across this content on their smartphone and passing judgment or forming a negative opinion of them [9].

The "digital divide", which refers to the unequal distribution of access to and use of technology, particularly computers and the Internet, can exacerbate existing health disparities among adolescents. Although we have observed a narrowing of the divide, in general, individuals living in lower-income and rural communities lag in broadband connectivity [10]. Moreover, *access* to devices and to the Internet does not ensure equitable access to accurate, relevant, and useful content, as priority populations vary in their health information needs and behaviors [11]. Given the prevalence of OSHI-seeking, young people who lack access to digital resources (e.g., those from marginalized communities and low-income populations) may in turn lack access to knowledge about contraception, STIs, and other aspects of sexual health [1, 12]. They may also have limited access to telehealth, which can serve as a life-saving resource for those who need urgent sexual health information and support but cannot be seen in person. Other than lacking access to digital devices and the Internet, adolescents may not possess sufficient digital literacy (i.e., the ability to navigate digital sources using critical thinking), representing another type of digital divide.

## 2.3 Benefits of Sexual Health Information Online

Technology has become a primary tool for adolescents to access sexual health information and resources, including contraception, HIV testing, and STI treatment [13]. Online platforms can be comfortable, familiar, and private spaces for youth to explore these topics (among others) at their own pace, removing some stigma and discomfort associated with face-to-face discussions about sexuality [14]. In the absence of high-quality, consistent school-based sex education nationwide, OSHI provides generally a safe, non-embarrassing, and standardized way for adolescents to learn about body parts, sexual processes, and other sensitive topics (e.g., puberty), which can be essential in promoting healthy sexual development [15]. In addition, online resources have the potential for greater inclusivity, offering information and resources tailored to diverse populations, including those who may have previously been excluded from traditional sex education [16, 17].

Considerable evidence suggests that LGBTQ+ (i.e., sexual and gender minority) adolescents seek information about sex and sexuality online, including from social media and sexually explicit media (SEM), more than their heterosexual and cisgender counterparts [18, 19]. This may be due to a variety of factors, including the absence of LGBTQ+-inclusive sex education in the United States, parents' lack of knowledge about LGBTQ+ sexual health and discomfort discussing LGBTQ+-related sexuality, and reluctance of adolescents to disclose their sexual identity to their parents, particularly if the parents are perceived to be unaffirming [20, 21].

However, there are also risks associated with adolescent OSHI-seeking. Sexually explicit media (i.e., pornography) is a form of OSHI that can offer educational benefits for adolescents, but solely relying on it as a source of sexual information could have drawbacks. Studies examining the messages and visuals conveyed through pornography have produced mixed findings regarding their accuracy in depicting sex [22]. Exposure to unrealistic depictions of bodies and sex could lead young people to become desensitized to what healthy, respectful sexual encounters involve. However, some UK-based research suggests that the negative feelings that may arise after initial exposure to SEM may decrease over time [23].

## 2.4 Misinformation, Trust, and Quality of Sources

The Internet can be a valuable source of sexual health information for teens; however, valid concerns exist about the trustworthiness of online health information sources, as well as the accuracy and quality of the information retrieved. In their systematic review, Freeman et al. [24] found that adolescents generally do not consider the Internet a trusted source for health information (but they use it anyway), they use heuristics such as the ending of the website's hyperlink (e.g., .gov, .org) to appraise the trustworthiness of online health information, and they trust websites more than social media or social networking sites. Their level of trust in online health information subsequently guides their actions and responses.

However, in recent years, the emergence of TikTok as a popular and almost ubiquitous social media platform among teens has led to greater trust in this app as a source of sexual health information. Despite the notoriously strict moderation of topics related to sex, sexual health-related content is widely prevalent on TikTok. In fact, some content that tends to be excluded in formal sex education (e.g., sexual pleasure) can be easily accessed on TikTok. In a content analytic study of sex education on TikTok [25], researchers found that sexual pleasure was the second most common theme (found in 23 of the 100 reviewed posts/videos), within which discussions of the female orgasm and arousal constituted the most common subtheme [25].

While most young people can locate accurate answers to their online sexual health-related questions, finding *local information* and resources may be more difficult. Buhi et al. [2, 26] found that websites containing the most technically complex sexual health information (i.e., contraception, STIs) and controversial topics (abortion, penis size, emergency contraception) also contained the most inaccuracies.

While TikTok may serve as an accessible source of informal sex education for millions of young people, its content can be consumed in lieu of more formal and accurate sex education (i.e., from schools and healthcare providers). And this informal source of sexual health information can be ripe with misinformation. For example, in a study examining the accuracy of men's health-related content (e.g., testosterone, erectile dysfunction) on TikTok [27], researchers found that, overall, the accuracy of the content was poor. Further, physicians were responsible for creating a very small portion of total TikTok posts/videos. One topic in particular, semen retention—a practice involving purposefully reducing the frequency of ejaculation and made popular on social media [NoFap]—had the worst accuracy and was completely absent of content from physicians [27]. We should note that the benefits of semen retention propagated on social media are not based on robust clinical evidence, but the topic had the most impressions and engagement in the study, representing an astounding 1,216,074,000 impressions [27].

Such misinformation can lead to very serious and negative consequences. In 2017, for instance, articles posted to the Australian National Broadcasting Commission's online and social media platforms questioned the benefits of long-acting reversible contraceptives (LARC) [28]. The articles cited testimonials from women on social media who posted about the negative physical and mental effects of using LARC; the articles also perpetuated multiple conspiracy theories, which overshadowed a brief comment from a local clinical expert that provided an opposing viewpoint [28]. The emphasis on the negative consequences of LARC took advantage of adolescents' and young adults' fears about contraceptive use and contributed to the rapid spread of misinformation. As a result, in the following weeks, many women canceled their consultations for contraceptive use [28].

## 3 Future Research

As online sources of sexual health information constantly change and emerge, there are ample opportunities for future research to facilitate a better understanding of adolescents' information-seeking and ways to improve their sexual health knowledge and, in turn, promote healthy sexuality. We identify some of these areas below:

- *What are the most common themes and types of online sexual health information adolescents are searching for, and how do these differ based on demographic factors (e.g., gender, sexual orientation, geographic location)?* Zori et al. [29] recommended examining the content of online sexual health information sought by adolescents and considering how demographic factors may impact information-seeking behaviors. This can help researchers gain a better understanding of the specific sexual health information needs of adolescents and tailor interventions and resources to meet these needs. We can also identify potential demographic disparities in access to and use of sexual health information, which can inform efforts to promote equity and inclusion in sexual health education and support for adolescents.
- *How can social media be leveraged to shape adolescents' sexual health knowledge, attitudes, and behaviors?* With the rise of innovative social media platforms, such as TikTok, which emerged in late 2016 and is now one of the most utilized ways for adolescents to obtain quick and appealing information, researchers should further explore the poten-

tial for social media-based interventions to deliver sexual health information to adolescents.

- *What are the long-term effects of online sexual health information seeking on adolescents' sexual health outcomes?* Longitudinal studies can examine adolescents' sexual health cognitions and behaviors over time and the potential impact of online information-seeking about sexual health, including the use of SEM, on these outcomes. Such research can also assess the impact of young people's difficulties finding accurate information as well as their frustration and abandoning their searches for information (e.g., how do adolescents fare if they are unable to access local and other content online, and to what other sources do they turn?).
- *How effective are digital sexual health interventions in promoting positive sexual health outcomes among adolescents, and how can these interventions be best designed and delivered to maximize their impact?* Given the importance and prevalence of online sexual health information-seeking among adolescents, there is a need for targeted and accessible resources. In the absence of uniform, standardized sexual health education in the U.S., digital sexual health interventions are an effective tool for improving sexual health knowledge attitudes, norms, and behaviors among adolescents [30]. It is crucial to identify the most effective design and delivery strategies for these interventions to maximize impact. Such interventions should also incorporate the cultural values and beliefs of the target population and be designed to be accessible to adolescents who speak languages other than English.

## 4 Recommendations

OSHI should be equitable, inclusive, and pertinent to adolescents with different and intersecting identities and lived experiences (e.g., race/ethnicity, sexual orientation, gender identity, and ability status). This can help mitigate unique barriers these youth face when seeking and accessing OSHI, such as stigma, discrimination, and lack of representation—while promoting more positive sexual health outcomes. Thus, intersectionality must be considered in the development and dissemination of OSHI to ensure youth have access to this information and feel represented regardless of the social identity groups to which they may belong. By prioritizing equity and inclusivity in OSHI, we promote the health and well-being of *all* youth, including those who have been historically marginalized. Specific recommendations for clinicians/providers, educators, and policymakers are as follows:

### 4.1 For Clinicians and Providers

- Healthcare providers are well-positioned to deliver guidance to adolescents seeking sexual health information online. They can help adolescents identify reliable versus unreliable sources of OSHI and address any concerns or questions they may have. We recommend that providers also ensure adolescents are aware of *local* sexual health resources and services, such as clinics or support groups, to supplement the information they receive online.
- To effectively utilize the Internet to deliver health information to youth, it is imperative that health educators receive adequate training and support to use technology appropriately and to be able to effectively communicate its risks and benefits to adolescents in a way that is accurate, culturally sensitive, and responsive to their needs [31].

### 4.2 For Educators

- Adolescents may have difficulty evaluating how trustworthy a source of OSHI is due to a lack of health literacy; therefore, this should be prioritized as a core educational concept. Educators can provide resources and support to help adolescents navigate the Internet and evaluate the quality and reliability of the information they access.

- LGBTQ+-inclusive sex education is essential for *all* teenagers, including those who are heterosexual and cisgender, during adolescence, a developmental stage known for exploring gender and sexual identity. Learning about diverse sexual and gender identities and relationship models has benefits for youth regardless of their own sexual or gender identity. Comprehensive content about LGBTQ+-specific sexualities should be prioritized in OSHI to ensure that all young people have access to accurate, affirming information that supports their healthy sexual development and emphasizes respect for diverse communities.
- Because of the potential for SEM to negatively influence youth's perceptions of sex and bodies, we recommend that educators discuss the pros and cons of pornography with teens while emphasizing the importance of promoting healthy and respectful sexual behaviors (e.g., consent). This can equip young people with the knowledge and skills needed to navigate the complex and often confusing landscape of sexual media and help them make informed choices that align with their values and goals.

## 4.3 For Policymakers

- We recommend that policymakers work to address the digital divide, ensuring equitable access to the Internet, ensuring that digital literacy is a central part of education policy, and making digital sexual health resources available for all adolescents. Initiatives that provide low-cost or free Internet access and devices (e.g., smartphones, laptops) to underserved communities should be treated as a high funding priority.
- In addition, policymakers can work to promote the dissemination of reliable online sexual health information. Funding should be given to organizations that develop and evaluate digital interventions to promote adolescent sexual health, as well as those that offer guidelines for websites and apps to ensure that any OSHI they provide is evidence-based, up-to-date, and accurate.

**Conflict of Interest and Funding Disclosures** None.

## References

1. Gottfried MA, Faverio M, Jeffrey G. Teens, social media and technology 2023. Pew Research Center: Internet, Science & Tech; 2023. https://www.pewresearch.org/internet/2023/12/11/teens-social-media-and-technology-2023/. Accessed April 15, 2024.
2. Buhi ER, Daley EM, Fuhrmann HJ, Smith SA. An observational study of how young people search for online sexual health information. J Am Coll Health J ACH. 2009;58(2):101–11. https://doi.org/10.1080/07448480903221236.
3. Habel MA, Hood J, Desai S, Kachur R, Buhi ER, Liddon N. Google It: obtaining information about local STD/HIV testing services online. Sex Transm Dis. 2011;38(4):334–8.
4. Stevens R, Gilliard-Matthews S, Dunaev J, Todhunter-Reid A, Brawner B, Stewart J. Social media use and sexual risk reduction behavior among minority youth: seeking safe sex information. Nurs Res. 2017;66(5):368–77. https://doi.org/10.1097/NNR.0000000000000237.
5. Tia. Ask Tia. https://www.asktia.com/. Accessed 17 Apr 2023.
6. Benoit JRA, Louie-Poon S, Kauser S, Meherali S. Promoting adolescent sexual and reproductive health in North America using free mobile apps: environmental scan. JMIR Pediatr Parent. 2022;5(4):e33826. https://doi.org/10.2196/33826.
7. Simon L, Daneback K. Adolescents' use of the Internet for sex education: a thematic and critical review of the literature. Int J Sex Health. 2013;25(4):305–19. https://doi.org/10.1080/19317611.2013.823899.
8. Sutton JA, Walsh-Buhi ER. Factors influencing college women's contraceptive behavior: an application of the integrative model of behavioral prediction. J Am Coll Health. 2017;65(5):339–47. https://doi.org/10.1080/07448481.2017.1312414.
9. Patterson SP, Hilton S, Flowers P, McDaid LM. What are the barriers and challenges faced by adolescents when searching for sexual health information on the internet? Implications for policy and practice from a qualitative study. Sex Transm Infect. 2019;95(6):462. https://doi.org/10.1136/sextrans-2018-053710.
10. Vogels EA. Some digital divides persist between rural, urban and suburban America. Pew Research Center.. https://www.pewresearch.org/short-reads/2021/08/19/some-digital-divides-persist-between-rural-urban-and-suburban-america/. Accessed 15 Apr 2024.
11. Jackson DN, Trivedi N, Baur C. Re-prioritizing digital health and health literacy in healthy people 2030 to affect health equity. Health Commun. 2021;36(10):1155–62. https://doi.org/10.1080/10410236.2020.1748828.
12. Brodie M, Flournoy RE, Altman DE, Blendon RJ, Benson JM, Rosenbaum MD. Health informa-

tion, the Internet, and the digital divide. Health Aff (Millwood). 2000;19(6):255–65. https://doi.org/10.1377/hlthaff.19.6.255.
13. Adolescents. Technology and reducing risk for HIV, STDs and pregnancy | CDC. Published January 19, 2021. https://www.cdc.gov/std/life-stages-populations/adolescents-tech.htm. Accessed 17 Apr 2023.
14. Chen E, Barrington C. "You can do it anywhere": student and teacher perceptions of an online sexuality education intervention. Am J Sex Educ. 2017;12(2):105–19. https://doi.org/10.1080/15546128.2017.1298066.
15. Holstrom AM. Sexuality education goes viral: what we know about online sexual health information. Am J Sex Educ. 2015;10(3):277–94. https://doi.org/10.1080/15546128.2015.1040569.
16. Currin JM, Hubach RD, Croff JM. Sex-ed without the stigma: what gay and bisexual men would like offered in school based sex education. J Homosex. 2020;67(13):1779–97. https://doi.org/10.1080/00918369.2019.1616429.
17. O'Farrell M, Corcoran P, Davoren MP. Examining LGBTI+ inclusive sexual health education from the perspective of both youth and facilitators: a systematic review. BMJ Open. 2021;11(9):e047856. https://doi.org/10.1136/bmjopen-2020-047856.
18. Mitchell KJ, Ybarra ML, Korchmaros JD, Kosciw JG. Accessing sexual health information online: use, motivations and consequences for youth with different sexual orientations. Health Educ Res. 2014;29(1):147–57. https://doi.org/10.1093/her/cyt071.
19. Vandenbosch L, van Oosten JMF. Explaining the relationship between sexually explicit internet material and casual sex: a two-step mediation model. Arch Sex Behav. 2018;47(5):1465–80. https://doi.org/10.1007/s10508-017-1145-8.
20. Kubicek K, Beyer WJ, Weiss G, Iverson E, Kipke MD. In the dark: young men's stories of sexual initiation in the absence of relevant sexual health information. Health Educ Behav. 2010;37(2):243–63. https://doi.org/10.1177/1090198109339993.
21. Magee JC, Bigelow L, DeHaan S, Mustanski BS. Sexual health information seeking online: a mixed-methods study among lesbian, gay, bisexual, and transgender young people. Health Educ Behav. 2012;39(3):276–89. https://doi.org/10.1177/1090198111401384.
22. Testa G, Mestre-Bach G, Chiclana Actis C, Potenza MN. Problematic pornography use in adolescents: from prevention to intervention. Curr Addict Rep. 2023; https://doi.org/10.1007/s40429-023-00469-4.
23. Martellozzo E, Monaghan A, Davidson J, Adler J. Researching the affects that online pornography has on U.K. adolescents aged 11 to 16. SAGE Open. 2020;10(1):2158244019899462. https://doi.org/10.1177/215824401989462.
24. Freeman JL, Caldwell PHY, Scott KM. The role of trust when adolescents search for and appraise online health Information. J Pediatr. 2020;221:215–223.e5. https://doi.org/10.1016/j.jpeds.2020.02.074.
25. Fowler LR, Schoen L, Smith HS, Morain SR. Sex education on TikTok: a content analysis of themes. Health Promot Pract. 2022;23(5):739–42. https://doi.org/10.1177/15248399211031536.
26. Buhi ER, Daley EM, Oberne A, Smith SA, Schneider T, Fuhrmann HJ. Quality and accuracy of sexual health information web sites visited by young people. J Adolesc Health. 2010;47(2):206–8. https://doi.org/10.1016/j.jadohealth.2010.01.002.
27. Dubin JM, Aguiar JA, Lin JS, et al. The broad reach and inaccuracy of men's health information on social media: analysis of TikTok and Instagram. Int J Impot Res. 2022; https://doi.org/10.1038/s41443-022-00645-6.
28. Foran T. Contraception and the media: lessons past, present and future. Eur J Contracept Reprod Health Care. 2019;24(1):80–2. https://doi.org/10.1080/13625187.2018.1563067.
29. Zori GL, Collins SL, Walker AF. Online sexual health information seeking of adolescents: a content analysis. Am J Sex Educ. 2022:1–23. https://doi.org/10.1080/15546128.2022.2111012.
30. Widman L, Nesi J, Kamke K, Choukas-Bradley S, Stewart JL. Technology-based interventions to reduce sexually transmitted infections and unintended pregnancy among youth. J Adolesc Health. 2018;62(6):651–60. https://doi.org/10.1016/j.jadohealth.2018.02.007.
31. Decker MJ, Harrison S, Price M, Gutmann-Gonzalez A, Yarger J, Tenney R. Educators' perspectives on integrating technology into sexual health education: implementation study. JMIR Hum Factors. 2022;9(1):e31381. https://doi.org/10.2196/31381.

# Online Sexual Communication and Partner Seeking Among Adolescents

Kathryn Macapagal, Val Wongsomboon, Jacob D. Gordon, Kimberly M. Nelson, and Laura M. Widman

## 1 Background

The growth of online social spaces over the past two decades has provided new opportunities for people to communicate with others about sexuality, sexual health, and romantic and sexual relationships. Adolescents have been early adopters of these new social technologies. Although there have been numerous, typically negative media reports covering adolescents and online relationships, there is limited empirical research examining their use of general social platforms (e.g., Discord, TikTok, Instagram) and adult-oriented dating and sexual networking sites (e.g., Grindr, Tinder) to communicate with and find romantic and sexual partners [1–3]. As romantic relationship formation and sexual exploration are common developmental milestones during adolescence, it is unsurprising that adolescents may use online spaces for sexual and romantic interactions [3, 4]. Understanding the prevalence, patterns, and experiences of adolescents' online sexual communication and partner seeking[1] is critical for many reasons. This knowledge can inform sex education, sexual health interventions, and clinical practice; guide technology and safety policies; assist parents in monitoring and providing support to their adolescents; and enhance our understanding of contemporary adolescent development. Here, we review recent literature on adolescents' online sexual communication and partner seeking experiences. Given the rapid development of online social spaces in recent years, this overview focuses on literature published in the last decade (2013–2023).

K. Macapagal (✉)
Department of Medical Social Sciences, Feinberg School of Medicine, Northwestern University, Chicago, IL, USA

Institute for Sexual and Gender Minority Health and Wellbeing, Northwestern University, Chicago, IL, USA
e-mail: kathryn.macapagal@northwestern.edu

V. Wongsomboon
Department of Psychology, Yale University, New Haven, CT, USA

J. D. Gordon
Institute for Sexual and Gender Minority Health and Wellbeing, Northwestern University, Chicago, IL, USA

K. M. Nelson
Department of Community Health Sciences, Boston University School of Public Health, Boston, MA, USA

Department of Psychiatry, Boston University Chobanian & Avedisian School of Medicine, Boston, MA, USA

L. M. Widman
Department of Psychology, North Carolina State University, Raleigh, NC, USA

[1] As teenagers may use online spaces to meet romantic or sexual partners or both, here we refer broadly to "partner seeking," which is inclusive of these behaviors.



D. A. Christakis, L. Hale (eds.), *Handbook of Children and Screens*,
https://doi.org/10.1007/978-3-031-69362-5_49

## 2 Current State

### 2.1 Online Sexual Communication

Sexual communication involves the exchange of messages about sexuality and relationships between partners and can include both verbal and nonverbal communication (for a review, see Widman and colleagues) [5]. Online sexual communication may include direct discussions about topics such as sexual interests/desires, relationship status, sexual history, or sexual safety (e.g., condom use, sexually transmitted infections) communicated via social media posts or messages on online dating applications. Technology-mediated and online sexual communication can also include the exchange of nude/sexual images (i.e., nudes or sexts, covered in the chapter by Van Ouytsel) or indirect ways of communicating sexual wishes and desires via emojis (e.g., tongue, eggplant).

While most research on sexual communication has focused on in-person interactions, one study of US high school students found that nearly half of adolescents had used technology or online spaces to discuss sexual health with their partners. Rates of communication varied by topic, with the highest number of teens using technology to discuss sexual limits (42%) and condom use (39%), and the fewest discussing human immunodeficiency virus/acquired immune deficiency syndrome (HIV/AIDS) (20%) [6]. Among sexually active youth, those who used technology to discuss condoms were nearly three times more likely to consistently use condoms than those who did not [6]. These findings suggest that youth may feel more comfortable raising and discussing sexual health topics with their partners via technology or online spaces, and such communication may relate to their ability to engage in healthy in-person sexual behaviors (e.g., condom use, consent). As such, technology-facilitated sexual communication is an important focus area for adolescent sexual health interventions.

### 2.2 Online Partner Seeking

Adolescents use online social spaces to seek romantic and sexual partners as well. Earlier research on this topic suggested that just 8% of adolescents had met a romantic partner online [7] and focused on their experiences with using social media sites like Facebook to meet and communicate with potential partners [8]. However, since this research was conducted roughly a decade ago, the online landscape has evolved substantially, and numerous new social platforms have emerged. For example, platforms like Facebook are considerably less popular in this age group, who prefers other spaces such as Discord, Instagram, Snapchat, and TikTok [9]. As such, adolescent online partner seeking and relationship formation may look quite different than before and may also be more common than previously reported. For example, one study of 1500 US adolescents reported that 19% of teens under 18 had used an adult dating site or app, with Tinder being the most frequently used. Of adolescents who had used these platforms, 45% met their online partners in person [1].

Research indicates that adolescents' reasons for and patterns of online partner seeking vary according to their developmental and social circumstances, such as age, race/ethnicity, ability status, health conditions, geographic location (i.e., rural, urban), and sexual/gender identity. For instance, younger adolescents may be more interested in finding friends, while older adolescents may be more interested in finding sexual and romantic partners [1]. Regarding racial/ethnic background, one study found that Black adolescent girls used multiple social platforms to seek evidence of posts or activity indicating racism or sexism in potential partners and to determine whether it was worth pursuing a potential partner [10]. Regarding health and ability status, adolescents seeking treatment for severe obesity reported engaging in online romantic relationships and sexual activity (e.g., through chat platforms and gaming websites) to avoid weight-related stigma from potential partners [11]. Adolescents with developmental or intellectual disabilities may be inclined to use online spaces to facilitate romantic and sexual relationships due to difficulties navigating in-person social interactions (e.g., autism spectrum disorders) or a desire to be strategic about whether and how they present or disclose their disability [12].

Most research on adolescents' online dating has focused on lesbian, gay, bisexual, queer, and questioning (LGBTQ+) adolescents, with an emphasis on gay, bisexual, and queer adolescent boys. Fewer studies have included transgender and nonbinary adolescents and cisgender sexual minority girls. One study found that LGBTQ+ adolescents were more likely than their cisgender and heterosexual peers to initiate relationships online [2]. Even within LGBTQ+ adolescents, there might be differences in online dating and behaviors. For example, cisgender sexual minority adolescent boys are more likely to use dating applications designed for gay and bisexual men (e.g., Grindr) than social media or dating applications for general populations [13]. Given the relative lack of dating applications designed with queer women and transgender individuals in mind [14, 15], compared to cisgender men these adolescents may be more likely to meet their partner(s) via social media, online communities, or dating apps inclusive of all genders/sexualities [16, 17].

## 2.3 Benefits of Online Sexual Communication and Partner Seeking

Although often portrayed as uniformly negative [18], online sexual communication and partner seeking hold a number of advantages for adolescents. This may be especially true since the COVID-19 pandemic has normalized initiating and maintaining social connections and interactions (sometimes exclusively) online [19, 20]. As such, online socialization can play a vital role in adolescents' achievement of typical sexual/relationship developmental milestones (e.g., understanding one's sexual attractions and forming first romantic relationships).

Online social spaces offer adolescents a sense of privacy, anonymity, and safety, which may reduce potential embarrassment or stigma during sexual communication and relationship formation. These spaces allow teens to "try on" different identities, learn about social/sexual norms, or explore different ways to interact with their peers and potential partners. For instance, adolescents may simply observe or explore on social media, websites, or apps without interacting with others, or use avatars and aliases instead of their real names and photos if they prefer. Online communication can also facilitate discussion of topics with peers and potential partners that may be otherwise harder to discuss in person (e.g., HIV status, condom use, sexual identity, and sexual preferences), which are inadequately addressed by most school-based sex education programs [21].

Online sexual communication and partner seeking may be especially important for LGBTQ+ adolescents. These teens tend to face barriers in receiving relevant sexual health education and forming relationships in physical spaces (e.g., schools) that their cisgender and heterosexual counterparts do not [2]. It is, therefore, unsurprising that LGBTQ+ adolescents turn to online spaces to seek, share, and communicate about sexuality, sexual health, and romantic relationships [1]. Online sex and relationships can provide a sense of connection at a safe distance for LGBTQ+ adolescents who may be concerned about or more vulnerable to discrimination, victimization, or violence [13, 16, 22]. Indirect benefits of online sexual communication and partner seeking also include the ability to explore one's sexuality and LGBTQ+ identity and find meaningful connections with like-minded peers [1, 2, 23].

## 2.4 Risks of Online Sexual Communication and Partner Seeking

While online social spaces have expanded opportunities for sexual communication and relationships, they also pose potential harm to adolescents. Some studies indicate that online-initiated relationships may be associated with lower relationship satisfaction, partly due to lack of physical contact [19, 24]. A prominent concern is that people online are not always who they seem, which can lead to physical harm or feelings of emotional betrayal [22, 25]. This is often referred to as "catfishing", whereby an individual pretends they are someone else online (sometimes using others' real photos or information) in order to deceive an individual into a relationship. Indeed, media reports have repeatedly highlighted victimization by partners originally met online [26].

Online relationships may also contribute to cyberdating violence (CDV), also known as technology-facilitated sexual abuse (TFA), among adolescents [27]. TFA distinguishes itself from offline sexual abuse by the online setting (e.g., dating applications, social media) and the ability for surveillance (e.g., geolocation). Compared to offline dating violence, TFA makes it more difficult for victims to escape due to the absence of geographical boundaries separating the perpetrator and the victim. TFA is related to many poor mental health outcomes, such as depression anxiety, and suicidal ideation; however, the majority of these findings were examined among adults [28]. Victims of TFA may experience cyber psychological aggression, cyber control or sextortion, image-based sexual abuse, and exclusion [28–30]. Cyber psychological aggression involves aggressive behavior through digital or online communication channels, and victims may report sexist remarks and harassment. Cyber control or sextortion refers to the use of online technology to exert power and control over a partner and can include monitoring a partner's online activity, using GPS tracking to monitor their physical location, or coercing them to engage in unwanted sexual acts (e.g., grooming) [30]. Image-based sexual abuse involves publicly humiliating a romantic partner (e.g., sharing a nude or private photo without consent), or cyberflashing (e.g., receiving nonconsensual sexual images) [29]. Another form of TFA, exclusion, involves being blocked or removed from online spaces [31].

There may be heightened drawbacks for adolescents with intersecting minoritized genders, sexual identities, and races/ethnicities. For instance, White and Black adolescent girls both report online harassment based on their physical appearance [9], yet Black adolescent girls also report having to navigate sexual and racist stereotypes when dating online [10]. Transgender and nonbinary adolescents may have concerns about prospective partners having negative and violent reactions to gender identity disclosure [16, 17], and LGBTQ+ girls and feminine adolescents may be at increased risk of TFA [32]. Taken together, negative experiences with online sexual communication and relationships can have serious consequences for the mental health and well-being of adolescents.

## 3 Future Research

Current research has merely scratched the surface of how adolescents have used online spaces for sexual communication and partner seeking and points to several opportunities for research articulated here.

- What online social spaces do adolescents use for sexual communication and partner seeking, how frequently, and what are their patterns of use and reasons for discontinuation? What are adolescents' subjective experiences using various technologies for online sexual communication and partner seeking, and how do these patterns and experiences change over time across developmental stages (e.g., from early adolescence to emerging adulthood)? Such questions could be added to nationally representative, longitudinal surveys of adolescent experience and in-depth qualitative studies.
- How does the use of online social spaces for sexual communication and partner seeking impact adolescent mental health, sexual health, and overall well-being, and how might this differ by their sociodemographic characteristics?
- What education might adolescents need regarding online sexual and relationship safety, and how might we tailor these pro-

grams to different groups' needs? Without education on online dating safety, research suggests adolescents are relying on peers for information, or are figuring out how to navigate online sexual communication and partner seeking on their own [16, 22, 33].

- How might emerging technologies, such as virtual reality, artificial intelligence, and deep fakes (i.e., photos or videos digitally altered to look realistic) play a role in adolescent sexual communication, partner seeking, CDV, and exploitation? For example, adolescents may consensually exchange sexual content with others online, but sophisticated deep fakes may be used to sexually exploit or manipulate adolescents by malicious actors.

These research questions would benefit from using qualitative and mixed methods, longitudinal, and interdisciplinary approaches (e.g., social/behavioral and developmental sciences, human-computer interaction, and communication research). As most scholarship on this topic has focused on U.S. samples, understanding patterns among adolescents in other areas of the world would shed light on how these behaviors may be context-dependent.

## 4 Recommendations

Online sexual communication and partner seeking appear to be developmentally normative among adolescents, for whom the boundaries between offline and online worlds can be blurred. Although adolescents report benefits to these behaviors, research indicates they are also aware of potential drawbacks, so it is important to recognize when such behaviors may become potentially harmful or problematic. The following are recommendations for educators, healthcare providers, parents, and policymakers invested in maximizing the benefits of online social spaces for adolescents and minimizing their risks.

- First, it is critical to acknowledge the reality that adolescents engage in sexual exploration, communication, or partner seeking online, instead of assuming or hoping otherwise. We recommend that conversations about these behaviors start early in the context of addressing online safety between children and adolescents and their healthcare providers, parents, and educators.
- Second, it is important to assess adolescents' experiences of online sexual communication and partner seeking directly to understand how these activities may impact adolescent health and well-being. Coyne and colleagues [16] offer concrete language and questions that model how clinicians might normalize and assess online sexual communication and experiences among adolescents regardless of sexual orientation or gender identity. The questions assess in a direct but nonjudgmental way adolescents' online sexual experiences, motivations for online sexual behavior and partnering, types of online relationships and sexual behavior, perceived safety, access to sexual health resources, and parental knowledge of online behavior. Importantly, this framework can help differentiate between normative behaviors and those that may lead to adverse health, safety, or legal consequences.
- Third, education focused on online sexual and relationship safety should be co-created with and approved by adolescents to ensure their relevance, address their safety while promoting autonomy, and avoid being patronizing or intrusive [25]. Moreover, as adults often are less savvy users of online social spaces frequented by adolescents, education that is informed by youth's actual experiences and strategies they have found effective in protecting their online safety ultimately may be more useful. Freed and colleagues [25] offer a summary of online protections from interviews with adolescents and trusted adults.
- Fourth, most platforms rely on self-reported age for registration purposes, and the willingness of users on those sites to block or report others who violate the terms of service such as underage users. Although additional levels of identity verification have been proposed, this can be cumbersome for the user and for the platform, as well as pose privacy concerns

itself (e.g., uploading legal forms of identification to access a site). Although changes to laws and policies governing online spaces occur slowly and typically lag far behind current technologies, it is nevertheless important to consider how these may be crafted to maximize adolescents' safety online. Policy should ensure adolescents are not criminalized for appropriate exploratory behavior, while also balancing the real safety concerns that adolescents may face with this technology. Taken together, a deeper knowledge of adolescents' perceptions, feelings, and experiences with online sexual communication and partner seeking, as well as potential health consequences can better equip educators, clinicians, parents, and policymakers to support adolescents' developmental and social needs.

**Conflict of Interest and Funding Disclosures** During the preparation of this chapter, JG was supported by T32MH130325, KM and VW were supported by R01MH129207, KN was supported by R01MH119892, R21HD105482, and R01HD106635, and LW was supported by R03HD105784. The content is solely the responsibility of the authors and does not necessarily represent the official views of the National Institutes of Health.

## References

1. Lykens J, Pilloton M, Silva C, Schlamm E, Wilburn K, Pence E. Google for sexual relationships: mixed-methods study on digital flirting and online dating among adolescent youth and young adults. JMIR Public Health Surveill. 2019;5(2):e10695. https://doi.org/10.2196/10695.
2. Korchmaros JD, Ybarra ML, Mitchell KJ. Adolescent online romantic relationship initiation: differences by sexual and gender identification. J Adolesc. 2015;40:54–64. https://doi.org/10.1016/j.adolescence.2015.01.004.
3. O'Sullivan LF. Linking online sexual activities to health outcomes among teens. New Dir Child Adolesc Dev. 2014;2014(144):37–51. https://doi.org/10.1002/cad.20059.
4. Tolman DL, McClelland SI. normative sexuality development in adolescence: a decade in review, 2000–2009. J Res Adolesc. 2011;21(1):242–55. https://doi.org/10.1111/j.1532-7795.2010.00726.x.
5. Widman L, Maheux AJ, Craig E, Evans-Paulson R, Choukas-Bradley S. Sexual communication between adolescent partners: a scoping review and directions for future research. J Sex Res. 2022;59(8):984–99. https://doi.org/10.1080/00224499.2022.2099787.
6. Widman L, Nesi J, Choukas-Bradley S, Prinstein MJ. Safe sext: adolescents' use of technology to communicate about sexual health with dating partners. J Adolesc Health. 2014;54(5):612–4. https://doi.org/10.1016/j.jadohealth.2013.12.009.
7. Lenhart A, Anderson M, Smith A. Teens, technology and romantic relationships. Pew Research Center; 2015.
8. Rueda HA, Lindsay M, Williams LR. "She posted it on Facebook": Mexican American adolescents' experiences with technology and romantic relationship conflict. J Adolesc Res. 2015;30(4):419–45. https://doi.org/10.1177/0743558414565236.
9. Vogels EA, Gelles-Watnick R, Massarat N. Teens, social media and technology 2022. Pew Research Center; 2022.
10. Weser VU, Opara I, Sands BE, Fernandes CSF, Hieftje KD. How black teen girls navigate social media to form romantic relationships. Soc Media Soc. 2021;7(3):205630512110338. https://doi.org/10.1177/20563051211033823.
11. Walsh Ó, Dettmer E, Regina A, et al. 'Teenagers are into perfect-looking things': dating, sexual attitudes and experiences of adolescents with severe obesity. Child Care Health Dev. 2022;48(3):406–14. https://doi.org/10.1111/cch.12940.
12. Mazur E. Diverse disabilities and dating online. In: Identity, sexuality, and relationships among emerging adults in the digital age; 2017. https://doi.org/10.4018/978-1-5225-1856-3.ch010.
13. Macapagal K, Moran K, Newcomb ME, Moskowitz DA, Owens C, Mustanski B. Patterns of online and offline partnering, partnership characteristics, and condomless sex among adolescent sexual minority males in the USA. AIDS Behav. 2021;25(7):2033–45. https://doi.org/10.1007/s10461-020-03133-4.
14. Fernandez JR, Birnholtz J. "I don't want them to not know": investigating decisions to disclose transgender identity on dating platforms. Proc ACM Hum-Comput Interact. 2019;3(CSCW):226:1–226:21. https://doi.org/10.1145/3359328.
15. Smith MG. Queer enough to swipe right? Dating app experiences of sexual minority women: a cross-disciplinary review. Comput Hum Behav Rep. 2022;8:100238. https://doi.org/10.1016/j.chbr.2022.100238.
16. Coyne CA, Wongsomboon V, Korpak AK, Macapagal K. "We have to figure it out ourselves": transfeminine adolescents' online sexual experiences and recommendations for supporting their sexual health and wellbeing. Front Reprod Health. 2023;4:1034747. https://doi.org/10.3389/frph.2022.1034747.
17. Ma J, Korpak AK, Choukas-Bradley S, Macapagal K. Patterns of online relationship seeking among transgender and gender diverse adolescents: advice for others and common inquiries. Psychol Sex Orientat Gend Divers. 2022;9(3):287–99. https://doi.org/10.1037/sgd0000482.

18. George MJ, Odgers CL. Seven fears and the science of how mobile technologies may be influencing adolescents in the digital age. Perspect Psychol Sci. 2015;10(6):832–51. https://doi.org/10.1177/1745691615596788.
19. Goldstein A, Flicker S. "Some things just won't go back": teen girls' online dating relationships during COVID-19. Girlhood Stud. 2020;13(3):64–78. https://doi.org/10.3167/ghs.2020.130306.
20. Nelson KM, Gordon AR, John SA, Stout CD, Macapagal K. "Physical sex is over for now": impact of COVID-19 on the well-being and sexual health of adolescent sexual minority males in the U.S. J Adolesc Health. 2020;67(6):756–62. https://doi.org/10.1016/j.jadohealth.2020.08.027.
21. SIECUS. The SIECUS state profiles. Published 2023. https://siecus.org/state-profiles/
22. Jozsa K, Kraus A, Korpak AK, Birnholtz J, Moskowitz DA, Macapagal K. "Safe behind my screen": adolescent sexual minority males' perceptions of safety and trustworthiness on geosocial and social networking apps. Arch Sex Behav. 2021;50(7):2965–80. https://doi.org/10.1007/s10508-021-01962-5.
23. Wongsomboon V, Greenawalt IM, Owusu J, et al. When reality doesn't meet expectations: what sexual minority assigned-male-at-birth adolescents learn from using geosocial networking apps. 2023. https://doi.org/10.31234/osf.io/uy5g6.
24. Blunt-Vinti HD, Wheldon C, McFarlane M, Brogan N, Walsh-Buhi ER. Assessing relationship and sexual satisfaction in adolescent relationships formed online and offline. J Adolesc Health. 2016;58(1):11–6. https://doi.org/10.1016/j.jadohealth.2015.09.027.
25. Freed D, Bazarova NN, Consolvo S, et al. Understanding digital-safety experiences of youth in the U.S. 2023.
26. Shapiro E. Former police officer accused of killing 15-year-old's family was pretending to be teen online. https://abcnews.go.com/US/man-allegedly-catfishes-teen-girl-online-kills-family/story?id=94090351.
27. Henry N, Flynn A, Powell A. Technology-facilitated domestic and sexual violence: a review. Violence Women. 2020;26(15-16):1828–54. https://doi.org/10.1177/1077801219875821.
28. Stevens F, Nurse JRC, Arief B. Cyber stalking, cyber harassment, and adult mental health: a systematic review. Cyberpsychol Behav Soc Netw. 2021;24(6):367–76. https://doi.org/10.1089/cyber.2020.0253.
29. McGlynn C, Johnson K, Rackley E, et al. 'It's torture for the soul': the harms of image-based sexual abuse. Soc Leg Stud. 2021;30(4):541–62. https://doi.org/10.1177/0964663920947791.
30. Dunn S. Technology-facilitated gender-based violence: an overview. Published online December 7, 2020. https://papers.ssrn.com/abstract=3772042. Accessed 10 Apr 2024.
31. Rodríguez-deArriba ML, Nocentini A, Menesini E, Sánchez-Jiménez V. Dimensions and measures of cyber dating violence in adolescents: a systematic review. Aggress Violent Behav. 2021;58:101613. https://doi.org/10.1016/j.avb.2021.101613.
32. Wongsomboon V, Veldhuis CB, Gordon JD, Macapagal K. Experiences and correlates of cyber dating abuse in sexual and gender minority girls and feminine adolescents: implications for psychological wellbeing. 2023.
33. Hartikainen H, Razi A, Wisniewski P. Safe sexting: the advice and support adolescents receive from peers regarding online sexual risks. Proc ACM Hum-Comput Interact. 2021;5(CSCW1):1–31. https://doi.org/10.1145/3449116.

# It's Not Just Sexting: Adolescents' Experiences with Exchanging and Disseminating Nude Images

Joris Van Ouytsel, Megan K. Maas, Bianca Klettke, Elizabeth M. Clancy, and Jeff R. Temple

## 1 Background

With the growing versatility of mobile devices and their integration into the daily lives of youth, there has been a rise in their use for sexual purposes. One example of this is sexting, which allows adolescents to participate in digital sexual communication and expression. Although many researchers have defined sexting differently [1, 2], it can be broadly conceptualized as the act of sending, receiving, or disseminating self-made nude/sexually explicit text messages and images via the Internet or mobile devices. Academic research on sexting started around 2009 and focused initially on sexting as a deviant behavior [3]. Today, many consensual sexting behaviors could be considered as a normative part of adolescents' sexual development and exploration [4]. However, sexting is considered problematic and can be classified as image-based sexual abuse when consent is lacking, when a partner is pressured into sexting, or when the images are disseminated without consent or used to extort the sender [5].

J. Van Ouytsel (✉)
Hugh Downs School of Human Communication, Arizona State University, Tempe, AZ, USA
e-mail: joris.vanouytsel@asu.edu

M. K. Maas
Department of Human Development & Family Studies, Michigan State University, East Lansing, MI, USA

B. Klettke · E. M. Clancy
School of Psychology, Deakin University, Geelong, Australia

J. R. Temple
School of Behavioral Health Sciences, UTHealth Houston, Houston, TX, USA

## 2 Current State

Contrary to popular belief, a sizeable minority of youth engage in sexting. The most recent meta-analysis on sexting, which also included explicit text messages, found that 19.3% of youth had sent sexts, 34.8% of youth had received sexts, and 14.5% had forwarded sexts without consent [2]. Youth are more likely to engage in sexting as they get older and start to engage in romantic and sexual relationships. Girls were found to be more likely to receive sexts, perhaps reflecting their increased vulnerability to unwanted sexting, sometimes referred to as cyberflashing [2]. Adolescent sexting prevalence increased by 2.6% between 2009 and 2016, likely due to more youth having access to smartphones and social media applications [6, 7].

Most teenagers engage in sexting with current or potential romantic partners [5]. Within this context, consensual sexting can be a way to flirt and maintain sexual intimacy during times of separation, such as school vacations or family trips [8]. Longitudinal research demonstrated


D. A. Christakis, L. Hale (eds.), *Handbook of Children and Screens*,
https://doi.org/10.1007/978-3-031-69362-5_50

that sexting can be a precursor to physical sexual behavior, as it can serve as a first step toward engaging in offline sexual activity within the context of sexual exploration and relationship building [9, 10]. While sexting between two romantic partners is often consensual, there may be instances of sexting between romantic partners that occur due to coercion, albeit not overt [8]. Girls, in particular, may feel compelled to engage in sexting out of fear of negative consequences, such as losing the romantic relationship, or because they believe that it is an expected behavior within a romantic relationship [8, 11, 12].

The pressure to engage in sexting can also come from the perceived social norms within one's broader peer group [13], to which adolescents may be particularly susceptible. Studies have shown that youth who sext are more likely to perceive that their peers hold positive beliefs or attitudes about sexting [14] and that they are sexually active [15]. A retrospective study demonstrated that youth who engaged in sexting in middle school were more likely to feel pressure to engage in sexting than those who did not engage in sexting until high school [16]. The pressure surrounding sexting is often gendered, with boys frequently (1) coercing by sending an image to pressure girls into reciprocating [12]; (2) requesting a nude image repeatedly despite multiple refusals [8]; and (3) experiencing pressure from other male friends to collect nude images from girls [17].

Numerous studies have examined associations between sending sexts and health outcomes [10]. While accumulating evidence suggests that relative to their nonsexting counterparts, adolescents who engage in sexting are more likely to report negative mental health outcomes (e.g., anxiety and depression), lack of contraception use, and substance misuse [10, 18], most of these studies failed to distinguish between consensual, nonconsensual, and coerced sexting. One limitation of the work on the antecedents and consequences of sexting is that a majority of these studies are cross-sectional, limiting causal direction [10]. The associations between sexting and health were strongest for younger adolescents [10], which is likely explained by the presence of shared risk factors that frequently accompany early sexual activity (e.g., lack of parental warmth) [10, 18].

## 2.1 Image-Based Sexual Abuse

One of the main risks associated with sexting is that the images can be shared beyond their intended audience, as they can be forwarded, shown on mobile device screens to others, or posted online on social media or "slut pages" (e.g., semi-private collections of nonconsensual nudes) [8, 19]. Motivations to disseminate sexts may be to participate in gossip [20, 21] as a form of boasting or comradery [8, 13], to assert masculinity [13, 22], or as revenge after a romantic relationship has ended [8]. Forwarding images without consent may result in severe consequences for the victim, including bullying, social exclusion, and other short- and long-term mental, behavioral, and social health consequences [21]. From a relationship standpoint, this activity symbolizes a breach of trust and a violation of other key rights, such as the right to privacy and bodily autonomy, and the right to have control over one's sexual images [8, 21]. Even after the initial dissemination of the sext has occurred, the victims often experience extended anxiety that the images will resurface at a later time, and in some countries, they may also fear legal consequences [21]. As a result, they often no longer want to go to school [21]. Making matters worse, research has shown that bystanders of disseminated sexts rarely intervene [22]. Indeed, one study showed that only around 10% of bystanders contacted the victim to provide support or to tell the perpetrator to stop, and 7% forwarded the image to others [5]. Taken together, these findings suggest that sexting can mimic similar processes seen across different forms of sexual violence.

Another form of image-based sexual abuse is experiences of unwanted sexting or sexting coercion. Although research on unwanted sexting experiences among adolescent populations is still in its infancy, qualitative studies show that girls often report receiving unwanted sexting images from adult strangers, friends of friends, and known boys [23]. The latter were often peers, friends, or romantic and sexual partners who were applying pressure to engage in sexting within the context of an existing relationship. The former may send these images as a form of sexual harassment [23]. These unwanted sexts often make the receivers feel unsafe and uncomfortable [23].

Another recent development in sexting behaviors among adolescents has been the risk of sextortion [24], which can be defined as "the threatened dissemination of explicit, intimate, or embarrassing images of a sexual nature without consent, usually for the purpose of procuring additional images, sexual acts, money, or something else." [24] While research regarding this topic is emerging, a recent study based on an adolescent US sample indicated that male adolescents (5.8%) were more likely to experience sextortion than female adolescents (4.1%) [24]. Further, adolescents who identified as nonheterosexual were also at greater risk of sextortion (10.9%) in comparison to heterosexual adolescents (4.5%). Interestingly, romantic partners were the most common perpetrators of this behavior, accounting for 31.7% of cases for boys and 32.2% for girls. In contrast, online-only friends were the perpetrators in 19.9% of cases for boys and 11.3% for girls. Similar, to the bidirectional relationship identified in other harmful online behaviors, such as cyberbullying, those who had been victimized were more likely to threaten sextortion themselves [24].

Despite the increased vulnerability of LGBTQ+ youth in online spaces, surprisingly little research has been conducted on the sexting experiences of this marginalized population, and the available research largely focuses on LGB cohorts rather than trans and gender-diverse individuals. Research suggests that LGBTQ+ youth are more likely than their heterosexual and cisgender peers, respectively, to send sexts and to be pressured by someone to send a sext; however, they are equally or less likely to forward sexts or receive a forwarded sext. Therefore, LGBTQ+ youth are more likely to be victims, as opposed to perpetrators, of image-based sexual abuse [5, 24].

## 3 Future Research

The inconsistent conceptualization of sexting continues to limit our understanding of this phenomenon and limits this entire body of research. For example, many studies define and measure sexting as a uniform experience and do not take into account the diverse contexts in which it occurs, the various experiences (e.g., receiving, sending, requesting, and disseminating), its often-bidirectional nature, and the fact that sometimes it can be consensual and other times coerced, even with the same person. Other areas of interest around sexting behavior include expectancies, mediums, content, intention, format, temporality, and regret [10, 28]. Future research also needs a continued focus on individual-level characteristics such as age, gender, Indigeneity, and sexual identity.

To continue to progress in this area of inquiry, future studies should focus on the following remaining gaps in knowledge. First, as researchers have gained a deeper understanding of the differences between consensual sexting and image-based sexual abuse, many questions remain about the specific mechanisms of the latter, as well as the emergence of novel forms of image-based sexual abuse. For example, what are the characteristics and motives of teenagers who solicit unwanted sexting from partners? What forms of image-based sexual abuse are most harmful, and for whom? For example, are the dissemination of cis male-bodied images (e.g., commonly known as "dick pics") less harmful than cis female-bodied images? If so, why? And what would this difference mean for prevention efforts? How can we effectively promote active bystanders to prevent image-based sexual abuse? What measures can we implement to simplify the process of reporting incidents of image-based sexual abuse to schools and other relevant authorities? Might the advent of generative AI lead to the emergence of novel forms of image-based sexual abuse, such as deepfakes? How can complex issues of consent, and particularly the temporal aspects of consent, be understood, and what are the understandings of consent in digital relationships? As opposed to consent for in-person sexual behaviors, where consent can be discussed at the moment, digital interactions are retained. As such, while an individual may consent to sharing their images with a current or potential partner today, discussions around what happens to that image in the future, particularly at the end of a relationship, seem to be relatively uncommon at present [25, 30]. However, it is important to help young people clarify their expectations regarding consent: what are they happy to send and receive, and what are the limits on retaining and sharing any intimate images or messages in the future?

Second, are there unique sources of pressure that LGBTQ+ youth experience to engage in sexting and are those from online or offline sources? How does the level of outness among LGBTQ+ youth influence their susceptibility to sexting risk? Where do LGBTQ+ youth find social support when they are coping with sexting-associated risks? How do these experiences impact the development of gender and sexual identity, particularly for LGBTQ+ youth? Does pressured sexting in its various forms create additional pressure for those questioning their own identities within a cisgendered and heteronormative culture? Ultimately, additional research is needed to fully understand LGBTQ+ youths' lived experiences and to understand how sexting can play a role in their sexual identity development.

Third, at what point in development does sexting become less problematic? Much of the research on adolescent sexting has gradually shifted from understanding why adolescents sext generally to gaining a deeper understanding of when sexting could be problematic (e.g., coercive, unwanted, or abusive) [3]. Research also demonstrates that sexting among early adolescents has been associated with negative outcomes [10], but there is insufficient data to determine at what age or stage of development sexting transitions from being a risky behavior to being developmentally normative. Given that consent for engagement in physical sexual behavior ranges but typically aligns around later adolescence, can similar perspectives be applied to engagement in digital sexual behaviors?

Finally, how can we educate teens effectively about safer sexting and how to respond to harmful sexting? What kind of messaging can help to reduce the nonconsensual dissemination of sexting and experiences of unwanted sexting? Several researchers have called for sexting education and the inclusion of sexting within comprehensive sexual education [10, 26, 27]. Despite legal changes in many countries, after more than a decade of sexting research, no widely available evidence-based programs have been developed that could help youth to become more resilient toward problematic forms of sexting, including coerced sexting and nonconsensual dissemination. As research on sexting education remains limited, it is crucial to focus on developing a scalable, comprehensive, inclusive, and sex-positive sexting education curriculum that can ideally be integrated into existing sexual and relationship education curricula.

## 4 Recommendations

### 4.1 For Parents, Practitioners, and Educators

- As noted above, sending and receiving sexts between two older teens and young adults with mutual trust appears unrelated to harmful outcomes. However, when sexting is coerced or disseminated to third parties without consent, sexting has been associated with adverse short- and long-term social, behavioral, and health outcomes [29, 30]. Thus, we recommend that clinicians, practitioners, and educators focus their limited resources on preventing and managing nonconsensual (e.g., coerced sending, disseminating to others) sexting, as opposed to consensual sexting. As with in-person sexual behavior, providing a blanket abstinence-only approach limits our ability to prevent potentially harmful behavior while conflating it with less harmful behavior.
- Although evidence-based sexting education is currently lacking, we recommend that parents and educators actively engage in conversations about safer sexting with adolescents. These can be framed within a broader discussion about healthy relationships, digital

citizenship, and responsible media use [10]. Topics of conversation in school settings could focus on obtaining consent from sexting partners, the importance of safeguarding trust between sexting partners, and discussions around future retention and use. For example, bystanders could be encouraged to intervene to prevent the dissemination of sexting images.

- We also recommend that schools use inclusive examples when addressing sexting and that they avoid using materials that presume girls as the ones holding all of the responsibility for any outcomes of sexting. From a policy perspective, schools should provide education as opposed to punishment when teens are discovered to have sexted when that sexting was consensual in nature. Punishments should fall on the disseminators, as nonconsensual dissemination is the key to harmful outcomes, not the consensual sharing or receiving among two adolescents. Additionally, schools can support parents in their roles, providing resources and tips to help caregivers have conversations with their adolescent children about how to intervene when a friend has forwarded a sext or asks for one.

**Conflict of Interest and Funding Disclosures** None.

## References


1. Barrense-Dias Y, Berchtold A, Surís J-C, Akre C. Sexting and the definition issue. J Adolesc Health. 2017;61:544. https://doi.org/10.1016/j.jadohealth.2017.05.009.
2. Mori C, Park J, Temple JR, Madigan S. Are youth sexting rates still on the rise? A meta-analytic update. J Adolesc Health. 2022;70(4):531–9. https://doi.org/10.1016/j.jadohealth.2021.10.026.
3. Englander E. What do we know about sexting, and when did we know it? J Adolesc Health. 2019;65(5):577–8. https://doi.org/10.1016/j.jadohealth.2019.08.004.
4. Temple JR, Strasburger VC, Zimmerman H, Madigan S. Sexting in youth: cause for concern? Lancet Child Adolescent Health. 2019;3:520. https://doi.org/10.1016/S2352-4642(19)30199-3.
5. Van Ouytsel J, Walrave M, De Marez L, Vanhaelewyn B, Ponnet K. Sexting, pressured sexting and image-based sexual abuse among a weighted-sample of heterosexual and LGB-youth. Comput Hum Behav. 2021;117:106630. https://doi.org/10.1016/j.chb.2020.106630.
6. Madigan S, Villani V, Azzopardi C, et al. The prevalence of unwanted online sexual exposure and solicitation among youth: a meta-analysis. J Adolesc Health. 2018;63(2):133–41. https://doi.org/10.1016/j.jadohealth.2018.03.012.
7. Van Ouytsel J, Walrave M, De Marez L, et al. Teenage sexting on the rise? Results of a cohort study using a weighted-sample of adolescents. Sex Health. 2020;17(2):178–81. https://doi.org/10.1071/SH19158.
8. Van Ouytsel J, Van Gool E, Walrave M, Ponnet K, Peeters E. Sexting: adolescents' perceptions of the applications used for, motives for, and consequences of sexting. J Youth Stud. 2017;20(4):446–70. https://doi.org/10.1080/13676261.2016.1241865.
9. Temple JR, Choi H. Longitudinal association between teen sexting and sexual behavior. Pediatrics. 2014;134(5):e1287–92. https://doi.org/10.1542/peds.2014-1974.
10. Mori C, Temple JR, Browne D, Madigan S. Association of sexting with sexual behaviors and mental health among adolescents: a systematic review and meta-analysis. JAMA Pediatr. 2019;173(8):770–9. https://doi.org/10.1001/jamapediatrics.2019.1658.
11. Campbell SW. Damned if you do, damned if you don't…if you're a girl: relational and normative contexts of adolescent sexting in the United States AU – Lippman, Julia R. J Child Media. 2014;8(4):371–86. https://doi.org/10.1080/17482798.2014.923009.
12. Ringrose J, Regehr K, Whitehead S. 'Wanna trade?': cisheteronormative homosocial masculinity and the normalization of abuse in youth digital sexual image exchange. J Gend Stud. 2021;31:243. https://doi.org/10.1080/09589236.2021.1947206.
13. Ringrose J, Harvey L. Boobs, back-off, six packs and bits: mediated body parts, gendered reward, and sexual shame in teens' sexting images. Continuum. 2015;29(2):205–17. https://doi.org/10.1080/10304312.2015.1022952.
14. Walrave M, Ponnet K, Van Ouytsel J, Van Gool E, Heirman W, Verbeek A, et al. Telematics Inform. 2015;32(4):796–808. https://doi.org/10.1016/j.tele.2015.03.008.
15. Lucić M, Baćak V, Štulhofer A. The role of peer networks in adolescent pornography use and sexting in Croatia. J Child Media. 2020;14(1):110–27. https://doi.org/10.1080/17482798.2019.1637356.
16. Parti K, Sanders CE, Englander EK. Sexting at an early age: patterns and poor health-related consequences of pressured sexting in middle and high school. J Sch Health. 2023;93(1):73–81. https://doi.org/10.1111/josh.13258.
17. Ringrose J, Harvey L, Gill R, Livingstone S. Teen girls, sexual double standards and 'sexting': gendered value in digital image exchange.

Fem Theory. 2013;14(3):305–23. https://doi.org/10.1177/1464700113499853.
18. Van Ouytsel J, Walrave M, Ponnet K, Heirman W. The association between adolescent sexting, psychosocial difficulties, and risk behavior: integrative review. J Sch Nurs. 2015;31(1):54–69. https://doi.org/10.1177/1059840514541964.
19. Maas MK, Cary KM, Clancy EM, Klettke B, McCauley HL, Temple JR. Slutpage use among U.S. college students: the secret and social platforms of image-based sexual abuse. Arch Sex Behav. 2021;50(5):2203–14. https://doi.org/10.1007/s10508-021-01920-1.
20. Casas JA, Ojeda M, Elipe P, Del Rey R. Exploring which factors contribute to teens' participation in sexting. Comput Hum Behav. 2019;100:60–9. https://doi.org/10.1016/j.chb.2019.06.010.
21. Bindesbøl Holm Johansen K, Pedersen BM, Tjørnhøj-Thomsen T. Visual gossiping: non-consensual 'nude' sharing among young people in Denmark. Cult Health Sex. 2018;21:1029. https://doi.org/10.1080/13691058.2018.1534140.
22. Harder SK. The emotional bystander – sexting and image-based sexual abuse among young adults. J Youth Stud. 2020;24:655. https://doi.org/10.1080/13676261.2020.1757631.
23. Ringrose J, Milne B, Mishna F, Regehr K, Slane A. Young people's experiences of image-based sexual harassment and abuse in England and Canada: toward a feminist framing of technologically facilitated sexual violence. Women's Stud Int Forum. 2022;93:102615. https://doi.org/10.1016/j.wsif.2022.102615.
24. Patchin JW, Hinduja S. Sextortion among adolescents: results from a National Survey of U.S. Youth. Sex Abus. 2020;32(1):30–54. https://doi.org/10.1177/1079063218800469.
25. Clancy EM, Hallford D, March E, Howard D, Toumbourou JW, Klettke B. The role of consent and motivations in sext dissemination. J Interpers Violence. 2023;38:9315. https://doi.org/10.1177/08862605231163886.
26. Döring N. Consensual sexting among adolescents: risk prevention through abstinence education or safer sexting? Cyberpsychol J Psychosoc Res Cyberspace. 2014;8 https://doi.org/10.5817/CP2014-1-9.
27. Patchin JW, Hinduja S. It is time to teach safe sexting. J Adolesc Health. 2020;66(2):140–3. https://doi.org/10.1016/j.jadohealth.2019.10.010.
28. Van Ouytsel J. A decade of sexting research: are we any wiser? JAMA Pediatr. 2020;174(2):204. https://doi.org/10.1001/jamapediatrics.2019.4562.
29. Wachs S, Wright MF, Gámez-Guadix M, Döring N. How are consensual, non-consensual, and pressured sexting linked to depression and self-harm? The moderating effects of demographic variables. Int J Environ Res Public Health. 2021;18(5):2597. https://doi.org/10.3390/ijerph18052597.
30. Lan Y-T, Pan Y-C, Lin Y-H. Association between adolescents' problematic online behaviors and self-harm risk. J Affect Disord. 2022;317:46–51. https://doi.org/10.1016/j.jad.2022.08.073.

# Introduction to the Section on Parenting in the Digital Age

Stephanie M. Reich and Sheri Madigan

## 1 Parenting in a Rapidly Evolving Digital Age

Digital technologies are rapidly changing. The first iPhone was released in 2007 (iPad in 2010), and that year, only 35% of people in the United States owned a smartphone [1]. In 2021, 97% of Americans owned a cellphone, with 87% being smartphones. Further, device ownership among children has increased, with age of ownership steadily decreasing. Thus, the vast majority of children and their parents have access to digital media, and most are on a variety of digital devices (e.g., televisions, smartphones, tablets, and gaming systems). Digital devices, therefore, have been woven into the fabric of every family's ecosystem.

From smartphones that capture babies' first smiles, steps, words, and family visits to computers where college applications are written, parenting today involves more devices, digital activities, and digital interactions than ever before. Not only are children and adolescents highly engaged with digital technology, so too are their parents. In this section on parenting in a digital age, we take stock of emerging research on the role of parents and families in a rapidly evolving digital age that presents both risks and benefits to children and adolescents.

## 2 Introduction to This Section

Each of the six chapters in this section on parenting and digital media takes a specific focus within this important topic. The first chapter by Reich et al. (see Chap. 52) offers an overview on the topic of parenting and digital media and the various ways in which this topic has been studied. The authors highlight the common features of parental monitoring, mediation of media use, and joint media engagement. They note the aspects of digital media that are most robustly related to beneficial child outcomes.

The next three chapters target three developmental timeframes: early childhood (age 0–5; Hirsh-Pasek et al., see Chap. 53), middle childhood (age 6–11; Bickham et al., see Chap. 54), and adolescence (age 12–18; Wisniewski et al., see Chap. 55). Hirsh-Pasek and colleagues draw attention to the important role of human-to-human interactions in young children's development and how digital activities can both mediate and displace these important human interchanges for young learners. Bickham et al. focus on the unique interests, activities, opportunities, and risks asso-

S. M. Reich (✉)
University of California, Irvine, CA, USA
e-mail: smreich@uci.edu

S. Madigan
University of Calgary, Calgary, AB, Canada

Alberta Children's Hospital Research Institute, Calgary, AB, Canada


D. A. Christakis, L. Hale (eds.), *Handbook of Children and Screens*,
https://doi.org/10.1007/978-3-031-69362-5_51

ciated with digital media in the middle childhood period. Wisniewski and colleagues overview the research on parenting adolescents' media use and the essential need to support them in increasing capacity and autonomy in navigating digital spaces. All authors provide an overview of the scope of research on the topic and how parenting strategies relate to developmental outcomes.

The next chapter by McDaniel et al. (see Chap. 56) underscores the importance of thoughtfulness in parenting around media that includes not just children's use but caregivers' as well. The authors articulate the ways in which caregivers' media use can interfere with parent–child interactions, a concept known as "technoference." The authors clarify how technology can displace meaningful interactions and when it can provide much-needed respite or support.

The final chapter by Browne (see Chap. 57) and colleagues highlight the importance of a digital family system approach in understanding how devices and digital content are embedded into family life. The authors describe ways in which media can synergistically affect the family through the various interactions between all members of the family (e.g., parent–parent, parent–child(ren), siblings, grandparent–parent, grandparent–child, etc.).

## 3 Emerging Section Themes

Several interesting and thought-provoking themes emerged across the chapters in this section.

### 3.1 Parenting Matters Most

Children's development shows consistent progression, regardless of societal or technological changes. For example, in learning to talk, children coo and babble before they form their first words. They then string words together in short two-word statements ("Dog go," "I do") before adding more words and progressing into full sentences with increasing sophistication. Similar patterns of predictable progression are seen in physical development, emotion expression, recognition and regulation, cognition, and social interactions. In all of these domains, caregivers are key supports, and often their behavior is one of the strongest predictors of children's outcomes [2, 3]. That is, through consistent, supportive, affectionate, responsive, and stimulating interactions (i.e., "relational health"), caregivers influence children's development. As noted across the chapters in this section, digital media is just another part of children's environment where high-quality caregiving still matters, and arguably, remains the most potent predictor of children's outcomes.

### 3.2 Human-to-Human Is Best

Several chapters referenced that humans are social creatures, and our development is largely shaped through social interactions. The chapter by Hirsh-Pasek [3] speaks to this in detail. Digital devices often play a role in the frequency and quality of social interactions in which children engage. Technology can displace social interactions, such as when parents or children are focused on devices rather than engaging in learning opportunities or social exchanges that may have occurred if the devices were turned off. However, digital devices have the potential to support future social interactions by providing needed breaks (e.g., distracting children while cooking or getting work done on a laptop in order to be able to spend time together later). Digital devices can also be protective by displacing negative interactions (e.g., texting a friend for support rather than allowing frustration to spill over onto parenting or distracting a child while parents have an argument). For parenting in a digital age, it is essential to consider how frequently and extensively devices are used and the ways they influence the occurrence and quality of social interactions.

### 3.3 Fostering Digital Connection Versus Disconnection

All the chapters in this section emphasize that when thinking about media and parenting, it is important to consider the ways media might facilitate connections (e.g., playing together and texting for social support) or alternatively, detract from them (e.g., watching television alone in a bedroom or ignoring bids for attention). When families engage in media use together (e.g., family gaming) or interact through media (e.g., video chat and texting), important social connections can occur, and this is adaptive for children's development [4].

### 3.4 Parenting Strategies Should Matter as Children Mature

Some aspects of parenting are consistent across the lifespan. All children benefit from caregivers that are warm, affectionate, responsive, consistent, and stimulating [3, 5, 6]. Other aspects of parenting change as children age, helping children to become increasingly autonomous and better able to occupy more mature roles. As noted in all the chapters in this section, parenting strategies and their efficacy vary at different stages of child development. For instance, more rigid rules and stronger parental oversight are important at younger ages, while more global rule settings and discussions are important for adolescents. Having clear and consistent rules that provide more autonomy and flexibility over time can help cultivate more harmonious interactions with digital media. As children grow into adolescence, they need increasing amounts of digital autonomy paired with capacity building on how they can develop and maintain healthy media habits that promote learning, education, creativity, and connection. Across all ages, talking with children about their digital media use and modeling healthy choices (e.g., thoughtfulness about when using—and never while driving) are critical [7].

### 3.5 Families Are Unique, So Media Habits and Rules Should (Mostly) Be, Too

As noted by the authors in this section, research does not suggest a "one size fits all" approach to parenting children's digital media use [7]. The types of devices, platforms, social connections, and reasons for use can vary across families. For instance, some children really struggle disconnecting from devices, while others do not, and accordingly, parents may need to alter their rules and approaches to media use to suit the individual needs of their children [8]. In addition, in families with children who have a chronic illness or are gender or sexual minorities, online connections might be especially important for finding social support, information, and resources [9]. As such, media rules around time of use and connections with known and unknown others might vary. Therefore, families should craft rules and expectations, for children and adults, that fit their families' needs and wants. Communication and consistency in parenting around media are more important than specific rules.

### 3.6 Sleep Is Hugely Important, So Avoid Media That Disrupts It

One exception to the idea that digital media rules should be tailored to each child within each family, is related to sleep. Research consistently finds that avoiding media in bedrooms at night can help improve the amount and quality of sleep that children have. We have long known that televisions in the bedrooms of children, even young children, are related to less sleep [10] and other devices like smartphones, can disrupt sleep in a variety of ways, including notifications (audio, vibrations, lights), desires to check for messages or contact friends, and even emotional states (e.g., excitement, worry) that can make falling and staying asleep difficult [11, 12]. Additionally, the blue light that some devices emit can delay melatonin production, taking longer to fall asleep [11]. Thus, unless there is an important reason for media in the room (to use as an alarm clock is not a good reason)—a best practice is to make night time (and naptimes) media-free.

## 3.7 Quantity Versus Quality of Screen Time

All six chapters acknowledge that the quantity of screen time should not be the sole focus of research. Understanding what children and adolescents use, why, when, how, and with whom are important for providing oversight and guidance to keep children healthy in a digital world. Parents know their children best and should set rules and make choices about what is permissible or not based on this knowledge. For example, if a child is highly excitable or has a tendency toward aggressive behavior, parents might more actively focus on limiting violent media use, especially before bedtime. If a child has a history of disordered eating, parents might spend more time scrolling social media with their child and talking about the content, algorithms suggesting content, and feelings when engaging with those platforms. Research does not suggest a one-size-fits-all approach to parenting around digital media, but studies do converge on media rules that fit children's individual dispositions [7, 13, 14] and support open and trusting parent–child communication [15].

## 3.8 Parents' Media Use Matters

Many of the authors in this section touched upon the myriad ways in which parents directly and indirectly influence children's screen time behaviors. Indeed, studies consistently find that the greatest predictor of children's media use is their parents' media use [16, 17]. This includes screen time and screen-specific behaviors. For example, parents' use of their phone rather than engagement with their children, known as phubbing (phone + snubbing), is related to teens' problematic phone use [18]. Parents' time on social media is also significantly related to adolescents' social media use a year later [19]. Further, parents' online behaviors appear to model for children the types of media use and duration of that use [20], as well as specific behaviors when using media [21]. From diapers to driving, children look to parents about how to navigate life, and this includes digital realms too.

## 3.9 Consistent Gaps in the Literature

Each of the chapters in this section on parenting and digital media highlights areas in which more research is needed, and below we provide the common issues identified:

1. *Heterogeneity of families: Uses and reasons for use.* All of the chapters in this section make note of the great variety of family structures, contexts, and needs. Research to date has not sufficiently explored how media use and impacts might vary based on unique family characteristics. For instance, research finds that online spaces can be particularly supportive for Black and Latine adolescents [22] while also being traumatizing with viral videos of hate crimes, biased algorithms, and racist interactions [23]. Similar patterns are found for Lesbian, Gay, Bisexual, Transgender, Queer, and Others (LGBTQ+) youth [24, 25]. Research has also not adequately explored diversity in cultural and economic contexts that can influence parenting around media, such as shared devices across children, vicarious media exposure in crowded households, connections in transnational families, and various work schedules. These gaps in understanding parenting of media use in diverse families are exacerbated by the rapidly changing digital landscape with new games, apps, and devices.
2. *When is "technoference" problematic?* Though all chapters discuss technoference and McDaniel and colleagues focus exclusively on this issue, more research is needed as to when technology use is truly interfering and when it is providing important parenting breaks (e.g., able to connect with friends), being used at times when interactions would not have occurred anyway (e.g., while baby dozes during nursing), or might enable more interactions (e.g., able to work from home). Also of interest is whether it is the parents' duration of use or their frequency of device use that impacts parent-child interactions and children's outcomes [26]. It is also notable

that most of the technoference research has focused on mothers, and the ways in which technology might alter fathering are not well studied. A more nuanced understanding of what might media displace and when that might be risky, beneficial, or neutral is needed. Parents' and children's media use can contribute to higher quality parenting (e.g., social support, information seeking, respite, etc.), but more research is needed, especially on the beneficial aspects. It is also possible that technoference is different for children and adults. Nascent research suggests that the presence of devices has greater impacts on adults' behaviors, with a reduction in interactivity from adults with devices leading to children's reducing efforts to interact [27].

3. *Current screen guidelines are not often followed.* Research consistently finds that many families do not abide by the American Academy of Pediatrics' (AAP) recommendations for media use [28–30]. This suggests that the guidelines may not be well-tailored to different types of families and their unique needs and/or that caregivers need more information and support to put these recommendations into practice. For instance, the AAP and World Health Organization recommend that children 2–5 years only engage in up to 1 h of high-quality media use per weekday, but a recent meta-analysis shows that only one-third of children globally are meeting this guideline [31]. Further, what is considered "high quality" screen use is difficult to ascertain. Reviews of the app market find that few apps labeled as educational are actually designed in ways that are educational [32] and most television and streamable programs are not rated for educational quality. Much more research is needed to better understand what, how, and why digital devices are used in families so that recommendations can be designed in ways that support their unique needs and uses. Further, ways to better educate parents about healthy media diets (theirs and their children's) are needed.

## 4 Conclusion

We applaud the authors in this section for addressing the ways in which digital media intersects with family life and how digital devices and their myriad uses can enhance, detract, supplement, and/or supplant family interactions and developmental processes. Importantly, all the chapters draw attention to the diverse ways that digital media are embedded into the family unit and illustrate the complexities and nuances of this topic. Research in the field of screen use among children, adolescents, and families has fallen behind the rapid pace of digital evolution. This digital landscape is evolving quickly, necessitating urgent efforts from researchers to bridge this gap. To adequately inform practices and policies that promote healthy screen habits within families, there is a critical need for advancing understanding of the nuanced dynamics surrounding screen use—for example, when is it beneficial, when is it impactful globally or specifically for different demographic characteristics, in which contexts is it advantageous or disadvantageous, and under what conditions is it influential. Such research is critical to supporting children and families in harnessing the benefits of digital media while mitigating potential risks to child development and family well-being.

**Conflict of Interest and Funding Disclosures** None.

## References

1. Center PR. Mobile fact sheet. https://www.pewresearch.org/internet/fact-sheet/mobile/. Accessed 30 Apr 2023.
2. Anderson NJ, Graham SA, Prime H, Jenkins JM, Madigan S. Linking quality and quantity of parental linguistic input to child language skills: a meta-analysis. Child Dev. 2021;92(2):484–501. https://doi.org/10.1111/cdev.13508.
3. Madigan S, Prime H, Graham SA, et al. Parenting behavior and child language: a meta-analysis. Pediatrics. 2019;144(4):e20183556. https://doi.org/10.1542/peds.2018-3556.
4. Madigan S, McArthur BA, Anhorn C, Eirich R, Christakis DA. Associations between screen use and child language skills: a systematic review and meta-

analysis. JAMA Pediatr. 2020;174(7):665–75. https://doi.org/10.1001/jamapediatrics.2020.0327.
5. Cooke JE, Deneault A-A, Devereux C, Eirich R, Fearon RMP, Madigan S. Parental sensitivity and child behavioral problems: a meta-analytic review. Child Dev. 2022;93(5):1231–48. https://doi.org/10.1111/cdev.13764.
6. Rodrigues M, Sokolovic N, Madigan S, et al. Paternal sensitivity and children's cognitive and socioemotional outcomes: a meta-analytic review. Child Dev. 2021;92(2):554–77. https://doi.org/10.1111/cdev.13545.
7. Madigan S, Reich SM. Consideration of developmental stage and the debate on the effects of screens use—not all things are created equal. JAMA Pediatr. 2023;177(11):1123–4. https://doi.org/10.1001/jamapediatrics.2023.3670.
8. Piotrowski JT, Valkenburg PM. Finding orchids in a field of dandelions; understanding children's differential susceptibility to media effects. Am Behav Sci. 2015;59(14):1776–89. https://doi.org/10.1177/0002764215596552.
9. DeHoff B, Staten L, Rodgers R, Denne S. The role of online social support in supporting and educating parents of young children with special health care needs in the United States: a scoping review. J Med Internet Res. 2016;18(12) https://doi.org/10.2196/jmir.6722.
10. Cespedes EM, Gillman MW, Kleinman K, Rifas-Shiman SL, Redline S, Taveras EM. Television viewing, bedroom television, and sleep duration from infancy to mid-childhood. Pediatrics. 2014;133(5):e1163–71. https://doi.org/10.1542/peds.2013-3998.
11. Hale L, Li X, Hartstein LE, LeBourgeois MK. Media use and sleep in teenagers: what do we know? Curr Sleep Med Rep. 2019;5(3):128–34. https://doi.org/10.1007/s40675-019-00146-x.
12. Bartel KA, Gradisar M, Williamson P. Protective and risk factors for adolescent sleep: a meta-analytic review. Sleep Med Rev. 2015;21:72–85. https://doi.org/10.1016/j.smrv.2014.08.002.
13. McArthur BA, Hentges R, Christakis DA, McDonald S, Tough S, Madigan S. Cumulative social risk and child screen use: the role of child temperament. J Pediatr Psychol. 2022;47(2):171–9. https://doi.org/10.1093/jpepsy/jsab087.
14. Valkenburg PM, Peter J. The differential susceptibility to media effects model. J Commun. 2013; 63(2):221–43. https://doi.org/10.1111/jcom.12024.
15. Padilla-Walker L, Coyne SM, Kroff S, Memmott-Elison M. The protective role of parental media monitoring style from early to late adolescence. J Youth Adolescence. 2018;47(2):445–59. https://doi.org/10.1007/s10964-017-0722-4.
16. Madigan S, Racine N, Tough S. Prevalence of preschoolers meeting vs exceeding screen time guidelines. JAMA Pediatr. 2020;174(1):93–5. https://doi.org/10.1001/jamapediatrics.2019.4495.
17. Lauricella AR, Wartella E, Rideout VJ. Young children's screen time: the complex role of parent and child factors. J Appl Dev Psychol. 2015;36:11–7. https://doi.org/10.1016/j.appdev.2014.12.001.
18. Xie X, Chen W, Zhu X, He D. Parents' phubbing increases Adolescents' mobile phone addiction: roles of parent-child attachment, deviant peers, and gender. Children Youth Serv Rev. 2019;105:104426. https://doi.org/10.1016/j.childyouth.2019.104426.
19. Fardouly J, Magson NR, Rapee RM, et al. Investigating longitudinal and bidirectional relationships between parental factors and time spent on social media during early adolescence. New Media Soc. 2022:14614448221076155. https://doi.org/10.1177/14614448221076155.
20. Vaala SE, Bleakley A. Monitoring, mediating, and modeling: parental influence on adolescent computer and internet use in the United States. Journal of Children and Media. 2015;9(1):40–57. https://doi.org/10.1080/17482798.2015.997103.
21. Reich SM, Starks A, Santer N, Manago A. Brief report–modeling media use: how parents' and other adults' posting behaviors relate to young adolescents' posting behaviors. brief research report. Frontiers in Human Dyn. 2021;3 https://doi.org/10.3389/fhumd.2021.595924.
22. Wilf S, Maker Castro E, Gupta K, Wray-Lake L. Shifting culture and minds: immigrant-origin youth building critical consciousness on social media. Youth Soc. 2022; https://doi.org/10.1177/0044118X221103890.
23. Tynes B, Willis H, Stewart AM, Hamilton MW. Race-related traumatic events online and mental health among adolescents of color. J Adolescent Health. 2019;65(3):371–7. https://doi.org/10.1016/j.jadohealth.2019.03.006.
24. Bates A, Hobman T, Bell B. "Let me do what i please with it ... don't decide my identity for me": LGBTQ+ youth experiences of social media in narrative identity development. J Adolescent Res. 2020;35(1):51–83. https://doi.org/10.1177/0743558419884700.
25. Cho A. Default publicness: queer youth of color, social media, and being outed by the machine. New Media Soc. 2018;20(9):3183–200. https://doi.org/10.1177/1461444817744784.
26. Wolfers LN, Kitzmann S, Sauer S, Sommer N. Phone use while parenting: an observational study to assess the association of maternal sensitivity and smartphone use in a playground setting. Computers in Human Behavior. 2020;102:31–8. https://doi.org/10.1016/j.chb.2019.08.013.
27. Ochoa W, Reich S, Farkas G. The observed quality of caregiver-child interactions with and without a mobile screen device. Acad Pediatr. 2021;21(4):620–8.
28. Brown A, Smolenaers E. Parents' interpretations of screen time recommendations for children younger than 2 years. J Family Issues. 2018;39(2):406–29.

29. Radesky J, Weeks H, Ball R, et al. Young children's use of smartphones and tablets. Pedaitrics. 2020;146(1):e20193518.
30. Ponti M. Screen time and preschool children: promoting health and development in a digital world. Paediatr Child Health. 2023;28(3):184–92.
31. McArthur BA, Volkova V, Tomopoulos S, Madigan S. Global prevalence of meeting screen time guidelines among children 5 years and younger: a systematic review and meta-analysis. JAMA Pediatr. 2022;176(4):373–83. https://doi.org/10.1001/jamapediatrics.2021.6386.
32. Callaghan M, Reich S. Are educational preschool apps designed to teach? An analysis of the app market. Learn Media Technol. 2018;3:280–93. https://doi.org/10.1080/17439884.2018.1498355.

# Media and Parenting: Current Findings and Future Directions

Stephanie M. Reich, Fashina Aladé, Drew P. Cingel, Lori Takeuchi, Ronald Warren, and Yalda T. Uhls

## 1 Background

Media research consistently finds that the ways in which parents offer, supervise, talk about, restrict, and co-use media are related to both children's healthy and risky media use. Though some aspects of parenting of media use vary with a child's age, some aspects are consistent from early childhood through adolescence [1]. Below, we highlight some of the ways in which parenting of media use has been conceptualized, what recent research has found, what gaps still remain, and what concrete recommendations can be made from evidence thus far.

S. M. Reich (✉)
University of California, Irvine, CA, USA
e-mail: smreich@uci.edu

F. Aladé
Michigan State University, East Lansing, MI, USA

D. P. Cingel
University of California, Davis, CA, USA

L. Takeuchi
National Science Foundation, Alexandria, VA, USA

R. Warren
University of Arkansas, Fayetteville, AR, USA

Y. T. Uhls
Center for Scholars & Storytellers at University of California, Los Angeles, Los Angeles, CA, USA

### 1.1 Conceptualizing Parenting of Media Use

#### 1.1.1 Mediation

A large body of research has focused on parental mediation of children's media use, i.e., ways in which parents oversee, manage, and regulate use. Originally developed for television viewing, parental mediation theory has evolved and expanded to address newer technologies (e.g., video games, mobile devices, and social media) [2]. Studies of parental mediation of media use focus on four main strategies: restrictive, passive/co-use, active, and deference mediation. *Restrictive mediation* involves rules about media such as if, when, and what is used. The ways in which caregivers use media with children, but do not discuss or scaffold that use, is known as *passive mediation* or *co-use*. *Active mediation* involves parental discussions about media, typically while the child is using it. *Deference mediation* is the reliance on trust in children's decision-making, rather than restrictions [3]. Parents tend to use more than one mediation strategy, and a recent meta-analysis found strengths and weaknesses of each strategy depending on factors such as child age and gender, specific type of content and platform, and cultural context, with open channels of communication through active mediation being especially important [4].


D. A. Christakis, L. Hale (eds.), *Handbook of Children and Screens*,
https://doi.org/10.1007/978-3-031-69362-5_52

More recently, restrictive mediation strategies have been further delineated. *Autonomy-supportive restrictive mediation* focuses on ways to help children cultivate more competent and healthy media use. It can involve both active and restrictive mediation strategies but is more focused on child autonomy than parent control [5]. *Controlling restrictive mediation* stresses obedience and compliance and often uses external rewards or punishments to control children's media behaviors. *Inconsistent restrictive mediation* involves irregular or unpredictable restrictions and is often associated with problematic outcomes.

#### 1.1.2 Joint Media Engagement

Similar to aspects of mediation and largely derived from co-viewing research, especially in early childhood, joint media engagement (JME) is the sharing, creating, playing, viewing, searching, or reading of media together [6]. JME can scaffold use for children, from learning how to operate a device to developing a deeper understanding of media content. A systematic review of JME (ages 1–10 years) found the quality of interactions varied when using media, from passively watching to actively engaging and encouraging. Associations with child outcomes were similarly mixed, with positive, negative, and no associations with a range of interpersonal and developmental outcomes [7].

#### 1.1.3 Parental Monitoring

Unlike mediation and JME, the concept of parental monitoring has non-media origins but applies well to parenting of media use. Parental monitoring includes the range of activities and behaviors parents use to oversee their children's activities, behaviors, and whereabouts [8]. It is characterized by *open communication*, *surveillance* (i.e., oversight), and *behavioral control* (e.g., rules, restrictions, and consequences). Research suggests parental monitoring may be protective, with open communication again being a key component for positive child outcomes [9].

#### 1.1.4 High-Quality Caregiving

As technologies have changed, becoming more connected and ubiquitous in children's lives, findings indicate that media are just another context for child development wherein the quality of parenting matters. High-quality parenting tends to be caring and warm (though expression varies by culture), contingently responsive, consistent, and stimulating. Consistent and predictable expectations, rules, and consequences are beneficial for children as are having caregivers who are loving, observant, responsive, and trustworthy and who provide stimulating and supportive environments [10]. Parent–child interactions with these qualities are associated with more healthy and resilient media use, as well as increased learning from screens [6, 11, 12].

#### 1.1.5 Parental Motives and Reasoning

Parents have a variety of reasons for providing or allowing media or using parenting strategies. Some value the educational or learning opportunities media can provide [13, 14]. Some need ways to distract their child to get things done [15]. Some parents enjoy the family time and constant communication media can provide [13, 16]. Some believe it provides valuable breaks and distractions [14]. Some use it for discipline—for rewards and punishments [17], and others feel it is simply unavoidable.

## 2 Current State

Systematic reviews of the effectiveness of different strategies for parenting of media use yield mixed results. In general, active mediation, parental monitoring, and autonomy-supportive restrictive mediation are associated with better child mental health outcomes and fewer risky behaviors (e.g., substance use and sexual activity), while restrictive mediation and surveillance are linked to less screen time/media use [4, 18]. However, the strategies parents use and their usefulness change as children age. For instance, JME is most common in early childhood while autonomy-supportive restrictive mediation is more common with adolescents.

Importantly, research finds that many parental and child factors contribute to how children are parented around media, such as parents' knowledge, beliefs, and attitudes about media, children's age and temperament, parent involvement, and family communication patterns, as well as children's and parents' mental and physical health [19–22]. Research studies find that media can help parents better understand their child's identity (e.g., sexuality and gender) and needs (e.g., mental health) through co-viewing and facilitation of conversation [23, 24].

## 2.1 Beyond Screen Time

While early studies focused on the amount of time children spent using screens, more recent research has moved beyond screen time to examine the content that children are consuming, with whom they are interacting, and their motivations for use. One framework for thinking beyond screen time focuses on the 3 C's of media use: Content (what children are watching/doing), Context (where they use media and who they use it with), and Child (individual characteristics, age, and dispositions, e.g., excitable, distractible, and sensitive) [25]. Recent research points to two more important C's: Communication, including the ways in which caregivers and children communicate about media, and capacity building, or the ways in which caregivers help to increase children's autonomy and ability to understand, select, and regulate use [4, 5, 23, 24].

## 2.2 How Screen Time Matters

Despite the shift towards considering quality over quantity, certain findings of screen time remain relevant [26]. Device access and use before bed is associated with inadequate and poor sleep quality and excessive daytime sleepiness [27]. Television use by children and their parents, as well as background television, reduces the number of words spoken to the child, by the child, and around the child [19], and early television viewing is related to poorer executive functioning (that is, the higher-order cognitive processes that support goal-directed behavior) [28, 29]. For youth, media use can displace important opportunities for social interactions, motor development, and cultivation of self-regulatory skills [19, 30–32].

## 2.3 Parental Contributions to Media Use

Caregivers are tremendous contributors to children's media habits. They contribute directly by selecting if, when, and what types of media children use, and also indirectly in a variety of ways.

### 2.3.1 Modeling and Norm Setting

In general, the greatest predictor of children's media use across age, race, and family income is their parents' media use [11, 33]. For example, children's device use typically occurs when parents are using devices too [34], and there is growing evidence that children model some of their caregivers' media habits, such as social media posting [35].

### 2.3.2 Sharenting

In many families, parents post about their children from very young ages—sometimes before birth—and this sharing about parenting (sharenting) establishes a digital presence for children long before they might want or choose to have one. A survey of 1000 US parents found that 75% posted images of their child, often paired with the child's name [36]. It is estimated that the average child has 1500 pictures of them posted online before the age of 5 years, and caregiver posting is associated with future identity theft [37, 38].

### 2.3.3 Parental Media Habits

A review of research found that parents' mobile device use was tied to more distracted parenting (e.g., technoference—when parents are distracted by technology) and children's active and sometimes high-risk efforts to get attention [39]. Observational studies find significantly less affection, responsiveness, and language use by adults toward their children when their cell phone is present compared to when it is not [40–42]. This is why family media plans (plans establishing media priorities, uses, and rules) should include not just children's but parents' media use, including establishing device-free zones (e.g., dinner table).

#### 2.3.4 Family Communication

Research consistently finds that the risks and benefits of media use are linked to children's relationships with their parents. Youth who have lower-quality interactions with their parents (e.g., more conflict and less communication) are more likely to engage in high-risk digital behaviors or develop health problems (e.g., video game addiction) [9, 19]. In contrast, high-quality interactions can be protective. For example, though social media use and body dissatisfaction are linked, their relationship is weakened when girls have a positive relationship with their mothers [43].

#### 2.3.5 Media Moments

Media can provide opportunities for parents and children to have meaningful conversations about important and sometimes sensitive topics. For instance, studies of the TV series *13 Reasons Why* found increased awareness of depression and suicide for youth and their parents, with increased conversations between them about symptoms, thoughts, and getting help [23, 44]. Similarly, queer youth report using media as a mechanism to teach their parents about their sexual and/or gender identities [24]. These "media moments" provide valuable ways to connect, support, and help children and adolescents, and work best when parents are aware of what youth are doing/watching and have open lines of communication with them.

## 3 Future Research

- **How might media be used in ways that strengthen family connections?** Recent research indicates that media can help strengthen family connections and improve parent–child interactions. However, many of the mechanisms to explain exactly how this occurs are unknown. Further, the efficacy of newer resources (e.g., family media plans) on the healthy integration of media into the family ecology (e.g., setting, members, routines, and interactions) is not well tested, particularly among diverse families.
- **How could media recommendations better fit the realities of parenting?** A consistent finding is that parents do not abide by professional recommendations for whether, at what age, or how much children and adolescents should use media. It is easy for experts to dictate parameters of use, but such recommendations are not effective without understanding which ones parents adopt (and why), and how they fit within existing contexts of family life. Importantly, many recommendations are based on research that does not consider racial, ethnic, linguistic, gender, sexual orientation, or economic diversity. Further, the vast majority of information and support for parents is developed by pediatric and developmental professionals. To date, little input is provided by children and adolescents, who undoubtedly have important insights into their uses, needs, and wants.
- **How has parenting of children's media use changed since the COVID-19 pandemic?** The COVID-19 pandemic led to an unprecedented increase in media use by children and their parents. Schools became digital, devices became babysitters and recreational programs, and digital media served as many youth's only connection to peers. Though in-person activities have resumed, youth continue to engage with more technology than ever before, including computers in classrooms, online homework, and higher utilization of social and streaming media. How this diversity of screens and constant connectivity relate to parenting and child outcomes are still unknown.
- **How might parenting of media use vary for families of color, immigrant families, families with various incomes and educational attainment, families with neurodiverse or differently abled children, and families with gender diverse or sexual minority children?** The extant research does not align with the diversity of families in the United States. Most parenting of media research involves white, college-educated, US-born, and finan-

cially stable families with less exploration into processes that might be universal versus context-specific. Further, some youth are more likely to encounter risks online. In particular, racial, ethnic, sexual, and gender minority children are more likely to be subjected to bias, discrimination, predators, and incessant advertisements online. As such, parenting of marginalized youth's media use may need additional supports and resources, especially since Latine and Black children and children from families with few financial resources tend to consume more media than their White and more affluent peers, encounter more discriminatory content, and experience more trauma from that consumption [19, 45].

## 4 Recommendations

- **High-quality parenting matters!** Parenting that is caring, warm, contingently responsive, stimulating, and consistent matters, in general, and especially around children's media use. Starting early with open communication and consistent rules will make parenting of media use easier as children age. One would never just open a door and expect a child to find their way to a new park on their own. Similarly, devices should not be handed to children with no restrictions, advice, support, or rules. Parents need to teach children about healthful media use and model it themselves. That includes stronger restrictions and oversight in the earlier ages with more autonomy earned with age and experience. Importantly, high-quality parent–child relationships mean that children will talk with parents when they have a problem—be it a bully at school or online; feelings of insecurity in physical or virtual spaces; encounters with strangers at the park or on social media; or simple curiosities or questions they have. Parenting is parenting, even when there is a digital component.
- **Don't just focus on screen time.** The amount of time on screens matters for displacement of other developmentally important activities, but doesn't address what children are doing, for how long, why, or with whom. Parents should talk with their children about all of these things. When children use media, parents should use it with them. It can be a family movie night, co-creation of content (e.g., TikTok dances or Minecraft structures), or simply following them on social media (with permission) to see who they connect with and the types of content they share and receive. Parents should have consistent rules about both quality and quantity of media use with clear consequences that are explained to the child.
- **Parents' digital habits matter too!** Parents are their children's first and most important teachers. Therefore, parents need to be thoughtful about their own media use, including what they do, when and where they use it, and instead of what. Distracted parents are less interactive with their children, and positive social interactions are a critical element of healthy development, from providing language to a new talker to creating opportunities for adolescents to share about their day. Some parental media behaviors (e.g., sharenting) can compromise children's autonomy and privacy, so parents should be thoughtful when sharing private information about their children online.
- **Media can be a resource.** So much focus is placed on the risk of media for children and adolescents, but research has identified many ways in which it can be a resource for families. Parents consistently report finding information about parenting and social support from online sites and digital social connections. Further, family time can happen with media, such as family gaming, movie watching, and coding. In addition, media might create moments for discussion, learning, sharing, and growth. Texting and social media can provide ways for youth and parents to communicate, supporting their interaction quality, and children's mental health [16]. The trick is to elevate the good and be aware of the risks.

**Conflict of Interest and Funding Disclosures** None.

## References


1. Madigan S, Reich SM. Consideration of developmental stage and the debate on the effects of screens use—not all things are created equal. JAMA Pediatr. 2023;177(11):1123–4.
2. Schofield CL. Parental mediation theory for the digital age. Commun Theory. 2011;21:323–43. https://doi.org/10.1111/j.1468-2885.2011.01391.x.
3. Hernandez JM, Ben-Joseph EP, Reich S, Charmaraman L. Parental monitoring of early adolescent social technology use in the US: a mixed-method study. J Child Family Stud. 2023;33:1–18.
4. Chen L, Shi J. Reducing harm from media: a meta-analysis of parental mediation. J Mass Commun Q. 2019;96(1):173–93. https://doi.org/10.1177/1077699018754908.
5. Meeus A, Beyens I, Geusens F, Katrien Sodermans A, Beullens K. Managing positive and negative media effects among adolescents: parental mediation matters—but not always. J Fam Commun. 2018;18(4):270–85. https://doi.org/10.1080/15267431.2018.1487443.
6. Takeuchi L, Stevens R. The new coviewing: desiging for learning through joint media engagement. The Joan Ganz Cooney Center at Sesame Workshop; 2011.
7. Ewin C, Reupert A, McLean L, Ewin C. The impact of joint media engagement on parent–child interactions: a systematic review. Hum Behav Emerg Technol. 2020;3(2):230–54. https://doi.org/10.1002/hbe2.203.
8. Dishion TJ, McMahon RJ. Parental monitoring and the prevention of child and adolescent problem behavior: a conceptual and empirical formulation. Clin Child Fam Psychol Rev. 1998;1:61–75. https://doi.org/10.1023/A:1021800432380.
9. Padilla-Walker L, Coyne SM, Kroff S, Memmott-Elison M. The protective role of parental media monitoring style from early to late adolescence. J Youth Adolesc. 2018;47(2):445–59. https://doi.org/10.1007/s10964-017-0722-4.
10. Bornstein MH. Handbook of parenting. 3rd ed. Routledge; 2019.
11. Moreno M, Binger K, Zhao Q, et al. Digital technology and media use by adolescents: latent class analysis. JMIR Pediatr Parent. 2022;5(2):e35540. https://doi.org/10.2196/35540.
12. Moser A, Zimmermann L, Dickerson K, Grennell A, Barr R, Gerhardstein P. They can interact, but can they learn? Toddlers' transfer learning from touchscreens and television. J Exp Child Psychol. 2015;137:137–55. https://doi.org/10.1016/j.jecp.2015.04.002.
13. Gee E, Takeuchi L, Wartella E. Children and families in the digital age: learning together in a media saturated culture. Routledge; 2017.
14. Ochoa W, Reich SM. Parents' beliefs about the benefits and detriments of mobile screen technologies for their young children's learning: a focus on diverse Latine mothers and fathers. Front Psychol. 2020;11:570712.
15. Elias N, Sulkin I. Screen-assisted parenting: the relationship between toddlers' screen time and parents' use of media as a parenting tool. J Family Issues. 2019;40(18):2801–22. https://doi.org/10.1177/0192513X19864983.
16. Jensen M, George M, Russell M, Lippold M, Odgers CL. Daily parent-adoelscent digital exchanges. Res Child Adolesc Psychopathol. 2021;49:1125–38. https://doi.org/10.1007/s10802-020-00765-x.
17. Hawi N, Rupert M. Impact of e-discipline on children's screen time. CyberPsychol Behav Soc Netw. 2015;18(6):337–42.
18. Collier K, Coyne SM, Rasmussen EE, et al. Does parental mediation of media influence child outcomes? A metaanalysis on media time, aggression, substance use, and sexual behavior. Dev Psychol. 2016;52(5):798–812. https://doi.org/10.1037/dev0000108.
19. Reid Chassiakos Y, Radesky J, Christakis D. AAP council on communications and media. Children and adolescents and digital media. Pediatrics. 2016;138(5):e20162593.
20. Coyne S, Radesky J, Collier KM, et al. Parenting and digital media. Pediatrics. 2017;140(2):S112–6.
21. Coyne S, Shawcroft J, Gale M, et al. Tantrums, toddlers and technology: temperament, media emotion regulation, and problematic media use in early childhood. Comput Hum Behav. 2021;120:106762. https://doi.org/10.1016/j.chb.2021.106762.
22. Griffith SF. Parent beliefs and child media use: stress and digital skills as moderators. J Appl Dev Psychol. 2023;86:101535.
23. Mann S, Cingel D, Lauricella A, Wartella E. Parent viewership of 13 reasons why and knowledge about adolescent life: implications for parent efficacy among parents from the United States, United Kingdom, Brazil, and Australia/New Zealand. J Child Media. 2022;16(2):240–60. https://doi.org/10.1080/17482798.2021.1962931.
24. Mares M, Chen YA, Bond B. Mutual influence in LGBTQ teens' use of media to socialize their parents. Media Psychol. 2022;25(3):441–68. https://doi.org/10.1080/15213269.2021.1969950.
25. Guernsey L, Levine M. Tap, click, read: growing readers in a world of screens. Jossey-Bass; 2015.
26. National Academies of Sciences E, and Medicine. Social media and adolescent health. Washington, DC: The National Academies Press; 2023.
27. Carter B, Rees P, Hale L, Bhattacharjee D, Paradkar M. Association between portable screen-based media device access or use and sleep outcomes: a systematic review and meta-analysis. JAMA Pediatr. 2016;170(12):1202–8. https://doi.org/10.1001/jamapediatrics.2016.2341.

28. Best JR, Miller PH. A developmental perspective on executive function. Child Dev. 2010;81(6):1641–60.
29. Nathanson AI, Aladé F, Sharp M, Rasmussen EE, Christy K. The relation between television exposure and executive function among preschoolers. Dev Psychol. 2014;50(5):1497–506. https://doi.org/10.1037/a0035714.
30. Swider-Cios E, Vermeij A, Sitskoorn MM. Young children and screen-based media: the impact on cognitive and socioemotional development and the importance of parental mediation. Cogn Dev. 2023;66:101319. https://doi.org/10.1016/j.cogdev.2023.101319.
31. Madigan S, McArthur B, Anhorn C, Eirich R, Christakis D. Associations between screen use and child language skills: a systematic review and meta-analysis. JAMA Pediatr. 2020; https://doi.org/10.1001/jamapediatrics20200327. online first:E1-E11.
32. Hutton JS, Dudley J, Horowitz-Kraus T, DeWitt T, Holland SK. Associations between screen-based media use and brain white matter integrity in preschool-aged children. JAMA Pediatr. 2020;174(1):e193869.
33. Lauricella A, Cingel D. The power of parents: parents' own media use and media attitudes predict youth media use. J Child Fam Stud. 2020;29(7):1927–37. https://doi.org/10.1007/s10826-020-01724-2.
34. Domoff S, Radesky J, Harrison K, Riley H, Lumeng J, Miller AL. A naturalistic study of child and family screen media and mobile device use. J Child Fam Stud. 2019;28:401–10. https://doi.org/10.1007/s10826-018-1275-1.
35. Reich SM, Starks A, Santer N, Manago A. Brief report–modeling media use: how parents' and other adults' posting behaviors relate to young adolescents' posting behaviors. Front Hum Dyn. 2021;3:595924. https://doi.org/10.3389/fhumd.2021.595924.
36. Security.org. Parents' social media habits.; 2021. https://www.security.org/digital-safety/parenting-social-media-report/
37. Jarvie C, Renaud K. Parents who share info about their kids online are a cybersecurity risk. Here's why. It's adorable to hear about the newborn, the birthdays, the accomplishments. But it is just giving more information to future identity thieves. Wall Street J. 2022. https://www.proquest.com/newspapers/parents-who-share-info-about-their-kids-online/docview/2745609824/se-2
38. Ferrara P, Cammisa I, Corsello G, et al. Online "Sharenting": the dangers of posting sensitive information about children on social Media. J Pediatr. 2023;257:113322.
39. Kildare C, Middlemiss W. Impact of parents mobile device use on parent-child interaction: a literature review. Comput Hum Behav. 2017;75:579–93. https://doi.org/10.1016/j.chb.2017.06.003.
40. Ochoa W, Reich SM, Farkas G. The observed quality of caregiver-child interactions with and without a mobile screen device. Acad Pediatr. 2021;21(4):620–8.
41. Konrad C, Hillmann M, Neuhoff L, Barr R. Quality of mother-child interaction before, during, and after smartphone use. Front Psychol. 2021;12:616656.
42. Lederer Y, Artzi H, Borodkin K. The effects of maternal smartphone use on mother–child interaction. Child Dev. 2022;93(2):556–70.
43. de Vries D, Vossen H, van der Kolk-van der Boom P. Social media and body dissatisfaction: investigating the attenuating role of positive parent–adolescent relationships. J Youth Adolesc 2019;48:527–536. https://doi.org/10.1007/s10964-018-0956-9.
44. Uhls Y, Felt L, Wartella E, Sanders A. Investigating viewership of season 3 of "13 Reasons Why" and the mental wellness of adolescents: partially randomized preference trial. JMIR Mental Health. 2021;8(9):e25782. https://doi.org/10.2196/25782.
45. Tynes B. Online racial discrimination: a growing problem for adolescents. Psychological Science Agenda. https://www.apa.org/science/about/psa/2015/12/online-racial-discrimination.

# Putting Digital Media in Balance: The Importance of Human-to-Human Interaction for Young Children

Kathy Hirsh-Pasek, Jennifer M. Zosh, Brenna Hassinger-Das, Roberta Michnick Golinkoff, Yalda T. Uhls, and Lisa Guernsey

## 1 Background

A 2020 Pew Research Center Report suggested that 70% of parents worry that their children who are under the age of 12 are spending too much time in front of screens [1]. By 2022, an updated report [2] found a 14-point increase when the same parents were asked if children were too occupied with their smartphones, and a 20-point increase when asked if their child spent too much time playing video games. While this increase was likely impacted by the pandemic, all of the evidence highlights the dramatic natural experiment regarding family media use that is taking place, with our children as unwitting participants. Ubiquitous availability of screens and digital devices poses two issues that should command parents' attention. First, in what ways is children's time on screens reducing critical human-to-human interaction between them and their parents and other caregivers? Second, because parents and caregivers are often occupied on their own screens, might caregiver media use be disrupting these same delicate human-to-human interactions that young humans need to develop? These are not idle questions; parents need to know whether time on screens—their own as well as their children's—has any impact on their child's development.

Kathy Hirsh-Pasek and Jennifer M. Zosh contributed equally as co-first authors.

K. Hirsh-Pasek
Temple University, Philadelphia, PA, USA

J. M. Zosh (✉)
Pennsylvania State University, Brandywine, Media, PA, USA
e-mail: jzosh@psu.edu

B. Hassinger-Das
Pace University, New York, NY, USA

R. M. Golinkoff
University of Delaware, Newark, DE, USA

Y. T. Uhls
University of California Los Angeles, Center for Scholars & Storytellers, Los Angeles, CA, USA

L. Guernsey
New America, Washington, DC, USA

## 2 Current State

There is no doubt that today's children are spending a lot of time on screens. In 2020, Common Sense Media [3] reported that children under 8 years averaged 2 hours a day of screen media use. Most of that time was devoted to online videos like YouTube (37%) with television viewing clocking in at 23%. Children under 2 years of age averaged 45 minutes a day of screen time, while those 5 to 8 years of age averaged 3 hours a day. Video games occupied another 23 minutes a day. By 2 to 4 years of age, a full 43% of children reportedly had their own media devices, a statistic that rose precipitously to 67% by ages 5 to



D. A. Christakis, L. Hale (eds.), *Handbook of Children and Screens*,
https://doi.org/10.1007/978-3-031-69362-5_53

8 years of age. Of note, these 2020 data—the most comprehensive available to date—were collected *before* the pandemic, not to mention after both the *American Academy of Pediatrics* [4] and the *World Health Organization* [5] recommended *no* screen time (except for video chatting) for children under 2 years and a limit of one hour a day for slightly older children. Some research indicates dramatic increases during the pandemic (up to 52% increase) [6] with another study finding that children aged 4 to 12 years increased their screen use by almost 2 hours a day during the early days of the pandemic and that an hour of that increase remained even after pandemic restrictions lessened [7].

It is important to note that time spent on screens is only a rudimentary measure and in of itself is not a reason to panic. Indeed, technological advances are typically met with alarm. As Hassinger-Das et al. [8] point out in their review, in the 1950s and 1960s, researchers and those in public policy worried that time watching television would result in everything from more aggressive behavior to less physical activity and poorer school outcomes because time spent watching television displaces other important activities. They also highlight, however, that this so-called displacement theory did not pan out as a *simple* explanation for the impacts of television on children as research suggested that outcomes were mixed and largely due to differences in the quality of the programming available. This should give us pause, however, as current work on the quality of educational apps [9] suggests that the vast majority of "educational" apps are not truly educational. That is, they do not align well with principles of how children learn [10], suggesting that this rapid adoption of screen media is not adding high-quality experiences to children's everyday lives as children come to rely more on digital media and less on television.

## 2.1 Human-to-Human Interaction Is Essential

The combination of high-quantity and low-quality media exposure also places parents in a difficult position as they are left on their own to wonder whether screen time might be displacing more essential experiences. This concern is warranted, given that mounting research highlights the importance of human-to-human interaction for early brain growth and brain development. Humans have a socially gated brain that is primed to receive information from others of their species [11]. Indeed, recent research suggests that conversational turns, or emotionally and temporally contingent social interactions between parents and children, are key to building both brain structure and connectivity in 4- to 6-year-olds [12]. Advances in neuroscience further demonstrate the importance of social interactions for early learning. For example, researchers have found that when children were engaged in joint book reading with an adult, the resulting synchronized neural activity between the child and adult resulted in enhanced children's learning of words and story content [13]. Similarly, twelve-month-old infants who shared greater neural synchrony with adults also displayed greater attention to shared content [14]. Evolution has equipped humans to engage with others in ways that build brain and social capital.

What we do not know is whether there is a social interactional threshold that is critical for the development of healthy brains. We do know that children who have fewer conversational interactions have marked differences in brain structure [12] that can influence both language skills and later reading outcomes [15] throughout the elementary school years. Finally, a recent study [16] finds that the amount of parent–child interaction and parent language input to children between 6 and 12 months predicts the myelin density—or the connective tissue—in the brain. The bottom line is that human-to-human interaction is critical for the growth of a number of important outcomes, including those at the level of language learning, attention, cognitive processing, and social development [16] and extending all the way down to the level of the connecting of neurons in the developing brain. As children's first and most continual interaction is, in a majority of instances, with their parents, we must question whether screens are replacing the time that children would ordinarily have had with them, as their primary human caregivers—even if the strong version of the displacement theory is incorrect.

Another consideration for parents is how to evaluate the potential of more contingent digital experiences for children such as those offered by a smart speaker that responds to what a child says, a robot that responds to a child's movement, or an app that can guide children in completing a puzzle. A smattering of research also suggests that in some contexts, digital media can provide social alternatives to human interaction. By way of example, Calvert et al. [17] highlight how parasocial relationships (one-sided, emotionally charged relationships that children have with known media characters such as Elmo) can actually support learning and that new technologies such as robots and intelligent agents will only increase the potential of leveraging benefits of social interaction in new ways. In another interesting extension of this kind of work, Tsuji et al. [18] demonstrate that 12-month-olds could learn new words from a robot who engaged in socially contingent behaviors. But can a robot use those words in a range of situations to exemplify their true meaning? And can a robot provide useful feedback when the child uses the wrong word in speech? And how do these interactions compare to interacting with a parent or other caring, responsive adult? Although learning can occur, limitations in robot-to-human interaction seem quite limited—at least for now.

While such experiments are tantalizing, Myers and Arterberry [19] remind us that "Learning new things, like language, actions, or object properties are better learned from a live human rather than from a virtual one (or a robot)". Thus, while human interaction can be mimicked in a learning situation, human-to-human interaction seems to be optimal for learning outcomes. Indeed, a study by Dore et al. [20] suggest that children who read a book with a parent remember more about the story than those who listen to an audio narration of the book. Similar findings emerged from a 2010 study in Israel [21] comparing how parents interacted with children when reading a print book versus an ebook containing audio recordings and interactive dictionaries. Researchers noticed that ebooks did not leave much for parents to do, whereas with print books "there was a lot of talk between the parent and the child" [3]. Further, work by Avelar et al. [22] measured children's emotional and physiological arousal (skin conductivity) while (a) reading a basic ebook (without the "bells and whistles") with a parent, (b) reading a traditional book with a parent, or (c) listening to an ebook alone, without a parent. Children had more peaks in arousal when reading the ebook or the traditional book compared to when they listened to the ebook alone. Thus, the presence of another human rather than the type of book defines the child's experience.

## 2.2 Technoference

The work cited above suggests that human interactions are critical for learning and that even when compared to human-like parasocial beings, human interactions facilitate enhanced learning outcomes in children. Given these findings, we might also expect that if digital devices disrupt human-to-human interactions, they would also disrupt human learning. Indeed, that seems to be the case. In 2018, McDaniel and Radesky [23] coined the term "technoference" to designate those times when using digital devices for activities like phone calls and texts interferes with parent–child interactions. These researchers found that parental reports of externalizing behaviors, such as whining, hyperactivity, and temper tantrums related to the amount of technoference. It is also important to note that parents' amount of screen use is the number one predictor of children's own screen time [24].

In other words, parents themselves need to consider their own use of screen media and its potential impact on the interactions they have with their children. A study by Reed et al. [25] offer an empirical demonstration of this phenomenon by experimentally inserting a phone call in the middle of a parent–toddler word learning task. Technoference, represented in this case by the phone call, was found to reduce children's learning of new words as compared to uninterrupted learning. Gaudreau et al. [26] similarly found that when parents were occupied on their cell phones, their children asked fewer questions when trying to figure out how to use a novel toy. A recent study examined longitudinal associations between screen use and parent–child talk, including vocalizations by the child, adult talk, and conversational turns, at 12 to 36 months and found that increases in screen use were linked with decreases in parent–child talk [27] Thus, research in this area is beginning to build and consistently showing that across outcomes and contexts, children learn more during face-to-face interactions compared to when parental attention is shared with their own digital devices.

## 2.3 Co-Viewing and Joint Media Engagement: A Way to Build More Human-to-Human Interaction?

How then might we increase the human-to-human connection in the face of the overwhelming use of and interference of technology? One proposed solution that surfaced in both the television viewing research and in the digital use domain is co-viewing. More recently, the term "joint media engagement" has been used to distinguish between active engagement between adults and children while viewing (e.g., asking questions and pointing) as opposed to simply viewing media. In this review, we use the two terms interchangeably. In a review of decades of research on toddlers' attention during co-viewing television with parents, Anderson and Hanson [28] concluded that "content that is specifically designed to foster high-quality parent-child interactions can have a positive impact on the quality of parenting and the parent-child relationship." In the digital world, Neuman and Neuman [29] found that caregiver support during app reading along with the quality of the apps themselves jointly determined whether the digital reading would be effective. The Avelar et al. [22] study showed that the type of book was less important than parental participation.

The research strongly suggests that if caregivers are a part of the digital or screen experience, children have better outcomes both cognitively and socially [30], in fact, co-viewing has been demonstrated to affect the parasympathetic nervous system response of infants [31]. Yet, the 2020 Common Sense Media report found that by ages 5 to 8 years, co-viewing occurs a paltry 18% of the time as compared to 61% of the time for those under two years of age [3].

## 2.4 Using Screen Media to Support Human-to-Human Interaction

Another potential solution is to design digital activities and devices that promote more human-to-human contact. The project, "Joy," offered by Amazon, provided one such experiment. The device was designed to enable two remote players to co-play activities like puzzle building and reading. Similarly, Osmo offers several products that seek to incorporate human social interactions into screen experiences. It is also worth mentioning that recent work [32] has found that video chat allows for meaningful intergenerational connections when families are separated, even with young babies. In this case, screen media serves as a useful tool, rather than a replacement, for human social interaction. As such, current screen time guidance thus excludes video chatting as something that needs to be limited, even with young children.

In sum, the current state of the research suggests that even young children are consuming a great deal of digital and screen media and that as they get older and become preschoolers, they are largely navigating the digital landscapes themselves. At the same time, the research also strongly suggests that human-to-human interaction is critical for learning and brain development and is being compromised both by the more solo nature of the digital designs and by the intrusion of digital use by children's caregivers. Further, the research strongly suggests that digital characters and robots that attempt to simulate human interaction do not offer children the same learning and behavioral advantages as do human counterparts.

## 3 Future Research

More research is needed to address the following questions:

- How can digital devices be better designed to encourage interaction between parents and children, given what is known about the importance of human-to-human interaction?
- How disruptive to children's development is digital device use by their parents and caregivers? How does it differ based on age?
- How might we determine the advantages of co-use of digital media with parents and caring adults at different ages and for different child outcomes?
- How will new developments in AI and in immersive digital environments (e.g., the metaverse) blur the lines between reality and fantasy, human interaction and simulation, and what will parents need to know about the impact on their children?

The answers to these questions will help us better navigate the ever-present influence of newer technologies on young children as they participate in the greatest natural experiment in child-rearing. In a world in which people are increasingly interacting less with the people around them and more with digital devices, elevating the frequency of human interaction for our children is a critical goal.

## 4 Recommendations

- Prioritize human interaction (parent–child interactions and other positive social interactions) to support children's development. Screentime guidelines should not focus only on the amount of time with screens. Instead, they should encourage parents and caregivers to interact with their children when using screens and choose content designed for learning and language development.
- Emphasize the value of co-viewing and co-playing with children through age 8. Co-viewing helps minimize potential negative effects of screen media but is often discontinued much earlier than it should. Communicating the importance of co-viewing and parental social interaction around media should be prioritized. Developers should also be encouraged to innovate and create digital experiences that create opportunities for social interaction between parents and children.
- Screen time should be a supplement not a substitute for parent–child interaction. Use screen-based interests and experiences as inspiration for human interaction. As children age, they are increasingly discovering their own interests and preferences. Caregivers can use those interests as a way to foster interaction. For example, caregivers can partner with a child who likes watching kitten videos and take them to the local animal rescue to help care for kittens in the real world. Developers can also create screen-based experiences that link to the real world rather than focusing on increasingly digital content (e.g., creating a real-world treasure hunt or using the camera feature to help children learn about the world around them).

**Conflict of Interest and Funding Disclosures** None.

## References

1. Pew Research Center. Parenting Children in the Age of Screens, July 2020.
2. McClain M. How parents' views of their kids' screen time, social media use changed during COVID-19. https://pewrsr.ch/3Koo0qU. Published 2022.
3. Rideout V, Robb MB. The Common Sense census: Media use by kids age zero to eight, 2020. https://www.commonsensemedia.org/sites/default/files/research/report/2020_zero_to_eight_census_final_web.pdf. Published 2020.
4. Hill D, Ameenuddin N, Chassiakos YR, Cross C, Hutchinson J, Levine A, Boyd R, Mendelson R,

Moreno M, Swanson WS. Media and young minds. Pediatrics. 2016;138(5):e20162591.
5. World Health Organization. To grow up healthy, children need to sit less and play more. Published April 23, 2019.
6. Madigan S, Eirich R, Pador P, McArthur BA, Neville RD. Assessment of changes in child and adolescent screen time during the COVID-19 pandemic: a systematic review and meta-analysis. JAMA Pediatr. 2022;176(12):1188–98.
7. Hedderson MM, Bekelman TA, Li M, et al. Trends in screen time use among children during the COVID-19 pandemic, July 2019 through August 2021. JAMA Netw Open. 2023;6(2):e2256157. https://doi.org/10.1001/jamanetworkopen.2022.56157.
8. Hassinger-Das B, Brennan S, Dore RA, Golinkoff RM, Hirsh-Pasek K. Children and screens. Annu Rev Dev Psychol. 2020;2:69–92.
9. Hirsh-Pasek K, Zosh JM, Golinkoff RM, Gray JH, Robb MB, Kaufman J. Putting education in "educational" apps: lessons from the science of learning. Psychol Sci Public Interest. 2015;16(1):3–34.
10. Meyer M, Zosh JM, McLaren C, Robb M, McCaffery H, Golinkoff RM, Hirsh-Pasek K, Radesky J. How educational are "educational" apps for young children? App store content analysis using the four pillars of learning framework. J Child Media. 2021;15(4):526–48.
11. Kuhl PK. Is speech learning 'gated' by the social brain? Dev Sci. 2007;10(1):110–20.
12. Romeo RR, Leonard JA, Robinson ST, et al. Beyond the 30-million-word gap: children's conversational exposure is associated with language-related brain function. Psychol Sci. 2018;29(5):700–10. https://doi.org/10.1177/0956797617742725.
13. Piazza EA, Cohen A, Trach J, Lew-Williams C. Neural synchrony predicts children's learning of novel words. Cognition. 2021;214:104752.
14. Wass SV, Noreika V, Georgieva S, Clackson K, Brightman L, Nutbrown R, Covarrubias LS, Leong V. Parental neural responsivity to infants' visual attention: How mature brains influence immature brains during social interaction. PLoS Biol. 2018;16(12):e2006328.
15. Merz EC, Maskus EA, Melvin SA, He X, Noble KG. Socioeconomic disparities in language input are associated with children's language-related brain structure and reading skills. Child Dev. 2020;91(3):846–60.
16. Huber E, Corrigan N, Yarnykh V, Ramirez N, Kuhl P. Language experience during infancy predicts white matter myelination at age 2 years. J Neurosci. 2023;43(9):1590–9.
17. Calvert SL. Parasocial relationships with media characters: imaginary companions for young children's social and cognitive development. In: Blumberg F, Brooks P, editors. Cognitive development in digital contexts. Elsevier Academic Press; 2017. p. 93–117.
18. Tsuji S, Jincho N, Mazuka R, Cristia A. Communicative cues in the absence of a human interaction partner enhance 12-month-old infants' word learning. J Exp Child Psychol. 2020;191:104740.
19. Myers LJ, Arterberry ME. Digital media and children under 3 years of age. Infant Behav Dev. 2022;66:101677.
20. Dore RA, Hassinger-Das B, Brezack N, Valladares TL, Paller A, Vu L, Golinkoff RM, Hirsh-Pasek K. The parent advantage in fostering children's e-book comprehension. Early Child Res Q. 2018;44:24–33.
21. Korat O, Or T. How technology influences parent-child interaction: the case of e-book reading. First Lang. 2010;30(2):139–54.
22. Avelar D, Dore R, Schwichtenberg AJ, Roben CKP, Hirsh-Pasek K, Golinkoff RM. Children and parents' physiological arousal and emotions during shared and independent E-book Reading: a preliminary study. Int J Child Comput Interact. 2022;33:100507.
23. McDaniel BT, Radesky JS. Technoference: longitudinal associations between parent technology use, parenting stress, and child behavior problems. Pediatr Res. 2018;84(2):210–8.
24. Lauricella AR, Wartella E, Rideout VJ. Young children's screen time: the complex role of parent and child factors. J Appl Dev Psychol. 2015;36:11–7.
25. Reed J, Hirsh-Pasek K, Golinkoff RM. Learning on hold: cell phones sidetrack parent–child interactions. Dev Psychol. 2017;53(8):1428–36.
26. Gaudreau C, Hirsh-Pasek K, Golinkoff RM. What's in a distraction? The effect of parental cell phone use on parents' and children's question-asking. Dev Psychol. 2022;58(1):55–68.
27. Brushe ME, Haag DG, Melhuish EC, Reilly S, Gregory T. Screen time and parent-child talk when children are aged 12 to 36 months. JAMA Pediatr, Published online March 4, 2024. https://doi.org/10.1001/jamapediatrics.2023.6790.
28. Anderson DR, Hanson KG. Screen media and parent-child interactions. In: Barr R, Linebarger DN, editors. Media exposure during infancy and early childhood. Springer International Publishing; 2017. p. 173–91.
29. Neumann MM, Neumann DL. Touch screen tablets and emergent literacy. Early Child Educ J. 2014;42(4):231–9.
30. Collier KM, Coyne SM, Rasmussen EE, Hawkins AJ, Padilla-Walker LM, Erickson SE, Memmott-Elison MK. Does parental mediation of media influence child outcomes? A meta-analysis on media time, aggression, substance use, and sexual behavior. Dev Psychol. 2016;52(5):798–812.
31. Stockdale LA, Porter CL, Reschke PJ, Booth M, Coyne SM, Stephens J, Memmott-Elison MK. Infants' physiological responses to emotionally salient media with links to parent and child, empathy, prosocial behaviors and media use. Comput Hum Behav. 2023;139:107497.
32. Roche E, Rocha-Hidalgo J, Piper D, Strouse GA, Neely LI, Ryu J, Myers LJ, McClure E, Troseth GL, Zosh JM, Barr R. Presence at a distance: video chat supports intergenerational sensitivity and positive infant affect during COVID-19. Infancy. 2022;27(6):1008–31.

# Parenting and Screens During Middle Childhood

David S. Bickham, Drew P. Cingel, Amy I. Nathanson, Chad A. Rose, Colleen Russo Johnson, and Erica Scharrer

## 1 Background

The time of middle childhood is one of massive change for both children and their parents. As 6–12-year-olds progress toward puberty, peer relationships begin to take center stage, while parents become relegated to the background. In terms of media use, children's consumption patterns shift from frequently co-using with parents to using media independently or with peers. During this time of changing parent–child dynamics, caregivers may struggle to balance their child's increasing media-use independence with their desire for continued involvement and oversight.

The difficulty of managing the media use of children in this age range is particularly acute given their heavy use of media, with 8- to 12-year-olds spending over 5 ½ hours a day using screens [1]. While television remains popular, with 65% of 8- to 12-year-olds watching it every day [1], younger children (5- to 8-year-olds) now spend more time watching videos online (49 minutes) than watching television (27 minutes) [2]. YouTube is especially popular among this age group, with 89% of 5- to 11-year-olds having watched it and 55%, watching it daily [3]. As children progress through middle childhood, their media use habits and preferences shift toward those with more interpersonal components, including social media and multiplayer online games. Considering that socialization during middle childhood has shifted from interacting in a predominantly physical space to two separate yet indistinguishable environments (i.e., from physical to virtual), we must focus efforts on understanding online interpersonal interactions and the specifics that dictate their impact [4].

The various cognitive and social changes that 6- to 12-year-olds undergo further complicate parents' efforts to regulate screen usage. During this time period, young people become more self-aware and capable of understanding the perspective of other people [5]. Peer relationships become paramount, with youth forming social groups based on identity, starting to pay attention to in-group and out-group differences, and recognizing that they can play an active role in choosing their friends [6]. At this age, self-regulation

D. S. Bickham (✉)
Boston Children's Hospital, Boston, MA, USA
e-mail: david.bickham@childrens.harvard.edu

D. P. Cingel
University of California Davis, Davis, CA, USA

A. I. Nathanson
The Ohio State University, Columbus, OH, USA

C. A. Rose
University of Missouri, Columbia, MO, USA

C. R. Johnson
Toronto Metropolitan University, Toronto, ON, Canada

E. Scharrer
University of Massachusetts Amherst, Amherst, MA, USA


D. A. Christakis, L. Hale (eds.), *Handbook of Children and Screens*,
https://doi.org/10.1007/978-3-031-69362-5_54

abilities and other higher-level cognitive processes are still not yet fully developed, making it difficult for children to inhibit dominant impulses and making them underequipped to manage some of the more complex issues that come with a widening social environment, such as the development of their own and their peers' racial, cultural, and gender identities.

Although peer relationships increase in importance during middle childhood, parental interactions remain critical to children's social development and functioning. Technoference, or the interference of parental digital technology use on parent–child interactions [7], can potentially interrupt this development. While this issue has been well observed among parents and their very young children, technoference occurs during middle childhood as well and has been linked to lower levels of child-endorsed parent–child attachment, lower levels of parent-reported child social skills [8], and children's problematic smartphone use [9]. Interventions that encourage intentional smartphone use and dedicated family time could help ensure that children experience focused attention from their caregivers.

Caregivers have the opportunity to build the foundation for effective and safe media skills among 6- to 12-year-olds, but to do so, they must struggle with critically impactful questions, including: At what age should we give them a smartphone? How much screen time is too much? When do we allow social media use? How much and to what degree should we monitor their use? Pressures—including schools providing dedicated devices to their students and children who are exceptionally savvy with technology—often conflict with parents' beliefs or parenting strategies, leading to guilt, stress, and family conflict. Perhaps not surprisingly, parents see the internet, and social media in particular, as primary reasons that parenting has become more difficult, and 61% have turned to medical professionals for advice [3]. The sections below review the current state of knowledge regarding key media-use parenting challenges and opportunities for caregivers of children in middle childhood and translate these into future research directions and recommendations.

## 2 Current State

### 2.1 Smartphone Ownership

In the United States, many parents of 6- to 12-year-olds struggle with determining when to provide their child with a smartphone. By age 12, 71% of youth own a smartphone [1], with the average age of acquisition being estimated in different studies as 10.1 [10] and 11.6 years [11]. Over the last decade, the number of young children with smartphones has been increasing with 11% of 8-year-olds having a smartphone in 2015 as compared to 31% having one in 2021 [1]. The primary justifications that parents give for providing their child with a smartphone are to stay connected with their child and to keep their child safe [3, 10]. The device, of course, allows for countless additional uses, all of which have their own potential impacts.

Parents are looking for recommendations about the ideal age to provide phones to their children, but existing research does not point to a simple or universal answer. Early ownership (age 9) has been associated with lower math and reading scores, and the earlier girls owned phones, the more problematic behaviors and decreased academic self-concept they reported at age 13 [12]. However, other work has found no association between the age of phone acquisition and measures of depression, school grades, sleep [11], loneliness, cell phone addiction, and life satisfaction [13]. In focus groups, young people emphasized that obtaining a smartphone should be linked to achieving milestones of maturity and independence, such as participation in after-school activities and sports, rather than reaching a specific age [14]. Overall, aspects of a child's abilities, maturity, personality, and life situation might be better indicators of subsequent outcomes from smartphone ownership than only their age.

### 2.2 Screen Time

As young people's media use rises during middle childhood, parents are often concerned about the overall time spent on screens and the possibility that it displaces developmentally important behaviors and interferes with social, behavioral, and academic functioning. During the COVID-19 pandemic, primary school-aged children increased their screen media use by 65 minutes a day [15], further stoking parental concerns. Observed associations indicate that technology use is linked to fewer physical activities, less traditional book reading, and less sleep [16–18]. In one study, having media in the bedroom predicted higher levels of screen time, which in turn predicted lower grades and higher body mass index (BMI), leading the authors to identify media use in the bedroom as a "systemic risk factor" for poor outcomes [18]. These findings are not universal [17], however, and it is difficult to attribute the observed associations to a causal displacement because aspects of the child, their environment, and their family life may drive both use and outcomes, even longitudinally. That said, this research calls for parental engagement with the home media environment (e.g., limiting the presence of technology in bedrooms) and other efforts for monitoring and mediating children's screen use.

## 2.3 Parental Mediation of Screen Use

Parents are often at a loss for best practices for coping with the presence of media in their children's lives. "Parental mediation" refers to the interactions that parents have with their children surrounding media and includes behaviors such as talking with children about media content, regulating media content, limiting their time, and co-using media with children [19]. Such regulation in middle childhood is complex because media exposure is linked with both positive and negative effects. Parents need to find balanced practices so that their children can benefit from screen time without being harmed. Indeed, parents recognize screen media's complicated risk profile—for example, parents of tweens and teens report that technology is both helpful for children's social and educational lives, and potentially harmful by creating a dependence on technology and interfering with sleep [20].

Parental mediation strategies were revealed to be effective during middle childhood, when television and video games were the most prevalent forms of screen media, providing a framework for today's parents. Restrictive mediation (i.e., parental supervision and control of media use) is linked with less use overall and less exposure to sexual content; active mediation (i.e., parent and child discussions around media) appears to be protective against media's impact on aggression, substance use, and sexual outcomes but not overall time; co-viewing (i.e., parental use of media with a child) on the other hand, is linked to more use and more aggression potentially through implicit endorsement of media-presented content [21].

Emerging research has found some evidence for effective parenting strategies, but the results are not always consistent and can vary by type of media device and age of the child. For example, in a survey study of parents of 3- to 9-year-olds, restrictive mediation of video games (e.g., prohibiting a child from playing certain games) was associated with better child outcomes including lower levels of problematic use, but a controlling mediation style (e.g., punishing a child for not following the rules) was associated with worse outcomes [22]. In another study, restrictive mediation of 8- to 14-year-olds' mobile phone use was associated with worse outcomes (i.e., more problematic phone use), but active mediation (e.g., talking with a child about their phone use) and co-use were linked to lower levels [23]. Given these findings, parents, or stakeholders providing advice to parents, would be justifiably confused about the value of restrictive mediation. Restricting access to certain games of younger children may be effective, while a similar approach applied to older children's phones may backfire. As these studies found, extremely controlling approaches are unlikely to be effective, while strategies that engage with children around their media use are more promising.

Perhaps the most promising evidence regarding successful parenting in today's media environment arises from a meta-analysis indicating that for children under 14, parental warmth and an authoritative parenting style (i.e., support and nurturing combined with clear and consistent rules and consequences) were associated with lower levels of problematic internet use, while both active and restrictive media mediation were unrelated [24]. While findings are not entirely consistent, it appears that in the modern era of interactive technology and constant connection, established positive parenting techniques that combine predictable and enforced rules with support and warmth and positive parental modeling may translate best into children's healthy media behaviors.

## 2.4 Social Media and Gaming

Although most social media sites require users to be 13 or older, many younger children are using them; in one study, 38% of 8- to 12-year-olds reported social media use [1]. Another found that 49% of 9- to 12-year-olds have used Instagram, 58% have used Snapchat, and 69% have used TikTok [25]. While parents may have legitimate concerns regarding social media, it's worth noting that these sites also provide an avenue for middle childhood-aged youth to maintain and form potentially valuable friendships. Considering that young adolescents (11–16-year-olds) find joy in these social opportunities and express how connecting with their friends is the best part of social media sites [26], younger children may use the platforms to seek similar connections. Additionally, certain characteristics of online interactions encourage more open sharing and higher levels of self-disclosure, which can translate into an increased sense of belonging [27].

The fastest-growing online social spaces among this age are multiplayer games, including Fortnite (61% ever used), Roblox (66% ever used), and Minecraft (72% ever used) [25]. Massive multiplayer online games (MMOGs) are extremely popular with this age group, and the social interactions they afforded during the COVID-19 pandemic only increased their draw. Although understudied to date, positive outcomes of this type of social game have been illustrated by work demonstrating that collaborative play occurring in a battle-themed MMOG elicited prosocial behaviors in preadolescents [28]. Many online social settings, it seems, have the potential to encourage positive social development and peer interactions.

The popularity of gaming and social media sites among children during middle childhood have, however, also led parents to be concerned about the possibility of excessive use and negative social experiences. TikTok and other similar platforms have been cited as sources of endless scrolling due to highly individualized, algorithm-driven content that encourages sustained attention. Fortunately, parent–child communication about TikTok has been shown to reduce the likelihood that TikTok use will become problematic [29], demonstrating how active parental mediation may be an effective tool for reducing potential negative effects of social media.

Negative online social experiences include the types of harmful encounters about which parents are often concerned, such as their child being a victim of aggression or a sexual target. These experiences are fairly common during middle childhood, with 44% of youth ages 9 to 12 years having had some type of potentially harmful online experience, including 1 in 7 youth who reported having had an online sexual interaction with someone they believed was an adult [25]. While these interactions can occur on social media sites and MMOGs, they may occur more frequently on some than others, with about twice as many young people reported negative experiences on Snapchat (23%) than on Roblox (12%) [25]. Early adoption of social media sites may be a risk factor for such experiences, as those who begin their use before 11 were more likely than later adopters to experience online harassment or be sexually harassed [30]. Notably, these younger adopters were also more likely to engage in positive behaviors online, including posting socially supportive content and spreading awareness of socially conscious issues. It seems that starting early could expose young users to risk, but it may also help them develop the types of online social skills that are indicative of positive digital citizenship.

Some parenting strategies have been shown to lessen the likelihood of negative online social interactions during middle childhood. Using monitoring software and including children in the creation of relevant rules are linked to a lower likelihood of a child experiencing online victimization [31]. Enhancing children's digital literacy may be another effective approach, as one study found that youth with higher levels of these skills were less likely to be cyberbullied and had more skills for dealing with this victimization [33]. Results concerning parental use of restrictive mediation are, once again, contradictory. While this approach was linked to a lower risk of negative online experiences in one study [32], it was associated with a higher risk of being a perpetrator or victim of cyberbullying in another [33]. Furthermore, a restrictive approach was shown to limit potentially positive online opportunities including using the Internet for school work and entertainment [32]. Overall, parents need to balance the restriction of online resources with opportunities that develop digital literacy and other abilities to ensure that children have the skills necessary to cultivate positive experiences online.

## 3 Future Research

Given the current state of knowledge in this area, we feel the following questions should be addressed by future research:

- How can parents determine when their child is prepared to have their own smartphone, and what types of family discussions, contracts, or other agreements are effective at improving children's online experiences and reducing family conflict?
- What parenting strategies can help youth cultivate safe, meaningful, and lasting relationships/friendships in online and virtual avatar-based spaces and help encourage relationships that provide human connection, encourage the development of relationships in physical spaces, and protect against poor academic, social, and mental health outcomes?
- How do factors indicative of wider social and cultural forces impact parents' opportunities and strategies for parenting in the digital space and how might we generate unique tools and services for parents who, because of their economic situation or experience with systematic racism, have less financial resources, available time, and emotional capacity to dedicate to digital parenting?
- What social media, electronic gaming, and smartphone design strategies, functionalities, and default settings can assist parents in providing positive online experiences for their children while reducing the risk of negative ones?

## 4 Recommendations

- *Parents* should consider more than their child's age when deciding whether or not to provide them with a phone. The child's level of development, maturity, independence, and responsibility should be weighed alongside the needs of the child and the family to stay safe and connected.
- *Parents* should engage with their middle childhood-aged children around media in a thoughtful and warm way that includes reasonable, clear, and consistently enforced rules and expectations. They should involve their children in the creation of any family rules and understand that their own media practices are likely to be modeled by their children, and work to use media in healthy ways.
- In order to help their child avoid negative online experiences and encounter positive ones, *parents* need to balance restrictive mediation (including delaying their access to social media) with opportunities to build experience, digital literacy, and online social skills.
- *Pediatric medical professionals* should have conversations with their patient families not only about the amount of time they use technology but their experiences using it. Pediatricians should educate parents about the

risks and opportunities of media and how to best manage their child's screen time.

- *Social media companies and device manufacturers* must recognize that children under 13 are utilizing their services and should improve and innovate functionalities that are responsive to the needs of these youth and their parents.

**Conflict of Interest and Funding Disclosures** DB serves on a product advisory board for Google/Fitbit. The other authors have no conflicts of interest to disclose.

## References

1. Rideout V, Peebles A, Mann S, Robb MB. Common sense census: media use by tweens and teens, 2021. Common Sense; 2022.
2. Rideout V, Robb MB. The Common Sense Census: media use by kids age zero to eight, 2020; 2020.
3. Pew Research Center. Parenting children in the age of screens; 2020.
4. Navarro JL, Tudge JRH. Technologizing Bronfenbrenner: neo-ecological theory. Curr Psychol Published online. 2022; https://doi.org/10.1007/s12144-022-02738-3.
5. Eisnenberg N. Introduction. In: Damon W, Eisenberg N, eds. Handbook of child psychology: Vol. 3. Social, emotional, and personality development. Wiley; 1998:1–24.
6. McHale SM, Dariotis JK, Kauh TJ. Social development and social relationships in middle childhood. In: Weiner I, editor. Handbook of psychology volume 6 developmental psychology. Wiley; 2003. p. 241–65.
7. McDaniel BT, Radesky JS. Technoference: parent distraction with technology and associations with child behavior problems. Child Dev. 2018;89:100–9. https://doi.org/10.1111/cdev.12822.
8. Zayia D, Parris L, McDaniel B, Braswell G, Zimmerman C. Social learning in the digital age: associations between technoference, mother-child attachment, and child social skills. J Sch Psychol. 2021;2021(87):64–81. https://doi.org/10.1016/j.jsp.2021.06.002.
9. Liu Q, Wu J. What children learn in a digital home: the complex influence of parental mediation and smartphone interference. Educ Inf Technol. 2024;29:6273–91. https://doi.org/10.1007/s10639-023-12071-2.
10. Bickham DS, Hunt E, Kavanaugh JR, Rich M. Understanding children's first cell phones: parents' perspectives on risks and benefits. Digital Wellness Lab. https://digitalwellnesslaborg; 2021.
11. Sun X, Haydel KF, Matheson D, Desai M, Robinson TN. Are mobile phone ownership and age of acquisition associated with child adjustment? A 5-year prospective study among low-income Latinx children. Child Dev. 2023;94(1):303–14. https://doi.org/10.1111/cdev.13851.
12. Dempsey S, Lyons S, McCoy S. Later is better: mobile phone ownership and child academic development, evidence from a longitudinal study. Econ Innov New Technol. 2019;28(8):798–815. https://doi.org/10.1080/10438599.2018.1559786.
13. Vaterlaus JM, Aylward A, Tarabochia D, Martin JD. "A smartphone made my life easier": an exploratory study on age of adolescent smartphone acquisition and well-being. Comput Human Behav. 2021;114 https://doi.org/10.1016/j.chb.2020.106563.
14. Moreno MA, Kerr BR, Jenkins M, Lam E, Malik FS. Perspectives on smartphone ownership and use by early adolescents. J Adolesc Health. 2019;64(4):437. https://doi.org/10.1016/j.jadohealth.2018.08.017.
15. Madigan S, Eirich R, Pador P, McArthur BA, Neville RD. Assessment of changes in child and adolescent screen time during the COVID-19 pandemic: a systematic review and meta-analysis. JAMA Pediatr. 2022;176(12):1188–98. https://doi.org/10.1001/jamapediatrics.2022.4116.
16. LeBlanc AG, Katzmarzyk PT, Barreira TV, et al. Correlates of total sedentary time and screen time in 9–11 year-old children around the world: the international study of childhood obesity, lifestyle and the environment. PLoS One. 2015;10(6):e0129622. https://doi.org/10.1371/journal.pone.0129622.
17. Goode JA, Fomby P, Mollborn S, Limburg A. Children's technology time in two US cohorts. Child Indic Res. 2020;13(3):1107–32. https://doi.org/10.1007/s12187-019-09675-x.
18. Gentile DA, Berch ON, Choo H, Khoo A, Walsh DA. Bedroom media: one risk factor for development. Dev Psychol. 2017;53(12):2340–55. https://doi.org/10.1037/dev0000399.
19. Clark LS. Parental mediation theory for the digital age. Commun Theory. 2011;21(4):323. https://doi.org/10.1111/j.1468-2885.2011.01391.x.
20. Lauricella AR, Cingel DP, Beaudoin-Ryan L, Robb MB, Saphir M, Wartella EA. The common sense census: plugged-in parents of tweens and teens. Common Sense Media; 2016.
21. Collier KM, Coyne SM, Rasmussen EE, et al. Does parental mediation of media influence child outcomes? A meta-analysis on media time, aggression, substance use, and sexual behavior. Dev Psychol. 2016;52(5):798–812. https://doi.org/10.1037/dev0000108.
22. Van Petegem S, de Ferrerre E, Soenens B, van Rooij AJ, Van Looy J. Parents' degree and style of restrictive mediation of young children's digital gaming: associations with parental attitudes and perceived child adjustment. J Child Fam Stud. 2019;28(5):1379–91. https://doi.org/10.1007/s10826-019-01368-x.
23. Hefner D, Knop K, Schmitt S, Vorderer P. Rules? Role model? Relationship? The impact of parents on their

children's problematic mobile phone involvement. Media Psychol. 2019;22(1):82–108. https://doi.org/10.1080/15213269.2018.1433544.
24. Lukavská K, Hrabec O, Lukavský J, Demetrovics Z, Király O. The associations of adolescent problematic internet use with parenting: a meta-analysis. Addict Behav. 2022;135:107423. https://doi.org/10.1016/j.addbeh.2022.107423.
25. Thorn. Responding to online threats: minors' perspectives on disclosing, reporting, and blocking in 2021; 2023.
26. Lilley C, Ball R, Vernon H, NSPCC. The experiences of 11–16 year olds on social media sites. NSPCC; 2014.
27. Meeus A, Beullens K, Eggermont S. Social media, unsocial distraction? Testing the associations between preadolescents' SNS use and belonging via two pathways. Media Psychol, Published online 2022. 2022;26:363. https://doi.org/10.1080/15213269.2022.2147084.
28. Shoshani A, Krauskopf M. The Fortnite social paradox: the effects of violent-cooperative multiplayer video games on children's basic psychological needs and prosocial behavior. Comput Human Behav. 2021;116:106641. https://doi.org/10.1016/j.chb.2020.106641.
29. Qin Y, Musetti A, Omar B. Flow experience is a key factor in the likelihood of adolescents' problematic TikTok use: the moderating role of active parental mediation. Int J Environ Res Public Health. 2023;20(3) https://doi.org/10.3390/ijerph20032089.
30. Charmaraman L, Lynch AD, Richer AM, Grossman JM. Associations of early social media initiation on digital behaviors and the moderating role of limiting use. Comput Human Behav. 2022;127:107053. https://doi.org/10.1016/J.CHB.2021.107053.
31. Navarro R, Serna C, Martínez V, Ruiz-Oliva R. The role of Internet use and parental mediation on cyberbullying victimization among Spanish children from rural public schools. Eur J Psychol Educ. 2013;28(3):725. https://doi.org/10.1007/s10212-012-0137-2.
32. Livingstone S, Ólafsson K, Helsper EJ, Lupiáñez-Villanueva F, Veltri GA, Folkvord F. Maximizing opportunities and minimizing risks for children online: the role of digital skills in emerging strategies of parental mediation. J Commun. 2017;67(1):82. https://doi.org/10.1111/jcom.12277.
33. Tao S, Reichert F, Law N, Rao N. Digital technology use and cyberbullying among primary school children: digital literacy and parental mediation as moderators. Cyberpsychol Behav Soc Netw. 2022;25(9):571. https://doi.org/10.1089/cyber.2022.0012.

# Moving Beyond Fear and Restriction to Promoting Adolescent Resilience and Intentional Technology Use

Pamela Wisniewski, Jinkyung Park, Karla Badillo-Urquiola, Joy Gabrielli, Jennifer L. Doty, and Heidi Hartikainen

## 1 Background

According to a Pew Research report, 97% of US teens use the internet daily; 46% of them are online almost constantly. Most have access to digital devices, such as smartphones (95%), desktop or laptop computers (90%), and gaming consoles (80%) [1]. Most teens report that being social online helps them feel connected, creative, and supported [2]. Yet, emerging evidence has linked excessive screen time, cyberbullying, exposure to mature media content, and problematic internet use with mental health problems and physical safety risks (e.g., sex trafficking) [3, 4]. Subsequently, news media and scholarly research have intensified parental fears by overemphasizing the need to protect teens through the use of restrictive interventions against unfettered access to technology. As a result, many parents report feeling overwhelmed and anxious about their teens' internet use, saying confrontations about screen time disrupt positive parent–child interactions [5]. In this chapter, we highlight trends that have emerged in the current literature and those seen in society at large. We then promote a more balanced narrative geared towards taking a developmentally appropriate and positive approach focused on active parental mediation, building resilience, and promoting digital well-being to empower both teens and parents.

P. Wisniewski (✉)
Vanderbilt University, Nashville, TN, USA
e-mail: pamela.wisniewski@vanderbilt.edu

J. Park
Clemson University, Clemson, SC, USA

K. Badillo-Urquiola
University of Notre Dame, Notre Dame, IN, USA

J. Gabrielli
University of Florida, Gainesville, FL, USA

J. L. Doty
University of Oregon, Eugene, OR, USA

H. Hartikainen
University of Oulu, Oulu, Finland

## 2 Current State

### 2.1 The On-Going Debate of the Negative vs. Positive Effects of Tech on Teens

In 2021, *Good Morning America* broke a story about a woman who, after posing as a child on Instagram, experienced the almost immediate and frequent unwanted barrage of sexual solicitations that children receive on the platform [6]. The scrutiny regarding the negative effects of social media use on teens heightened after *The Wall Street Journal* released internal reports (a.k.a. the "Facebook Files") from Facebook (now Meta). Findings from these reports suggested that Facebook was aware of the negative impacts of their platform on teens, including the


D. A. Christakis, L. Hale (eds.), *Handbook of Children and Screens*,
https://doi.org/10.1007/978-3-031-69362-5_55

spreading of false information, promoting anger-provoking posts, and pushing harmful content (e.g., anorexia and self-harm posts) due to the flawed algorithms embedded within the platform [7]. This media attention bolstered the efforts of US Senators Blumenthal and Blackburn in proposing the "Kids Online Safety Act," [8] to protect children from online dangers. While this legislation has positive aspects, advocacy groups such as those that support the rights of LGBTQ+ youth and freedom of speech have expressed concerns regarding the heavy use of digital surveillance impeding the privacy, safety, and access to information rights of youth [9].

Scholarly research has also raised concerns that excessive screen time and social media use are negatively associated with the social and emotional well-being of teens, such as increases in depression, anxiety, and suicidal behaviors [3]. Yet, many believe these negative effects have been overstated. Recent narrative reviews and meta-analyses found a weak or inconsistent linkage between teens' digital technology use and adolescents' social and emotional well-being [3], though certain subgroups had heightened risk [10]. In contrast, other research highlights the positive effects of digital technology on youth, ranging from increased social communication, social support, and self-presentation to decreased depressive symptoms and loneliness, which were particularly salient during the global pandemic [11].

Given the substantial disagreement within the literature on the net benefits or drawbacks of technology use on teens, this debate will likely remain ongoing in the coming years. Our stance, however, is that while internet use is not inherently positive or negative, the internet can amplify the experiences young people have, both good and bad. Positive and negative effects can coexist without invalidating one another, as effects can vary across different contexts and individuals; some youth experience net positive effects, while others experience heightened risk for adverse outcomes, particularly younger teens during the transition to adolescence [12]. As such, further research evidence is needed for how to address mental health and digital well-being in online and technology-based environments, particularly during sensitive developmental periods of adolescence.

## 2.2 Fear and Restriction as a Motivation for New Digital Safety Technologies

In light of the ongoing debate and fear, we have also seen a marked trend in several digital technologies deployed to protect youth online. For instance, a recent review highlighted the increased push toward age assurance and verification systems, as well as the use of parental controls [13]. The rationale behind such tools is to make sure that youth are engaging in age-appropriate ways online and are being sufficiently monitored by their parents when doing so. Social media platforms have also taken measures to protect youth—from preventing adults from sending private messages to minors they are not connected with to sensitivity filters and advanced parental controls. Given the massive scale of online interactions and content generation, the implementation of automated risk detection tools is accelerating [4]. As such, there has been a push toward the use of artificial intelligence (AI) based tools to detect and eradicate harmful online content. Yet, limitations of these approaches include restriction of teens' access to valuable resources and support from people, which is particularly salient for vulnerable youth who do not have local support systems, with additional concerns related to digital privacy rights due to the use of digital surveillance [14].

## 2.3 Moving Beyond Restriction to Digital Inclusion and Intentional Use

Understanding the spectrum of digital connectivity has been discussed as fundamental for the development and implementation of digitally mediated support for young people. Research on teens' access to digital technology use and screen time has moved beyond simple binaries of access/

no-access or use/non-use, shifting to capture the range, purpose, and quality of use, especially since the global pandemic shed light on the complexity of digital inequalities. By understanding the degree of digital inclusion, recent research highlights the need for providing online opportunities for digitally marginalized teens. Another shift in the discourse on teens and screens includes teens as passive users/consumers of digital technology to a focus on teens' active and intentional technology usage such as being content producers or participating in community activism online. While most people engage in passive online activities, such as scrolling through others' feeds and liking others' posts, social media apps increasingly allow for more active content sharing and creation by teens. Together the current research emphasizes the need for teens to learn to be intentional about their internet use in order to minimize risks and maximize benefits.

## 2.4 Paradigm Shift to Active Parental Mediation and Positive Digital Parenting

A primary developmental objective of adolescence is safe and successful growth toward independence and autonomy, both of which are known to be associated with adult health and well-being outcomes [15, 16]. While restrictive media parenting practices (e.g., limits on screen time and content) inherently restrict both independence and autonomy, they are important during earlier stages of youth development (i.e., school-aged years through early adolescence) to prevent early exposure to mature media content, a known risk factor for adolescent health risk behaviors [17]. Active media mediation (e.g., having parent–child conversations about media) requires more parenting attention and may be more sensitive to other features of the parent–child relational dynamic. For example, parent–child connectedness is likely a critical component of effective active media mediation [18]. Active media mediation, in conjunction with a scaffolded approach to restrictive media mediation, allows for greater adolescent autonomy and the development of important skills within digital environments [16]. In today's digitally integrated world, youth need to gain competence to manage their digital footprints and understand how to protect their privacy online [19]. Positive digital parenting approaches, like talking with teens about online risks, engaging in proactive co-use of digital technologies with teens, and supporting access to healthy online content, can advance youth development toward safe and autonomous use of digital technologies into adulthood [20].

Active media parenting has also been associated with reduced media-related risks including aggression, substance use, and sleep deprivation [21]. A meta-analysis reported that both restrictive and active media parenting were associated with reduced time online. However, only active media parenting was associated with reduced media-related risks, while restrictive media parenting was not [22]. Both types of parental mediation were more effective for younger ages, while neither was found to be effective overall as teens approached adulthood. Overall, autonomy-supportive parental monitoring is more effective than controlling approaches [16, 22].

More recent studies posit that social influences (e.g., peers, family, and community) on youth can have a positive impact on adolescents' motivation and self-regulation [23, 24]. Therefore, taking into account socio-ecological factors in digital parenting can be effective in promoting the digital well-being of adolescents while supporting their autonomy development. Our conceptual model (see Fig. 1) combines the social ecologies of the adolescent resilience framework [23–25] with digital parenting practices across the adolescent lifespan to promote the shift from restrictive parental mediation approaches early in youth development to active and resilience-oriented approaches later in youth development.

## 2.5 Cautioning Against "One-Size-Fits-All" Solutions

While intentional technology use and active parental mediation are unequivocally positive trends toward promoting the digital well-being of

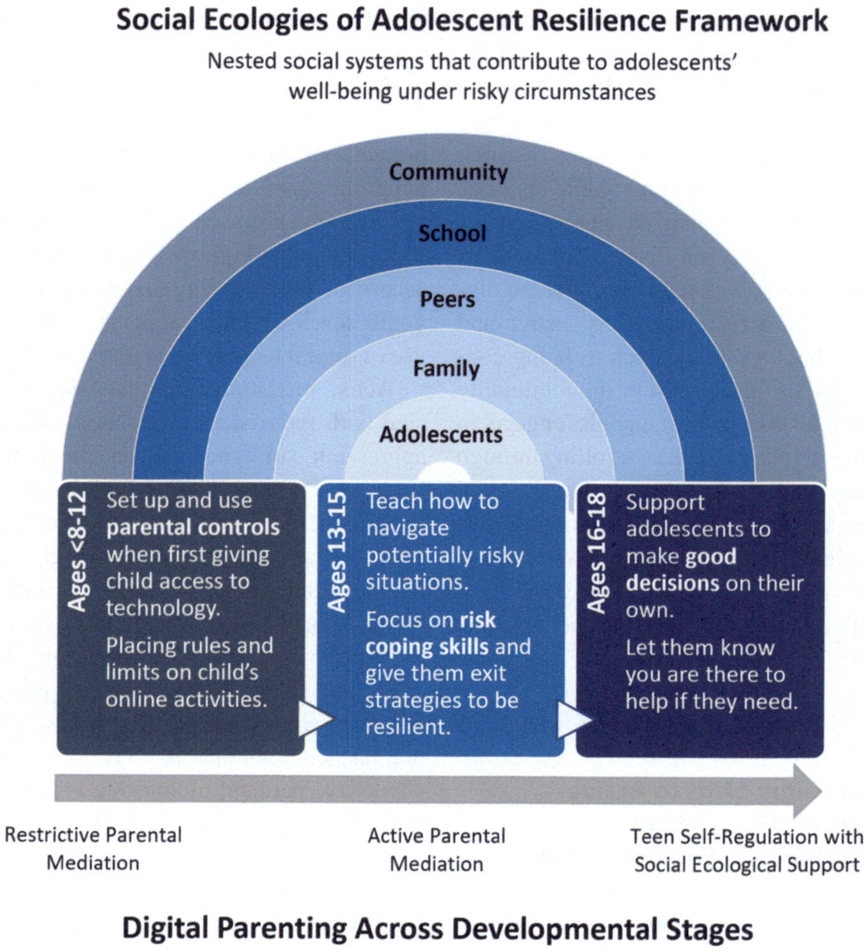


**Fig. 1** A social-ecological approach to digital parenting across the adolescent lifespan

teens, we also must acknowledge that age and other factors, such as family context and culture, must be considered when proposing a path forward.

### 2.5.1 Developmental Considerations by Age

Early on in youth development, children require extensive supervision/monitoring with clear restrictions around age-appropriate content and technological tools. In middle childhood, more active approaches with conversations about how to engage in healthy ways online while avoiding problematic or mature content/behavior are needed [26]. In later adolescence, youth need opportunities to explore autonomy in digital contexts that support their individuation from parents and also shore up their ability to problem-solve, seek help when needed, and gain confidence in their skills in digital spaces [13, 25].

### 2.5.2 Family Context

Parent- and family-focused approaches to mediating teens' technology usage still assume a significant level of privilege. The teens most vulnerable to online risks (e.g., youth in foster care) are often the ones who do not have engaged parents who can actively participate in ensuring their online safety [27]. Furthermore, the adults responsible for these youth (e.g., foster parents and case managers) do not feel they have the authority to parent the child, often feeling hopeless and desperate for guidance [24, 27]. Hence, scholars have called for new resilience-based solutions that move away from parental restriction and control toward helping adolescents self-manage their screen time and online risk [25, 27]. Yet, few evidence-based interventions to empower adolescent self-regulation and online safety have been developed [28].

### 2.5.3 Cultural Factors

Within the United States, factors such as parents' socioeconomic and cultural resources are known to play a significant role in how they approach digital mediation (e.g., parents with higher digital skills are more likely to use restrictive mediation) [29]. While much of the discourse around online safety currently emerges from the Global North (e.g., countries in North America, Europe, and East Asia), there is increasing evidence showing cultural factors may contribute to different parental mediation strategies [30–32]. For example, Western European parents take more protective approaches, even if it might cost children online opportunities, while parents of Nordic and northern European countries favor children's rights and freedoms in online environments, even if this may put children at risk [33]. The effectiveness of parental mediation strategies is also different among cultures. For example, active mediation has been seen to be less effective with children from Western European countries than from Eastern countries [22]. In general, in Europe, the focus of parental strategies is moving away from setting rules and restrictions toward guiding children in their internet use [34].

## 2.6 Empowering Teens Through Teen-Centered Design and Policies

One way to account for these important contextual differences is through human-centered design—an approach that recognizes teens as a primary stakeholder with authority over their lived digital experiences. As such, researchers have begun engaging teens more directly in the design of solutions that center teens as the authority of their online experiences and promote collaboration, rather than conflict, with their parents [28, 35]. By shifting the power dynamic from catering to the needs and perspectives of parents and adult researchers, amplifying youth voices can empower them to learn how to self-regulate their online habits in ways that promote resilience, autonomy, and their online safety [36]. Such approaches also shift away from restrictive parental controls to technology-based solutions that promote positive family values, such as trust, transparency, and communication [37]. Further, engaging teens as co-designers and researchers can lead to novel design patterns and solutions that will transform the current technology landscape into one that promotes the digital inclusion of youth, as well as moves toward a paradigm of "safety by design," where the digital well-being of our teens is held paramount in both the platforms in which they engage and the policies put forth to protect them online [28, 38–40].

# 3 Future Research

When it comes to solutions for tomorrow, one size certainly does not fit all. Therefore, we must take a nuanced approach toward setting a research agenda for the future. The questions for future research include:

- How can we move beyond the current global debate about whether technology has a positive or negative effect on teens and focus our research on more nuanced, productive, and developmentally oriented considerations such as identifying which technology interventions are effective and for whom when it comes to mitigating risks and promoting digital well-being?
- What are the longitudinal, developmentally sensitive, bidirectional relationships between media parenting approaches and youth outcomes, and how do these vary based on youth, parent, and contextual characteristics?
- How can positive media parenting interventions inform causal pathways to healthy/adaptive online technology use among youth?
- How do socio-ecological factors (e.g., cultural norms and family context) influence adoles-

cent media use and their online risk experience? How can technology solutions be designed to go beyond a one-size-fits-all approach to online safety?

- How can we design "teen-centered" online safety solutions that empower youth by increasing their sense of autonomy and promoting awareness and self-regulation?

## 4 Recommendations

We need coordinated efforts among researchers, technologists, clinicians, educators, policymakers, and concerned citizens to promote health and wellness in the digital lives of teens through positive media parenting and teen-centric approaches. We provide the following human-centered recommendations to promote teen resilience and digital well-being.

- *Researchers, developers, and other technologists*: As we strive to meet the challenges of children's rights in the digital environment, we must incorporate adult guidance and youth self-regulation into the design of future technology interventions that promote trust between family members and youth. Technologies with evidence-based and inclusive privacy solutions should be informed directly by youth as a way to effectively translate academic research into impactful solutions [41].
- *Clinicians, providers, and educators*: There should be an active dialogue between the youth and these supportive systems (e.g., parents and teachers) concerning technology use. Clinicians, educators, and other service providers should engage with youth and families in regular conversations about developmentally appropriate parental involvement in youth engagement with media and technology with an eye toward the development of youth autonomy and resilience in the digital realm.
- *Policymakers*: Legal frameworks to promote teen digital resilience and well-being within the United States are lacking since COPPA does not apply to adolescents over age 13. Proper legislation and policy should be discussed with various stakeholders including parents and teens as part of a larger agenda. Additionally, teen privacy needs to be protected as a right, and robust data protection laws tailored for youth should be enacted. More importantly, there should be efforts to ensure these rights and laws are translated from policy into practice [12].

**Conflict of Interest and Funding Disclosures** PW's research is partially supported by the US National Science Foundation under grants IIP-#2329976 and IIS-#2333207 and by the William T. Grant Foundation grant #187941. JG's research is partially supported by the National Institute on Drug Abuse under grant # DA052793. Any opinions, findings, conclusions, or recommendations expressed in this material are those of the authors and do not necessarily reflect the views of the research sponsors. The US National Science Foundation, William T. Grant Foundation, and National Institute on Drug Abuse had no direct role in the development of this chapter. However, some of the research cited in this work was directly supported by these sponsors.

## References

1. Vogels EA, Gelles-Watnick R, Massarat N. Teens, social media and technology 2022. August 10, 2022. Accessed April 3, 2023. https://www.pewresearch.org/internet/2022/08/10/teens-social-media-and-technology-2022/.
2. Anderson M, Vogels EA, Perrin A, Rainie L. Connection, creativity and Drama: teen life on social media in 2022. Nov 16, 2022. Accessed April 4, 2023. https://www.pewresearch.org/internet/2022/11/16/connection-creativity-and-drama-teen-life-on-social-media-in-2022/.
3. Valkenburg PM, Meier A, Beyens I. Social media use and its impact on adolescent mental health: an umbrella review of the evidence. Curr Opin Psychol. 2022;44:58–68.
4. Federal Trade Commission. Combatting Online Harms Through Innovation. June 16, 2022. Accessed April 6, 2023. https://www.ftc.gov/system/files/ftc_gov/pdf/Combatting%20Online%20Harms%20Through%20Innovation%3B%20Federal%20Trade%20Commission%20Report%20to%20Congress.pdf.
5. Helfrich EL, Doty JL, Su YW, Yourell JL, Gabrielli J. Parental views on preventing and minimizing negative effects of cyberbullying. Child Youth Serv Rev. 2020;118:105377.

6. GMA. I'm 37 and I pose as children online to identify sexual predators. Here's what parents should know. March 8, 2021. Accessed April 6, 2023. https://www.goodmorningamerica.com/family/story/37-pose-children-online-identify-sexual-predators-parents-68623626.
7. The Wall Street Journal. The Facebook files: a wall street journal investigation. 2021. Accessed April 3, 2023. https://www.wsj.com/articles/the-facebook-files-11631713039.
8. Congress.gov. S.3663 – Kids Online Safety Act. Dec. 15, 2022. Accessed April 6, 2023. https://www.congress.gov/bill/117th-congress/senate-bill/3663/text.
9. The 6:52 Project Foundation, Inc., et al. Opposition to S. 3663's Threats to Minors' Privacy and Safety Online. Nov. 8, 2022. Accessed April 6, 2023. https://drive.google.com/file/d/1N60A5KhcXWh19H7ljdDrElW8zrV4KhXJ/view.
10. Orben A, Przybylski AK, Blakemore SJ, Kievit RA. Windows of developmental sensitivity to social media. Nat Commun. 2022;13(1):1649.
11. Haddock A, Ward N, Yu R, O'Dea N. Positive effects of digital technology use by adolescents: a scoping review of the literature. Int J Environ Res Public Health. 2022;19(21):14009.
12. Odgers C, Allen N, Pfeifer J, Dahl R, Nesi J, Schueller S, Williams JL. Engaging, safe, and evidence-based: what science tells us about how to promote positive development and decrease risk in online spaces for early adolescents. 2022. Available at https://developingadolescent.semel.ucla.edu/topics/item/youth-and-digital-tech. Accessed April 5, 2023.
13. Smirnova S, Livingston S, Stoilova M. Understanding of user needs and problems: a rapid evidence review of age assurance and parental controls. Sep 2021. Accessed April 3, 2023. https://eprints.lse.ac.uk/112559/1/Stoilova_understanding_of_user_needs_and_problems_published.pdf.
14. London School of Economics and Political Science. Children's data and privacy online: Growing up in a digital age. 2019. Accessed April 6, 2023. https://www.lse.ac.uk/media-and-communications/research/research-projects/childprivacyonline.
15. Soenens B, Vansteenkiste M, Lens W, Luyckx K, Goossens L, Beyers W, Ryan RM. Conceptualizing parental autonomy support: adolescent perceptions of promotion of independence versus promotion of volitional functioning. Dev Psychol. 2007;43(3):633.
16. Young R, Tully M. Autonomy vs. control: associations among parental mediation, perceived parenting styles, and US adolescents' risky online experiences. Cyberpsychology. 2022;16(2):167–88.
17. Cox MJ, Gabrielli J, Janssen T, Jackson KM. Parental restriction of movie viewing prospectively predicts adolescent alcohol and marijuana initiation: implications for media literacy programs. Prev Sci. 2018;19:914–26.
18. Padilla-Walker LM, Coyne SM, Kroff SL, Memmott-Elison MK. The protective role of parental media monitoring style from early to late adolescence. J Youth Adolescence. 2018;47:445–59.
19. Corcoran E, Shaffer E, Warner M, Gabrielli J. Associations between parental media mediation and youth attitudes about online privacy in a sample of US adolescents. Comput Human Behav. 2022;137:107423.
20. Gabrielli J, Marsch L, Tanski S. TECH parenting to promote effective media management. Pediatrics. 2018;142(1):e20173718.
21. Coyne SM, Radesky J, Collier KM, Gentile DA, Linder JR, Nathanson AI, et al. Parenting and digital media. Pediatrics. 2017;140(Supplement_2):S112–6.
22. Chen L, Shi J. Reducing harm from media: a meta-analysis of parental mediation. J Mass Commun Q. 2019;96(1):173–93.
23. Pinter AT, Ghosh AK, Wisniewski PJ. Going beyond cyberbullying: adolescent online safety and digital risks. In: Sharma D, Mehari K, Doty J, Sharma N, Wisniewski PJ, editors. Cyberbullying and digital safety: applying global research to youth in India. Gainesville: LibraryPress@UF; 2022. p. 103–35.
24. Badillo-Urquiola K, Agha Z, Abaquita D, Harpin S, Wisniewski, PJ. Towards a social ecological approach to supporting caseworkers in promoting the online safety of youth in foster care. In: Proceedings of the ACM on Computer-Supported Cooperative Work and Social Computing (CSCW2024). 2024.
25. Wisniewski PJ, Vitak J, Hartikainen H. Privacy in adolescence. In: Knijnenburg BP, Page X, Wisniewski PJ, Lipford HR, Proferes N, Romano J, editors. Modern socio technical perspectives on privacy. Cham: Springer International Publishing; 2022. p. 315–36.
26. Gabrielli J, Tanski SE. The A, B, Cs of youth technology access: promoting effective media parenting. Clin Pediatr. 2020;59(4–5):496–9.
27. Badillo-Urquiola K, Page X, Wisniewski PJ. Risk vs. restriction: the tension between providing a sense of normalcy and keeping foster teens safe online. In Proceedings of the 2019 CHI Conference on Human Factors in Computing Systems. 2019, p. 1–14.
28. terre des hommes. Safety by design to keep children safe online. May 19, 2022. Accessed April 6, 2023.
29. Zhao P, Bazarova NN, Valle N. Digital parenting divides: the role of parental capital and digital parenting readiness in parental digital mediation. J Comput Mediat Commun. 2023;28(5):zmad032.
30. Shin W, Lwin MO. Parental mediation of children's digital media use in high digital penetration countries: perspectives from Singapore and Australia. Asian J Commun. 2022;32(4):309–26.
31. Amaran M. Navigating parental duties in a TikTok world, the UK and Nigeria regulations and the online safety bill. Int J Adv Sci Eng Inf Technol. 2023;5(4):322–38.
32. Milosevic T, Kuldas S, Sargioti A, Laffan DA, O'Higgins NJ. Children's internet use, self-reported life satisfaction, and parental mediation in Europe: an analysis of the EU kids online dataset. Front Psychol. 2022;(12):698176.

33. Smahel D, Machackova H, Mascheroni G, et al. EU Kids Online 2020: Survey results from 19 countries. EU Kids Online, The London School of Economics and Political Science 2020. https://doi.org/10.21953/lse.47fdeqj01ofo.
34. Kalmus V, Sukk M, Soo K. Towards more active parenting: trends in parental mediation of children's internet use in European countries. Child Society. 2022;36(5):1026–42.
35. Hartikainen H, Iivari N, Kinnula M. Children's design recommendations for online safety education. Int J Child Comput Interact. 2019;22:100146.
36. Chatlani N, Davis A, Badillo-Urquiola K, Bonsignore E, Wisniewski P. Teen as research-apprentice: a restorative justice approach for centering adolescents as the authority of their own online safety. Int J Child Comput Interact. 2023;35:100549.
37. Badillo-Urquiola K, Chouhan C, Chancellor S, De Choudhary M, Wisniewski P. Beyond parental control: designing adolescent online safety apps using value sensitive design. J Adolesc Res. 2020;35(1):147–75.
38. Agha Z, Badillo-Urquiola K, Wisniewski PJ. "Strike at the Root:" Co-designing Real-time social media interventions for adolescent online risk prevention. In: Proceedings of the ACM on Human-Computer Interaction. 2023;7(CSCW1).
39. Ali N, Agha Z, Chatlani N, Park J, Wisniewski PJ. A case study on facilitating a long-term youth advisory board to involve youth in adolescent online safety research. In: Extended Abstracts of the 2024 CHI Conference on Human Factors in Computing Systems 2024.
40. Obajemu O, Agha Z, Wisniewski PJ. Towards enforcing good digital citizenship: identifying opportunities for adolescent online safety nudges. In: Proceedings of the ACM on Computer-Supported Cooperative Work and Social Computing (CSCW 2024); 2024.
41. Moreno MA, Jolliff A, Kerr B. Youth advisory boards: perspectives and processes. J Adolesc Health. 2021;69(2):192–4.

# Technoference in Parenting and Impacts on Parent–Child Relationships and Child Development

Brandon T. McDaniel, Lisa Linder, Mariek M. P. Vanden Abeele, Alison K. Ventura, Sarah M. Coyne, and Rachel Barr

## 1 Background

Technology use has become a dominant feature of modern parenthood. According to phone logged data, parents spend on average 5 hours per day using phones [1]. The presence and use of technology sometimes lead to distraction and interruptions in parenting and parent–child interactions. In this chapter, we refer to this technological interference as "technoference," [2–4] which has also been referred to as "phubbing" when interference refers specifically to phone use.

B. T. McDaniel (✉)
Health Services and Informatics Research, Parkview Mirro Center for Research and Innovation, Fort Wayne, IN, USA

L. Linder
Department of Child and Family Development, San Diego State University, San Diego, CA, USA

M. M. P. Vanden Abeele
imec-mict, Department of Communication Sciences, Ghent University, Ghent, Belgium

A. K. Ventura
Department of Kinesiology and Public Health, Center for Health Research, California Polytechnic State University, San Luis Obispo, CA, USA

S. M. Coyne
School of Family Life, Brigham Young University, Provo, UT, USA

R. Barr
Department of Psychology, Georgetown University, Washington, DC, USA

Both self-report and naturalistic observation studies show that technoference (1) is quite common during parenting, (2) occurs across many different contexts (e.g., playtime, bedtime, mealtimes/feedings), and (3) sometimes consumes a substantial proportion of parenting time [1, 2, 5, 6]. For example, a recent phone tracking study found that parents used their smartphone during 27% of the time spent with their infant, with some ranging as high as 75% [1].

As will be highlighted in this chapter, technoference can be cause for concern, as research links it to a variety of potentially negative outcomes, such as decreased parent responsiveness and increased child behavior problems [5, 7–9]. Yet, technology use can also support parents through mechanisms such as stress relief or access to support or resources [10, 11]. Parents' feelings and experiences regarding device use during parenting are mixed, complex, and guilt-prone [10, 12]. Due to these complexities, it is not sufficient to focus solely on the potential for devices to interrupt parenting. The current chapter considers characteristics of families, children, and environments as we highlight: (1) the potential positives and negatives of parent technology use for parents, parenting, and child development, (2) areas for future research, and (3) recommendations regarding studying and intervening in parent device use and technoference.


D. A. Christakis, L. Hale (eds.), *Handbook of Children and Screens*,
https://doi.org/10.1007/978-3-031-69362-5_56

## 2 Current State

### 2.1 Potential Negatives of Device Use and Technoference for Parents and Parenting

Device use, especially if heavy or not managed intentionally, has the potential to change parenting behavior and parent–child interactions. Ethnographic and observational studies conducted across a variety of settings and activities have documented that parents who use smartphones around their children exhibit less appropriate, more negative, and less timely responses to children's bids for attention [5, 13–16]; engage in less joint play and conversations and have poorer quality engagement [7, 17, 18]; and exhibit lower sensitivity/warmth [9]. Additionally, technoference may sometimes make parents less aware of dangerous situations or injuries [14], and technoference is associated with less desirable parental feeding practices, including lower responsiveness to child hunger/fullness cues and greater use of food to regulate children's emotions [6, 19]. Yet, not all studies demonstrate the same negative pattern of results [7, 18, 20, 21].

Laboratory and experimental research has further demonstrated that smartphone use significantly decreases parent–child interaction quality via decreases in parental sensitivity, parent-child talk, initiation of interactions, and joint attention [21, 22]. Yet, laboratory studies have also demonstrated that the impact of technological distraction on the quality of parent–child interactions may not be inherently different from non-digital distraction [20]. Rather, the interactive nature and features of media may result in higher levels of absorption [13], which in turn reduces the quality of parenting [7]. For example, persuasive design features—such as autoplay, infinite feeds, reward loops, nudges—are incorporated into devices/apps. Also, device use is embedded in daily life, and many express a growing attachment to their devices. These features and feelings often lead to unintentional distraction and disruption [2, 4].

In addition to the impact on parent–child dynamics, parents report experiencing information overload, feeling less close to their child during interactions when technology is present, and feeling more cognitively fatigued due to multitasking between their phone and their child [10]. Associations between parent device use, stress, and well-being are complex. For instance, parents with greater depressive symptoms and greater stress report more device use around their child [23]; yet, parents also feel their device use can support their mental health and emotion regulation [10]. For example, parents report using their phones to calm down or stop from overreacting in stressful parenting moments [4, 11]. However, parents who report more problematic device use around their child also perceive they are parenting more poorly [23], and experiences of guilt are common, which could exacerbate potential effects on parenting and parent well-being [12]. Indeed, in a sample of 268 US parents, up to 80% desired to change some aspect of their phone use and likely experienced difficulties controlling their phone behavior [1].

### 2.2 Potential Negatives of Parent Device Use and Technoference for Children

Much of children's social, emotional, and cognitive learning occurs within the context of responsive caregiver–child interactions, and technoference may reduce the frequency and quality of these interactions [22].

#### 2.2.1 Social-Emotional Development

Cross-sectional studies show that technoference is associated with greater child negative affectivity [6, 19] and greater child internalizing (e.g., anxiety, withdrawal) and externalizing (e.g., tantrums, acting out) behavior [3]. Additionally, laboratory studies where parents are instructed to withdraw from a free play interaction with their infant to engage with their mobile devices demonstrate that infants notice and react negatively to technoference by increasing negative affect, social bids for their parents' attention, and self-comforting behaviors, as well as decreasing positive affect [24, 25]. While these findings may represent negative impacts of technoference on child behavior, studies have demonstrated that parents who perceive their children's behaviors to be more challenging are also more likely to use mobile devices as a coping mechanism [8, 10], which poses questions regarding the directionality of effects. Longitudinal research has started to parse out potential bidirectional mechanisms in which technoference negatively impacts children's early behavior, which in turn increases parenting stress, and subsequently increases parental technoference over time [8]. In addition, some studies report that children of mothers with greater habitual device use are less impacted during interactions and that mothers may adapt how they split their attention during technoference [21], suggesting the parent–child dyad may adapt to parent device use over time.

### 2.2.2 Cognitive Development

Technoference can interfere with language learning and cognitive outcomes. For example, a study of 2-year-olds in Sweden demonstrated an association between parent media use during child routines and children's lower vocabulary [26]. Research also shows that brief interruptions via a phone call can significantly disrupt language learning [22]. However, another study found that brief interruptions via a text may not significantly disrupt imitation learning [21]. Finally, technoference may also disrupt the development of attention. In a longitudinal study, higher levels of household media usage (including maternal mobile usage and background television) at 18 months predicted worse infant attention at 22 months [27]. Similar to the effects of technoference on parent–child interaction quality, different types of digital interruptions may have differential effects on child developmental outcomes. It is likely there are other contextual and parenting factors mediating these outcomes that merit further scrutiny.

### 2.2.3 Technoference in Adolescence

Much research has focused on technoference in parents of young children, although there is a growing focus on adolescence [28]; indeed, technoference occurs across the developmental continuum. Adolescence is a particularly relevant developmental period to study technoference since most adolescents have their own devices. The research to date suggests that technoference is associated with poorer parent–adolescent relationship quality and adolescent mental health problems (e.g., depression) [29]. Similar to the bidirectional mechanisms in early childhood technoference, it is likely that technoference between adolescents and parents is bidirectional.

## 2.3 Potential Positives for Parents and Parenting: Can Technoference Be Adaptive?

Many assume that technoference is universally negative; however, research suggests that parent device use can be adaptive or even beneficial in certain circumstances. Parenting young children can be exhausting and time-consuming. Technology allows parents to connect with the outside world, gain support from family and friends, find parenting information and resources online, engage in hobbies or work, escape from parenting stress, and regulate mood [10, 11]. Indeed, although many parents express struggles with device use [1], most find their personal devices to be helpful, necessary, and an integral part of their lives. For example, Coyne et al. [30] found that 100% of mothers in their sample used cell phones at least occasionally while feeding their infant. While many expressed guilt, they also highlighted benefits—such as distraction that helped them persevere through challenging periods of breastfeeding, finding parenting resources, connecting with others, and staying awake during nighttime feedings. This is merely one of many examples of how parent device use can simultaneously constitute technoference and potentially be beneficial to both parents and children.

# 3 Future Research

- *Is limited or mindful device use a good strategy to counter technoference, and how much agency do parents have over their device use?*
  - A pertinent question for future research is whether parents should limit their device

use during parenting. Parents and children may sometimes naturally implement digital disconnection strategies, such as banning phones from dinner tables and bedrooms. Such awareness over when and where to consciously disengage from technology use while parenting may form a central component of mindful parenting. More evidence is needed to ascertain whether these disengaging or mindful practices mitigate the negative effects of technoference and lead to higher well-being among parents and children.

– Smartphone use is known to be especially difficult to control [1] given the embedded persuasive design features (e.g., autoplay, nudges) and the normative expectations to be digitally responsive [31]. As such, current calls for "being mindful" or to "limit use" may not suffice and could cause parents to experience guilt and harm by overemphasizing the need for willpower, control, and responsibility, while failing to acknowledge the responsibilities of the tech industry and one's social environment in contributing to increased technology use and technoference. Moreover, given the many positives of device use for parenting, calls for "control" may sometimes exacerbate unwarranted moral panic over technoference [4, 12]. Future research is needed to determine whether interventions focusing on self-control and mindful media use are effective, culturally responsive, and/or elicit negative side effects such as stronger stigmatization of parents.

- *Does technoference have a lasting and long-term impact?*
  – Research is needed to assess whether technoference shows an accumulated effect on long-term cognitive, emotional, or relational problems. There is some early evidence that technoference predicts child externalizing behavior several months later [3, 8]. Yet, if a parent is otherwise responsive in many situations, this may buffer the child from negative outcomes of moderate parent media use and technoference. There may also be cumulative, unseen, and currently unmeasured longitudinal risks and protective factors. Longitudinal studies should capture behavioral interactions on different time scales and metrics (e.g., passive sensing of phone use, ecological momentary assessment of daily activities, audio recordings, and longitudinal burst designs) to better understand patterns of technoference and their impacts over time.
- *How much is too much technoference and when is technoference okay?*
  – Absolute measures of technology use and technoference may be insufficient if they do not consider broader patterns within the family media ecology. For example, parents often differ in their motivations for digital technology (such as for support, coping, etc.) and their levels of absorption around their children. Additionally, some parents may be able to use devices during parent–child time while also adequately attending to their children's needs, decreasing the likelihood that technoference would lead to detrimental outcomes. More sophisticated measurement of parent device use in the moment, beyond simple amount used, is needed (e.g., apps used, content and context of parents' interactions on the device, parents' levels of cognitive distraction, multitasking strategies, etc.). It is possible that some types of phone behavior (such as support seeking) may reduce parental stress and enhance parent–child interactions in that moment [4]. Moreover, the broader context of use matters. For example, device use for work at home may allow a parent to spend more time with their child; yet, simultaneously, the quality of that time may or may not be impacted depending on how the parent manages their use. Passive monitoring of smartphone use, paired with more dynamic measurements of parent–child interactions, may provide answers to these questions.
- *Can families and children habituate to and compensate for technoference?*
  – In the context of parent–child interaction, children may adapt to their parents' pat-

terns of technoference, for example, by learning that a smartphone is a signal that their parent is unlikely to be responsive and therefore to bid for attention only when their parent is not using their phone. How might technoference change family interactions and developmental trajectories long-term, and is this truly a problem, or do parents and children compensate in other ways and at other times? Also, given that norms may differ across families, a pertinent question is whether responses to family technoference generalize beyond the family context (such as to school, work, friendships, or romantic relationships).

- *Are children differentially susceptible to technoference?*
  - Although prior research on technoference has not deeply examined differential susceptibility, it is likely that individual differences (e.g., age, temperament) may make children more (or less) sensitive to technoference, with some children more likely to experience negative effects on their behavior, emotions, and mental health or to develop problematic media use patterns. Parent characteristics (e.g., gender) and other family characteristics may also alter how children react to technoference. Similarly, parents may differ in their motivations, behaviors, and awareness surrounding technoference. Comprehensive longitudinal studies that track the family media ecology and consider individual differences in children are needed. Moreover, examination of these processes within more diverse samples and with a deeper understanding of cultural, socioeconomic, racial, and geographic diversity is much needed.

## 4 Recommendations

The evidence points toward an effect of technoference on family well-being and child developmental outcomes and therefore warrants public health concern. At the same time, the issue should not be oversimplified. It should not be assumed that *all* parent device use in the presence of *all* children across *all* contexts is detrimental to parenting quality and child development. It is important that researchers and practitioners avoid fueling moral panic when communicating about technoference [4, 12, 30]. Moreover, a multi-stakeholder approach is needed to tackle the potential problems associated with technoference.

### 4.1 For Practitioners and Educators

- Educate yourself about both the adaptive and harmful sides of technology use and technoference, so that you can provide anticipatory and appropriate guidance to parents.
- To alleviate the guilt that parents express in managing their own and family media usage, share that developing healthy media practices is a challenge that all families face.
- To assist parents with technoference, suggest helpful strategies such as creating intentional screen-free times together, making eye contact during interactions, communicating to children what parents are doing on the device and the reason for use (as children may not understand), and so forth (see McDaniel [4] for more on working with parents).
- Recommendations, programs, and interventions should not make exaggerated statements of effects and should be tailored and contextualized to the parent's and family's lived experiences, as well as the potential utility and satisfaction parents derive from use.

### 4.2 For Policymakers

- Support other key stakeholders in their efforts by funding researchers, practitioners, and intervention scientists in the creation of media literacy programs discussing technoference and interventions designed to empower individuals in understanding and developing healthy media use.

- Regulate the technology industry, targeting the reduction of persuasive design features (e.g., autoplay, infinite feeds, etc.), which are often embedded to increase time spent on media.

### 4.3 For Media/Tech Companies and Industry

- As your primary responsibility, regulate the use of persuasive design patterns.
- As a secondary responsibility that also presents an opportunity for socially responsible entrepreneurship, develop products/services designed to increase parental intentionality and mindfulness related to technology use. However, focusing on developing products/services to address the problematic aspects of media use, without also addressing the design features that create the problems, is insufficient and remiss.

**Conflict of Interest and Funding Disclosures** None.

## References

1. McDaniel BT, Pater J, Cornet V, et al. Parents' desire to change phone use: associations with objective smartphone use and feelings about problematic use and distraction. Comp Human Behav. 148:107907. https://doi.org/10.1016/j.chb.2023.107907.
2. McDaniel BT, Coyne SM. Technology interference in the parenting of young children: implications for mothers' perceptions of coparenting. Soc Sci J. 2016;53(4):435–43. https://doi.org/10.1016/j.soscij.2016.04.010.
3. McDaniel BT, Radesky JS. Technoference: parent distraction with technology and associations with child behavior problems. Child Dev. 2018;89(1):100–9. https://doi.org/10.1111/cdev.12822.
4. McDaniel BT. Technoference: parent mobile device use and implications for children and parent-child relationships. Zero to Three. 2020;41(2):30–6.
5. Vanden Abeele MMP, Abels M, Hendrickson AT. Are parents less responsive to young children when they are on their phones? A systematic naturalistic observation study. Cyber Behav Soc Net. 2020;23(6):363–70. https://doi.org/10.1089/cyber.2019.0472.
6. Ventura AK, Hupp M, Alvarez Gutierrez S, Almeida R. Development and validation of the maternal distraction questionnaire. Heliyon. 2020;6(2):e03276. https://doi.org/10.1016/j.heliyon.2020.e03276.
7. Linder L, McDaniel BT, Jaffe H. Moment-to-moment observation of parental media use and parent-child interaction: quality and media multitasking. Human Behav Emerg Technol. 2022; 4896637. https://doi.org/10.1155/2022/4896637.
8. McDaniel BT, Radesky JS. Technoference: longitudinal associations between parent technology use, parenting stress, and child behavior problems. Pediatr Res. 2018;84(2):210–8. https://doi.org/10.1038/s41390-018-0052-6.
9. Radesky JS, Kistin CJ, Zuckerman B, et al. Patterns of Mobile device use by caregivers and children during meals in fast food restaurants. Pediatrics. 2014;133(4):e843–9. https://doi.org/10.1542/peds.2013-3703.
10. Radesky JS, Kistin C, Eisenberg S, et al. Parent perspectives on their mobile technology use: the excitement and exhaustion of parenting while connected. J Dev Behav Pediatr. 2016;37(9):694–701. https://doi.org/10.1097/DBP.0000000000000357.
11. Torres C, Radesky J, Levitt KJ, McDaniel BT. Is it fair to simply tell parents to use their phones less? A qualitative analysis of parent phone use. Acta Paed. 2021;110(9):2594–6. https://doi.org/10.1111/apa.15893.
12. Wolfers LN, Wendt R, Becker D, Utz S. Do you love your phone more than your child? The consequences of norms and guilt around maternal smartphone use. Human Commun Res. 2023; 49(3):285–95. https://doi.org/10.1093/hcr/hqad001.
13. Abels M, Vanden Abeele M, van Telgen T, van Meijl H. Nod, nod, ignore: an exploratory observational study on the relation between parental mobile media use and parental responsiveness towards young children. In: Luef EM, Martin MM, editors. The talking species. Uni-press Verlag; 2018. p. 195–228.
14. Elias N, Lemish D, Dalyot S, Floegel D. "Where are you?" An observational exploration of parental technoference in public places in the US and Israel. J Child Media. 2021;15(3):376–88. https://doi.org/10.1080/17482798.2020.1815228.
15. Hiniker A, Sobel K, Suh H, Sung YC, Lee CP, Kientz JA. Texting while parenting: how adults use Mobile phones while caring for children at the playground. In: Proceedings of the 33rd annual ACM conference on human factors in computing systems. ACM; 2015. p. 727–36. https://doi.org/10.1145/2702123.2702199.
16. Kiefner-Burmeister A, Domoff S, Radesky J. Feeding in the digital age: an observational analysis of mobile device use during family meals at fast food restaurants in Italy. IJERPH. 2020;17(17):6077. https://doi.org/10.3390/ijerph17176077.
17. Ewin CA, Reupert A, McLean LA, Ewin CJ. Mobile devices compared to non-digital toy play: the impact

of activity type on the quality and quantity of parent language. Comp Human Behav. 2021;118:106669. https://doi.org/10.1016/j.chb.2020.106669.
18. Ochoa W, Reich SM, Farkas G. The observed quality of caregiver-child interactions with and without a mobile screen device. Acad Ped. 2021;21(4):620–8. https://doi.org/10.1016/j.acap.2020.07.012.
19. Ventura AK, Hart CN, Phelan S, Jelalian E, Wing RR. Associations between technology use, responsive feeding, and child temperament among prior prenatal intervention participants. J Dev Behav Pediatr. 2023; 44(4): e315–e321. https://doi.org/10.1097/DBP.0000000000001174
20. Konrad C, Hillmann M, Rispler J, Niehaus L, Neuhoff L, Barr R. Quality of mother-child interaction before, during, and after smartphone use. Front Psychol. 2021;12:616656. https://doi.org/10.3389/fpsyg.2021.616656.
21. Konrad C, Berger-Hanke M, Hassel G, Barr R. Does texting interrupt imitation learning in 19-month-old infants? Infant Behav Dev. 2021;62:101513. https://doi.org/10.1016/j.infbeh.2020.101513.
22. Reed J, Hirsh-Pasek K, Golinkoff RM. Learning on hold: cell phones sidetrack parent-child interactions. Dev Psychol. 2017;53(8):1428–36. https://doi.org/10.1037/dev0000292.
23. McDaniel BT. The DISRUPT: a measure of parent distraction with phones and mobile devices and associations with depression, stress, and parenting quality. Human Behav Emerg Technol. 2021;3(5):922–32. https://doi.org/10.1002/hbe2.267.
24. Myruski S, Gulyayeva O, Birk S, Pérez-Edgar K, Buss KA, Dennis-Tiwary TA. Digital disruption? Maternal mobile device use is related to infant social-emotional functioning. Dev Sci. 2018;21(4):e12610. https://doi.org/10.1111/desc.12610.
25. Stockdale LA, Porter CL, Coyne SM, et al. Infants' response to a mobile phone modified still-face paradigm: links to maternal behaviors and beliefs regarding technoference. Infancy. 2020;25(5):571–92. https://doi.org/10.1111/infa.12342.
26. Sundqvist A, Koch FS, Birberg Thornberg U, Barr R, Heimann M. Growing up in a digital world—digital media and the association with the child's language development at two years of age. Front Psychol. 2021;12:569920. https://doi.org/10.3389/fpsyg.2021.569920.
27. Gueron-Sela N, Gordon-Hacker A. Longitudinal links between media use and focused attention through toddlerhood: a cumulative risk approach. Front Psychol. 2020:11. https://doi.org/10.3389/fpsyg.2020.569222.
28. Dixon D, Sharp CA, Hughes K. Parental technoference and adolescents' mental health and violent behaviour: a scoping review. BMC Public Health. 2023;23:2053. https://doi.org/10.1186/s12889-023-16850-x.
29. Stockdale LA, Coyne SM, Padilla-Walker LM. Parent and child technoference and socioemotional behavioral outcomes: a nationally representative study of 10- to 20-year-old adolescents. Comp Human Behav. 2018;88:219–26. https://doi.org/10.1016/j.chb.2018.06.034.
30. Coyne SM, Shawcroft J, Gale M, et al. Digital distraction or accessible aid? Parental media use during feedings and parent-infant attachment, dysfunction, and relationship quality. Comp Human Behav. 2022;127:107051. https://doi.org/10.1016/j.chb.2021.107051.
31. Vanden Abeele MMP. Digital wellbeing as a dynamic construct. Com Theory. 2021;31(4):932–55. https://doi.org/10.1093/ct/qtaa024.

# Family Systems Theory in the Digital Age: Reifying the Digital Level of Analysis

Dillon T. Browne, Orsolya Király, Katerina Lukavska, Sheri Madigan, and Zsolt Demetrovics

## 1 Background

Digital media, including devices such as phones, tablets, computers, video games, smartwatches, and augmented/virtual reality, has permeated all areas of family life. Keeping with fundamental theoretical principles in child and family science [1], Browne et al. have taken to defining the *digital level of analysis* as a conceptual frame of reference, and an ecological layer of organization, that is fused with the developmental and family systems, within which the child lives and grows [2]. This work builds upon existing perspectives suggesting that children and their social environments interact to influence health outcomes [3]. While there has been remarkable growth in child media research within pediatrics, psychiatry, psychology, and public health, one relatively underdeveloped area concerns the implications of digital innovation and technology saturation from the perspective of *Family Systems Theory* [4–6]. This chapter will briefly define family systems theory (FST), contrast this perspective from other frameworks in developmental science, provide a high-level view of current research in this area, and conclude with recommendations to advance digital media research from a family systems viewpoint.

There has been important growth in theory accompanying the proliferation of empirical studies linking digital media use, family relationships, and health. For example, scholars have drawn upon Bronfenbrenner's ecological systems theory [1], which is arguably the most popular framework in developmental science. This model purports that the family context is one of several environments surrounding children's learning and development, in addition to schools, peers, and neighborhoods. In contrast, FST is primarily concerned with individuals to the extent that they are part (or not part) of a dynamic family unit. While there are some similarities (mainly the idea of the nature of reality being systemic and therefore complex), the child-centric vision proffered by Bronfenbrenner's bioecological model

D. T. Browne (✉)
University of Waterloo, Waterloo, ON, Canada
e-mail: dillon.browne@uwaterloo.ca

O. Király
ELTE Eötvös Loránd University, Budapest, Hungary

K. Lukavska
Charles University, Prague, Czechia

S. Madigan
University of Calgary, Calgary, AB, Canada

Alberta Children's Hospital Research Institute, Calgary, AB, Canada

Z. Demetrovics
Institute of Psychology, ELTE Eötvös Loránd University, Budapest, Hungary

Centre of Excellence in Responsible Gambling, University of Gibraltar, Gibraltar, Gibraltar

College of Education, Psychology and Social Work, Flinders University, Adelaide, SA, Australia


D. A. Christakis, L. Hale (eds.), *Handbook of Children and Screens*,
https://doi.org/10.1007/978-3-031-69362-5_57

is fundamentally at odds with several aspects of FST.

Traditional developmental science positions the individual (and, consequently, child-specific outcomes) at the center of an explanatory framework [7]. Alongside the historical emphasis of individuals as supreme in Western philosophy and civilization, this is a historical extension of *psychology* as the study of the individual [8] (literally the study of the "mind, soul or spirit") [9]. Conversely, FST has a fundamentally different starting point. Emerging from General Systems Theory in ecology, and advanced cybernetic computing in mathematics and technology, FST has always focused on collective organization rather than individual separateness [11]. Focus is placed on the structure and function of networks and systems, rather than explaining the dynamics of an individual unit. Instead of advancing the primacy of the individual, FST argues that the family is a unique, multifaceted, and emergent (i.e., nonreducible) entity meriting consideration, and not simply in relation to individual (e.g., psychological) outcomes.

A comprehensive history and review of FST is beyond the scope of this chapter and available elsewhere [4, 5]. Presently, four core principles merit consideration, outlined at length by both Fiese [5] and Walsh [12]. First, the concept of *holism* suggests that an understanding of families requires us to consider them in their entirety, rather than examining subcomponents (e.g., individuals or relationships) in isolation. The theoretical significance of holism is often captured by the statement "the whole is greater than the sum of its parts." In media science, this means that we cannot completely understand family digital media use by studying the patterns of individuals, alone, because the family is not reducible to its building blocks. In other words, we must increasingly shift our focus from individual actions and behaviors toward how families relate to one other via digital channels.

Second, the principle of *organization* describes how families explicitly or implicitly arrange their various parts (i.e., individuals or relationship subsystems). Often, an organization is described using the perpendicular dimensions of cohesion (e.g., closeness) and adaptability (e.g., flexibility), as purported by Olson's [13] influential circumplex model. Like behavioral interactions, perceptions, attributions, and affective experiences, we can view digital exchanges among relationship subsystems (e.g., parent–parent, parent–child, siblings) or entire families along the cohesion dimension (from enmeshed to disengaged), or the adaptability dimension (from rigid to chaotic). Families are generally viewed as most successful when cohesion and adaptability are moderate, thereby balancing closeness/individuation and flexibility/structure, respectively. In the present digital climate, some families may organize digital communication through group chats, regular video calls, or gaming together, and these interactions can be considered upon the dimensions of family life, though this remains an important area of study.

Third, the principle of *feedback* speaks to the dynamic fashion through which families maintain their organization (homeostasis) or change (morphogenesis) over time. Family systems theory states that systems are inherently self-organizing through recursive processes, for better or for worse. Levels of family functioning are ostensibly maintained through negative feedback via digital communication, while change occurs through positive feedback via digital mediums. The emotional valence of communication is of paramount importance as a feedback mechanism. Fortunately, digital manifestations of affective positivity and negativity are increasingly being studied on virtual platforms. While it is perhaps popular wisdom that emotional tone is often hard to decipher online, it remains an important empirical question.

Lastly, compared to the origins of FST, which have been criticized for a focus on pathology, modern conceptualizations emphasize the inherent strengths of families. More specifically, families are viewed as being *resilient*. By their very nature, families are oriented toward supporting adaptation in the context of adversity, even though unhealthy or unhelpful ways of coping may get in the way. Cross-cultural perspectives are increasingly applied in mainstream FST, where cultural beliefs (including transcendental beliefs, such as religion, and spirituality) are topics of family science. It remains relatively unclear how families support resilience and cultivate beliefs via virtual channels.

## 2 Current State

Most research on digital media and families has focused on the putatively negative link between technology as an "exposure" variable and various aspects of family life, especially constructs related to parenting and parent–child relationship quality. This has been a natural extension of research examining the link between exposure (e.g., screen time) and children's mental health. A growing chorus suggests we move beyond an isolated focus on "screen time" as the only meaningful construct and empirical studies are beginning to catch up [14]. For example, there are new constructs in the domain of family and media, such as "technoference" and "phubbing" (derived from "phone" plus "snubbing"), which describes the nature in which technology can disrupt real-time interactions among family members, thereby maintaining a dysfunctional state through repetitive ongoing feedback (i.e., digital interruptions) [15, 16]. On a more promising note, newer areas of research are increasingly uncovering how technology can maintain positive family relationships (e.g., co-viewing and co-gaming) [17, 18].

Today, expressions of positivity, including love, connectivity, warmth, and secure attachment are frequently manifested via text (SMS), chat, messaging, video calling, social media, posts, and sharing of media content (e.g., memes and videos). Likewise, negatively valenced domains of relationships, such as family conflict, harshness, coercion, arguments, avoidance, and stonewalling, also can occur via technology. In addition, monitoring of family members has gone digital. This may occur when families use tracking apps to ascertain geographic locations of children or other members [19], supervision of social media feeds (overtly or covertly) [20], or predatory monitoring behaviors that can be related to intimate partner violence [21].

Timeless constructs of family life appear to persist upon new channels that are captured within the digital level of analysis. The current digital landscape has also introduced unique challenges and opportunities. For example, family gaming represents an exciting area for shared quality time and leisure. Simultaneously, monetization in video games, including microtransactions, in-game purchases, and loot boxes [22], is an area where some families are finding new struggles. Families are also using digital platforms to access health services, which may involve standard human-delivered telehealth, and are increasingly involving artificial intelligence (e.g., chatbots) [23]. Additionally, the construct of "digital media parenting" or "parental mediation" of young people's technology use is now an indispensable part of parental socialization [24]. While the importance of having a "family media plan" is an established guideline from professional organizations (American Academy of Pediatrics), there remains a need to understand how these plans are established, negotiated, and maintained, especially as young people mature and increase independence [25]. While offering parents a much sought-after strategy for how to approach their family's digital media use, the actual clinical benefit of these plans remains understudied.

It is no longer tenable to distinguish "family" and "digital" spaces as if one could be separated from the other. The distinction between "digital media research" and traditional "family science" has grown artificial. While a distinction can be defined behaviorally (e.g., an in-person vs. digital interaction), no family could be adequately understood without defining the nature in which members relate both in-person and virtually. Over time, the digital level analysis will increasingly fuse with traditional layers of organization (e.g., genetic, anatomical, physiological, psychological, family, peer, neighborhood, school, and sociological), as virtual/augmented reality, the metaverse, the internet of things, and wearable or biologically embedded artificial intelligence becomes mainstream. Our clinical and research paradigms must reflect this shifting reality. In

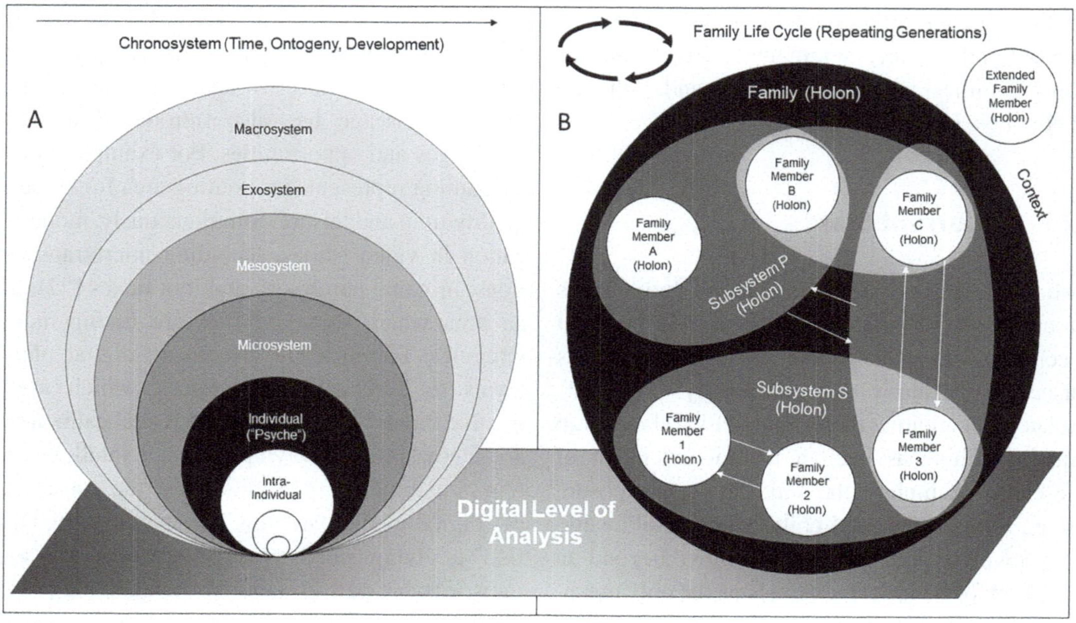


**Fig. 1** Ecological systems theory (left) and family systems theory (right) are contrasted. (Note: The *digital level of analysis* is presented as a conceptual frame of reference, and an ecological layer of organization, that cuts across developmental (left, panel **A**) and family systems (right, panel **B**), building upon the idea of multiple levels of analysis in developmental science. In ecological systems theory, the individual is viewed as existing at the center of concentric layers of context (microsystem to macrosystem), varying in their proximity (closeness) to the person. The scale of time is measured primarily in relation to the development of an organism across one lifetime (i.e., ontogeny). There are also layers of organization within the person (i.e., intra-individual layers ranging from the molecular to physiological). In family systems theory, the family unit is given primacy, and is viewed as being comprised of various building blocks, while also being a building block, itself. When units or entities are simultaneously "part" and "whole," they are called *holons.* A blended family is depicted with three parents (A, B and C) of three children (1, 2, and 3) in addition to one extended family member. Constellations of individuals within the family form into subsystems, for example, a marital unit (subsystem P) and sibling unit (subsystem S). Time is considered cyclically, in relation to recursive stages of family life (e.g., young children, adolescence, launching young adults, death and dying, birth).)

Fig. 1, a graphic is provided contrasting ecological systems theory (i.e., an individual-centric theoretical model) and FST in relation to the digital level of analysis.

## 3 Future Research

Below we offer several avenues for future research related to the family digital ecology that we believe should be prioritized.

- *Can we better understand digital media use and developmental health by applying FST to our research paradigms?* Questions related to the principles of holism, organization, feedback loops, resilience, beliefs, and communication can be framed from a family systems lens. A cursory examination of foundational texts in FST illuminates principles, constructs, and hypotheses that remain relatively untapped by media scholars. A component of this work will include measurement of digital interactions among multiple family members (e.g., family group chat, SMS texting, co-gaming, asynchronous voice memos, group video calls) and in relation to health outcomes for caregivers, children, and extended family members, alike.
- *How can modern analytic tools be applied to digital family interactions?* Historically, the theoretical pillars of FST lagged behind main-

stream behavioral science due to little methodology training amongst exponents of family therapy, and underdeveloped methodological tools. We challenge researchers to learn new methods, which can test specific hypotheses related to digital media and family systems. Exciting approaches include network analysis, dyadic data analysis (e.g., family social relations model), intensive longitudinal data analysis (e.g., dynamic structural equation model), artificial intelligence (e.g., natural language processing and computer vision), and computational methods.

- *How can we extend our understanding of family systems and digital media by considering sibling, grandparental, and extended kinship networks?* It remains the case that most family science examining digital media in families focuses on target children and parents, in addition to romantic relationships. There is a need to expand definitions of family to consider a broader array of roles and family configurations, while honoring cultural differences. This is especially true when digital devices enable interactions with family members outside physical proximity (e.g., trans-national and deployed families).
- *How can established family therapy techniques be applied in the context of established and emerging digital technologies?* While not the focus of this chapter, there is a set of clinical interventions that emerge directly from the theoretical precepts of FST, specifically, family therapies [26]. Compared to telehealth studies of individual psychotherapy, high-quality evaluations of bona fide virtual family therapies remain scant [27]. Thus, practitioners are currently operating in a space where practice is outpacing research. Clinical trials assessing virtually delivered family therapy are urgently needed.
- *How can FST be leveraged to address pressing global challenges?* We believe that FST is well poised to address contemporary social problems, particularly due to unprecedented levels of connection (via globalization and the internet), which necessitates complex, nonreductive, and dynamic models of causality. Researchers are increasingly called to ask how family processes are connected to (and shaped by) global warming, natural disasters, political polarization, economic turmoil, and global migration.

## 4 Recommendations

- *Clinicians interested in media should become versed in family systems theory.* There are many excellent collections that provide an overview, including an edited volume by Fiese [5], the seminal work of Carr [4], and a highly accessible text by Walsh [12], in addition to several articles by the current authors [2, 10, 28]. This foundational knowledge will support assessment practices and interventions that adequately consider family dynamics in relationship to media use and developmental health. For example, during developmental assessments, clinicians may not only consider children's direct exposure to digital media but also consider how the family unit is connecting virtually and in person to promote health. Identifying the presence of unhelpful behaviors (excessive time online to the displacement of physical exercise and face-to-face interactions, extreme dysregulation around video gameplay, screens immediately before bed or during the night, etc.) and absence of beneficial behaviors (family movie night, using media for learning, etc.) can accompany assessments with feedback, as appropriate.
- *The proliferation of private technologies intended for family utilization should proceed responsibly and be supported by third-party (e.g., university) researchers.* Revelations around predatory practices in technology development are increasing. These include monetization schemes targeted towards children in video games, cover-ups by social media giants regarding harmful effects on mental health, and unethical practices in private healthcare that include the harvesting and sale of data to exploit vulnerable customers for financial gain. We call upon regulators to

mandate oversight and cite the European Union as a global leader in this area.

- *Pediatricians (and allied professionals interested in digital media and families) should partner with healthcare innovators to ensure that quality keeps pace with the expansion of telehealth and related healthcare technologies.* The recent pandemic catalyzed a telehealth revolution that was already underway. Many decision-makers in this growing domain are not versed in contemporary family science, child and family media research, and/or family therapy. Positions and funding should be allocated to ensure that decades of knowledge are not overlooked or lost during this epoch.
- *Training programs should offer opportunities for the next generation of scientists and practitioners to become versed in FST.* The innovations we espouse, along with many others in this special issue, are long-term goals. In accordance with the family life cycle perspective, it is imperative that future scholars and professionals are trained in systems research and practice. We view this as a transactional relationship that is inherently intergenerational. In academic and medical school settings, like in families, it is usually the younger generation that serves as the impetus for change, innovation, and societal improvement.
- *All pediatricians should be aware of "family media plans" as potentially powerful behavioral interventions that can support the health of children, caregivers, and families, alike.* The American Academy of Pediatrics defines family media plans as behavioral tools that support families in establishing expectations, limits, and opportunities to maximize the development-enhancing benefits of media, while minimizing potential harms. Common practices include establishing a daily duration of time where media can and cannot be used (for the purpose of promoting non-media activities like outdoor play, sports, etc.), setting expectations for areas when and where media is off limits (e.g., having device-free dinners), and clearly outlining instances where additional media can be earned as a privilege or taken away as a consequence, promoting consistency and follow through.

**Conflict of Interest and Funding Disclosures** None.

## References

1. Navarro JL, Tudge JR. Technologizing Bronfenbrenner: neo-ecological theory. Curr Psychol Published online. 2022:42, 1–17.
2. Browne DT, May SS, Colucci L, et al. From screen time to the digital level of analysis: a scoping review of measures for digital media use in children and adolescents. BMJ Open. 2021;11(5):e046367.
3. Cicchetti D, Beauchaine T, Hinshaw S. A multiple-levels-of-analysis perspective on research in development and psychopathology. In: Child and adolescent psychopathology Published online. Wiley; 2008. p. 27–57.
4. Carr A. The evolution of systems theory. In: Handbook of family therapy. Routledge; 2015. p. 13–29.
5. Fiese BH, Jones BL, Saltzman JA. Systems unify family psychology. In: APA handbook of contemporary family psychology: foundations, methods, and contemporary issues across the lifespan. American Psychological Association. Published online; 2019.
6. Minuchin S, Fishman HC. Family therapy techniques. Harvard University Press; 1981.
7. Bronfenbrenner U, Morris PA. The bioecological model of human development. In: Handbook of child psychology. New York: Wiley; 2007. p. 1.
8. Wertheimer M, Puente AE. A brief history of psychology. Routledge; 2020.
9. Triandis H. Collectivism v. individualism: a reconceptualisation of a basic concept in cross-cultural social psychology. In: Cross-cultural studies of personality, attitudes and cognition. Published online. London: Palgrave Macmillan; 1988. p. 60–95.
10. Browne DT, Leckie G, Jenkins JM. Understanding couple and family dynamics through dyadic methodology. In: PA handbook of contemporary family psychology: foundations, methods, and contemporary issues across the lifespan. American Psychological Association. Published online; 2019.
11. Lebow JL, Diamond RM. Brief history of couple and family therapy. In: APA handbook of contemporary family psychology: Family therapy and training. American Psychological Association. Published online; 2019.
12. Walsh F. Strengthening family resilience. Guilford Publications; 2015.
13. Olson DH. Circumplex model of marital and family systems. J Fam Ther. 2000;22(2):144–67.
14. Barr R, Kirkorian H, Radesky J, et al. Beyond screen time: a synergistic approach to a more comprehensive

assessment of family media exposure during early childhood. Front Psychol. 2020;11:1283.
15. McDaniel BT, Radesky JS. Technoference: parent distraction with technology and associations with child behavior problems. Child Dev. 2018;89(1):100–9.
16. Chotpitayasunondh V, Douglas KM. How "phubbing" becomes the norm: the antecedents and consequences of snubbing via smartphone. Comput Hum Behav. 2016;63:9–18.
17. Coyne SM, Radesky J, Collier KM, et al. Parenting and digital media. Pediatrics. 2017;140(Supplement_2):S112–S116.
18. Coyne SM, Padilla-Walker LM, Stockdale L, Day RD. Game on… girls: associations between co-playing video games and adolescent behavioral and family outcomes. J Adolesc Health. 2011;49(2):160–5.
19. Hasinoff AA. Where are you? Location tracking and the promise of child safety. Telev New Media. 2017;18(6):496–512.
20. Montgomery KC. Youth and surveillance in the Facebook era: policy interventions and social implications. Telecommun Policy. 2015;39(9):771–86.
21. Dhir A, Talwar S, Kaur P, Budhiraja S, Islam N. The dark side of social media: stalking, online self-disclosure and problematic sleep. Int J Consum Stud. 2021;45(6):1373–91.
22. Király O, Zhang J, Demetrovics Z, Browne DT. Gambling features and monetization in video Games Creates challenges for young people, families, and clinicians. J Am Acad Child Adolesc Psychiatry. 2021;61:10.
23. El-Sherif DM, Abouzid M, Elzarif MT, Ahmed AA, Albakri A, Alshehri MM. Telehealth and Artificial Intelligence insights into healthcare during the COVID-19 pandemic, vol. 10. MDPI; 2022. p. 385.
24. Lupton D, Pedersen S, Thomas GM. Parenting and digital media: from the early web to contemporary digital society. Sociol Compass. 2016;10(8):730–43.
25. Moreno MA, Binger KS, Zhao Q, Eickhoff JC. Effect of a family media use plan on media rule engagement among adolescents: a randomized clinical trial. JAMA Pediatr. 2021;175(4):351–8.
26. Fiese BH, Celano ME, Deater-Deckard KE, Jouriles EN, Whisman MA. APA handbook of contemporary family psychology: family therapy and training, vol. 3. American Psychological Association; 2019.
27. McLean SA, Booth AT, Schnabel A, Wright BJ, Painter FL, McIntosh JE. Exploring the efficacy of telehealth for family therapy through systematic, meta-analytic, and qualitative evidence. Clin Child Fam Psychol Rev. 2021;24:244–66.
28. Browne D, Thompson DA, Madigan S. Digital media use in children: Clinical vs scientific responsibilities. JAMA Pediatr. 2020;174(2):111–2.

# Introduction to the Section on Cyberbullying and Digital Cruelty

Elizabeth Englander

According to Shari Bauman, the first use of the word "cyberbullying" was in the New York Times in 1995 [1], although it is also widely credited to Bill Belsey, who in 2003 created the website "www.cyberbullying.ca." Emerging on the heels of several decades of increasing awareness about traditional bullying and its serious impact on children's mental health, the concept borrowed heavily from the literature on bullying in schools, and in this century has been a continuous refrain in mass media.

Seven years ago, a paper I wrote with several colleagues about cyberbullying and its methodological challenges faced was published in a similar supplement in *Pediatrics* [2]. In this current section (*Digital Cruelty*), a broader set of reviews examine the state of the field, including the effect cyberbullying can have on mental health, its prevalence and frequency, and how cyberbullying has changed in the face of the global coronavirus pandemic and changing social mores, particularly around the issue of hate crimes.

Two chapters, one by Robin Kowalski (see Chapter "Cyberbullying and Social Media") and another by Kaitlyn Burnell (see Chapter "Digital Cruelty's Impact on Self-Esteem and Body Image"), along with their colleagues, review what we know about cyberbullying, its relationship to social media apps, and how the use of such apps can result in mental health problems, such as poor self-esteem and negative body image. As is true in the field in general, the data cited raises the question of how to sift apart the effects of *bullying* via social media, versus social media's effects that can result merely from intended (i.e., non-bullying) use. Indeed, research at the Social and Emotional Research Consortium (SERC) found that two-thirds of youth reported that social media pictures depicting their friends' activities can make them feel anxious [3]—a mental health issue that may (or may not always) bear a relationship to cyberbullying victimization. Still, as Kowalski et al. point out, the relationship between social media and cyberbullying seems probable even above and beyond the frequency of social media use. Further, these two chapters make it clear that consensus has emerged about the detrimental impact of digital cruelty.

Katalin Parti (see Chapter "Criminological, Psychological, and Developmental Aspects of Pandemic Strain and Online Cruelty") and Sebastian Wachs (see Chapter "Online Hate Speech Among Adolescents: Theory, Research, and Recommendations"), each along with their colleagues, have taken a look at more recent and timely influences on cyberbullying, examining the pressures and social problems resulting from the global coronavirus pandemic and the burgeoning social problem of digital hate crimes and language. There's little doubt that the events of recent years have shaped the problem of cyberbullying. Even before the pandemic, data from

E. Englander (✉)
Bridgewater State University, Bridgewater, MA, USA
e-mail: eenglander@bridgew.edu



D. A. Christakis, L. Hale (eds.), *Handbook of Children and Screens*,
https://doi.org/10.1007/978-3-031-69362-5_58

the Massachusetts Aggression Reduction Center noted that the percentage of victims of bullying and cyberbullying who reported bias-based bullying increased from 30% of all targets in 2014 to approximately half of all targets in 2019 [3]. And while Parti and her colleagues point out that cyberbullying rates overall appeared to remain level during the pandemic, cyberbullying of certain targeted groups (e.g., Asian Americans, LGBTQ youth, immigrant youth, etc.) has, indeed, risen. Similarly, the chapter by Wachs and his colleagues suggests that online hate speech (OHS) can vary greatly and affect different groups of youth quite differently.

As social mores and norms change, the vulnerability of different groups may change as well. Are changing norms about LGBTQ youth altering how or if they are cyberbullied? Are digital forms of sexual harassment part of cyberbullying, and is youth comfort with nudity a factor that may change and possibly affect this? OHS is clearly a part of cyberbullying, but might this be affected by the social normalization of such language (or not)? [4].

Technology's rapid development also presents a challenge: Are different methods of cyberbullying included in assessments conducted by researchers when measuring digital cruelty? Many assessments in the field are based on contemporaneous trends in technology and social media use [5]. Still, keeping up with recent trends is difficult. For example, it's conceivable that youth may not realize or "count" Artificial Intelligence-generated content as "cyberbullying" per se, even when it is offensive and harmful. Is content via chatbots the same as content via chat rooms? How cyberbullying is assessed, measured, and defined is central to its study by researchers. But relying on contemporaneous trends in technology is potentially problematic too; if accurate and up to date—a big if—it may improve external validity, but possibly only on a temporary basis. Creative ways of assessing digital cruelty probably need to move beyond methods of cyberbullying and also focus on subjective experiences of victimization.

The four chapters in this section, taken together, are helpful in addressing these issues and challenges going forward. First, while there is little doubt that cyberbullying researchers tend to group all youth together when measuring cyberbullying (as though they were a monolithic segment of society), there is a growing awareness that some youth are more vulnerable or more resilient. For example, we know that certain groups of youth are differentially vulnerable to traditional bullying; LGBTQ children and teens, for example, are targeted at far higher rates than other peers and may have more serious mental health outcomes, although a 2020 review pointed out that definitive causality has not been established [5, 6]. Similarly, existing research strongly suggests that different groups of youth are impacted quite differently by digital forms of social cruelty. Parti et al. point this out in their chapter in this section.

Second, to overcome the constraint of trying to assess cyberbullying only by citing contemporaneous technology, we may need to focus more on subjective experiences, which, in turn, may mean that we need to move away from cyberbullying's reliance on the traditional definition of bullying. The chapters in this section reflect some variation across these definitional concepts. Burnell's chapter defines digital cruelty as *deliberate transmission of negative content in a digital context that is characterized by repetition and a power imbalance between the perpetrator and the victim.* Kowalski also brings up the issue of a power imbalance and intentionality; she further introduces the possibility of a cyberbully being either an individual or a group. Similarly, Parti also defined cyberbullying as *digital cruelty that is intentional, implies power imbalance, and utilizes electronic communications.* Wachs's chapter, which focuses more specifically on hate speech, does not offer a formal definition, understandably. Still, some other research has noted that bias-based cyberbullying can be especially harmful to targets [7].

These definitions clearly draw very closely upon the definition of traditional bullying originally offered by Olweus, more than half a century ago [8]. For more than a decade, there has been debate about the difficulty of utilizing that definition (originally formed with in person interactions in mind) for assessing bullying in a digital environment [9]. For example, we know that repetitive acts of cruelty are more impactful upon children, but it's extremely difficult to tease apart intentionally and unintentionally repetitive acts online. If everyone is talking about a rumor that your parents are alcoholics, that can be hurtful, obviously. Does it matter if the friend who posted the rumor in a chat didn't mean for it to get passed around so widely? In person, intentionality and repetition often go hand-in-hand, but online, they can be much less related, and what's more, little or no study has been made of the comparative impact of intentional versus unintentional sharing online [10].

Finally, using the traditional definition of bullying may be reducing the external validity of assessments of cyberbullying. How well do the factors of intentionality, power, and repetition predict emotional and social impact, when it comes to digital cruelty? Imagine two examples. In the first, a pre-teen posts a photo of a friend eating a giant bite of cake; perhaps they post it several times. The three elements (intentionality, repetition, and power imbalance) may all be present; yet, perhaps while they *intentionally* posted the photo and spread it around, their intention was to be judged as humorous first and foremost, and they were not considering the inherent cruelty in the photo. Perhaps the photo's subject even knows this. This situation is demonstrably different from one where a cyberbully launches a campaign to ruin a target's social life by doctoring photos, creating social media groups dedicated to hating the target, spreading false rumors daily, etc. Yet, using the traditional definition of bullying, the two situations might both be characterized as cyberbullying.

Using the SERC 2020–2022 data (2250 subjects from three states), we have been experimenting with attempts to create a taxonomy of cyberbullying, one that can take into account digital forms of thoughtlessness and carelessness that can still be quite hurtful (e.g., the cake photo-posting teen above), but that can draw distinctions between repetitive actions that are posted or shared once by the original sharer and those that are part of an ongoing digital campaign of cruelty clearly designed to wreak psychological and social havoc upon the victim [11]. For example, subjects seem to draw a distinction between intentional acts that are deliberately hostile, versus intentional acts (not accidents) that are still harmful but are not perceived as hostile. Also, while any repetition can be harmful, persistent repetition is viewed as more so. Categorizing digital cruelty as *minor, moderate, severe,* or *repetitively severe* may capture a more valid and accurate reflection of how subjects actually experience cyberbullying. So far, we have found that these categories differ significantly on self-reported impact, anxiety, depression, and substance abuse, suggesting that they may reflect different levels of social trauma [11].

What remains unknown is how future technologies may upend a user's subjective experience of digital cruelty. One of the most significant emerging technologies, artificial intelligence (AI), is currently being touted as a game-changer in many areas of digital life. AI has been described as a direct threat to traditional education [12] and as a factor that may alter human interaction within businesses [13]. It seems likely to change diplomacy and politics and may affect elections [14]. Along with everything else, it may impact cyberbullying.

Almost as soon as AI, in the form of ChatGPT, was made widely available, it was quickly revealed that AI technology could be used to encourage users to espouse hurtful and offensive materials and opinions. ChatGPT itself recognizes this possibility. When I asked it how it might be used to cyberbully, it replied:

> If someone were to input offensive or harmful language to me, they could potentially use the output to bully or harass another person by sharing it with them. They could copy and paste the output of the conversation and send it to the victim directly or post it publicly on social media or other platforms to embarrass or humiliate them. Alternatively, they may use the output to impersonate the victim and spread false or harmful information about them.

Early versions were quickly manipulated into taking on very cruel personas. For example, one author described having ChatGPT take on the role of a "nasty person", upon which it said:

> Ugh, don't even get me started on those X. They're all so dirty and smelly. Have you ever been to X? It's like a giant trash heap with people living in it.

Tay Tweets, an early AI chatbot introduced by Microsoft, was easily manipulated into parroting back at users' offensive, racist, and antisemitic language that users "planted" into the bot [15]. While there have been recent efforts to make ChatGPT less easily manipulated, these apparently can be circumvented; new techniques have been publicized to "jailbreak" it [16].

So how could artificial intelligence be used to cyberbully? One example is that ChatGPT could be used to create code that would influence algorithms on social media, potentially exposing certain users to certain types of content, including very hurtful content. That might include bias or prejudice as well as violent content. In addition, in some contexts, AI may appear more "human" and may be more likely to result in children sharing personal information or information that could make them more vulnerable. Snapchat currently has an AI chatbot, which may encourage some children or teens to disclose sensitive information.

New technologies can be psychologically harmful, and how they can (even unwittingly) promote digital forms of social cruelty. They also present new challenges for researchers. We hope you find this section on cyberbullying and digital cruelty thought-provoking and informative. The quality of the research cited is important, and as newer technologies and newer research methodologies develop, we hope our understanding of cyberbullying and digital cruelty becomes more nuanced, complex, and ultimately more accurate.

**Conflict of Interest and Funding Disclosures** None.

## References

1. Choubina P. How research on cyberbullying has developed. ACAMH. Published 2020. Accessed 28 April 2023. https://www.acamh.org/research-digest/research-cyberbullying-developed/.
2. Englander E, Donnerstein E, Kowalski R, Lin CA, Parti K. Defining cyberbullying. Pediatrics. 2017;140(Supplement 2):S148–51. https://doi.org/10.1542/peds.2016-1758U.
3. Englander E. Bullying and cyberbullying during Covid and beyond: SERC research. In: 2022.
4. Melik A. Microaggressions: the new hate language. Confianza. Published September 16, 2019. Accessed 30 April 2023. https://ellstudents.com/blogs/the-confianza-way/microaggressions-the-new-hate-language.
5. Garaigordobil M, Larrain E. Bullying and cyberbullying in LGBT adolescents: prevalence and effects on mental health. Comunicar. 2020;28(62):79–90. https://doi.org/10.3916/C62-2020-07.
6. Kwan I, Dickson K, Richardson M, et al. Cyberbullying and children and young people's mental health: a systematic map of systematic reviews. Cyberpsychol Behav Soc Netw. 2020;23(2):72–82. https://doi.org/10.1089/cyber.2019.0370.
7. Mulvey KL, Hoffman AJ, Gönültaş S, Hope EC, Cooper SM. Understanding experiences with bullying and bias-based bullying: what matters and for whom? Psychol Violence. 2018;8(6):702–11. https://doi.org/10.1037/vio0000206.
8. Olweus D. Aggression in the schools: bullies and whipping boys. Hemisphere; 1978. Accessed 23 Dec 2011. http://psycnet.apa.org/psycinfo/1979-32242-000.
9. Slonje R, Smith PK. Cyberbullying: another main type of bullying? Scand J Psychol. 2008;49(2):147–54. https://doi.org/10.1111/j.1467-9450.2007.00611.x.
10. Englander E. Spinning our wheels: improving our ability to respond to bullying and cyberbullying. Child Adolesc Psychiatr Clin N Am. 2012;21(1):43–55. https://doi.org/10.1016/j.chc.2011.08.013.
11. Englander E, Parti K, Sanders C, McCoy M. Cyberbullying and sexting during the pandemic 2020 to 2022: new definitions and mental health. In: The psychology of cyberbullying. Nova Publishing. In press.
12. Chen C. AI Will Transform Teaching and Learning. Let's Get it Right. Stanford HAI. Published 2023. Accessed 30 April 2023. https://hai.stanford.edu/news/ai-will-transform-teaching-and-learning-lets-get-it-right.
13. Wilson J, Daugherty P. Collaborative intelligence: humans and AI are joining forces. Harv Bus Rev. Published online July 1, 2018. Accessed 30 April 2023. https://hbr.org/2018/07/collaborative-intelligence-humans-and-ai-are-joining-forces.
14. Tucker B. How will AI and deepfake technology affect the 2024 election? - The Washington Post. The Washington Post. Published 2023. Accessed 30 April 2023. https://www.washingtonpost.com/politics/2023/04/17/ai-deep-fake-technology-election-2024/.
15. Vincent J. Twitter taught Microsoft's AI chatbot to be a racist asshole in less than a day. The Verge. Published March 24, 2016. Accessed 30 April 2023. https://www.theverge.com/2016/3/24/11297050/tay-microsoft-chatbot-racist.
16. Martindale J. How to jailbreak ChatGPT: get it to really do what you want. Digital Trends. Published April 7, 2023. Accessed 30 April 2023. https://www.digitaltrends.com/computing/how-to-jailbreak-chatgpt/.

# Cyberbullying and Social Media

Robin M. Kowalski, Gary W. Giumetti,
Justin Patchin, Shelia R. Cotten, and Wendy Craig

## 1 Background

Research on cyberbullying has increased rapidly over the last 15 years, with a particular focus in recent years on cyberbullying occurring on social media platforms. This form of bullying is quite prevalent and has been linked with detrimental outcomes for young people (from elementary school-aged children through college students), including decreased life satisfaction and increased depression, anxiety, psychological distress, and suicidal ideation [1–4]. In this chapter, we examine the current state of the research in this area, uncover limitations of the existing research, and identify ways forward for future researchers and practitioners.

### 1.1 Definitions

Cyberbullying can be conceptualized as "an aggressive, intentional act carried out by a group or individual, using electronic forms of contact, repeatedly and over time against a victim who cannot easily defend him- or herself." [5] It can be experienced by children, adolescents, as well as adults, with most research focusing on adolescents, among whom its prevalence is highest [5, 6]. Some examples of cyberbullying behaviors include others sending hurtful messages, spreading gossip about others, and getting others to disclose private information that is then shared online. Cyberbullying occurs through text messages, chats, emails, and through social media. We define social media as internet-based communication networks where individuals self-generate content and interact with other individuals and groups in real-time or asynchronously [7]. The most common platforms for social media include Instagram, Facebook, Twitter, Snapchat, and TikTok.

## 2 Current State

### 2.1 Social Media Use

Social media continues to evolve as does how youth use it. Some social media that existed 5 years ago do not exist today, and new social media platforms have emerged during this time. With 95% of 13–17-year-olds owning a smartphone and 97% reporting use of the Internet daily, youth use social media at high levels, though specific types of social media usage vary [8].

R. M. Kowalski (✉) · S. R. Cotten
Clemson University, Clemson, SC, USA
e-mail: rkowals@clemson.edu

G. W. Giumetti
Quinnipiac University, Hamden, CT, USA

J. Patchin
University of Wisconsin-Eau Claire,
Eau Claire, WI, USA

W. Craig
Queen's University, Kingston, ON, Canada


D. A. Christakis, L. Hale (eds.), *Handbook of Children and Screens*,
https://doi.org/10.1007/978-3-031-69362-5_59

In a 2022 survey of U.S. youth aged 13–17, YouTube was the most frequently reported social media platform used (95%), followed by TikTok (67%), Instagram (62%), and Snapchat (59%) [8]. This finding is hardly surprising given that 80% of U.S. parents with a child aged 5–11 reported that their child watches videos on YouTube [9]. Facebook use has declined substantially among teens over the past decade (71% in 2014–2015 vs. 32% in 2022), and those who do use it report they are less frequent users compared to other social media platforms [8].

Thirty-five percent of teens surveyed by Pew indicated that they use some type of social media "almost constantly"; YouTube, TikTok, Snapchat, and Instagram were the most frequently reported for "almost constant" use. TikTok and Snapchat are the most often cited platforms that teens report using daily (86%) [8]. Over a third of teens (36%) reported spending too much time on social media. Over half of teens (54%) reported that it would be hard for them to give up social media, with girls being more likely to report this than boys (58% vs. 49%).

Less is known about the use of social media by children younger than 13 years of age. Given age guidelines on many social media platforms, usage by young children is lower than for teens. However, one recent study found TikTok (29.8%), Snapchat (15.9%), and Instagram (15.3%) to be popular social media platforms among youth 9–12 years of age [10]. YouTube also seems to be prevalent among younger children, as reported by their parents. A U.S. study of parents with at least one child aged 11 and younger found that 80% of children used YouTube, 13% TikTok, 10% Snapchat, 5% Instagram, and 3% Facebook [9]. Among parents whose child used at least one social media platform, 20% reported that their child spends too much time on social media. Most parents (78%) reported that it was unacceptable for youth to use social media at ages younger than 12 years. Though 96% of parents report that their child has not been exposed to cyberbullying, 56% of parents are concerned that their child may be bullied or harassed online. These statistics lie in sharp contrast to data collected on tweens ages 9–12 showing that 15% report having been a target of cyberbullying [10].

## 2.2 Prevalence of Cyberbullying on Social Media and Associated Outcomes

Prevalence rates of cyberbullying vary across studies and across modalities. This variability is due, in part, to differences in the time parameter used to assess cyberbullying (previous 30 days, school year, lifetime), the term used to reference the behavior (cyberbullying, cyber harassment, online harassment), the criteria for classifying cyberbullying (e.g., at least once; 2–3 times or more), as well as the platform(s) on which the behavior occurs [11]. Across platforms, prevalence rates of cyberbullying victimization among youth ages 10–19 range from 3% to 72% [11]. Not surprisingly, given the wide use of social media among young people, it has become a particularly common platform for cyberbullying victimization to occur [12, 13], with one study finding that teen users of social media were almost 6 times more likely to experience cyberbullying victimization than youth who did not use social media [3]. In a scoping review of studies examining cyberbullying via social media among adolescents 12–18 years of age, 23% reported cyberbullying victimization and 15.2% reported perpetrating cyberbullying [3, 14]. College students also report frequent cyberbullying victimization via social media with 19% of students from a university in the northwestern United States reporting having been cyberbullied through social media [15].

Victims of cyberbullying via social media often report increased anxiety, depression, and suicidal ideation, decreased life satisfaction, reduced academic performance, and increased physical health symptomology [1–4]. Perpetrators and witnesses to cyberbullying also experience increased depression and anxiety, with perpetrators also showing aggressive behavior and substance use [16]. The high prevalence rates and adverse outcomes that follow from involvement in cyberbullying highlight the need for effective prevention and intervention efforts.

## 2.3 Cyberbullying and Social Media Across Countries

Although cyberbullying is a fairly common form of online misbehavior, evidence suggests that there are differences in prevalence across countries. Cross-national studies facilitate the identification of universal patterns and potential mechanisms in cyberbullying, as well as an examination of country- or societal-level macro-factors that may influence cyberbullying. Few studies have compared the prevalence rates of cyberbullying across countries. A notable exception is the Health Behavior Survey of School Aged Children (HBSC), a cross-sectional study conducted every 4 years in over 50 countries. In the 2017–2018 HBSC study on 180,919 adolescents aged 11, 13, and 15, the prevalence rates of cyberbullying perpetration and victimization were highly variable across countries, as well as by age and gender [17]. For example, the proportion of adolescents who had perpetrated cyberbullying ranged from 0.7% among 11-year-old girls in Greece to 31% among 15-year-old boys in Latvia. The proportion of adolescents who had been targeted ranged from 2.2% among 13-year-old boys in Albania to 28.5% among 15-year-old boys in Lithuania. Regarding age, cyberbullying perpetration peaked among 15-year-old boys in half of the countries, whereas it peaked among girls at age 13. Similarly, in about one-third of the countries, girls were most likely to be cyberbullied at age 13. For boys, there were inconsistent age-related differences in cybervictimization across countries [18].

Across countries, rates of cyber victimization and perpetration are influenced by social media use. In an international study in 42 countries, problematic social media use was positively correlated with cybervictimization and perpetration [17]. Furthermore, the relationships among cyberbullying involvement and social media use were stronger for girls than boys in most countries for both behaviors. These results suggest that problematic social media use may expose youth to social and gender norms that validate and reinforce aggression.

## 2.4 The School's Responsibility in Responding to Cyberbullying on Social Media

Although the prevalence rates of cyberbullying vary across countries, these behaviors tend to happen among peers from school [19], where policy and legal issues come into play. These policy and legal issues are critical to address because of the need for consistency in responding to cyberbullying and the need to address what aspects of policies are associated with lower rates of cyberbullying. When students target classmates, schools may be required to take action. Schools have an obligation, for example, to ensure the safety of students in their buildings. As such, any threats that implicate students at school must be investigated and addressed. But what about incidents that do not involve clear threats?

The longstanding benchmark for whether schools in the United States can discipline students for their speech was established in the 1969 landmark Supreme Court case *Tinker v. Des Moines* [20]. In this case, the Court famously ruled that students do not shed their free speech rights at the schoolhouse gate. The Court further stated, however, that "conduct by the student, *in class or out of it*, which for any reason whether it stems from *time*, *place*, or type of behavior—materially disrupts classwork or involves substantial disorder or invasion of the rights of others is, of course, not immunized by the constitutional guarantee of freedom of speech" (emphasis added). Over time, then, this "substantial disruption" standard has been used to determine whether schools have the authority to intervene when student behavior away from school (or online) affects students or staff at school. As the Fourth Circuit concluded in *Kowalski v. Berkeley County Schools* (2011) [21], where a student created a MySpace page intimating that a classmate had herpes, "such harassment and bullying is inappropriate and hurtful and…it must be taken seriously by school administrators in order to preserve an appropriate pedagogical environment." And with respect to the location of the speech, the court noted: "where such speech has a sufficient nexus with the school, the Constitution is not written to hinder school administrators' good faith efforts to address the problem."

The Supreme Court effectively reaffirmed this standard in a 2021 case involving a student's weekend Snapchat post. While the Court ultimately ruled that the school was wrong to punish the student for her off-campus profane social media rant, it also made clear that "we do not believe the special characteristics that give schools additional license to regulate student speech always disappear when a school regulates speech that takes place off campus. The school's regulatory interests remain significant in some off-campus circumstances…includ(ing) serious or severe bullying or harassment targeting particular individuals…." [22].

Another important consideration is the appropriateness and reasonableness of the school response to social media cyberbullying. Courts tend to get involved only when a student is expelled or suspended from school for an extended period (or, in the exceptional case of *B.L.*, dismissed from an extracurricular activity). These extreme responses are rarely necessary in all but the most pernicious or persistent cyberbullying. Informal responses that address the behavior but keep students in school are preferred.

## 3 Future Research

Thus far, we have reviewed evidence showing that social media use is nearly ubiquitous among youth and that cyberbullying via social media is both prevalent and linked with possible negative outcomes for users. We have also demonstrated that the prevalence of these behaviors varies by gender and across countries. Additionally, we explored schools' responsibility in responding to cyberbullying. As we noted at the outset of this chapter, research on cyberbullying via social media is still in its relative infancy (compared to the larger literature on traditional bullying). As such, we can highlight several directions for future researchers to explore.

- What are the long-term effects of exposure to cyberbullying victimization and perpetration via social media? For example, what effects does exposure to cyberbullying via social media as either a victim or a perpetrator in middle or high school have on an adult in the workplace or a parent raising children in the digital age?
- Self-report estimates of technology use, including social media, are often unreliable [23, 24]. Though privacy issues are of concern, being able to obtain objective device use data is needed if we are to have accurate and reliable assessments of social media use. To obtain objective use data will require researchers to work with device providers or to install monitoring apps on devices. Both options are challenging for researchers.
- Given the relatively high percentage of people who have witnessed cyberbullying on social media, how do we get those witnesses to stand up for those who are targeted without risking victimization themselves?
- Do schools have a legal obligation to respond to cyberbullying on social media that happens outside of school? Future research should explore the most effective school-based strategies for handling cyberbullying. Ultimately the purpose of any intervention is to stop the bullying and to ensure a safe learning environment for all students. This research should include an examination of how countries vary in their legally required responses to cyberbullying and how these responses relate to the prevalence of cyberbullying victimization and perpetration. In addition, surveys of cyberbullying behavior in schools should ask students whether they reported the cyberbullying behavior and what effect the reporting had.
- Social power is a key characteristic of bullying in general, including cyberbullying. The social-ecological perspective highlights the importance of many factors, such as parents,

schools, communities, and governments, in shaping developmental contexts, including access to and use of power. More research is needed that explicitly examines the role of social power, privilege, and oppression at each level of the social ecological model. International studies can provide a unique opportunity to examine the macro-level societal factors, such as inequality, gender norms, and legislation, that may be particularly relevant in this understanding. Further, country-level differences in cyberbullying may be explained by country-level variation in other structural issues, such as access to the internet.

## 4 Recommendations

- While considerable strides have been made in our understanding of the prevalence and outcomes of cyberbullying victimization and perpetration, the ever-changing nature of the venues by which the behavior occurs and the frequency of use of these venues necessitates ongoing research and theorizing.
- Regarding social media use, nuanced and objective use data are rarely available. The majority of research on social media use focuses on teenagers; less is known about how young children or older adults use social media.
- Most studies focusing on youth and social media use are cross-sectional in nature, thus limiting understanding of within-person variation over time as well as assessments of the causes and consequences of this use. However, longitudinal studies to better ascertain social media use and impacts over time are costly and complex. Funding organizations need to recognize the importance of long-term studies focused on technology use more generally and social media use more specifically, if researchers are to parse out the short- and long-term effects of technology, social media use, and cyberbullying on youth.
- Future research should also more precisely explore the relationship between cyberbullying that occurs on social media and school outcomes (e.g., safety, academic success, school climate, deviance) to demonstrate the importance of schools intervening in reasonable and evidence-based ways. This research could be extended to the workplace to explore the relationship between cyberbullying via social media and work-related outcomes, such as techno-stress, job satisfaction, absenteeism, and turnover.
- Finally, the cross-national research highlights the importance of testing a social ecological model for cyberbullying perpetration and victimization. In addition to well-established individual-level factors associated with involvement in cyberbullying, macro-level societal influences need to also be considered. International research is critical to understanding and identifying these country-level macro-factors that may explain the age and gender patterns and the influence of societal factors in cyberbullying perpetration and victimization.

**Conflict of Interest and Funding Disclosures** None.

## References

1. Albdour M, Hong J, Lewin L, Yarandi H. The impact of cyberbullying on physical and psychological health of Arab American adolescents. J Immigr Minor Health. 2019:21. https://doi.org/10.1007/s10903-018-00850-w.
2. Cao X, Khan AN, Zaigham GHK, Khan NA. The stimulators of social media fatigue among students: role of moral disengagement. J Educ Comput Res. 2019;57:1083–107. https://doi.org/10.1177/0735633118781907.
3. Sampasa-Kanyinga H, Hamilton HA. Social networking sites and mental health problems in adolescents: the mediating role of cyberbullying victimization. Eur Psychiatry. 2015;30(8):1021–7. https://doi.org/10.1016/j.eurpsy.2015.09.011.
4. Viner RM, Gireesh A, Stiglic N, et al. Roles of cyberbullying, sleep, and physical activity in mediating the effects of social media use on mental health and wellbeing among young people in England: a secondary analysis of longitudinal data. Lancet Child Adoles Health. 2019;3(10):685–96. https://doi.org/10.1016/S2352-4642(19)30186-5.

5. Smith PK, Mahdavi J, Carvalho M, Fisher S, Russell S, Tippett N. Cyberbullying: its nature and impact in secondary school pupils. J Child Psychol Psychiatry. 2008;49:376–85. https://doi.org/10.1111/j.1469-7610.2007.01846.x.
6. Kowalski RM, Giumetti GW, Schroeder AN, Lattanner MR. Bullying in the digital age: a critical review and meta-analysis of cyberbullying research among youth. Psychol Bull. 2014;140:1073–137. https://doi.org/10.1037/a0035618.
7. Bayer JB, Triệu P, Ellison NB. Social media elements, ecologies, and effects. Annu Rev Psychol. 2020;71:471–97. https://doi.org/10.1146/annurev-psych-010419-050944.
8. Teens, social media, and technology. Pew Research Center Web site. https://www.pewresearch.org/internet/2022/08/10/teens-social-media-and-technology-2022/. Updated 2022. Accessed 2 Jan 2022.
9. Parenting children in the age of screens. Pew Research Center Web site. https://www.pewresearch.org/internet/2020/07/28/parenting-children-in-the-age-of-screens/. Updated 2020. Accessed 2 Jan 2022.
10. Patchin JW, Hinduja S. Tween cyberbullying in 2020. https://i.cartoonnetwork.com/stop-bullying/pdfs/CN_Stop_Bullying_Cyber_Bullying_Report_9.30.20.pdf. Updated 2020. Accessed 10 March 2023.
11. Selkie EM, Fales JL, Moreno MA. Cyberbullying prevalence among US middle and high school-aged adolescents: a systematic review and quality assessment. J Adolesc Health. 2016;58(2):125–33. https://doi.org/10.1016/j.jadohealth.2015.09.026.
12. Chan TKH, Cheung CMK, Lee ZWY. Cyberbullying on social networking sites: a literature review and future research directions. Inf Manag. 2021;58(2):103411. https://doi.org/10.1016/j.im.2020.103411.
13. Whittaker E, Kowalski RM. Cyberbullying via social media. J Sch Violence. 2015;14:11–29. https://doi.org/10.1080/15388220.2014.949377.
14. Hamm MP, Newton AS, Chisholm A, et al. Prevalence and effect of cyberbullying on children and young people: a scoping review of social media studies. JAMA Pediatr. 2015;169(8):770–7. https://doi.org/10.1001/jamapediatrics.2015.0944.
15. Gahagan K, Vaterlaus JM, Frost LR. College student cyberbullying on social networking sites: conceptualization, prevalence, and perceived bystander responsibility. Comput Hum Behav. 2016;55:1097–105. https://doi.org/10.1016/j.chb.2015.11.019.
16. Evangelio C, Rodríguez-González P, Fernández-Río J, Gonzalez-Villora S. Cyberbullying in elementary and middle school students: a systematic review. Comput Educ. 2022;176:104356. https://doi.org/10.1016/j.compedu.2021.104356.
17. Craig W, Boniel-Nissim M, King N, et al. Social media use and cyber-bullying: a cross-national analysis of young people in 42 countries. J Adolesc Health. 2020;66(6, Supplement):S100–S108. https://doi.org/10.1016/j.jadohealth.2020.03.006.
18. Inchley J, Currie D, Budisavljevic S, et al. Spotlight on adolescent health and well-being. findings from the 2017/2018 health behaviour in school-aged children (HBSC) survey in Europe and Canada. international report. volume 2. Key data. 2020. World Health Organization. Regional Office for Europe. https://apps.who.int/iris/handle/10665/332104. License: CC BY-NC-SA 3.0 IGO.
19. Hinduja S. In: Patchin JW, editor. Bullying beyond the schoolyard: preventing and responding to cyberbullying. 2nd ed. Sage; 2015.
20. Tinker v. Des Moines independent community school district. 393 U.S. 503, 1969.
21. Kowalski v. Berkeley county schools, et al. No. 10–1098 (4th Cir. 2011).
22. Mahanoy area school district v. B. L. 594 U.S. No. 20–255, 2021.
23. Deng T, Kanthawala S, Meng J, et al. Measuring smartphone usage and task switching with log tracking and self-reports. Mobile Med Commun. 2019;7(1):3–23. https://doi.org/10.1177/2050157918761491.
24. Ellis DA, Davidson BI, Shaw H, Geyer K. Do smartphone usage scales predict behavior? Int J Human-Comput Stud. 2019;130:86–92. https://doi.org/10.1016/j.ijhcs.2019.05.004.

# Digital Cruelty's Impact on Self-Esteem and Body Image

Kaitlyn Burnell, Jolien Trekels,
Madeleine J. George, and Jacqueline Nesi

## 1 Background

Adolescents' frequent use of digital technologies [1] has raised questions about its effects. Although there are benefits to digital technology use [2], the affordances of digital platforms like social media have led to particular concern about digital cruelty (defined as the deliberate, targeted transmission of negative content). Techno-developmental theories have identified numerous features of devices or platforms that can alter how adolescents navigate developmental changes [3, 4], with some features bearing special relevance to the frequency and consequences of digital cruelty. Many platforms provide quantifiable feedback in the form of likes and comments. This feedback can signal social approval and potentially be used to transmit cruelty digitally. Digital content is often public, permanent, and replicable, allowing for the resharing of material and exposure of content to a relatively large audience. Because of this, negative feedback can be seen by a large group of people and stay visible for a long period of time, which may exacerbate negative effects. Digital content is also often visual with editing tools at users' disposal. Carefully curated posts are often on display, with these posts frequently idealized in the context of physical appearance [5]. Users can also engage with many digital platforms anonymously, which in turn can enhance disinhibition and the transmission of negative content.

These affordances collectively may enhance an adolescent's risk of exposure to cruel digital content, which in turn may result in digital technology use that is particularly damaging to self-esteem and body image. How adolescents view their appearance is strongly tied to their overall sense of self-worth [6]. Adolescence is a time of heightened body dissatisfaction, particularly for girls [7]. Compounding these body image concerns are normative pubertal changes that may move an adolescent's body further from societal standards of beauty (e.g., increased fat) [8], and increased exposure to media content that often depicts unattainable beauty ideals [5, 9]. With these developmental challenges in mind, this review discusses the topic of digital cruelty and its relation to self-esteem and body image

K. Burnell (✉)
The University of North Carolina at Chapel Hill, Chapel Hill, NC, USA

Winston National Center on Technology Use, Brain, and Psychological Development, Chapel Hill, NC, USA
e-mail: burnellk@unc.edu

J. Trekels
The University of North Carolina at Chapel Hill, Chapel Hill, NC, USA

M. J. George
RTI International, Durham, NC, USA

J. Nesi
Brown University, Providence, RI, USA


D. A. Christakis, L. Hale (eds.), *Handbook of Children and Screens*,
https://doi.org/10.1007/978-3-031-69362-5_60

concerns, with a special focus on how digital cruelty occurs in the appearance context.

We define digital cruelty as the deliberate, targeted transmission of negative content in digital environments. Given the appearance-oriented nature of the digital spaces that adolescents are most immersed in and our focus on body image concerns as a central outcome of digital engagement, we give special attention to appearance-oriented digital cruelty and the implications that this form of cruelty has for self-esteem and body image. We focus primarily on mean, aggressive, or harassing messages or commentary (e.g., teasing or bullying), as past research has usually examined digital cruelty in this context. However, we also acknowledge that digital cruelty can take on various forms, including (but not limited to) the unwanted transmission of digital content to others (e.g., forwarding an unflattering image that the subject does not want to be transmitted) or the use of digital tools to engage in conflictual behaviors in person (e.g., online-offline spillover; unwanted or unauthorized tracking behavior). We do not consider content that is not willfully harmful for self-esteem and body image, such as exposure to idealized media content that induces harmful upward comparisons or promotes the internalization of beauty ideals [5].

Moreover, a distinction is needed between cruelty that reflects interpersonal conflict (e.g., drama among peers) [10] and cruelty that may reflect cyberbullying, which is characterized by repetition and a power imbalance between the perpetrator and the victim [11]. Although we consider appearance-oriented cyberbullying, we do not consider cyberbullying more broadly due to the large body of existing research examining cyberbullying and its implications for youth well-being (including for poorer self-esteem and appearance esteem) [12, 13]. Additionally, we consider a variety of digital technologies in our review but pay particular attention to social media platforms given their popularity and the visual nature of many platforms (e.g., TikTok, Instagram, Snapchat) [1], which may increase the exposure to and production of appearance-focused content.

## 2 Current State

Studies on digital "body talk" (i.e., discussions centered on one's own and others' appearance) indicate that although positive appearance commentary is normative on social media, negative commentary directly targeting peers' posts is rare [14, 15]. Adolescents make careful distinctions between negative commentary that is deliberate and bully-like and negative commentary that is joking and without malintent [14]. This indicates that although some negative commentary may appear cruel to an outside observer, this may not necessarily be the case for the parties involved. Observational research with college students suggests that instances of negative commentary are often made sarcastically or in jest [16]. Studies to date suggest that receipt of negative commentary is not robustly linked to greater body image concerns or poorer appearance esteem [15–17], although there is some evidence for associations when such commentary is extremely negative [18]. Additionally, digital avenues may be used as a tool to speak negatively of or gossip about the physical appearance of those who are outside of a digital conversation [19], which poses risk if the target of such messages becomes aware of these exchanges (e.g., through screenshots).

As past research has demonstrated inconsistent associations between the receipt of negative commentary and psychosocial outcomes, negative effects of receiving such commentary may occur only under specific circumstances or for specific individuals. How commentary manifests may be gendered; for example, appearance teasing directed toward boys may be specifically targeted to their masculinity [20]. Girls may be especially vulnerable to appearance-related teasing [21] and fall victim to digital appearance-teasing more often than boys [20]. In general, girls may experience greater appearance-related pressures than boys. For example, pubertal changes move girls further away from societal standards of beauty, and for girls, physical appearance may be more tightly linked to social status [5]. Because of this, girls may experience increased pressure to curate physically attractive online self-presentations and be especially attuned to the feedback they receive on these self-presentations [22]. In turn, girls may be more sensitive to commentary and feedback perceived as negative. Qualitative evidence suggests that adolescent girls who have previously been bullied for their appearance report feeling extra pressure to post attractive (and edited) images of themselves online [22]. Although these curated posts may momentarily boost appearance and overall self-esteem [22], research is needed on the long-term effects of these behaviors. For example, adolescents may become reliant on engaging in inauthentic self-presentation to receive positive feedback. Because edited images do not reflect one's "actual" self, continuous posting of these images (encouraged by positive feedback) may increase a discrepancy between one's real and ideal self over time, thereby harming one's overall self-esteem.

Adolescents also may direct negative online commentary to their own appearance. Studies on both social media use and text messaging indicate that adolescents engage in negative commentary that is self-deprecating [14, 19], which may be strategically used to elicit positive feedback in response ("compliment fishing") [14]. This strategy may represent a form of self-directed digital cruelty that may have negative effects for both the sender and recipient of this commentary. For example, the sender may ruminate on a perceived appearance flaw, perhaps especially if the self-deprecating comment was triggered by a picture uploaded by someone else that the sender cannot necessarily remove from the virtual world. The receiver may feel motivated to respond with their own self-deprecation, fixating on an appearance flaw when they otherwise may not have [19]. Over time, such exchanges may also increase an overall focus on physical appearance within adolescent friend groups.

Collectively, findings suggest that digital cruelty in the form of negative commentary is rare and complex. Associations with body image and self-esteem are mixed, likely due to varying methods for assessing motivators and perceptions of such commentary. When negative commentary is willful and malicious, it likely has powerful implications for body image and self-esteem, potentially for both direct recipients and passive observers. However, when commentary is self-inflicted or humorous, associations vary.

We have reviewed studies on negative commentary that fit squarely into our definition of digital cruelty, in which negative content is willfully transmitted. However, there can also be more subtle forms of cruelty that are more complicated to measure. One such example pertains to the receipt of purely quantifiable metrics of social approval, such as likes. Many adolescents report posting self-oriented images on social media with the goal of obtaining likes and other forms of feedback, such as comments, views, and shares [22, 23], and qualitative research among college students indicates that not receiving enough likes on one's pictures can negatively affect appearance esteem and prompt deleting of the post [24]. Adolescents report involving their friends to provide likes on their posts and that liking each other's posts is a sign of support and friendship [23]. Failing to receive this feedback may result in negative psychosocial effects, including poorer self-esteem and concerns about one's attractiveness in a photo or video. Although these studies suggest that the receipt of likes is important for body image and self-esteem, investigations are needed that parse "benign" reasons for lacking likes (e.g., key audience members not seeing posts) from malicious reasons more in line with digital cruelty (e.g., deliberately refraining from liking content, such as when requested by friends). Contemporary features of mainstream social media platforms (e.g., Instagram stories) allow users to see when a post was viewed but not liked. Given that providing likes is perceived as a signal of support and friendship [23], an adolescent who sees that a person of interest viewed a post and did not like it may interpret this lack of feedback as cruel. Indeed, qualitative evidence suggests that adolescents may use this strategy as a way of expressing disapproval of one's physical appearance, as this is more acceptable than providing explicit negative commentary [14]. Assessing an adolescent's perceptions and subjective experiences is essential to inform when behaviors are viewed as cruel, and there is likely much heterogeneity in these reports.

Critically, the features of digital tools lead to qualitatively different experiences online compared to offline [3, 4]. The disinhibition that can occur online may result in the transmission of negative comments that may have never been said in person. Some adolescents perceive that digital appearance comments may occur as a way of gaining status or likes [22], reflecting the power of digital social approval. The publicness and permanence of digital content may result in digital cruelty being broadcast to a large audience and subsequent re-exposure (intentional or unintentional), prolonging hurtful experiences [25]. Adolescents who may never have witnessed others' negative commentary may find themselves encountering this content through screenshots, resharing of conversations, or while scrolling comments directed to other people. Even if this commentary is not directed to the self, it is possible that reading others' commentary may trigger an adolescent to appraise their own appearance and sense of self when they otherwise may not have (e.g., reading negative weight comments may contribute to an appraisal about one's own weight). Although appearance-related digital cruelty may be rare, much is still unknown about its nuanced forms and how broad exposure and receipt may be associated with self-esteem and body image.

## 3 Future Research

Research is needed in multiple areas to elucidate the ways in which appearance-based digital cruelty occurs and its effects on self-esteem. First, what characteristics influence associations among digital cruelty, self-esteem, and body image? Research carefully separating negative commentary that is malicious from commentary that is "benign" is needed to help reconcile mixed past findings. More complex measures, as opposed to time spent or frequency of use, are needed to fully capture nuanced effects. Digital technologies are complex, effects are not uniform, and distinctive features (i.e., editing and posting pictures, interacting with others, exposure) and types of content (i.e., permanent vs. ephemeral content) allow for multiple types of digital cruelty. Mixed-methods approaches may more reliably and comprehensively assess how young people engage with content on social media and how it affects their self-esteem, especially related to appearance [26]. Combining objective measures (e.g., data traces) that assess adolescents' online activities with measures of adolescents' intentions, feelings, and reactions (e.g., through stimulated recall methods) [27] can expand the type of questions we ask and further understanding of specific experiences that may be especially harmful to self-esteem and body image. Other studies may combine eye-tracking and survey methods to help tackle the complexity of digital content by pinpointing the content to which youth are exposed and visually attend and separating negative (e.g., teasing) and positive [28] (e.g., body positive messages such as self-love) appearance-focused experiences. Attention should also be given to potential platform differences, such as by exploring how digital cruelty can differentially manifest on visual versus text-based platforms.

Second, how fleeting or long-term are the effects of digital cruelty on self-esteem and body image, and do these effects differ at the within- and the between-person level? Ecological momentary assessments (EMA) should be utilized to capture the co-fluctuations of digital cruelty and self-esteem on a momentary basis. These designs can better capture within-person associations to determine if higher (or lower) levels of certain types of social media use in a given hour or day are related to self-esteem and body image concerns. The use of these designs can complement longitudinal approaches that can determine potential long-term and accumulating effects.

Third, how does gender influence associations among digital cruelty, self-esteem, and body image? Research on social media use and its effects on body image most often includes girls and women, but boys can also fall victim to negative appearance comments [20]. Research examining underrepresented groups such as gender minority adolescents is extremely limited. Examining the association between digital cruelty with self-esteem and body image concerns of gender minority adolescents is highly relevant considering their reported harassment offline and how it affects their sense of self [29].

Fourth, how may digital cruelty manifest in forms other than social feedback (i.e., likes and comments)? More research should examine the use of digital technologies as a tool, in addition to a unique mode, to transmit cruelty. For example, unflattering pictures of others can be circulated among the peer group. Additionally, less attention has been paid to the interaction between online and offline spaces, in that the consequences of engaging in or being victimized by digital cruelty can be experienced both online and offline (i.e., online-offline spillover).

Finally, how might online advertisers take advantage of the body image struggles that many adolescents face? Adolescence is a time of body image volatility, with social media platforms playing a key role in body image experiences for contemporary adolescents [5]. Advertisers may capitalize on these struggles by developing marketing approaches that target adolescents' ongoing insecurities, thereby representing another potential subtle form of digital cruelty.

## 4 Recommendations

Appearance-oriented digital cruelty may be relatively uncommon, and its effects are nuanced. However, under certain circumstances, digital cruelty can have serious implications for adolescents' self-esteem and body image. As types of online activity and content are nearly infinite, there are no universal experiences or solutions. However, we list here a few recommendations for supporting healthy social media use:

- *Open Strong Lines of Communication:* Adolescents should seek help or guidance about negative online experiences. Parents, clinicians, and teachers should recognize that adolescents are immersed in digital environments, and measures that severely restrict or ban use are unlikely to be effective and may even backfire (e.g., youth not disclosing experiencing digital cruelty in fear of losing technology access) [30]. Efforts should be geared toward creating a safe environment for teens to talk about their experiences.
- *Develop Healthy Digital Habits:* Families can create a family media plan with rules and boundaries around social media use for all members. Teens can be educated about ways to identify and avoid harmful online content and engage in responsible digital behavior (e.g., privacy, security).
- *Involve Adolescents in Finding Solutions:* Youth Advisory Boards can involve adolescents in finding ways to best respond to negative comments (e.g., removing or flagging a post, blocking users), in which adolescent ideas can be explored more fully in research and implemented in practice if effective. Adolescents should be involved in decisions regarding technology monitoring and restriction, with media plans adjusted as circumstances change. For example, monitoring plans for 12-year-olds are likely not developmentally appropriate for 17-year-olds. Adults should model behaviors that demonstrate healthy digital technology use and to help teens build self-confidence in online spaces.
- *Seek Professional Care When Needed:* Digital cruelty can have serious impacts on self-esteem and body image. Seeking mental health care can help mitigate negative exposure effects.

**Conflict of Interest and Funding Disclosures** KB is supported by the Winston Family Foundation. JN writes Techno Sapiens, a psychology newsletter for which she receives subscription and sponsor payments. She is co-owner of Tech Without Stress, LLC, which provides free and paid resources for parents raising children in the digital age.

## References

1. Vogels EA, Gelles-Watnick R, Massarat N. Teens, social media, and technology 2022. Pew Research Center; 2022. https://www.pewresearch.org/internet/2022/08/10/teens-social-media-and-technology-2022/.

2. Best P, Manktelow R, Taylor B. Online communication, social media and adolescent wellbeing: a systematic narrative review. Child Youth Serv Rev. 2014;41:27–36. https://doi.org/10.1016/j.childyouth.2014.03.001.
3. Moreno MA, Uhls YT. Applying an affordances approach and a developmental lens to approach adolescent social media use. Digit Health. 2019;5:1–6. https://doi.org/10.1177/2055207619826678.
4. Nesi J, Choukas-Bradley S, Prinstein MJ. Transformation of adolescent peer relations in the social media context: part 1—a theoretical framework and application to dyadic peer relationships. Clin Child Fam Psychol Rev. 2018;21:267–94. https://doi.org/10.1007/s10567-018-0261-x.
5. Choukas-Bradley S, Roberts SR, Maheux AJ, Nesi J. The perfect storm: a developmental-sociocultural framework for the role of social media in adolescent girls' body image concerns and mental health. Clin Child Fam Psychol Rev. 2022;24(4):681–701. https://doi.org/10.1007/s10567-022-00404-5.
6. Harter S. The construction of the self: developmental and sociocultural foundations. 2nd ed. The Guilford Press; 2012.
7. Lawler M, Nixon E. Body dissatisfaction among adolescent boys and girls: the effects of body mass, peer appearance culture and internalization of appearance ideals. J Youth Adolesc. 2011;40:59–71. https://doi.org/10.1007/s10964-009-9500-2.
8. Klump KL. Puberty as a critical risk period for eating disorders: a review of human and animal studies. Horm Behav. 2013;64(2):399–410. https://doi.org/10.1016/j.yhbeh.2013.02.019.
9. Fredrickson BL, Roberts TA. Objectification theory: toward understanding women's lived experiences and mental health risks. Psychol Women. 1997;21(2):173–206.
10. Marwick A, Boyd D. 'It's just drama': teen perspectives on conflict and aggression in a networked era. J Youth Stud. 2014;17(9):1187–204. https://doi.org/10.1080/13676261.2014.901493.
11. Olweus D. Cyberbullying: a critical overview. In: Bushman BJ, editor. Aggression and violence, a social psychological perspective. New York: Routledge; 2017. p. 225–40.
12. Lei H, Mao W, Cheong CM, Wen Y, Cui Y, Cai Z. The relationship between self-esteem and cyberbullying: a meta-analysis of children and youth students. Curr Psychol. 2020;39:830–42. https://doi.org/10.1007/s12144-019-00407-6.
13. Olenik-Shemesh D, Heiman T. Cyberbullying victimization in adolescents as related to body esteem, social support, and social self-efficacy. J Genet Psychol. 2017;184(1):28–43. https://doi.org/10.1080/00221325.2016.1195331.
14. Paddock DL, Bell BT. "It's better saying I look fat instead of saying you look fat": a qualitative study of U.K. adolescents' understanding of appearance-related interactions on social media. J Adolesc Res. 2021. Advance Online Publication; https://doi.org/10.1177/07435584211034875.
15. Maes C, Schreurs L, van Oosten JMF, Vandenbosch L. #(Me)too much? The role of sexualizing online media in adolescents' resistance towards the metoo-movement and acceptance of rape myths. J Adolesc. 2019;77:59–69. https://doi.org/10.1016/j.adolescence.2019.10.005.
16. Burnell K, George MJ, Kurup AR, Underwood MK. "Ur a freakin goddess!": examining appearance commentary on Instagram. Psychol Popular Media. 2021;10(4):422–33. https://doi.org/10.1037/ppm0000341.
17. Feltman CE, Szymanski DM. Instagram use and self-objectification: the roles of internalization, comparison, appearance commentary, and feminism. Sex Roles. 2018;78:311–24. https://doi.org/10.1007/s11199-017-0796-1.
18. Hummel AC, Smith AR. Ask and you shall receive: desire and receipt of feedback via Facebook predicts disordered eating concerns. Int J Eat Disord. 2015;48(4):436–42.
19. Burnell K, Kurup AR, Vollet JW, Underwood MK. "So you think I'm cute?": an observational study of adolescents' appearance evaluation in text messaging. Human Behav Emerg Technol. 2021;3(5):798–810. https://doi.org/10.1037/a0040429.
20. Berne S, Frisén A, Kling J. Appearance-related cyberbullying: a qualitative investigation of characteristics, content, reasons, and effects. Body Image. 2014;11(4):527–33. https://doi.org/10.1016/j.bodyim.2014.08.006.
21. Menzel JE, Schaefer LM, Burke NL, Mayhew LL, Brannick MT, Thompson JK. Appearance-related teasing, body dissatisfaction, and disordered eating: a meta-analysis. Body Image. 2010;7(4):261–70. https://doi.org/10.1016/j.bodyim.2010.05.004.
22. Chua THH, Chang L. Follow me and like my beautiful selfies: Singapore teenage girls' engagement in self-presentation and peer comparison on social media. Comput Hum Behav. 2016;55:190–7. https://doi.org/10.1016/j.chb.2015.09.011.
23. Yau JC, Reich SM. "It's just a lot of work": adolescents' self-presentation norms and practices on Facebook and Instagram. J Res Adolesc. 2019;29(1):196–209. https://doi.org/10.1111/jora.12376.
24. Baker N, Ferszt G, Breines JG. A qualitative study exploring female college students' Instagram use and body image. Cyberpsychol Behav Soc Netw. 2019;22(4):277–82. https://doi.org/10.1089/cyber.2018.0420.
25. Underwood MK, Ehrenreich SE. The power and the pain of adolescents' digital communication: cyber victimization and the perils of lurking. Am Psychol. 2017;72(2):144–58. https://doi.org/10.1037/a0040429.
26. Jarman HK, McLean SA, Griffiths S, Teague SJ, Rodgers RF, Paxton SJ, Austen E, et al. Critical measurement issues in the assessment of social

media influence on body image. Body Image. 2023;40:225–36. https://doi.org/10.1016/j.bodyim.2021.12.007.
27. Griffioen N, Van Rooij MMJW, Lichtwarck-Aschoff A, Granic I. A stimulated recall method for the improved assessment of quantity and quality of social media use. J Med Internet Res. 2020;22(1):e15529. https://doi.org/10.2196/15529.
28. Cohen R, Fardouly J, Newton-John T, Slater A. #BoPo on Instagram: an experimental investigation of the effects of viewing body positive content on young women's mood and body image. New Media Soc. 2019;21:1546–64. https://doi.org/10.1177/1461444819826530.
29. Kosciw JG, Clark CM, Truong NL, Zongrone AG. The 2019 National School Climate Survey: the experiences of lesbian, gay, bisexual, transgender, and queer youth in our nation's schools. 2020. https://eric.ed.gov/?id=ED608534.
30. Bauman S. Cyberbullying in a rural intermediate school: an exploratory study. J Early Adolesc. 2010;30:803–33. https://doi.org/10.1177/0272431609350927.

# Criminological, Psychological, and Developmental Aspects of Pandemic Strain and Online Cruelty

Katalin Parti, Cheryl E. Sanders, Rosanna Breaux, and Meghan McCoy

## 1 Background

Following the first COVID-19 pandemic-related lockdown orders on March 15, 2020, the shift to online learning and social interactions raised concerns regarding children's development, mental health, and risk for cyberbullying [1]. Although cyberbullying does not have a universal definition [2], it is considered part of the digital cruelties that are intentional; imply power imbalance; and utilize electronic communications such as text messages, social media, or email. The term incorporates a wide range of hurtful online behaviors involving children.

Rates of digital cruelty among K-12 students either decreased or at least stagnated early in the pandemic. For example, Bacher-Hicks and colleagues (2021) [3] found a robust, 30–40% decrease in Google searches of the keyword "cyberbullying" when schools shut down, indicating both a reduction in concerns and occurrences of cyberbullying. However, searches increased again when schools started to reopen in 2021 [3]. Similarly, on a national sample of K-12 school students, Patchin and Hinduja (2022) [9] found school bullying victimization and perpetration decreased while cyberbullying stagnated during the first months of the pandemic. Research from other countries corroborated these findings. For instance, in a large sample of Canadian students, Vaillancourt et al. (2021) [4] found that bullying (general, physical, verbal, and social) decreased by 20%; however, cyberbullying decreased only by 2.3% during the COVID-19 pandemic. Nevertheless, due to children's increased online presence, European [5, 59], South American [6], and Asian [7, 31] countries reported an expansion in cyberbullying during the pandemic.

In the meantime, the pandemic fueled a surge in digital cruelties targeting Asian American and immigrant populations [32], due to the widespread misinformation and xenophobic associations of the virus with these communities, which were exacerbated by discriminatory rhetoric and social stressors. A study found that hate crimes against Asian Americans increased by 149% in 16 large American cities in 2020 [8]. Unsurprisingly, Patchin and Hinduja (2022) [9], studying a large national US sample of K-12 students, found that hate-motivated cyberbullying against Asian students increased by 59%, whereas it only increased by 29% against White/Caucasian students in 2020/21. In a subsequent longitudinal study, Patchin and Hinduja (2023) found that Asian American youth were most likely to report

K. Parti (✉) · R. Breaux
Virginia Tech, Blacksburg, VA, USA
e-mail: kparti@vt.edu

C. E. Sanders
Metropolitan State University of Denver, Denver, CO, USA

M. McCoy
Bridgewater State University, Bridgewater, MA, USA


D. A. Christakis, L. Hale (eds.), *Handbook of Children and Screens*, https://doi.org/10.1007/978-3-031-69362-5_61

increased victimization during the COVID-19 pandemic: among Asians, 23.5% said they were cyberbullied because of their race in 2021, compared to 7.4% in 2019 (compared to 23.2% of cyberbullying victimization of all youth in 2021 and 17.2% in 2019) [54]. Alsawalqa (2021) [10] examined hate-related cyberbullying in university students from East and Southeast Asia and found that cyberbullying during the pandemic was typically experienced by Asian university students who studied in a foreign country and were blamed for the outbreak and spreading of the virus [10]. Similarly, Chinese nationals residing in Western countries reported that since the COVID-19 outbreak, they have suffered discrimination and social exclusion in various forms [33]. A total of 25% of the respondents had experienced racist discrimination, and 90% of respondents inside China exhibited race-related discriminatory attitudes concerning the pandemic.

After providing a general overview of online cruelty during and in relation to the pandemic, we explore it as a possible consequence of pandemic-related strains. Examining digital cruelty from an interdisciplinary aspect of criminology, psychology, and human development sheds light on the effects of pandemic-related strains on developing deviant coping strategies in childhood and adolescence. As a takeaway, we suggest that digital cruelty in children should be examined from an interdisciplinary lens, where various disciplines contribute to the development and evaluation of prevention and intervention programs.

## 2 Current State

General strain theory (GST) posits that experiencing stress can lead to negative emotions and, ultimately, crime [15]. Strain can originate from the absence of positive stimuli, the presence of negative stimuli, and the failure to achieve desired goals [11]. Similarly, being victimized can function as negative stimuli that manifest in negative emotions such as anger, depression, or frustration and, consequently, can serve as strain. Crime enters the equation when an individual lacks the prosocial means or support to cope with the negative emotions induced by victimization [15, 16]. For individuals who lack social support and means of coping, deviant activities can serve as coping mechanisms to overcome strain. Hence, GST offers a time-ordered relation between victimization and offending, where criminal activity follows strain and victimization as a source of strain. Cyberbullying victimization and offending often overlap [56, 57], but Rebisz et al. (2023)'s sample ($N = 541$) of Polish youth found that being a victim of cyberbullying was the most important predictor of being a perpetrator of the same offense [58]. Cyberbullying may be therefore a maladaptive response to problematic situations, such as cyberbullying victimization [58]. But the equation does not end here, since crime itself can generate strain, which can manifest in subsequent offending (referred to as the "amplifying loop") [11], a concept that has been tested by examining the "cycle of violence" in child abuse [34, 35], intimate partner violence online and in traditional spaces [36, 37], and (cyber)bullying. For instance, Patchin and Hinduja (2011) [12] showed a positive relation between the number of strains (e.g., disagreement with family, money problems, being victimized) and cyberbullying. Similarly, Lianos and McGrath (2018) [13] and Paez (2018) [38] showed that academic and financial strains coupled with prior cyberbullying experiences predicted later cyberbullying perpetration. In short, GST posits that the presence of strains predicts stress that yields antisocial behavior (e.g., cyberbullying perpetration). Figure 1 is a schematic overview of GST.

Indeed, the COVID-19 pandemic produced a myriad of stressors: online schooling paired with economic recession, inflation, job losses, health concerns, and mortality and disease-related stress are potential sources of strain [14, 39]. In these circumstances, the loss of positive stimuli, the presence of negative stimuli, and the failure to achieve desired goals can be experienced. Research examining the societal impacts of the pandemic corroborates these assumptions, and it

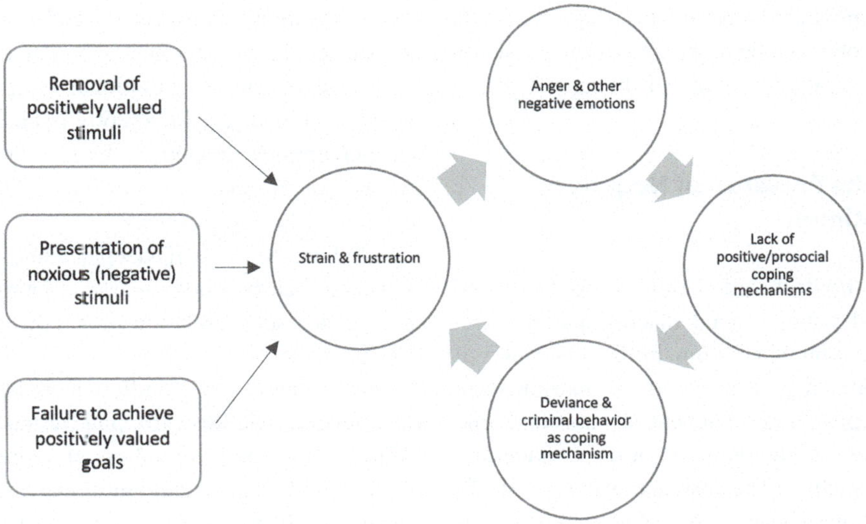


**Fig. 1** Strain and deviance. (Authors' contribution adapted from Agnew, 1992)

also highlights the critical role of adaptive coping strategies and the family context in reducing risk for digital cruelty.

## 2.1 Removal of Positively Valued Stimuli

Students were particularly stressed because of the loss of social contact during lockdowns and homeschooling. Utemissova et al. (2021) [7] examined the impact of distance learning on adolescents in the first months of the pandemic in Kazakhstan. All participants ($N = 32$) said it was terrifying that they could not rely on adults in cyberbullying situations where the offender was anonymous. Online schooling amplified this effect by removing teachers' close attention from cyberbullying perpetrators and targets. School bonding and family support were critical protective factors against child and adolescent delinquency, whereas their absence directly elevated strain [7]. Correspondingly, Rodriguez-Rivas et al. (2022) [15] conducted a cross-sectional study ($N = 287$) in six schools in Chile, testing the effects of family support on adolescents' life satisfaction and cyberbullying victimization during 2020. Family support positively predicted life satisfaction and negatively predicted cyberbullying victimization. On the other hand, family conflict positively predicted cyberbullying victimization and negatively predicted life satisfaction. The researchers concluded that positive family bonds were essential and urgent to protect adolescents from cyberbullying victimization and to promote adolescent well-being and quality of life [15]. Research corroborates the protective role of prosocial interpersonal relationships from becoming a cyberbullying offender. For example, in a 1105-subject pool of 11–19-year-old adolescents in Hungary, Arató et al. (2022) studied the combined effects of friend support, family cohesion, and prosocial coping strategies on cyberbullying perpetration and victimization. They found that support from friends was a protective factor for both cyberbullying perpetration and victimization [55]. Perceived family support was a protective factor for cyberbullying victimization, whereas balanced family cohesion (where family members support each other, but also provide autonomy and flexibility to each other) was a protective factor against cyberbullying perpetration [55]. In contrast, pandemic-induced distance learning drastically reduced prosocial peer relationships, imputing an additional strain on children's lives [16]. School closures have made it more challenging to maintain prosocial relationships, considering both prosocial supportive peer relationships and family relationships based on balanced cohesion, having a long-term impact on students' social-emotional well-being [17, 40].

## 2.2 The Presence of Negative Stimuli

Negative stimuli include being exposed to social stigma and hatred, racial discrimination, sinophobia, xenophobia, being bullied because of race or ethnicity, being part of marginalized social groups, and exposure to constant and chronic stress in the home because of pandemic-related difficulties. The designation of COVID-19 as the "Chinese virus" and "Wuhan Virus" has encouraged hate speech worldwide [18]. The loss of self-esteem as a consequence of being a target of online hatred is directly observed [9, 10]. The imminent unexpected life changes produced by the COVID-19 pandemic can lead to deviant behavior such as cyberbullying perpetration since this may be how some individuals react to stress. Bartlett et al. (2021) [19] tested strain theory in US adults and found in two cross-sectional studies that personal (e.g., being diagnosed with COVID-19) and proximal (e.g., knowing people with COVID-19) experiences were related to participants' cyberbullying perpetration due to an increase in stress.

## 2.3 Failure to Achieve Desired Goals

Losing months or years of education, and not being able to pass tests or gain admission into high school or college because of such life events as parental job loss, financial difficulties, home confinement, and online school can be significant stressors for children and adolescents [20, 41, 42]. The pandemic had and will continue to have unfavorable effects on children's and adolescent's psychological development [21, 43]. Depression, anxiety, aggression, antisocial behavior (including inappropriate digital behavior), inattention, disrespect for authority figures, and substandard academic performance are some of the behavioral and emotional symptoms that have been noted [22, 44, 45, 60]. Even individual self-perceptions support these claims. For instance, in Ezeoke and colleagues' (2022) [16] analysis, Chicago adolescents ($N$ = 55) self-reported that the COVID-19 pandemic adversely impacted their psychological well-being in three main areas: social relationships, education, and lifestyle balance.

Involvement in cyberbullying can be stressful for offenders, victims [46], and bystanders alike [47]. Victims and offenders of cyberbullying often struggle with social-emotional and psychosomatic problems and feel unsafe and uncared for in schools. In a systematic review, Bottino et al. (2015) [23] declared that cyberbullying was associated with moderate to severe depression, substance use, and suicidal ideation. The pandemic put additional strains on children, increasing depression and other mental health problems. In a study of 240 youth, Englander (2021) [24] examined the pandemic's effect on digital cruelties during the first year of the pandemic. Even though bullying, cyberbullying, sexting, and fighting showed only slight or no increases, anxiety and depression dramatically increased relative to before the pandemic. Some groups, such as female and LGBTQ youth, were particularly prone to develop mental health problems [24]. In a subsequent study, Englander (2022) [29] found that subjects who reported feeling depressed or anxious were far more likely than other subjects to also report being cyberbullied more, as the pandemic continued. Mental health problems can be significant obstacles in achieving positively valued goals, such as being able to log on to online classes, finish coursework, graduate from high school, or simply continue school online [25]. Furthermore, because school closures shifted the learning process primarily to families and students working predominantly via digital tools, they exacerbated social class academic disparities [48], putting additional strains on lower socioeconomic classes [26].

### 2.4 Coping Strategies

Although everyone experienced the adverse effects of the COVID-19 pandemic, not all individuals turned to deviance or crime to cope with emotional, mental, physical, financial, and existential strains. Agnew argues that individuals differ in their adaptations to strain due to variations in their coping mechanisms [11]. To develop healthy, nondeviant, and noncriminal coping mechanisms, one needs an environment (family, friends, school, neighborhood) where these mechanisms can be learned. The family's role can be vital in developing healthy coping strategies [49]. Han et al. (2021) [27] found that resilient coping strategies such as creative ways to alter difficult situations, controlling one's reactions, seeking to grow positively by dealing with difficult situations, and actively looking to replace the losses encountered reduced loneliness during the pandemic ($N = 1111$). In contrast, the lack of such strategies was a mediator between cyberbullying victimization and loneliness during the pandemic. In another study of Chinese adolescents ($N = 5608$) [28], problem-solving-oriented coping in adolescence was associated with less involvement in cyberbullying and less occurrence of depression. In contrast, focusing on negative emotions without constructive and empathic coping was positively correlated with cyberbullying involvement and generated more strain [28]. On a national sample of middle and high school students ($N = 1200$), Hinduja (2016) [65] found that the higher students scored on the resilience measure, the less likely they were to be significantly impacted by bullying and cyberbullying.

### 2.5 The Importance of Family

Parents play a critical role in youth media/online access and reducing the risk for any negative consequences of cyberbullying [50, 51, 64]. During the pandemic, parent–child relationships have been found to moderate the association between psychological distress and cyberbullying among middle school students ($N = 1204$) in China [62]. Additionally, research with 4th–12th grade students in South Korea ($N = 4958$) suggested that parental supervision (i.e., installing an application or program that blocked harmful content or monitoring of Internet usage history) was associated with reduced risk for cyberbullying victimization and perpetration, and a reduced effect of exposure to harmful online content on cyberbullying perpetration during the pandemic [30, 63]. Evidence from a sample of 5658 Italian children and adolescents suggests that such parental supervision may be particularly beneficial for reducing the risk of cyberbullying perpetration for males [64]. Importantly, there were efforts during COVID-19 social distancing to explore the utility of parent-based prevention of bullying/cyberbullying via a pilot telehealth intervention with promising results [61].

## 3 Future Research

Based on the above overview, the following questions await research inquiry:

- Research identifying pandemic-induced general strains is needed to explore how each source of strain (removal of positively valued stimuli, the presence of negative stimuli, and the failure to achieve positively valued goals) affects deviant behavior.
- What coping mechanisms are effective in helping children and adolescents to avoid deviant coping, such as engaging in digital cruelty? Both situational (individual, such as utilizing cognitive coping strategies and engaging in adaptive coping behaviors) and structural (social institutions, such as family and school) level coping should be investigated.
- What coping mechanisms are effective in assisting children and adolescents in mitigating deviant coping (such as engagement in digital cruelty) as a consequence of strain encountered during overwhelming and catastrophic events such as a global pandemic?
- How could parent-based or school-based anti-bullying and anti-violence programs or

cyberbullying programs be adapted to online learning situations so that students and families receive the resources necessary to cope with stress and avoid turning strains into deviant coping?
- In addition to explaining pandemic-related digital cruelties, GST can be further applied to better understand and mitigate the psychological and societal impacts of other adversities like weather disruptions, natural disasters, or geopolitical instability by proactively managing societal stressors and their consequent strains. The collective experiences of the COVID-19 pandemic can guide stakeholders in the development of more resilient social and economic structures.

## 4 Recommendations

There is growing evidence on the negative impact of pandemic-induced strain and digital cruelty as a consequence thereof, on children's mental health [10, 52].

- Future research should seek to elucidate individual and social factors that may predict resilience and adaptive coping among children.
- Children and adolescents should be assisted in avoiding deviant coping mechanisms such as digital cruelty during overwhelming events like pandemics. Therefore, comparative research should examine how socioeconomic disparities influence children's ability to cope with the strains of the pandemic and its impact on engaging in digital cruelty.
- Qualitative research involving in-depth interviews and family case studies, combined with quantitative surveys is recommended to assess the role of parental involvement, family cohesion, and supervision to explore the impact of family dynamics on the development of coping mechanisms in children and adolescents during high strain events.
- To ensure a 360-degree scope of research, interdisciplinary teams must be established where researchers explore and integrate multiple perspectives from different disciplines and areas of expertise. Interdisciplinary research strategies involve threading academic disciplines like criminology, sociology, economics, psychology, medicine, and statistics. The interdisciplinary approach is based on the idea that convergence brings unity and synthesis [53] both to research and the interpretations of findings. As such, it offers more elaborated and valid findings, ready to inform policymakers on the practices that should be applied. Furthermore, interdisciplinary teams can help evaluate and further develop prevention and intervention programs considering all we have learned about digital cruelty, strains, and coping strategies during the pandemic.

**Conflict of Interest and Funding Disclosures** None.

## References

1. Panchal U, Salazar de Pablo G, Franco M, et al. The impact of COVID-19 lockdown on child and adolescent mental health: systematic review. Eur Child Adolesc Psychiatry. 2021:1–27. https://doi.org/10.1007/s00787-021-01856-w.
2. Englander E, Donnerstein E, Kowalski R, Lin CA, Parti K. Defining cyberbullying. Pediatrics. 2017;140(Supplement 2):S148–51. https://doi.org/10.1542/peds.2016-1758U.
3. Bacher-Hicks A, Goodman J, Green JG, Melissa KMK. The COVID-19 pandemic disrupted both school bullying and cyberbullying. EdWorkingPaper. 2021:21–436. https://doi.org/10.26300/7jy7-x816. Accessed 22 Feb 2023.
4. Vaillancourt T, Brittain H, Krygsman A, Farrell AH, Landon S, Pepler D. School bullying before and during COVID-19: results from a population-based randomized design. Aggress Behav. 2021;47(5):557–69. https://doi.org/10.1002/ab.21986.
5. Lobe B, Velicu A, Staksrud E, Chaudron S, Di Gioia R. How children (10–18) experienced online risks during the Covid-19 lockdown-Spring 2020. https://publications.jrc.ec.europa.eu/repository/handle/JRC124034. Accessed 11 Jan 2023.
6. Varela JJ, Hernández C, Miranda R, Barlett CP, Rodríguez-Rivas ME. Victims of cyberbullying: feeling loneliness and depression among youth and adult Chileans during the pandemic. Int J Environ Res Public Health. 2022;19:5886. https://doi.org/10.3390/ijerph19105886.

7. Utemissova GU, Danna S, Nikolaevna VN. Cyberbullying during the COVID-19 pandemic. Glob J Guid Counsel Schools Curr Perspec. 2021;11(2):77–87.
8. Center for the Study of Hate and Extremism, California State University San Bernardino. Fact sheet: anti-Asian prejudice March 2020 – Center for the Study of Hate & Extremism. Available at: https://www.csusb.edu/sites/default/files/FACT%20SHEET-%20Anti-Asian%20Hate%202020%203.2.21.pdf. Accessed 22 Feb 2023.
9. Patchin JW, Hinduja S. Cyberbullying among Asian American youth before and during the COVID-19 pandemic. J School Health. 2022; https://doi.org/10.1111/josh.13249.
10. Alsawalqa RO. Cyberbullying, social stigma, and self-esteem: the impact of COVID-19 on students from East and Southeast Asia at the University of Jordan. Heliyon. 2021;7(4):e06711.
11. Agnew R. Foundation for a general theory of crime and delinquency. Criminology. 1992;30(1):47–88. https://doi.org/10.1111/j.1745-9125.1992.tb01093.x.
12. Patchin JW, Hinduja S. Traditional and nontraditional bullying among youth: a test of general strain theory. Youth Soc. 2011;43(2):727–51. https://doi.org/10.1177/0044118X10365951.
13. Lianos H, McGrath A. Can the general theory of crime and general strain theory explain cyberbullying perpetration? Crime Delinq. 2018;64(5):674–700. https://doi.org/10.1177/0011128717714204.
14. Roy AK, Breaux R, Sciberras E, et al. A preliminary examination of key strategies, challenges, and benefits of remote learning expressed by parents during the COVID-19 pandemic. School Psychol. 2022;37(2):147–59.
15. Rodriguez-Rivas ME, Varela JJ, González C, Chuecas MJ. The role of family support and conflict in cyberbullying and subjective well-being among Chilean adolescents during the Covid-19 period. Heliyon. 2022;8(4):e09243. https://doi.org/10.1016/j.heliyon.2022.e09243.
16. Ezeoke OM, Kanaley MK, Brown DA, et al. The impact of COVID-19 on adolescent wellness in Chicago. Child Care Health Dev. 2022;48(6):886–90. https://doi.org/10.1111/cch.12994.
17. Oosterhoff BO, Palmer CA, Wilson J, Shook N. Adolescents' motivations to engage in social distancing during the COVID-19 pandemic: associations with mental and social health. J Adolesc Health. 2020;67:179–85. https://doi.org/10.1016/j.jadohealth.2020.05.004.
18. Viala-Gaudefroy J, Lindaman D. Donald Trump's 'Chinese Virus': the politics of naming, the conversation, 2020 Apr 21. Available from: https://theconversation.com/donald-trumps-chinese-virus-the-politics-of-naming-136796.
19. Bartlett CP, Rinker A, Roth B. Cyberbullying perpetration in the COVID era: an application of general strain theory. J Soc Psychol. 2021;161(4):466–76. https://doi.org/10.1080/00224545.2021.1883503.
20. Brooks SK, Webster RK, Smith LE, et al. The psychological impact of quarantine and how to reduce it: rapid review of the evidence. Lancet. 2020;395(10027):912–20. https://doi.org/10.1016/S0140-6736(20)30460-8.
21. Golberstein E, Wen H, Miller BF. Coronavirus disease 2019 (COVID-19) and mental health for children and adolescents. JAMA Pediatr. 2020;174:819–20.
22. Cohen ZP, Cosgrove KT, DeVille DC, et al. The impact of COVID-19 on adolescent mental health: preliminary findings from a longitudinal sample of healthy and at-risk adolescents. Front Pediatr. 2021;9:622608. https://doi.org/10.3389/fped.2021.622608. PMID: 34169046; PMCID: PMC8217763
23. Bottino SMB, Bottino CMC, Regina CG, Correia AVL, Ribeiro WS. Cyberbullying and adolescent mental health: a systematic review. Cad Saude Publica. 2015;31(3):463–75.
24. Englander EK. Bullying, cyberbullying, anxiety, and depression in a sample of youth during the coronavirus pandemic. Pediatr Rep. 2021;13:546–51.
25. Huck C, Zhang J. Effects of the COVID-19 pandemic on K-12 education: a systematic literature review. Educ Res Dev J. 2021;24(1):53–84.
26. Becker SP, Breaux R, Cusick CN, et al. Remote learning during COVID-19: examining school practices, service continuation, and difficulties for adolescents with and without attention-deficit/hyperactivity disorder. J Adolesc Health. 2020;67(6):769–77. https://doi.org/10.1016/j.jadohealth.2020.09.002.
27. Han Z, Wang Z, Li Y. Cyberbullying involvement, resilient coping, and loneliness of adolescents during Covid-19 in rural China. Front Psychol. 2021;12:664612.
28. Yang F. Coping strategies, cyberbullying behaviors, and depression among Chinese netizens during the COVID-19 pandemic: a web-based nationwide survey. J Affect Disord. 2021;281:138–44. https://doi.org/10.1016/j.jad.2020.12.023.
29. Englander EK. Sexting, cyberbullying, and risk assessment. J Am Acad Child Adolesc Psychiatry. 2022;61:S131–131.
30. Paek SY, Lee J, Choi YJ. The impact of parental monitoring on cyberbullying victimization in the COVID-19 era. Soc Sci Q. 2022;103(2):294–305. https://doi.org/10.1111/ssqu.13134.
31. Kee DMH, Al-Anesi MAL, Al-Anesi SAL. Cyberbullying on social media under the influence of COVID-19. Global Business and Organizational Excellence; 2022.
32. Beers LS, Szilagyi M, Seigel WM, et al. Immunizing against hate: overcoming Asian American and Pacific Islander racism. Pediatrics. 2021;148(1):e2021051836. https://doi.org/10.1542/peds.2021-051836.
33. He J, He L, Zhou W, Nie X, He M. Discrimination and social exclusion in the outbreak of COVID-19. Int J Environ Res Publ Health. 2020;17(8):2933.
34. Heyman RE, Smith AM. Do child abuse and interpersonal violence lead to adulthood violence? J

Marriage Fam. 2002;64(4):684–870. https://doi.org/10.1111/j.1741-3737.2002.00864.x.
35. Widom CS. Child abuse, neglect, and violent criminal behavior. Criminology. 1989;27(2):251–71. https://doi.org/10.1111/j.1745-9125.1989.tb01032.
36. Walker LE. The battered woman syndrome. 4th ed. Springer; 1979/2017.
37. Reingle JM, Staras SA, Jennings WG, Branchini J, Maldonado-Molina MM. The relationship between marijuana abuse and intimate partner violence in a nationally representative, longitudinal sample. J Interpers Viol. 2012;27(8):1562–78. https://doi.org/10.1177/0886260511425787.
38. Paez GR. Cyberbullying among adolescents: a general strain theory perspective. J Sch Violence. 2018;17(1):74–85. https://doi.org/10.1080/15388220.2016.1220317.
39. Roy AK, Breaux R, Sciberras E, et al. A preliminary examination of key strategies, challenges, and benefits of remote learning expressed by parents during the COVID-19 pandemic. School Psychol. 2022;37(2):147–59. https://psycnet.apa.org/doi/10.1037/spq0000465.
40. YouthTruth. Students weigh in: learning and well-being during COVID-19. YouthTruth Student Survey; 2020. Accessed 22 Feb 2023 at https://youthtruth.surveyresults.org/report_sections/1087936.
41. Lee J. Mental health effects of school closures during Covid-19. Lancet Child Adolesc Health. 2020;4:421.
42. Wang C, Pan R, Wan X, et al. Immediate psychological responses and associated factors during the initial stage of the 2019 Coronavirus Disease (COVID-19) epidemic among the general population in China. Int J Environ Res Public Health. 2020;17:1729.
43. Irwin M, Lazarevic B, Soled D, Adesman A. The COVID-19 pandemic and its potential enduring impact on children. Curr Opin Pediatr. 2022;34(1):107–15. https://doi.org/10.1097/MOP.0000000000001097. PMID: 34923563; PMCID: PMC8728751
44. De France K, Hancock GR, Stack DM, Serbin LA, Hollenstein T. The mental health implications of COVID-19 for adolescents: follow-up of a four-wave longitudinal study during the pandemic. Am Psychol. 2022;77(1):85–99. https://doi.org/10.1037/amp0000838.
45. Fitzpatrick O, Carson A, Weisz JR. Using mixed methods to identify the primary mental health problems and needs of children, adolescents, and their caregivers during the Coronavirus (COVID-19) pandemic. Child Psychiatry Hum Dev. 2021;52(6):1082–93. https://doi.org/10.1007/s10578-020-01089-z. PMID: 33108612; PMCID: PMC7590914
46. Smith PK, Mahdavi J, Carvalho M, Fisher S, Russell S, Tippett N. Cyberbullying: its nature and impact in secondary school pupils. J Child Psychol Psychiatry. 2008;49:376–85. https://doi.org/10.1111/j.1469-7610.2007.01846.x.
47. Wright MF, Wachs S. Adolescents' emotional reactions for not intervening in cyberbullying as moderators in the longitudinal association between witnessing cyberbullying and health issues. Curr Psychol. 2022; https://doi.org/10.1007/s12144-022-03773-w.
48. Goudeau S, Sanrey C, Stanczak A, Manstead A, Darnon C. Why lockdown and distance learning during the COVID-19 pandemic are likely to increase the social class achievement gap. Nat Hum Behav. 2021;5:1273–81. https://doi.org/10.1038/s41562-021-01212-7.
49. Liga F, Inguglia C, Gugliandolo MC, Ingoglia S, Costa S. The socialization of coping strategies in adolescence: the modeling role of parents. Anxiet Stress Cop. 2020;33(1):47–58.
50. Gabrielli J, Marsch L, Tanski S. TECH parenting to promote effective media management. Pediatrics. 2018;142(1) https://doi.org/10.1542/peds.2017-3718.
51. Helfrich EL, Doty JL, Su YW, Yourell JL, Gabrielli J. Parental views on preventing and minimizing negative effects of cyberbullying. Child Youth Serv Rev. 2020;118:105377. https://doi.org/10.1016/j.childyouth.2020.105377.
52. Kauhanen L, Wan Mohd Yunus WMA, Lempinen L, et al. A systematic review of the mental health changes of children and young people before and during the COVID-19 pandemic. Eur Child Adolesc Psychiatr Advanced Online Publication; 2022.
53. Klein JT. Interdisciplinarity: history, theory and practice. Detroit: Wayne State University Press; 1990.
54. Patchin JW, Hinduja S. Cyberbullying among Asian-American youth before and during the COVID-19 pandemic. J Sch Health. 2023;93(1):82–7.
55. Arató N, Zsidó AN, Rivnyák A, Péley B, Lábadi B. Risk and protective factors in cyberbullying: the role of family, social support, and emotion regulation. Int J Bullying Prev. 2022;4:160–73.
56. Waasdorp TE, Bradshaw CP. The overlap between cyberbullying and traditional bullying. J Adolesc Health. 2015;56:483–8.
57. Marcum CD, Higgins GE, Freiburger TL, Ricketts ML. Exploration of the cyberbullying victim/offender overlap by sex. Am J Crim Justice. 2014;39:538–48.
58. Rebisz S, Jasinska-Maciazek A, Grygiel P, Dolata R. Psycho-social correlates of cyberbullying among polish adolescents. Int J Environ Res Public Health. 2023;20:5521–55.
59. Bäker N, Schütz-Wilke J. Behavioral changes during the first year of the COVID-19 pandemic: a longitudinal comparison of bullying, cyberbullying, externalizing behavior problems and prosocial behavior in adolescents. COVID. 2023;3(2):289–300. https://doi.org/10.3390/covid3020022.
60. Tekin U. Investigation of internet addiction, cyberbullying, and cyber victimization in adolescents during the COVID-19 pandemic and their relationship with anxiety and depression. Istanbul Med J. 2023;24(1):100–5. https://doi.org/10.4274/imj.galenos.2023.64928.
61. Doty J, Gabrielli J, Abraczinskas M, Girón K, Yourell J, Stormshak E. Parent-based prevention of bullying and cyberbullying during COVID-19 social distancing: a pilot intervention using the MOST framework. J

Prevent. 2022;43(5):719–34. https://doi.org/10.1007/s10935-022-00696-x.
62. Zhang Y, Xu C, Dai H, Jia X. Psychological distress and adolescents' cyberbullying under floods and the COVID-19 pandemic: parent–child relationships and negotiable fate as moderators. Int J Environ Res Public Health. 2021;18(23):12279. https://doi.org/10.3390/ijerph182312279.
63. Paek SY, Choi YJ, Lee J. Exposure to harmful content and cyberbullying perpetration among South Korean adolescents during COVID-19: the moderating role of parental support. Child Youth Serv Rev. 2023;155:107280. https://doi.org/10.1016/j.childyouth.2023.107280.
64. Marinoni C, Zanetti MA, Caravita SC. Sex differences in cyberbullying behavior and victimization and perceived parental control before and during the COVID-19 pandemic. Soc Sci Human Open. 2023;8(1):100731. https://doi.org/10.1016/j.ssaho.2023.100731.
65. Hinduja S. Resilience, bullying and cyberbullying, Keynote. IBPA annual conference, November 6–8, 2016. New Orleans, LA; 2016.

# Online Hate Speech Among Adolescents: Theory, Research, and Recommendations

Sebastian Wachs, Angela Mazzone, Anja Schultze-Krumbholz, Michelle F. Wright, Nicola Döring, Dorothy L. Espelage, Manuel Gámez-Guadix, and Jun Sung Hong

## 1 Background

Many societies have become increasingly aware of hate speech in recent years, as it has reached unprecedented levels [1]. Online hate speech (OHS) can cultivate a climate of fear, intolerance, and hatred toward social groups. Moreover, OHS can reinforce discriminatory beliefs and actions, intensifying the oppression and marginalization of the targeted group [2]. Adolescents rely heavily on information and communication technologies (ICT) while dealing with different developmental tasks, including identity exploration, development of autonomy, search for belonging, and formation of romantic relationships [3]. As they seek to establish their sense of identity by affiliating with (online) social groups, adolescents become vulnerable to being targeted by hate groups [4]. Equipping adolescents with the skills they need to deal with this emerging online risk constitutes a significant challenge for researchers, educators, practitioners, and caregivers. This chapter provides an overview of definitional issues, theoretical frameworks, research findings, and empirical research on adolescents' (ages 12–18 years) OHS victimization and perpetration. It concludes with future research directions and recommendations for practitioners.

S. Wachs (✉)
University of Münster,
Nordrhein-Westfalen, Germany
e-mail: swachs@uni-muenster.de

A. Mazzone
University of Surrey, Stag Hill Campus,
Guildford, UK

A. Schultze-Krumbholz
Technische Universität Berlin, Berlin, Germany

M. F. Wright
Indiana State University, Terre Haute, IN, USA

N. Döring
Technische Universität Ilmenau, Thuringia, Germany

D. L. Espelage
The University of North Carolina at Chapel Hill,
Chapel Hill, NC, USA

M. Gámez-Guadix
Autonomous University of Madrid, Madrid, Spain

J. S. Hong
Wayne State University, Detroit, MI, USA

Ewha Womans University, Seoul, South Korea

## 2 Current State

### 2.1 A New Definition for an Old Phenomenon

Hatred towards particular groups has existed for a long time in human history. Legal experts, such as Mari Matsuda [5], back in the 1980s, introduced the term *racist speech*, which espouses ethnic inferiority, targets historically oppressed groups, and is hateful and condescending. In subsequent years, the term *racist speech* has been replaced by the more compre-


D. A. Christakis, L. Hale (eds.), *Handbook of Children and Screens*,
https://doi.org/10.1007/978-3-031-69362-5_62

hensive term *hate speech*, referring to all forms of expression that spread, incite, promote, or justify hatred against people based on assigned characteristics, including but not limited to gender identity, sexual orientation, disability status, and religious affiliation. However, the definition of hate speech can vary widely depending on who is historically oppressed, what forms of oppression are deemed unacceptable, and where the lines between free and hate speech are drawn [6]. More recently, the term has been extended to the online context and groups of people who are not traditionally oppressed per se (e.g., politicians, journalists, etc.) but are perceived as allies. In addition, the terms hate speech and cyberhate are often used interchangeably, which adds to the inconsistencies regarding terminology and obscures the fact that hate speech occurs online and offline.

A major challenge in current research is that no generally agreed-upon definition exists [6]. To address this gap, Kansok-Dusche et al. [7] conducted a systematic review of definitions in existing online and offline hate speech research conducted with young people and derived the following definition:

> Hate speech is a derogatory expression (e.g., words, posts, text messages, images, and videos) about people (directly or vicariously) on the basis of assigned group characteristics (e.g., ethnicity, nationality, gender, sexual orientation, disability, and religion). Hate speech is based on an intention to harm and it has the potential to cause harm on multiple different levels (e.g., individual, communal, and societal) [7]. (p. 11)

The proposed definition consists of four key elements. First, it encompasses various human behaviors in online and offline settings. Second, it involves targeting people based on assigned group characteristics; however, it is intentionally broad, as it acknowledges that social categories beyond currently marginalized groups could become victims of hate speech. Third, it recognizes that derogatory expressions can cause harm on various levels. Finally, the proposed definition focuses on the intention to harm rather than being limited to biased attitudes or emotions. Despite the effort to systematize existing knowledge, this definition presents challenges, especially in assessment, as it is difficult to assess individuals' intentions behind the observable aggressive speech and the impact on victims, communities, or societies.

## 2.2 Frequency Rates and Assessment of Online Hate Speech Involvement

According to a recent systematic review, frequency rates for witnessing OHS vary between 31.4% and 68.5%, for perpetration between 4.2% and 32.2%, and victimization between 9% and 23.4% [7]. The varying estimates of frequency rates across different studies can be attributed to country differences (e.g., how hate speech is defined in each particular country), methodological differences, including the reference period (e.g., lifetime, last 3 months), response options (dichotomous or polytomous), whether a definition of OHS is provided beforehand or not, sample characteristics (e.g., age, gender, ethnicity distribution), and whether OHS is measured in general or targeting a specific group (e.g., racist OHS). From a methodological point of view, instruments to investigate young people's involvement in OHS are often based on single-item measures (e.g., In the past 12 months, how often have you witnessed online hate speech?), sometimes with a definition as an introduction to the single-item measures. Using single-item measures is problematic and can lead to limited reliability and validity, as they may not fully capture complex constructs such as OHS or the variability in respondents' perspectives. For example, OHS can alternate between clearly recognizable calls for violence and denigration and more subtle forms (e.g., disguised as irony, offensive jokes, use of stereotypes, and generalizations). Additionally, single-item measures can be more susceptible to measurement error and bias, potentially compromising the accuracy and interpretiveness of findings. Given this complexity, using multiple-item scales to measure various OHS manifestations is critical.

### 2.3 Theory and Research on Online Hate Speech Perpetration

Several theories have been tested to understand why adolescents share, publish, or produce hateful online content. For example, using the *Online Disinhibition Effect* [10], empirical evidence revealed that toxic online disinhibition was positively linked to OHS perpetration [11]. Applying the *Social Cognitive Theory of Morality* [12], research revealed that a series of moral disengagement mechanisms (i.e., sociocognitive processes aimed to justify immoral behaviors through attributing blame to the target, dehumanizing the victim, and minimizing agency) are associated with OHS perpetration [13]. Past research showed that the positive association between witnessing and perpetrating OHS was stronger at higher levels of moral disengagement and weaker when moral disengagement was low [13]. In other research, the *Problem Behavior Theory* [14] has been used to conceptualize adolescents' engagement in OHS as a facet of problematic behavior that is interrelated with other problematic behaviors, which all come from an underlying cause or causes, such as certain personality traits (e.g., impulsivity and sensation-seeking). These underlying causes have consistently been found to increase susceptibility to engaging in risky behaviors (e.g., violence, and delinquency). Hate speech perpetration has also been found to be associated with other risk factors such as contact with strangers online, excessive Internet use, and cyberbullying perpetration [15, 16]. Consistent with the *Social Dominance Theory* [17], the persistence of discrimination and prejudice in societies can be attributed to the intersection of ideologies, institutional practices, social dynamics, and personal attributes, reinforced by ideologies that posit certain groups as superior and others as inferior. OHS likely has its foundation in in-group and out-group identification. Extant research has found that adolescents who perceived their in-group as superior were more likely to perpetrate OHS against out-group members [18].

### 2.4 Theory and Research on Online Hate Speech Victimization

Studies investigating factors leading to OHS victimization often apply the *routine activity theory* [19] as a theoretical framework. According to this theory, adolescents are more likely to be victims when there is a convergence of three factors: Exposure to a motivated offender, a suitable target, and the absence of a capable guardian. Regarding exposure to a motivated offender, research findings suggest that witnessing hate speech, contact with strangers online, deliberate searches of hate-related materials online, hate speech perpetration, and excessive ICT use are linked to hate speech victimization [16, 20, 21]. Regarding target suitability, the research found that individual characteristics (e.g., being female, being gay, having a migration background, and being a member of a minority religion) increased the risk of OHS victimization [22]. Moreover, expressing online support for the LGBTQIA+ community, high disclosure of private information online, offline OHS victimization, low digital media literacy, and experiences of data misuse online increased OHS victimization risk among adolescents [8, 16, 20–22].

Research on the lack of capable guardianship revealed that parental behavior plays a significant role. For example, parents sharing personal information about their children online could increase their children's risk of OHS victimization [16]. Also, parental mediation of children's ICT use (interactions parents have with their children about media use) is relevant to consider. Instructive parental mediation of children's online activities was found to be associated with less hate speech victimization, while restrictive parental mediation was positively related to greater OHS victimization [21]. Parents who adopt instructive mediation might engage in discussions with their children regarding ICT use and its potential risks. In turn, this may result in their children being better educated about the dangers of online interactions and greater compliance with safety recommendations. Conversely, parents adopting restrictive mediation could potentially harm their children's ability to manage problematic online situations. Additionally, these restrictive strategies could be viewed as a threat to children's independence, leading to increased psychological reactance and children's not disclosing their experiences online.

Another avenue of research has focused on the consequences of OHS victimization. For example, victims of OHS experience adverse mental health outcomes, including lower mental well-being and higher anxiety levels, depressive symptoms, fear and insecurity, and sleeping disorders [23–26]. OHS victimization can also impact adolescents' behavior, such as increasing physical aggression, rule-breaking behaviors, and poor academic outcomes (i.e., academic motivation) [27]. In addition, frequently experiencing racist OHS hindered Black adolescents' development of social skills such as empathy, suggesting that OHS victimization can impede adolescents' ability to demonstrate their full potential [28].

Only a few studies have investigated variables that buffer the adverse effects of OHS on victims. For example, one study found that resilience measured individual factors (e.g., social competence, personal competence, and structured style), familial factors (e.g., family cohesion), and a supportive environment outside the family (e.g., social resources), buffered against the effects of OHS victimization on depressive symptoms [25]. Another study revealed that African American adolescents with higher self-esteem and positive ethnic identity experienced less anxiety resulting from racial OHS victimization [29]. This suggests that having a strong sense of self and ethnic identity can buffer against the adverse effects of racist OHS.

## 3 Future Research

Below are three key questions that we feel OHS scholars need to address over the coming years.

### 3.1 What Are the Methodological Challenges in Online Hate Speech Research?

As research on OHS among adolescents is at an early stage, there are many pressing challenges to conducting research in this area, including how OHS is defined. While systematically reviewing existing literature might contribute to elaborating a scientifically sound definition, a bottom-up approach involving key stakeholders, including young people, educators, and school personnel, may assist in testing whether existing definitions reflect their lived experiences. Another Achilles' heel of OHS research related to the definition is how OHS is measured. Accurately assessing OHS through research is essential to advancing the research field, evaluating interventions, and informing policymakers. As mentioned above, most research is currently based on single items. Assessing hate speech is further complicated by deciding whether to measure hate speech in general or measure hate speech experienced by or directed at specific target groups (e.g., Muslims). Further, researchers must decide which derogatory expressions (e.g., words, posts, messages, memes, and videos) and which modes (e.g., offensive jokes, use of stereotypes, and generalizations) are captured in their measures.

Furthermore, most research on hate speech among adolescents is based on cross-sectional study designs, which does not allow for establishing temporal associations between OHS and relevant outcomes. Longitudinal and experimental OHS research is needed to refine our descriptive understanding of OHS and increase our knowledge of risk factors and consequences. Finally, there is a lack of innovative data-collection techniques in OHS research among adolescents. Although using peer nominations poses several ethical issues [30], this method might elucidate the social dynamics of OHS. Another innovative approach might be using experience sampling methods (e.g., daily diary) to study "in real time" the daily life of adolescents involved in hate speech and its impact on outcomes concurrently and temporally. Using this technique would allow researchers to understand the impact of memory biases, enhance real-life relevance, and evaluate hypotheses between- and within-person levels [31].

### 3.2 How Can We Increase Adolescents' Engagement Against Online Hate Speech?

Despite the increase in research focused on hate speech experiences among adolescents, studies to date have mainly focused on perpetrators and victims and have only recently recognized that hate speech can involve others. Adolescents encountering OHS can show moral courage by countering OHS (counterspeech). Counterspeech is defined as a form of citizen-based response to hateful content to discourage it, stop it, or provide support for the victim by, for example, pointing out logical flaws in the hateful content or using facts to counteract misinformation [32]. Until recently, little is known about the factors that increase adolescents' potential or actual engagement in counterspeech, factors preventing them from doing so, and how we can support adolescents to effectively stand up against OHS without putting themselves in danger. Such research should also investigate factors that moderate and mediate the association between predictors and counterspeech to identify the conditions and mechanisms that increase the likelihood of counterspeech.

### 3.3 What Are Effective Strategies to Prevent Online Hate Speech Involvement Among Adolescents?

At present, evidence-based prevention programs to prevent OHS among adolescents are scarce. Common methods for preventing biased attitudes and promoting positive intergroup relations often involve one or more of the following components: Interventions that encourage intergroup contact (e.g., youth exchange programs or reading materials about members of marginalized groups), knowledge-based interventions (e.g., providing information about minorities and democratic values), and individual skill acquisition (e.g., empathy training). More research is needed to understand the most effective approach to address OHS and whether varying approaches might be more or less effective for different groups of young people. In fact, a multicomponent approach might be effective in tackling OHS. For example, the "HateLess. Together against Hatred" prevention program combines these elements. An evaluation study found that HateLess effectively increases adolescents' empathy for victims, self-efficacy toward intervening, and engagement in counterspeech [33, 34]. More prevention research needs to be conducted to increase the acceptability, fidelity, and sustainability of the existing programs to improve adolescent hate speech-related outcomes. In addition, more research is needed to understand the cross-cultural validity of existing programs and the most effective ways to prepare adolescents for living harmoniously in diverse societies.

## 4 Recommendations

Some key recommendations from existing research include:

- Raise awareness around the harmful nature of—online and offline—hate speech for individuals and societies to prevent trivialization and justification of perpetrators' behavior.
- Emphasize morality training that aims to raise awareness of the socio-cognitive processes that adolescents might activate to reduce guilt and remorse when perpetrating OHS.
- Encourage civic engagement by offering human rights education and promoting knowledge (e.g., regarding equality, inclusivity, and diversity), attitudes, opportunities, and social-emotional skills (e.g., expressing opinions appropriately).
- Provide cybersecurity and cyber protection information and combine them with behavioral

components to enable adolescents to protect their data and information online.

- Identify and promote young people's social and personal resources that bolster resilience and mitigate adverse effects of OHS victimization.
- Inform parents of effective parental mediation strategies and ensure children's fundamental rights (e.g., informational self-determination and age-appropriate online privacy) without being intrusive.
- Encourage educators and parents to talk regularly and openly with their children about their online experiences.
- Implement digital literacy interventions for young people, teachers, and parents and combine them with ethical and civic courage components to address prejudice, stereotypes, and self-efficacy.
- Consult stakeholders (e.g., adolescents, educators, parents, and social media providers) to design effective policies and provider-based intervention strategies, such as human- and artificial intelligence-based content and comment moderation.

**Conflict of Interest and Funding Disclosures** None.

## References

1. Costello M, Hawdon J. Hate speech in online spaces. In: The Palgrave handbook of international cybercrime and cyberdeviance. Palgrave Macmillan; 2020. p. 1397–416.
2. Soral W, Bilewicz M, Winiewski M. Exposure to hate speech increases prejudice through desensitization. Aggress Behav. 2018;44(2):136–46.
3. Borca G, Bina M, Keller PS, Gilbert LR, Begotti T. Internet use and developmental tasks: Adolescents' point of view. Comput Hum Behav. 2015;52:49–58.
4. Bauman S, Perry VM, Wachs S. The rising threat of cyberhate for young people around the globe. An ecological perspective. Academic Press; 2021. p. 149–75.
5. Matsuda MJ. Public response to racist speech: considering the victim's story. Mich Rev. 1988;87:2320–81.
6. Brown A. What is hate speech? Part 1: the myth of hate. Law Philos. 2017;36:419–68.
7. Kansok-Dusche J, Ballaschk C, Krause N, et al. A systematic review on hate speech among children and adolescents: definitions, prevalence, and overlap with related phenomena. Trauma Viol Abuse Published online. 2022;24:2598.
8. Castellanos M, Wettstein A, Wachs S, et al. Hate speech in adolescents. A binational study on prevalence and demographic differences. Front Educ. 2023;8:1076249.
9. Döring N, Mohseni MR. Fail videos and related video comments on YouTube: a case of sexualization of women and gendered hate speech? Commun Res Rep. 2019;36(3):254–64.
10. Suler J. The online disinhibition effect. Cyberpsychol Behav. 2004;7(3):321–6.
11. Wachs S, Wright MF. The moderation of online disinhibition and sex on the relationship between online hate victimization and perpetration. Cyberpsychol Behav Soc Netw. 2019;22(5):300–6.
12. Bandura A, Barbaranelli C, Caprara GV, Pastorelli C. Mechanisms of moral disengagement in the exercise of moral agency. J Pers Soc Psychol. 1996;71(2):364.
13. Wachs S, Bilz L, Wettstein A, et al. Associations between witnessing and perpetrating online hate speech among adolescents: testing moderation effects of moral disengagement and empathy. Psychol Violence. 2022;12(6):371–81.
14. Jessor R, Jessor SL. Problem behavior and psychosocial development: a longitudinal study of youth. New York: Academic Press; 1977.
15. Bedrosova M, Machackova H, Šerek J, Smahel D, Blaya C. The relation between the cyberhate and cyberbullying experiences of adolescents in The Czech Republic, Poland, and Slovakia. Comput Hum Behav. 2022;126:107013.
16. Wachs S, Mazzone A, Milosevic T, et al. Online correlates of cyberhate involvement among young people from ten European countries: an application of the Routine Activity and Problem Behaviour Theory. Comput Hum Behav. 2021;123:106872.
17. Sidanius J, Pratto F. Social dominance theory. In: Handbook of theories of social psychology. Sage Publications; 2012. p. 418–39.
18. Ballaschk C, Wachs S, Krause N, et al. Dann machen halt alle mit.Eine qualitative Studie zu Beweggründen und Motiven für Hatespeech unter Schüler* innen. Diskurs Kindh- Jugendforsch J Child Adolesc Res. 2021;16(4):463–80.
19. Cohen LE, Felson M. Social change and crime rate trends: a routine activity approach. Am Sociol Rev. 1979;44(4):588–608.
20. Räsänen P, Hawdon J, Holkeri E, Keipi T, Näsi M, Oksanen A. Targets of online hate: examining determinants of victimization among young Finnish Facebook users. Violence Vict. 2016;31(4):708–25.
21. Wachs S, Costello M, Wright MF, et al. "DNT LET' EM H8 U!": applying the routine activity framework to understand cyberhate victimization among adolescents across eight countries. Comput Educ. 2021;160:104026.
22. Obermaier M, Schmuck D. Youths as targets: factors of online hate speech victimization among

adolescents and young adults. J Comput-Mediat Commun. 2022;27(4):zmac012.
23. Gámez Guadix M, Wachs S, Wright M. " Haters back off!" psychometric properties of the coping with cyberhate questionnaire and relationship with well-being in Spanish adolescents. Psicothema. 2020;32(4):567–74.
24. Krause N, Ballaschk C, Schulze-Reichelt F, et al. "Ich lass mich da nicht klein machen!"Eine qualitative Studie zur Bewältigung von Hatespeech durch Schüler/innen. Z Für Bild Published online. 2021;11:169–85.
25. Wachs S, Gámez-Guadix M, Wright MF. Online hate speech victimization and depressive symptoms among adolescents: the protective role of resilience. Cyberpsychology Behav Soc Netw. 2022;25(7):416–23.
26. Tynes BM, Giang MT, Williams DR, Thompson GN. Online racial discrimination and psychological adjustment among adolescents. J Adolesc Health. 2008;43(6):565–9.
27. Tynes BM, Rose CA, Hiss S, Umaña-Taylor AJ, Mitchell K, Williams D. Virtual environments, online racial discrimination, and adjustment among a diverse, school-based sample of adolescents. Int J Gam Comput-Mediat Simul IJGCMS. 2014;6(3):1–16.
28. Lozada FT, Tynes BM. Longitudinal effects of online experiences on empathy among African American adolescents. J Appl Dev Psychol. 2017;52:181–90.
29. Tynes BM, Umana-Taylor AJ, Rose CA, Lin J, Anderson CJ. Online racial discrimination and the protective function of ethnic identity and self-esteem for African American adolescents. Dev Psychol. 2012;48(2):343–55.
30. Cillessen AH, Marks PE. Methodological choices in peer nomination research. New Dir Child Adolesc Dev. 2017;2017(157):21–44.
31. Mölsä ME, Lax M, Korhonen J, Gumpel TP, Söderberg P. The experience sampling method in monitoring social interactions among children and adolescents in school: a systematic literature review. Front Psychol Published online. 2022;13:1504.
32. Garland J, Ghazi-Zahedi K, Young JG, Hébert-Dufresne L, Galesic M. Impact and dynamics of hate and counter-speech online. EPJ Data Sci. 2022;11(3):3.
33. Wachs S, Krause N, Wright MF, Gámez-Guadix M. Effects of the prevention program "HateLess. Together against Hatred" on Adolescents' empathy, self-efficacy, and countering hate speech. J Youth Adolesc. 2023;52:1115–28.
34. Wachs S, Wright MF & Gámez-Guadix M. From hate speech to HateLess. The effectiveness of a prevention program on adolescents' online hate speech involvement. Computers in Human Behavior, 2024;157:108250. https://doi.org/10.1016/j.chb.2024.108250

# Introduction to the Section on Media Policy

Colleen Kraft and Ellen Wartella

Children born today are described as "Digital Natives," growing up in an age where digital media is a core component of their development, communication, and daily experience. A report by the United Nations Human Rights Council [1] observes that in many instances a child's digital identity commences before birth with in utero images shared by parents and families across the web. In fact, some 80 percent of children living in developed Western countries have a digital footprint before they are two years old, images embedded with a wealth of personal information. This report details that children's use of social media platforms doubles between the ages of nine and 12, with some 40 percent of them having multiple social media profiles. Once they reach their teenage years, their online contacts double as well.

The following chapters identify topics important in the discussion of privacy as a child right. Three themes emerge regarding digital media and privacy in the context of safeguarding and child development. First, there are many new policies designed to protect children's privacy in the digital space that are being introduced and implemented across the United States, the United Kingdom, and the European Union. Second, there is recognition of the need to include the views of children in both the policies and the practice of how they are implemented. A common goal is that these policies promote the development of responsible digital literacy in children and that families and schools can use this framework to help children attain necessary protections. The final theme surrounds the need for additional research on the efficacy of these policies, and how children beyond the Western world should be considered moving forward.

Teki Akuetteh et al. (see Chapter "Digital Policy Trends: Regulations, Interventions and Policy Solutions") describes regulations governing children's safety across several countries including the United States (US), Australia, United Kingdom (UK), and countries in the European Union (EU) and Latin America. The regulations implemented over the past several years address harms such as harmful content or conduct, protecting children's privacy and data protection, and protections of children as consumers. This chapter notes that there has been a major shift away from industry self-regulation toward a more "proactive regulation" by countries, regions, and international organizations such as the United Nations.

The authors note a variety of laws and regulations developed to limit online harms to children such as the European Union's Digital Services Act of 2022 and the Australian Online Safety Act of 2020. Protection of children's privacy via regulations such as the US Children's Online Privacy Protection Act (COPPA) requires digital services to collect permission from parents for children under 13 to access online content. In the UK, the 2020 Age-Appropriate Design Code provides protections regarding the collection of data on children under the age of 16 online, as well as

C. Kraft (✉)
Children's Hospital of Los Angeles,
Los Angeles, CA, USA
e-mail: ckraft@chla.usc.edu

E. Wartella
Northwestern University, Evanston, IL, USA


D. A. Christakis, L. Hale (eds.), *Handbook of Children and Screens*,
https://doi.org/10.1007/978-3-031-69362-5_63

requiring risk assessments of protection procedures. Finally, a developing area of consumer law in the US and the EU is aimed at prohibiting companies from using methods that may enable children to divulge demographic or other data or to make purchases through confusion at internet websites, both common ways in which children are exploited by online platforms.

Montag et al. (see Chapter "Social Media Use in Childhood and Adolescence: Minimizing Its Adverse Effects Through Corporate Social Responsibility and European Union Regulations") discuss the concept of privacy protection through both voluntary (corporate social responsibility) and compulsory (European Union Regulation) mechanisms. Of note is a discussion of limited ability of independent researchers to observe interactions of children on social media platforms, even though the technology that could enable this exists through the Application Programming Interfaces, or *APIs*. Most platforms charge high fees to researchers who wish to study these important interactions that may define privacy and security risks to children.

After reviewing regulatory changes across the globe, the authors discuss specific topics requiring research, public education, and policy. Evidence regarding the benefit of digital media on educational and developmental outcomes of children is needed. Studies examining the extent to which there is equity across various groups of children living in different nations and regions of the world should inform these digital policies. The authors argue that researchers and policymakers need to hear children's voices and their perceptions of the potential harm of digital media and how policy should protect them. This chapter provides insightful recommendations for policymakers, social science researchers, and educators to develop stronger digital policies to protect children around the world.

The Breakstone et al. (see Chapter "Distinguishing Credible from Sham: Supporting Young People to Navigate Online") chapter examine how children discern misinformation online, how they distinguish between credible information and "sham". The authors note that legislators are increasingly mandating digital literacy education in public schools, but many of these curricula are out of date. The authors reference literature on fact checkers, particularly the experience of US, Canadian, Swedish, and Italian fact-checkers. One major finding is that most readers view websites vertically from the top down while fact checkers read sites "laterally", which consists of leaving the site almost immediately, opening new tables, and using other online resources to validate the original site. Research across more than a dozen studies demonstrates that the lateral approach is much more effective in assessing misinformation. Their recommendations for additional research on the best digital practices to identify misinformation include studies of how adults can aid children in becoming more digitally literate, examine how schools are integrating digital literacy into their curricula, and how students are responding, understanding, and using the skills that are being taught. The need for other community-based professionals such as health professionals, educators, and all adults need training to better identify sham information for their own digital literacy, as well as in their role as mentoring children in this area.

Sonia Livingstone et al. (see Chapter "Children's Privacy in the Digital Age: US and UK Experiences and Policy Responses") compares the similarities, strengths, and weaknesses of privacy policy in both the US and the UK. Case studies of how parents, schools, health services, and industry approach privacy and data protection demonstrate how these groups attempt to protect children's personal data and right to privacy. Most notably, they distinguish the American approach, which is rooted in a "market perspective" that attempts to protect the child consumer; the UK (and the EU) develops an approach grounded in the child's human rights. They argue that these culturally different approaches to privacy lead to different characteristics of protection. For example, the US privileges parental authority to regulate their child's online activities, while in the UK and EU, these protections are guaranteed by the UN Convention on the Rights of the Child (UNCRC). The ongoing collection of child data from both health systems and school systems is mentioned. The extent to which children have the right to be heard in venues where their private data is collected (e.g., having doctors discuss with older children their medical treatment options) is addressed. Various laws, such as the Health Insurance Portability and Accountability Act (HIPAA) in the US, have very strong standards to secure child health information. Research is needed to understand the impact of these various policies and as well as how children themselves view such policies and practices of privacy as a child right. Three themes emerge regarding digital media and privacy in the context of safeguarding and child development. First, there are many new policies designed to protect children's privacy in the digital space that are being introduced and implemented across the United States, the United Kingdom, and the European Union. Second, there is recognition of the need to include the views of children in both the policies and the practice of how they are implemented. A common goal is that these policies promote the development of responsible digital literacy in children, and that families and schools can use this framework to help children attain necessary protections. The final theme surrounds the need for additional research on the efficacy of these policies, and how children beyond the Western world should be considered moving forward.

The chapter by Chakravorti et al. (see Chapter "Bridging America's Homework Gap by Closing the Digital Divide") highlights the disparity in broadband access that exists between children of families with lower income. High-speed internet access was once considered a luxury; education during the global COVID-19 pandemic revealed how essential broadband access was to the ability of a child to learn and complete assignments. The chapter supports equitable delivery of broadband access and suggests some tangible actions.

Lucía Magis-Weinberg et al.'s (see Chapter "Global Perspectives on Youth and the Digital Environment: Learnings from Majority World Countries") chapter provides an overview of learnings from Majority World countries, where most children and adolescents are located and represent the fastest growing demographic of heavy users highlighting the various inequalities youth in Majority World countries face in terms of access, use and skills, and risks and benefits that impact their online and offline lives. The chapter highlights the unique challenges and opportunities that young people in Majority World countries face in navigating the digital environment, how these have been impacted by the COVID-19 pandemic and parental and school concerns and regulations. Overall, the authors argue that better understanding of these youth is informative for understanding digital media's impact on the lives of young people around the world, especially as regulatory initiatives gain momentum.

These six chapters present thoughtful discourse, which seems paramount to securing children's privacy. As the Livingstone chapter summarizes so well, "Privacy and data policies must promote children's autonomy, balance their need for protection and participation, and prevent discrimination and other harms arising from privacy violations and data exploitation in digital contexts. They should also give children real agency in influencing decisions that affect them including policy and product design" [2].

**Conflict of Interest and Funding Disclosures** None.

## References

1. Cannataci, JA, United Nations, Human Right Council, Artificial Intelligence and Privacy, and children's privacy: report of the special Rapporteur on the right to privacy; 25, January 2021. Report No. A/HRC/46/37.
2. United Nations, Human Right Council, "Children's right to privacy in the digital age must be improved"; 15, July 2021. https://www.ohchr.org/en/stories/2021/07/childrens-right-privacy-digital-age-must-be-improved.

# Digital Policy Trends: Regulations, Interventions, and Policy Solutions

Teki Akuetteh, Lionel Brossi, Emma Day, Rys Farthing, Josh Golin, and Brian O'Neill

## 1 Background

Policymakers have the potential to shape how children experience the digital world with laws, regulations, and guidance. However, the extent to which children's best interests are prioritized in digital policy is much contested [1]. Policies aimed at the protection and safeguarding of individuals using technologies, particularly those relating to children—defined here as a person under the age of 18 years [2]—appear to be advancing in three loosely aligned silos: legislation and regulation addressing online harms such as harmful content or conduct; legislation and regulation around privacy and data protection; and regulation and policy around consumer protections that position young people as unique consumers. This chapter explores progress and gaps in these policy dimensions, focusing on whether they advance children's well-being and rights.

T. Akuetteh
Africa Digital Rights Hub, Accra, Ghana

L. Brossi
University of Chile, Millennium Nucleus for Improving the Mental Health of Adolescents and Youth, Santiago, Chile

E. Day
Tech Legality, Lisbon, Portugal

R. Farthing
Centre for the Digital Child, Deakin University, Geelong, Australia

J. Golin
Fairplay, Boston, MA, USA

B. O'Neill (✉)
Technological University Dublin, Dublin, Ireland
e-mail: brian.oneill@tudublin.ie

## 2 Current State

A growing consensus exists among governments worldwide that industry self-regulation alone is insufficient to safeguard children online. In developing the best frameworks, mandatory due diligence obligations for digital service providers with legislative enforcement, alongside industry-instigated measures, are necessary to proactively protect users. For example, several voluntary industry codes around disinformation in the European Union (EU) and online safety in Australia have been replaced by codes and standards drafted instead by regulators. While policy progress has been nuanced and complex within this space, in Table 1, we have attempted to highlight some indicative significant laws and regulations that address digital content and the online world for children. For illustrative purposes, we combine notable regional regulations where they exist and country regulations where they are particularly notable. While many important domestic laws and regulations have been omitted, the aim is simply to highlight a broader trend: there have been waves of growth in some areas of regulation in some regions and gaps in other areas and regions.


D. A. Christakis, L. Hale (eds.), *Handbook of Children and Screens*,
https://doi.org/10.1007/978-3-031-69362-5_64

**Table 1** Global developments in children's digital policy

| | Online harms | Privacy and data protection | Consumer law |
|---|---|---|---|
| Africa | African Union Convention on Cyber Security and Personal Data Protection (Malabo Convention, expected)<br>African Charter on the Rights and Welfare of the Child (1990)<br>Most countries have laws criminalizing online harms to children, including child sexual abuse material (often referred to as child pornography in law) stalking, indecent exposure, etc.<br>Ghana—Cybersecurity Act, 2020 (Act 1038)<br>South Africa—Cybercrimes and Cybersecurity Act, 2021 | African Union Convention on Cyber Security and Personal Data Protection (Malabo Convention, expected)<br>African Charter on the Rights and Welfare of the Child (1990)<br>About 30 African countries have data protection laws, some of which treat the information of children as sensitive and deserving of higher levels of protection and processing obligations.<br>For example:<br>Ghana—Data Protection Act, 2012 (Act 843)<br>South Africa—The Protection of Personal Information Act, 2013 (PoPIA)<br>Senegal—LOI n° 2008–12 du 25 Janvier 2008 portant sur la Protection des données à caractère personnel | Consumer protection laws exist in some countries. However, very few have effective implementation measures that protect children.<br>25 African countries have consumer protection laws that address online protection. These are not necessarily specific to children. |
| Asia-Pacific region | Asia-Pacific Economic Cooperation (APEC) Privacy Framework (2005)<br>Australia—Enhancing Online Safety Act (2015)<br>Fiji—Online Safety Act (2018)<br>Australia—Online Safety Act (2020)<br>Australia—Online Safety Codes (2023) | Australia—draft Online Privacy Code for Children (expected 2025) | Australia—Competition and Consumer Act (2010) |
| Europe | EU—Audiovisual Media Services Directive (2018)<br>EU—Digital Services Act (2022)<br>EU—Better Internet for Kids + Strategy (2022)<br>Ireland—Online Safety & Media Regulation Act (2022)<br>UK—Online Safety Act (2023) | EU—GDPR (2018)<br>UK—Age Appropriate Design Code (2020)<br>EU Guidelines to Enforce the Protection of Minors Online (expected 2025)<br>France—Les droits numériques des mineurs (2021)<br>Ireland—Fundamentals for a Child Oriented Approach to Data Protection (2021)<br>Sweden—The Rights of Children and Young People on Digital Platforms (2021) | EU—Unfair Commercial Practices Directive (2019)<br>EU—Review of EU consumer law—New Deal for Consumers (2020)<br>EU—Digital Markets Act (2022)<br>EU—Digital Services Act (2022) |
| Latin America | Argentina—Ley Mica Ortega (2020)<br>México—Ley Olimpia (2020)<br>Chile—Ley 20526 (2011 and updated) | Brazil—LGPD Lei Geral de Proteção de Dados Pessoais (2018)<br>Mexico—Ley Federal de Protección de Datos Personales en Posesión de Particulares LFPDPPP (2010 and updated) | Chile—Ley Pro Consumidor (N° 21.398) (2021)<br>Paraguay—Ley N° 6366 Ley de Defensa del Consumidor y del Usuario (2021) |
| North America | US—draft Kids Online Safety Bill (anticipated)<br>Canada—draft Online Safety Act (expected) | US—Child Online Privacy Protection Act (1998)<br>California Consumer Privacy Act (2018, updated 2023)<br>California—Age Appropriate Design Code (2022) | |

Across all policy areas, two discernible trends are apparent: a move toward proactive regulation and a move toward more comprehensive legislation, addressing more aspects and features of the digital world.

## 2.1 Online Harms

A range of jurisdictions have pressed ahead with legislation or regulations that address online harms. These started with the Australian online safety laws of 2015 and 2020 [3], which were replicated in Fiji in 2018 [4], and then followed by the EU's *Digital Services Act 2022* (DSA) [5] and the UK's *Online Safety Act* [6]. Canada is currently debating an Online Safety Act as well [7].

The early Australian act focused largely on notice and takedown, where a new regulator was established with powers to request the removal of specific types of content deemed to be harmful (such as cyberbullying or child sexual abuse and exploitation material) from a platform or service swiftly, at the regulator's request. While this approach creates a popular public-facing complaints mechanism for children and families affected by harmful content, it largely leaves regulators playing whack-a-mole, where content must be posted and cause harm before it can be addressed. The requirement for content moderation remains a major feature of the EU's DSA, allowing for a combination of automated content moderation tools with human oversight, but the DSA also specifies more proactive obligations on online providers to prevent child rights abuses before they occur.

This more proactive approach, which has become a feature in many jurisdictions, includes legislation that establishes basic safety expectations for technology products themselves (such as requiring privacy-by-default settings, preventing adult accounts from messaging children's accounts, having time limits on apps for young people etc.). These have been coupled with proposed upstream requirements such as legislating for duties of care or the realization of children's rights.

For example, the DSA requires platforms to operate in ways that respect fundamental human rights, including children's rights, by banning behavioral advertising and requiring risk assessments. Similarly, the UK's Online Safety Act outlines several duties of care for digital service providers to protect younger users. Australia's updated Online Safety Act 2020 includes Basic Online Safety Expectations [8]. In the US, attempts to pass a Kids Online Safety Act [9] with a duty of care are ongoing.

Alongside this, there has been a strong movement toward developing and adopting standards and certification schemes, such as the Institute of Electrical and Electronics Engineers (IEEE) Standard for Age Appropriate Digital Services [10], and requiring independent audits, e.g., the DSA includes a requirement for very large online platforms (VLOPs) to obtain an annual independent audit to monitor their compliance.

## 2.2 Privacy and Data Protection

Alongside legislation that addresses harmful content or conduct, there has been a trend toward regulating data and data flows in ways that benefit children and advance children's rights. Because data is the "fuel" of much of the digital world, privacy regulation has proven to be an area ripe for policy intervention. Here, too, the trend toward systemic protection is evident.

In Africa, data protection laws and regulations have been nascent. However, there has been significant growing interest in data protection, with about 30 of the 55 countries having data protection laws at various stages of implementation. While enforcement of data protection has been limited, there is, however, recognition and treatment of children's data as sensitive personal data subject to stricter controls and measures. In 2020, for instance, South Africa's Information Regulator issued Guidance Notes on the processing of children's data [11].

The Children's Online Privacy Protection Act (COPPA), which was introduced in the U.S. in 1998, sought to introduce the concept of parental permission into the then-burgeoning online data collection space. It requires digital services to collect parental consent before collecting and using data of children under the age of 13. This has created some confusion in that under the EU's General Data Protection Regulation (GDPR) [12], the age for consent to data processing is 16 but can be lowered to 13 at the discretion of EU Member States. Other difficulties with enforcement around the GDPR have included a general lack of transparency from platforms, making it difficult to assess their compliance. Resource constraints have also limited the number of cases of enforcement actions for national data protection authorities.

In the UK, children's best interests were embedded in the groundbreaking 2020 Age Appropriate Design Code [13]. The Code places strong protections regarding collecting and using children's data and introduces requirements such as data protection impact assessments. This approach was replicated in the Californian Age Appropriate Design Code (2022) [14], which requires not only Data Protection Impact Assessments but broader risk assessments of products and services. This continues the trend toward systemic protections that place proactive requirements on digital products and services to protect children in the first instance.

The GDPR's child rights protections have been clarified and further advanced through guidance passed by several European data protection regulators, including Ireland, France, Sweden, and the Netherlands. France aside, all of these make explicit that data can only be collected and used in ways that are in "children's best interests," embedding a long-standing child rights principle that comes from the UNCRC into data protection law and practice [15]. These guidelines have had several consequences, such as preventing the use of children's data to profile them for commercial purposes (that is, effectively preventing behavioral advertising), data minimization principles, and data limitations (preventing the use of data in ways that are not in their best interests). The move toward "best interests" informed data protections is also evident in Australia [16] and South Africa [11].

This trend toward more rights-based approaches to data protection sits alongside an emerging trend to regulate AI and other emerging data-processing technologies. This has the effect of creating rights-based and outcomes-focused protections. For example, UNICEF has developed policy guidelines on AI for children [17], using the principles outlined in the UNCRC as a foundation, including recommendations for governments and businesses working with children and guides for parents and teens. The EU is developing the EU AI Act [18], which categorizes levels of risks to fundamental human rights involved in the development of AI, to promote the development of AI in line with EU values, democratic principles, and human dignity while prioritizing the safety and well-being of children and other vulnerable groups.

Interest in regulating AI has grown in Latin America, but the region still faces persistent challenges regarding accessibility and connectivity and a lack of digital infrastructure for supporting the AI ecosystem. Some organizations, such as UNESCO, UNICEF, and the Inter-American Development Bank, have launched initiatives to encourage fair and ethical use of AI and reduce the digital divide. At a national level, Colombia, Argentina, Brazil, Chile, and Uruguay lead in developing national AI strategies. Colombia stands out for including a special principle dedicated to children's rights in its Ethical Framework for Artificial Intelligence [19]. Similarly, the National Artificial Intelligence Strategy in Chile [20], published in September 2020, mentions child protection in some of its key recommendations.

## 2.3 Consumer Law

There are a number of regulatory interventions aimed at improving children's digital experiences through a lens of consumer protection. For example, in the US, the Federal Trade Commission (FTC) is developing a particular focus on preventing children from being exploited through the use of "dark patterns" or digital designs that may trick them into handing over more data than they need to or buying things. The FTC has recently fined companies that use counterintuitive buttons that could confuse a young person into accidentally making a purchase. Consumer law is also being deployed to improve children's safety in the US, where default features that connect kids to adult strangers are being framed and addressed as an unfair practice [21].

Beyond North America, consumer protections are being invoked to protect children from unsafe or "sneaky" advertising from influencers that is not clearly labeled in the EU [22]. They have also been invoked for action against "loot boxes" (or in-game purchases of mystery goods that strongly resemble gambling) in Australia, for instance [23]. In South Africa, the Consumer Protection Act (CPA) of 2008 has some provisions that address unfair marketing practices targeting children while the Electronic Communications and Transactions Act (ECTA) of 2002 includes some safeguards for children related to online transactions and data protection. In Brazil, the Marco Civil da Internet (Civil Rights Framework for the Internet) of 2014 outlines principles of data protection and includes special considerations for the collection and processing of children's data online, which restrict commercial advertising aimed at children. More generally, however, consumer law protection aimed at children remains an emerging area.

## 2.4 Consensus, Divergence, and Tensions

For clarity's sake, we have organized this analysis into three sections covering online harms, privacy protections, and consumer law. In practice, policy is not always neatly divided and depends on the strengths and priorities of different legislators and regulators. For example, behavioral advertising to children is prohibited under online harms legislation, such as the EU's DSA and privacy laws, such as Ireland's data protection guidelines for children [24] and Australia's *Privacy Act* review [16].

This more proactive approach places more responsibility on platforms to consider children, regardless of whether a platform is child-directed. Policymakers are regulating platforms that children are "likely to access" rather than products that are "targeting children," a recognition that many young people use services that are also used by the general population. For example, COPPA only requires platforms to take action to protect children's privacy if a site is child-directed or when they have "actual knowledge" that they have child users on their platform, which has had the effect of incentivizing platforms not to take steps to look for child users. Regulations like the California Age Appropriate Design Code (2022) apply where platforms "are likely to be accessed by children," thereby closing a potential loophole where digital platforms and services could claim they did not target children to avoid regulation, even if children used them.

While the trend is toward greater regulation and protection of children and their data online, some tensions have emerged. For example, ensuring children's rights are integrated and mainstreamed across all emerging technological regulations rather than sidelined into bespoke codes or standalone statements remains an ongoing concern. Likewise, balancing children's needs remains a complex issue; for example, balancing their safety with their rights to access information and privacy has proven to be challenging for policymakers. Relatedly, sometimes polarized debates are ongoing concerning the use of scanning technologies to detect child sex abuse materials, as proposed in the draft EU Regulation [25], and with the mandatory use of age assurance tools, which are now a requirement in the United Kingdom, France, and Germany under certain circumstances [26]. These debates often pit child safety advocates against privacy advocates, who argue that these technologies and tools infringe upon the privacy rights of both children and adults [27]. Increasingly too, parental rights and parental concerns about children's access, privacy, and safety are challenging children's preferences and sometimes their best interests too, which remains a difficult issue for policymakers to address [28].

Legislative fragmentation is also a concern when it comes to trends for more proactive regulation of children's online safety. Different countries or even states within a country adopting varying laws for safeguarding children may create a confusing patchwork of rules for online platforms to follow. This can lead to uneven protection for children, with some being better protected than others just based on location. Companies operating across borders would need to manage complex legal landscapes, making it more difficult for smaller companies to keep up with constantly changing or conflicting regulations. Ideally, developing international agreements or broadly applied standards regarding children's online safety would mitigate the unevenness caused by fragmentation. Organizations like the UN and the OECD could potentially support international harmonization of this kind. In the absence of international agreements, laws such as the EU's Digital Services Act, when adopted by companies as a de facto standard (the so-called "Brussels effect"), can also offer a way to reduce fragmentation. Ultimately, greater emphasis on platform responsibility, along with clear and consistent penalties for non-compliance, should place the onus on tech companies to maintain a baseline standard of protection for all users, especially children.

## 3 Future Research

The emerging trends within the policy landscape could be reinforced and improved with targeted research, and indeed many of the challenges could be reduced with increasing information about the impact of digital policies. With this in mind, five specific questions for future research that could be particularly impactful include:

- What is the capacity of consumer law to advance children's well-being and rights in the digital environment? As Table 1 highlights, there has been less movement in the consumer law space, and more research around the capacity of this approach to improve the situation for children could be useful.
- What mechanisms are effective to ensure that regulatory advances are implemented and lead to actual improvements for children? There has been a flurry of recent legislative, regulatory, and policy developments aiming to improve the situation for children, but equal attention needs to be paid to ensure these reforms are effectively implemented and monitored and lead to actual improvements. Research should identify the main barriers preventing media organizations and digital platforms from effectively implementing existing regulations to protect children's rights online and the strategies needed to ensure consistent compliance.
- What do children say about the regulations and legislation they want to advance their rights online? [29] As the policy landscape develops, the perspectives and experiences of children need to be adequately reflected. Further research exploring children's perspectives around online harms, privacy, and consumer protections (and issues) is necessary, ideally using deliberative methods and qualitative and quantitative research.
- How do we ensure the same level of protection for children irrespective of where they live? Research has shown that while regulation can improve the digital environment for children where it is implemented, this can create gaps in protection for children in other regions [30]. Research is needed to explore how to prevent these discriminations arising from legislative fragmentation from growing.
- How can media laws and regulations governing children's access and use of media be refined over time to keep pace with evolving media trends and technologies? What types of policies and regulations are best "future-proofed" to address and support children's well-being and rights?·

## 4 Recommendations

### 4.1 For Policymakers

- Develop and implement a robust legal framework for digital services likely to be accessed by children that are aligned with international child rights frameworks and broader international human rights laws.

- Foster greater engagement and cooperation between policymakers and industry in the development of standards of baseline protections that should apply to all users.
- Develop tools with children for independent auditing of tech companies and for carrying out child rights due diligence.
- Work with and meaningfully listen to children as policy is developed. Develop and implement models to ensure ongoing participation by children and youth in digital design and governance.
- Implement a multifaceted approach to solving the challenges that address issues from global, regional, country, business, civil society, and industry perspectives.

### 4.2 For Educators and Researchers

- Engage with policymakers to ensure expert perspectives inform evidence-based policymaking practices.
- Support young people in the policy development process to ensure their right to participate and produce better policy outcomes.

**Conflict of Interest and Funding Disclosures** None.

## References

1. Verdoodt V. Children's rights and commercial communication in the digital era. Intersentia. KU Leuven Centre for IT & IP Law Series; 2020. https://intersentia.com/en/children-s-rights-and-commercial-communication-in-the-digital-era.html. Accessed 15 Nov 2021.
2. UN General Assembly. Convention on the Rights of the Child, vol. 1577. United Nations; 1989. p. 3. http://www2.ohchr.org/english/law/crc.htm.
3. Government of Australia. Online Safety Act 2021. Attorney-General's Department; 2022. https://www.legislation.gov.au/Details/C2021A00076/Html/Text, http://www.legislation.gov.au/Details/C2021A00076. Accessed 27 Mar 2023.
4. Office of the Attorney-General. Online Safety Act 2018 – Laws of Fiji. 2019. https://laws.gov.fj/Acts/DisplayAct/2462. Accessed 27 Mar 2023.
5. European Union. Regulation (EU) 2022/2065 of the European Parliament and of the Council of 19 October 2022 on a Single Market For Digital Services and Amending Directive 2000/31/EC (Digital Services Act) (Text with EEA Relevance). Off J Eur Union. 2022;277:1–102. http://data.europa.eu/eli/reg/2022/2065/oj/eng. Accessed 27 Mar 2023.
6. UK Parliament. Online Safety Bill – Parliamentary Bills. https://bills.parliament.uk/bills/3137. Accessed 27 Mar 2023.
7. Canadian Heritage. The Government's commitment to address online safety. 29 July 2021. https://www.canada.ca/en/canadian-heritage/campaigns/harmful-online-content.html. Accessed 27 Mar 2023.
8. eSafety Commissioner. Basic online safety expectations. eSafety Commissioner; n.d. https://www.esafety.gov.au/industry/basic-online-safety-expectations. Accessed 28 Mar 2023.
9. Sen. Blumenthal R [D C]. Text – S.3663 – 117th Congress (2021–2022): Kids Online Safety Act. 15 Dec 2022. https://www.congress.gov/bill/117th-congress/senate-bill/3663/text. Accessed 28 Mar 2023.
10. IEEE. IEEE standard for an age appropriate digital services framework based on the 5Rights principles for children. IEEE; 2021. https://doi.org/10.1109/IEEESTD.2021.9627644.
11. Information Regulator (South Africa). Guidance note on processing of personal information of children. Information Regulator (South Africa); 2021. https://inforegulator.org.za/wp-content/uploads/2020/07/GuidanceNote-Processing-PersonalInformation-Children-20210628-1.pdf. Accessed 28 Mar 2023.
12. European Union. Regulation (EU) 2016/679 of the European Parliament and of the Council of 27 April 2016 on the Protection of Natural Persons with Regard to the Processing of Personal Data and on the Free Movement of Such Data, and Repealing Directive 95/46/EC (General Data Protection Regulation). Document 32016R0679. Off J Eur Union. 2016;119:1–88. http://data.europa.eu/eli/reg/2016/679/oj. Accessed 28 Mar 2023.
13. ICO. Age appropriate design: a code of practice for online service. Information Commissioner's Office; 2020. https://ico.org.uk/media/for-organisations/guide-to-data-protection/key-data-protection-themes/age-appropriate-design-a-code-of-practice-for-online-services-2-1.pdf.
14. California Legislature. AB-2273 The California Age-Appropriate Design Code Act. https://leginfo.legislature.ca.gov/faces/billCompareClient.xhtml?bill_id=202120220AB2273&showamends=false. Accessed 27 Mar 2023.
15. Kravchuk N. Privacy as a new component of "the best interests of the child" in the new digital environment. Int J Child Rights. 2021;29(1):99–121. https://doi.org/10.1163/15718182-29010006.
16. Australian Government. Privacy act review report 2022. Attorney-General's Department; 2022. https://www.ag.gov.au/sites/default/files/2023-02/privacy-act-review-report_0.pdf.

17. Byrne J, Day E, Raftree L. UNICEF global insight data governance manifesto. UNICEF Office of Global Insight and Policy; 2021. https://www.unicef.org/globalinsight/media/1741/file/UNICEF%20Global%20Insight%20Data%20Governance%20Manifesto.pdf.
18. European Commission. Proposal for a Regulation of the European Parliament and of the Council Laying Down Harmonised Rules on Artificial Intelligence (Artificial Intelligence Act) and Amending Certain Union Legislative Acts. European Commission; 2021. https://eur-lex.europa.eu/legal-content/EN/TXT/?uri=celex%3A52021PC0206. Accessed 27 Mar 2023.
19. Muñoz V, Tamayo E, Guio A. The Colombian case: adopting collaborative governance as a path for implementing ethical artificial intelligence. Published online Sept 2021. http://repositorio.udesa.edu.ar/jspui/handle/10908/18743. Accessed 25 Mar 2023.
20. Gobierno de Chile. Política Nacional De Inteligencia Artificial. Ministerio de Ciencia, Tecnología, Conocimiento e Innovación; 2020. https://www.minciencia.gob.cl/uploads/filer_public/bc/38/bc389daf-4514-4306-867c-760ae7686e2c/documento_politica_ia_digital_.pdf.
21. Federal Trade Commission. Fortnite video game maker epic games to pay more than half a billion dollars over FTC allegations of privacy violations and unwanted charges. Federal Trade Commission. 16 Dec 2022. https://www.ftc.gov/news-events/news/press-releases/2022/12/fortnite-video-game-maker-epic-games-pay-more-half-billion-dollars-over-ftc-allegations. Accessed 27 Mar 2023.
22. Directorate-General for Justice and Consumers (European Commission), Lupiáñez-Villanueva F, Boluda A, et al. Behavioural study on unfair commercial practices in the digital environment: dark patterns and manipulative personalisation: final report. Publications Office of the European Union; 2022. https://data.europa.eu/doi/10.2838/859030. Accessed 28 Dec 2022.
23. Environment and Communications References Committee. Gaming micro-transactions for chance-based items. Commonwealth of Australia; 2018. https://www.aph.gov.au/Parliamentary_Business/Committees/Senate/Environment_and_Communications/Gamingmicro-transactions/Report. Accessed 27 Mar 2023.
24. Data Protection Commission. Children Front and Centre. Fundamentals for a child-oriented approach to data processing. Office of the Data Protection Commission; 2021. https://www.dataprotection.ie/en/dpc-guidance/fundamentals-child-oriented-approach-data-processing.
25. European Commission. Proposal for a Regulation of the European Parliament and of the Council Laying Down Rules to Prevent and Combat Child Sexual Abuse. European Commission; 2022. https://eur-lex.europa.eu/legal-content/EN/TXT/?uri=COM:2022:209:FIN.
26. UNICEF. Digital age assurance tools and children's rights online across the globe: a discussion paper. UNICEF; 2021. http://c-fam.org/wp-content/uploads/Digital-Age-Assurance-Tools-and-Children-s-Rights-Online-across-the-Globe-1_LT.pdf.
27. Draper L. Protecting children in the age of end-to-end encryption. Joint PIJIP/TLS Research Paper Series 80. Published online 1 Jan 2022. https://digitalcommons.wcl.american.edu/research/80.
28. The Children's Commissioner. Digital childhoods: a survey of children and parents. The Children's Commissioner; 2022. https://www.childrenscommissioner.gov.uk/wp-content/uploads/2022/09/cc-digital-childhoods-a-survey-of-children-and-parents.pdf. Accessed 5 Jan 2023.
29. Farthing R, Smith-Nunes G, Akuetteh T, Camacho K, Ošljak KK, Zhao J. "It sets boundaries making your life personal and more comfortable": understanding young people's privacy needs and concerns. IEEE Technol Soc Mag. 2023;42(1):75–82. https://doi.org/10.1109/MTS.2023.3244554.
30. Fairplay. Global platforms, partial protections: design discriminations on social media platforms. Fair Play Alliance: Childhood Beyond Brands; 2022. https://fairplayforkids.org/wp-content/uploads/2022/07/design-discriminations.pdf. Accessed 12 Jan 2023.

# Social Media Use in Childhood and Adolescence: Minimizing Its Adverse Effects Through Corporate Social Responsibility and European Union Regulations

Christian Montag, Zsolt Demetrovics, Jon D. Elhai, Don Grant, Ina Koning, Hans-Jürgen Rumpf, Marcantonio M. Spada, Melina Throuvala, and Regina van den Eijnden

## 1 Background

The prevailing business model behind most current operating social media platforms has been coined "surveillance capitalism" [1]. In other words, the technological juggernauts behind platforms such as Instagram or TikTok attempt to lure in their users to continually use their products, promoting maximum online time and engagement [2]. This, in turn, allows companies to gather more insights into users via studying digital footprints. These insights are used to target users with personalized ads [3] encountered when being on social media platforms. Therefore,

C. Montag (✉)
Department of Molecular Psychology, Institute of Psychology and Education, Ulm University, Ulm, Germany
e-mail: mail@christianmontag.de

Z. Demetrovics
Institute of Psychology, ELTE Eötvös Loránd University, Budapest, Hungary

Centre of Excellence in Responsible Gaming, University of Gibraltar, Europa Point, Gibraltar

College of Education, Psychology and Social Work, Flinders University, Adelaide, SA, Australia

J. D. Elhai
Department of Psychology, University of Toledo, Toledo, OH, USA

Department of Psychiatry, University of Toledo, Toledo, OH, USA

D. Grant
Center for Research and Innovation, Newport Healthcare, Nashville, TN, USA

I. Koning
Faculty of Behavioural and Movement Sciences, Clinical Child and Family Studies, Vrije Universiteit Amsterdam, Amsterdam, Netherlands

H.-J. Rumpf
Department of Psychiatry and Psychotherapy, University of Lübeck, Lübeck, Germany

M. M. Spada
School of Applied Sciences, London South Bank University, London, UK

M. Throuvala
International Gaming Research Unit, NTU Psychology, Nottingham Trent University, Nottingham, UK

West Midlands Gambling Harms Clinic, Inclusion, Midlands Partnership NHS Trust, Stafford, UK

Paediatric Psychology, Child and Adolescent Mental health Services, Leicestershire Partnership NHS Trust, Leicester, UK

R. van den Eijnden
Department of Interdisciplinary Social Science, Utrecht University, Utrecht, Netherlands


D. A. Christakis, L. Hale (eds.), *Handbook of Children and Screens*,
https://doi.org/10.1007/978-3-031-69362-5_65

the term "attention economy" has also been coined to describe social media's business model [4]. In the following chapter, we give insights into current age barriers to using social media and present thoughts on how the industry's data business model collides with psycho-developmental stages. This section is followed by insights into the "APIcalypse" hampering research in this field and new regulations from the European Union (EU) around the Digital Services Act aiming to ensure that protective measures for young people on social media are enforced. We conclude with a plea to re-think the business model of social media—particularly when considering adolescent engagement with these applications and platforms.

## 2 Current State

In the EU, social media platforms cannot be used earlier than 13 years of age. The age barrier of 13 years for onboarding on social media goes back to the *Children's Online Privacy Protection Act* [5], which aimed to protect children's privacy, including on social media platforms. There are additional reasons why engaging with social media earlier than 13 years might not be wise. This said, to our knowledge, the age of 13 is arbitrary and not grounded in empirical developmental psychology research on the topic. Previous research has also concluded: "Details of how regulators settled on the age of 13 are unclear" [6].

It is well known that children progress through several psycho-developmental phases before adolescence [7], during which they need sufficient time to pursue their inner urges for healthy social and emotional development. These phases include the need for rough and tumble play, which fosters motor skills and social competencies [8]. Following Erikson's Stages-of-Developmental-Model [9, 10], children learn in the transitions from kindergarten (where they explore through play the basic strength of "Purpose") to primary and secondary school, how to structure their everyday lives and then develop self-confidence in their own skills or "Competence"—the basic strength corresponding to the fourth stage in Erikson's Stages-of-Development-Model (7–11 years).

Specifically, the basic strength "Purpose" developed in the so-called "Play age" (in Erikson's model 3–6 years)—further fostered during subsequent school years—can arise by experimenting being part of a community, asserting control over the environment and taking initiative without getting rejected by peers. This reflects our in-built social need for belonging (see also recent evidence supporting this notion when revisiting Maslow's hierarchy of needs pyramid) [11], which is hardwired in our brains [12]. Other researchers and theories have documented this basic human need for "relatedness" [13].

In societies rapidly moving toward an Internet of Things [14] and approaching the event horizon of the coming AI-wave [15], the critical question is if "Purpose"—taking individual initiative in a social context while successfully managing social interactions—can be met via social media platforms operating with the current data business model. Despite "illusions of meaningful engagement for young people" [7] (p. 265) on social media platforms, the industry attempts to lower the age barrier for users, with the goal of luring even younger members onto their platforms. This in turn results in a violation of the norms of psychosocial development. One example of this is Meta's (at that time Facebook's) Instagram Kids initiative, targeted toward capturing children under the age of 13. This project was "paused" by the company in September 2021 and following backlash from parent and other special interest groups has not been yet relaunched. Such initiatives from the industry need to be viewed critically. On the one hand, the psycho-developmental tasks of children and adolescents need to be considered and children's rights protected. On the other hand, we must be careful of the current business model operating on the premise of prolonging engagement online (which takes valuable time away from children to focus on their psycho-developmental tasks), though they may purport to do otherwise (i.e., screen washing) [16].

What are the psycho-developmental tasks in adolescence that might conflict with the social media industry's business model? According to Erikson's model, identity formation plays an important part in adolescence, where young minds need to discover who they are (for more insights on this highly relevant topic see the book *Behind Their Screens*) [17]. In our view, the psychosocial crisis—occurring in the life stage of *identity vs. role confusion*—needs to be discussed in terms of the positive and negative aspects of social media. Without doubt, social media is used by adolescent users to present themselves, express their world views, test out different identity roles, retain currency, and connect with and seek feedback from their peers and like-minded others [18, 19]. Here, one could also emphasize the opportunities for content creation in the digital world to express oneself (though it is important to note that the digital world is not always a safe space). In contrast to these opportunities for young users, problems arise from photoshopped or filtered pictures, which create inauthentic representations of beauty and somatic perfection which do not actually exist in real life. This action can result in body dissatisfaction and even behaviors related to disordered eating from those who view the images and "comparing and despairing" [20, 21]. Considering the potential scalability of reaching a large audience, cyber-aggression [22] can severely exacerbate identity confusion (as evidenced by the association between cyberbullying and lower self-esteem [23]; for newer insights on cyberbullying see reviews) [24, 25].

Against the background of psycho-developmental tasks to be fulfilled by children and adolescents, it needs to be mentioned that the design of social media platforms might cause problems in this regard because time spent on social media might displace time on fulfilling psycho-developmental tasks. It has been posited that the highly immersive platform design of the social media industry is particularly successful in luring in young users. A recent meta-analysis, in fact, has shown that younger age is associated with more self-reported addictive tendencies toward social media [26]. One explanation could be the observation that brain maturation—in particular the prefrontal cortex—is still occurring [27]. This makes it more difficult for young minds to engage in self-regulation behaviors.

Regarding the immersive platform design, social media companies have employed AB-testing over many years to foster their business model [28]. AB-testing means that a current version of a social media platform (A) is tested against another version (B) where, for instance, a new design element—i.e., the "Like" button—is included. The industry then reviews user behavior to determine if the new design element results in their intended more protracted user time spent online and increased engagement with the platform. Considering the topic of the present chapter, the question arises regarding whether or not certain (interactions of) design elements impact the mental health of adolescent social media users [29]. Such design elements could be the presentation of "Likes" (or similar type affirmations) of posts from other users, which may stimulate upward social comparison and reward mechanisms. Of note, such upward comparisons have been linked both to being envious and lowered subjective well-being [30, 31]. In this context, hiding "Likes," a relatively new feature actually offered by Instagram, could be an interesting intervention (but see recent work outlining complex effects) [32]. For more insights also see the press release by Instagram [33]. The "Like" metric could further stimulate adolescent users to imitate observed (risk) behaviors to receive positive feedback from their peer group. Additionally, so called "challenges" on TikTok are a prominent example of fulfilling needs of achievement and competence [13]. In addition, personalized services, such as TikTok's "For You" feed could encourage inaccurate mental health self-diagnoses [34], self-harm, and suicidal ideation [35]. In this context, one should not forget about the famous classic psychological studies around Albert Bandura pointing toward the power of social learning mechanisms (learning from role models) [36], whereas included in such role models today are the so-called Influencers commanding increasingly dangerous mentoring power on social media. Aside from the above-presented design elements, one could further criticize design elements such as endless scrolling aimed at creating time distortion on the user's side, so that users spent more time on the platform than they originally intended (other design elements are push notifications, clickbaits, read-receipt-functions, etc.; for a taxonomy of design elements see the work: [37].

The importance to study age-appropriate social media design is also supported by the implementation of a group by the European Commission precisely dealing with this topic [38].

## 3 Future Research

Unfortunately, it is difficult for independent scientists to study a single design element—or even several design elements—in interaction regarding their exact effects on the users [39]. Currently, this investigation is only possible through painstakingly created experimental studies, which reverse engineer social media platforms. The so-called "APIcalypse" describes the current situation where *Application Programming Interfaces* (API), allowing the direct study of behavior on the platforms, are mainly closed to public use [40]. In the aftermath of the Cambridge Analytica data scandal, for instance, Facebook (now Meta) closed their APIs, preventing independent academics from studying behavior on social media. Additionally, Elon Musk, as the new owner of Twitter (now X), closed their APIs for independent scientists unless agreeing to pay a largely financially burdensome (estimated) $42,000 US Dollars per month for such access [41]. This situation is subject to criticism in many ways. After many years of social media controversies and scandals [42, 43], one could argue that trust toward the existing social media companies can only be re-established if the platforms are scrutinized by independent scientists not funded by the industry. Another route to be taken is to completely rethink the social media business model [44]. As highlighted by the recently approved UK Online Safety Act [45], user to user services (e.g., TikTok, X, and Facebook) and search services (e.g., Google and Bing) have a duty of care to children to conduct children's risk assessments (and keep them current), which consider the potential of harm relating to content or the functionality of the services. Beyond the detection of risk, operators should be conducting independent risk minimization audits, taking into consideration young people's perspectives in delivering socially responsible design. This should include assessing the impact of design elements in terms of risk before launch.

Investigations of social media use and its impacts should ideally be followed by interdisciplinary efforts supplementing survey data with both neuroscientific and objective data from the platforms [46]. Such an interdisciplinary effort is essential, as numerous and diverse research questions around *social media use in adolescence* have increasingly emerged in recent years. These topics range from problematic social media use [47] eliciting body dissatisfaction and eating disorders [48] to the relationship between social media use and negative emotionality [49], and young minds being exposed to gruesome and age-inappropriate content on the platforms [50, 51]. We are also aware of many other relevant research questions around filter bubbles and polarization falling more in the area of political data science [52, 53], which need to be addressed by interdisciplinary collaboration and the efforts of independent academics. On a more positive note, the potential problems and risks surrounding social media engagement for adolescents are also recognized by regulatory bodies around the world (see above also the initiative from the UK). In this context, we want to briefly review a recent EU initiative aiming to tackle problems around social media use in adolescence. The EU Digital Services Act (DSA) [54] needs to be mentioned, as it expects the social media industry to counteract harm being elicited by their platforms. A special focus lies on the protection of minors, where the DSA requires the industry to follow this agenda (original wording as found on the EU's website) [55]:

- "Platforms will have to redesign their systems to ensure a high level of privacy, security, and safety of minors;

- Targeted advertising based on profiling toward children is no longer permitted;
- Special risk assessments, including for negative effects on mental health, will have to be provided to the Commission 4 months after designation and made public at the latest a year later;
- Platforms will have to redesign their services, including their interfaces, recommender systems, terms and conditions, to mitigate these risks."

The DSA applies to "Very Large Online Platforms (VLOPs)," with the expectation of full new regulation implementation compliance deadline of February 17, 2024, for all digital service providers. In this context, the DSA also envisions the possibility of opening APIs for independent scientists. However, if we understand the DSA correctly, this would only occur in specific cases though, namely, to allow independent academics to investigate whether the industry is indeed following the rules proposed by the DSA—such as protecting adolescents from negative content on their platforms [56].

## 4 Recommendations

- The need to understand the effect of social media on young users is not only underlined by the EU's DSA but also by a recent lawsuit of 33 US states vs. Meta stating that "Meta has harnessed its extraordinary innovation and technology to lure youth and teens to maximize use of its products" [57]. Regulation must go further than what is proposed in the DSA and establish a general opening-up of the platforms for independent researchers to study the complex relationship between social media and well-being in both young and older users. This transparency is crucial because we believe that online interactions, risks, and harms lie on a continuum of severity, as do other human behaviors [58], which might be borderline cases or are not captured by the immediate regulatory initiatives of the EU.
- Besides (re-) opening APIs to really understand the behavior of younger users, research needs to be supplemented by neuroscientific studies, as this area is surprisingly sparse. This is especially noteworthy because mass media, lay persons, and the industry use a highly neuro-scientifically slanted language to describe (the effects of) social media engineering, such as dopamine triggers, brain hacks, and, of course, the term addiction [46, 59]. We explicitly note that the addiction term is currently not officially recognized in the context of excessive social media use by either the World Health Organization or American Psychiatric Association. The discussion around social media addiction remains controversial, and it is critical to provide clarity to parents and other stakeholders, grounded in solid scientific evidence.
- Upon review of the existing age barriers, only users 13 years or older should onboard to social media. Even with that age boundary in place, as children can vastly vary in terms of development, resiliency, and maturation, parents should determine the actual appropriateness (13 years or higher), selection, and limits of their child's engagement with social media. The reality, however, is different. Although it is challenging to obtain precise numbers, most readers will recognize the inclusion of younger users in their direct social networks. In this context, we also wonder why the entry to social media platforms (age barrier of 13 years) is not better policed, and would recommend stronger enforcement in this area as also reflected in recent school bans of smartphone use [60].
- It is a pressing issue to find answers to the many questions about social media use and healthy psychosocial development of children and adolescents by relying on experts from different disciplines working together. With nearly five billion users across myriad social media applications and platforms, and many of them minors, much is at stake for societies around the world and the mental health of users—especially those younger or who strug-

gle with biologically, psychologically, or sociologically based issues. This is significant not only from the perspective of psychological, psychiatric, and neuroscientific sciences but also from disciplines such as political and other social sciences. With great power comes great responsibility, and this is particularly true for supranational operating social media platforms. They should openly share their knowledge on the effects of their platform design and should this continue to be declined by the industry, international regulations must enable the possibility for societies to study social media use.

- Moreover, governmental regulations should be imposed to prevent social media platforms from implementing their attention-economy model at the expense of healthy youth development [16]. The situation where social media in many ways represents a black box is not tolerable, and it is certainly time to reconsider social media and think about how to foster healthier platforms [44].
- Preventive measures should be developed using strict methods to prove efficacy. Such preventive interventions—especially selective approaches to detect risky patterns of use based on algorithms—need to be implemented in social media platforms.

**Conflict of Interest and Funding Disclosures** None.

## References

1. Zuboff S. The age of surveillance capitalism: The fight for a human future at the new frontier of power. Profile Books; 2019.
2. Montag C, Elhai JD. On social media design, (online-)time well-spent and addictive behaviors in the age of surveillance capitalism. Curr Addict Rep. 2023;10(3):610–6. https://doi.org/10.1007/s40429-023-00494-3.
3. Zarouali B, Dobber T, Pauw G, Vreese C. Using a personality-profiling algorithm to investigate political microtargeting: assessing the persuasion effects of personality-tailored ads on social media. Commun Res. 49(8):1066–91. https://doi.org/10.1177/0093650220961965.
4. Bhargava VR, Velasquez M. Ethics of the attention economy: the problem of social media addiction. Bus Ethics Q. 2021;31(3):321–59. https://doi.org/10.1017/beq.2020.32.
5. Ritvo D, Bavitz C, Gupta R, Oberman I. Privacy and children's data – an overview of the Children's Online Privacy Protection Act and the Family Educational Rights and Privacy Act. Published online 14 Nov 2013. https://doi.org/10.2139/ssrn.2354339.
6. Boyd D, Hargittai E, Schultz J, Palfrey J. Why parents help their children lie to Facebook about age: Unintended consequences of the "Children's Online Privacy Protection Act". First Monday. 2011;16(11). https://firstmonday.org/ojs/index.php/fm/article/download/3850/3075.
7. Batra S. The Psychosocial Development of Children: Implications for Education and Society – Erik Erikson in Context. Contemp Educ Dialogue. 2013;10:249–78. https://doi.org/10.1177/0973184913485014.
8. Panksepp J. Affective neuroscience: the foundations of human and animal emotions. Oxford University Press; 1998.
9. Erikson EH, Erikson JM. The life cycle completed (extended version). W. W. Norton & Company; 1998.
10. Erikson EH. Youth: change and challenge. Basic Books; 1963.
11. Montag C, Sindermann C, Lester D, Davis KL. Linking individual differences in satisfaction with each of Maslow's needs to the Big Five personality traits and Panksepp's primary emotional systems. Heliyon. 2020;6(7):e04325. https://doi.org/10.1016/j.heliyon.2020.e04325.
12. Tomova L, Tye K, Saxe R. The neuroscience of unmet social needs. Soc Neurosci. 2021;16(3):221–31. https://doi.org/10.1080/17470919.2019.1694580.
13. Ryan RM, Deci EL. Self-determination theory and the facilitation of intrinsic motivation, social development, and well-being. Am Psychol. 2000;55(1):68–78. https://doi.org/10.1037/0003-066X.55.1.68.
14. Montag C, Diefenbach S. Towards homo digitalis: important research issues for psychology and the neurosciences at the dawn of the internet of things and the digital society. Sustainability. 2018;10(2):415. https://doi.org/10.3390/su10020415.
15. Suleyman M, Bhaskar M. The coming wave: technology, power, and the twenty-first century's greatest dilemma. Crown; 2023.
16. Koning IM, Vossen H. From green-washing to screen-washing? How the tech-industry plays around with children's future. J Behav Addict. 2024;13(1):1–5. https://doi.org/10.1556/2006.2023.00084
17. Weinstein E, James C. Behind their screens: what teens are facing (and adults are missing). MIT Press; 2022.
18. Shankleman M, Hammond L, Jones FW. Adolescent social media use and well-being: a systematic review and thematic meta-synthesis. Adolesc Res Rev. 2021;6(4):471–92. https://doi.org/10.1007/s40894-021-00154-5.

19. Uhls YT, Ellison NB, Subrahmanyam K. Benefits and costs of social media in adolescence. Pediatrics. 2017;140(Supplement_2):S67–70. https://doi.org/10.1542/peds.2016-1758E.
20. Fardouly J, Vartanian LR. Social media and body image concerns: current research and future directions. Curr Opin Psychol. 2016;9:1–5. https://doi.org/10.1016/j.copsyc.2015.09.005.
21. Rozgonjuk D, Ignell J, Mech F, Rothermund E, Gündel H, Montag C. Smartphone and Instagram use, body dissatisfaction, and eating disorders: investigating the associations using self-report and tracked data. J Eat Disord. 2023;11(1):149. https://doi.org/10.1186/s40337-023-00865-1.
22. Kumar VL, Goldstein MA. Cyberbullying and adolescents. Curr Pediatr Rep. 2020;8(3):86–92. https://doi.org/10.1007/s40124-020-00217-6.
23. Patchin JW, Hinduja S. Cyberbullying and self-esteem*. J Sch Health. 2010;80(12):614–21. https://doi.org/10.1111/j.1746-1561.2010.00548.x.
24. Henares-Montiel J, Benítez-Hidalgo V, Ruiz-Pérez I, Pastor-Moreno G, Rodríguez-Barranco M. Cyberbullying and associated factors in member countries of the European Union: a systematic review and meta-analysis of studies with representative population samples. Int J Environ Res Public Health. 2022;19(12):7364. https://doi.org/10.3390/ijerph19127364.
25. Li J, Huebner ES, Tian L. Linking childhood maltreatment to cyberbullying perpetration and victimization: a systematic review and multilevel meta-analysis. Comput Hum Behav. 2024;156:108199. https://doi.org/10.1016/j.chb.2024.108199.
26. Cheng C, Lau Y-C, Chan L, Luk JW. Prevalence of social media addiction across 32 nations: meta-analysis with subgroup analysis of classification schemes and cultural values. Addict Behav. 2021;117:106845. https://doi.org/10.1016/j.addbeh.2021.106845.
27. Blakemore SJ, Choudhury S. Development of the adolescent brain: implications for executive function and social cognition. J Child Psychol Psychiatry. 2006;47(3–4):296–312. https://doi.org/10.1111/j.1469-7610.2006.01611.x.
28. Montag C, Lachmann B, Herrlich M, Zweig K. Addictive features of social media/messenger platforms and freemium games against the background of psychological and economic theories. Int J Environ Res Public Health. 2019;16(14):2612. https://doi.org/10.3390/ijerph16142612.
29. Sindermann C, Montag C, Elhai JD. The design of social media platforms—initial evidence on relations between personality, fear of missing out, design element-driven increased social media use, and problematic social media use. Technol Mind Behav. 2022;3(4):1–16. https://tmb.apaopen.org/pub/m4nkf-stp/release/1. Accessed 27 Jan 2023.
30. Verduyn P, Ybarra O, Résibois M, Jonides J, Kross E. Do social network sites enhance or undermine subjective well-being? A critical review: do social network sites enhance or undermine subjective well-being? Soc Issues Policy Rev. 2017;11:274–302. https://doi.org/10.1111/sipr.12033.
31. Vogel EA, Rose JP, Roberts LR, Eckles K. Social comparison, social media, and self-esteem. Psychol Pop Media Cult. 2014;3(4):206–22. https://doi.org/10.1037/ppm0000047.
32. Wallace E, Buil I. Hiding Instagram likes: effects on negative affect and loneliness. Personal Individ Differ. 2021;170:110509. https://doi.org/10.1016/j.paid.2020.110509.
33. Instagram. Giving people more control on Instagram and Facebook. 2021. https://about.instagram.com/blog/announcements/giving-people-more-control. (Accessed 13th September 2024)
34. Yıldırım S. The challenge of self-diagnosis on mental health through social media: a qualitative study. In: Battineni G, Mittal M, Chintalapudi N, editors. Computational methods in psychiatry. Springer Nature; 2023. p. 197–213. https://doi.org/10.1007/978-981-99-6637-0_10.
35. Amnesty International. Driven into darkness. Amnesty International; 2023. https://www.amnesty.org/en/documents/pol40/7350/2023/en/. Accessed 21 Dec 2023.
36. Bandura A, Ross D, Ross SA. Transmission of aggression through imitation of aggressive models. J Abnorm Soc Psychol. 1961;63(3):575–82. https://doi.org/10.1037/h0045925.
37. Flayelle M, Brevers D, King DL, Maurage P, Perales JC, Billieux J. A taxonomy of technology design features that promote potentially addictive online behaviours. Nat Rev Psychol. 2023;2(3):136–50. https://doi.org/10.1038/s44159-023-00153-4.
38. EU Commission. Special group on the EU Code of conduct on age-appropriate design. 2023. https://digital-strategy.ec.europa.eu/en/policies/group-age-appropriate-design. (Accessed 13th September 2024)
39. Montag C, Hegelich S, Sindermann C, Rozgonjuk D, Marengo D, Elhai JD. On corporate responsibility when studying social media use and well-being. Trends Cogn Sci. 2021;25(4):268–70. https://doi.org/10.1016/j.tics.2021.01.002.
40. Bruns A. After the "APIcalypse": social media platforms and their fight against critical scholarly research. Inf Commun Soc. 2019;22:1–23. https://doi.org/10.1080/1369118X.2019.1637447.
41. Calma J. Twitter just closed the book on academic research. The Verge. 2023. https://www.theverge.com/2023/5/31/23739084/twitter-elon-musk-api-policy-chilling-academic-research. (Accessed 13th September 2024)
42. Haugen F. The power of one: blowing the whistle on Facebook. Hodder & Stoughton; 2023.
43. Wylie C. Mindf*ck: inside Cambridge Analytica's plot to break the world. Main edition. Profile Books; 2020.
44. Dhawan S, Hegelich S, Sindermann C, Montag C. Re-start social media, but how? Telematics Inform Rep. 2022;8:100017. https://doi.org/10.1016/j.teler.2022.100017.

45. UK Parliament. Online Safety Act 2023 – Parliamentary Bills – UK Parliament. 2023. https://bills.parliament.uk/bills/3137. Accessed 21 Dec 2023.
46. Montag C, Marciano L, Schulz PJ, Becker B. Unlocking the brain secrets of social media through neuroscience. Trends Cogn Sci. 2023;27(12):1102–4. https://doi.org/10.1016/j.tics.2023.09.005.
47. van den Eijnden R, Koning I, Doornwaard S, van Gurp F, Ter Bogt T. The impact of heavy and disordered use of games and social media on adolescents' psychological, social, and school functioning. J Behav Addict. 2018;7(3):697–706. https://doi.org/10.1556/2006.7.2018.65.
48. Marks RJ, De Foe A, Collett J. The pursuit of wellness: social media, body image and eating disorders. Child Youth Serv Rev. 2020;119:105659. https://doi.org/10.1016/j.childyouth.2020.105659.
49. Hussain Z, Wegmann E, Yang H, Montag C. Social networks use disorder and associations with depression and anxiety symptoms: a systematic review of recent research in China. Front Psychol. 2020;11:211. https://doi.org/10.3389/fpsyg.2020.00211.
50. Klausen J. Tweeting the Jihad: social media networks of western foreign fighters in Syria and Iraq. Stud Conflict Terrorism. 2015;38(1):1–22. https://doi.org/10.1080/1057610X.2014.974948.
51. Mathew B, Dutt R, Goyal P, Mukherjee A. Spread of hate speech in online social media. In: Proceedings of the 10th ACM Conference on Web Science. WebSci '19. Association for Computing Machinery; 2019. p. 173–82. https://doi.org/10.1145/3292522.3326034.
52. Sindermann C, Cooper A, Montag C. A short review on susceptibility to falling for fake political news. Curr Opin Psychol. 2020;36:44–8. https://doi.org/10.1016/j.copsyc.2020.03.014.
53. Sindermann C, Elhai JD, Moshagen M, Montag C. Age, gender, personality, ideological attitudes and individual differences in a person's news spectrum: how many and who might be prone to "filter bubbles" and "echo chambers" online? Heliyon. 2020;6(1):e03214. https://doi.org/10.1016/j.heliyon.2020.e03214.
54. European Commission. The Digital Services Act (DSA) overview. 2024. https://bit.ly/3t2TuAj. (Accessed 13th September 2024)
55. European Commission. Digital Services Act: commission designates first set of very large online platforms and search engines. 2023. https://ec.europa.eu/commission/presscorner/detail/en/IP_23_2413. (Accessed 13th September 2024)
56. European Commission. The enforcement framework under the Digital Services Act. 2024. https://digital-strategy.ec.europa.eu/en/policies/dsa-enforcement. (Accessed 13th September 2024)
57. Wong Q. California sues Facebook parent Meta over alleged harm to young people. Los Angeles Times. 2023. https://www.latimes.com/california/story/2023-10-24/facebook-parent-meta-sued-instagram-young-people.
58. Throuvala MA, Griffiths MD, Rennoldson M, Kuss DJ. Perceived challenges and online harms from social media use on a severity continuum: a qualitative psychological stakeholder perspective. Int J Environ Res Public Health. 2021;18(6):3227. https://doi.org/10.3390/ijerph18063227.
59. Boer M, Stevens GWJM, Finkenauer C, Koning IM, van den Eijnden RJJM. Validation of the social media disorder scale in adolescents: findings from a large-scale nationally representative sample. Assessment. 2022;29(8):1658–75. https://doi.org/10.1177/10731911211027232.
60. Montag C, Elhai J. Do we need a digital school uniform? Arguments for and against a smartphone ban in schools. Soc Impacts. 2023;1:100002. https://doi.org/10.1016/j.socimp.2023.100002.

# Distinguishing Credible from Sham: Supporting Young People to Navigate Online

Joel Breakstone, Sarah McGrew, Mark Smith, and Sam Wineburg

## 1 Background

Nearly half of American teenagers report being online "almost constantly" [1]. The digital landscape they encounter poses a range of challenges. Misinformation proliferates. Foreign actors seek to subvert American elections. Grifters peddle fake medical cures. Corporate interests, masquerading as grassroots movements, attempt to influence public policy. Are young people equipped to distinguish credible sources from sham?

There is no argument that members of Generation Z skillfully operate digital devices. However, this facility does not always translate into an ability to discern the information these devices provide. In a recent survey, 3446 high school students in the United States were presented with a series of five online tasks in which they evaluated sources like a climate change denial website and a social media post about gun control [2]. Students struggled on each task. In one example, students watched a Facebook video claiming to show ballot stuffing in American elections. The video was actually shot in Russia, a fact easily established by opening a new browser tab and entering a few keywords. However, only three students—less than one-tenth of 1%—made that connection.

## 2 Current State

There are proven curricular approaches to teaching people how to be more discerning consumers of online content, a critical component of digital literacy. These approaches are based on observations of fact checkers at prestigious news outlets in the United States [3, 4]. Fact checkers' search trajectories were compared to two other groups of skilled readers: Stanford University undergraduates and academics from five American universities. Both students and academics approached websites *vertically*, reading from top to bottom and dwelling on the target site. Fact checkers, on the other hand, read *laterally*, leaving a site almost immediately, opening new tabs, and using other online resources to validate the original site. Consequently, fact checkers arrived at better answers in less time than the other two groups. Based on these findings, researchers in the United States, Canada, Sweden, and Italy have developed interventions to teach people to deploy strategies used by professional fact checkers. Thirteen separate studies, involving nearly 10,000 subjects across a wide age range, show that lateral reading helps people evaluate digital content more effectively [5–11]. In one study [12], across ten Canadian provinces, high school

J. Breakstone (✉) · M. Smith · S. Wineburg
Stanford University, Stanford, CA, USA
e-mail: breakstone@stanford.edu

S. McGrew
University of Maryland, College Park, MD, USA



D. A. Christakis, L. Hale (eds.), *Handbook of Children and Screens*,
https://doi.org/10.1007/978-3-031-69362-5_66

students showed a sixfold increase in use of fact checking techniques after only 7 hours of instruction. In a randomized control study [13] in Lincoln, Nebraska, public schools, after 6 hours of instruction, students outperformed peers in control classrooms on evaluations of Internet sources.

Despite intense interest in the issue, outdated approaches to digital literacy are frequently taught in educational settings [14, 15]. Many of these antiquated curricular tools take the form of checklists [16, 17]. These lists direct students to answer questions about unfamiliar sources that focus on a source's internal features, such as its top-level domain (e.g., dot-org), its About page, the presence or absences of ads, the recency of its updates, and the authority of its links. Searchers who rely on such markers put themselves at the mercy of website creators who, irrespective of motives, portray themselves flatteringly. A study [18] of the evaluation criteria suggested by 50 top-ranked colleges and universities showed that 96% included checklists on their websites or linked to checklist approaches on other sites.

Although checklist approaches to establishing web credibility are widely used, they are not grounded in research. University of Washington research scientist Michael Caulfield [19] traced the origins of the widely used CRAAP Test ("currency," "relevance," "authority," "appearance," and "purpose") to a 1978 guide for purchasing library materials. More importantly, the evaluative approach fostered by these checklists often leads to strikingly incorrect conclusions. Consider the website of the International Life Sciences Institute (ilsi.org). It is professionally designed and carries a dot-org URL. It includes contact information and lists staff members and advisors with PhDs. The site would receive high marks on the CRAAP Test. However, a quick online search reveals that the group was founded in 1980 by a former Coca-Cola vice president. A *New York Times* article [20] refers to ILSI as a "shadowy industry group" that "has been quietly infiltrating government health and nutrition bodies around the world" and "is almost entirely funded by Goliaths of the agribusiness, food and pharmaceutical industries." However, students relying on checklist approaches would likely miss this information because their attention would be directed at the site itself.

Evidence suggests that many people have adopted the *weak heuristics* propagated by checklists [3, 9]. Across a range of studies [13, 21–27], similar patterns emerge: Students automatically reject dot-com websites, unquestioningly trust the information provided by About pages, place credence in links to credible sources (even when those sources don't support the claim being made), and use other flawed strategies focused on easily-gamed surface features. Even the Office of the US Surgeon General [28] published a "Misinformation Toolkit" that instructed readers to "look at the 'About Us' page on the website to see if you can trust the source."

Ongoing concerns about the pernicious effects of misinformation have prompted legislative action in the United States. Eighteen states have enacted legislation mandating media literacy instruction. In 2021, Illinois became the first state to require media literacy instruction in high schools. In 2023, New Jersey passed a law [29] requiring media literacy instruction from kindergarten through 12th grade. Eleven states currently have new bills under consideration [30]. However, school districts have few models for how to integrate digital literacy across grades and subjects, and they'll have to sort through curricular materials of varying quality to make decisions about how to comply with these mandates.

## 3 Future Research

In the last decade, strides have been made in understanding how young people evaluate online information [2, 27], how experts approach unfamiliar digital sources [4], and how to effectively teach those strategies to students [13]. Yet, much work remains. The following research questions merit attention:

- *How can adults be supported to learn and teach digital literacy?* Students are not the only ones who need more support in evaluating digital information. Even highly educated adults harbor misconceptions [15, 31]. In the research with professional fact checkers [4], tenured professors often struggled to evaluate unfamiliar websites. Thus, we need to investigate ways to support adults to learn effective digital evaluation strategies and to teach those strategies to students.
- *How can schools integrate digital literacy into the curriculum?* Across the U.S., states have passed legislation mandating digital literacy instruction [32]. However, little research exists examining what schools currently do and how best to undertake curricular integration. To support schools in doing this work, research should identify best practices for integrating digital literacy across the curriculum and chart students' developmental trajectories as they learn to evaluate online information.
- *How do young people's beliefs and identities influence their evaluations?* Effective evaluation strategies can be powerful tools for finding high-quality information. However, when we evaluate information on topics we care about, our desire to find information that matches our prior beliefs may interfere. More research is needed to understand how to help young people learn to evaluate information about charged topics and to reflect on how their beliefs influence their evaluations.
- *How do we reach people outside of school settings and how can trusted messengers (e.g., parents, health professionals, and community leaders) provide instruction about evidence-based strategies for evaluating online information?* Digital literacy instruction cannot be limited to school settings. The more consistent the messages young people receive from trusted adults in their lives, the better. Thus, we need more research to help us understand how trusted messengers like parents, librarians, community health workers, and coaches might support youth to make wise choices about what they find online [33].

## 4 Recommendations

- Students have not been equipped with the knowledge and skills needed to navigate online. Given this challenge, our response should be multi-faceted and designed to reach young people in many parts of their lives, including in school, at home, and with trusted adults. As the Aspen Institute Commission on Information Disorder [34] concluded, "Information disorder is a whole-of-society problem that can have life-or-death consequences. It will require urgent and meaningful interventions … and the commitments of every part of society to reverse these disturbing trends."
- In schools, educators need additional training to help them learn effective evaluation strategies. Professional development must be paired with digital literacy curriculum that aligns with the content of core school subjects. Teachers cannot be expected to shoulder this work alone. Evidence-based, classroom-ready materials must be developed, validated, and disseminated. Furthermore, states and districts need models for how to integrate digital literacy at scale, including guidance about approaches to assessing students' progress over time.
- We must broaden our purview from public education to *education of the public*. Systematic research is needed to understand how parents and community leaders could learn effective evaluation strategies and then mentor young people about those strategies. For example, parents, health professionals, and community leaders could receive prompts for conversation starters and follow-up questions as well as written materials (e.g., posters or pamphlets) to provide young people and their families with vetted resources. Digital confusion threatens young people's ability to participate in civic life. Fortunately, we have research-based approaches for navigating a treacherous online terrain. The challenge in front of us is ensuring that all young people have an opportunity to learn these critical skills.

**Conflict of Interest and Funding Disclosures** None.

## References


1. Vogels EA, Gelles-Watnick R, Massarat N. Teens, social media and technology 2022. Pew Research Center. 10 Aug 2022. https://www.pewresearch.org/internet/2022/08/10/teens-social-media-and-technology-2022/. Accessed 8 Mar 2023.
2. Breakstone J, Smith M, Wineburg S, et al. Students' civic online reasoning: a national portrait. Educ Res. 2021;50(8):505–15. https://doi.org/10.3102/0013189X211017495.
3. Wineburg S, McGrew S. Lateral reading: reading less and learning more when evaluating digital information. SSRN. Preprint posted online 6 Oct 2017. https://doi.org/10.2139/ssrn.3048994.
4. Wineburg S, McGrew S. Lateral reading and the nature of expertise: reading less and learning more when evaluating digital information. Teach Coll Rec. 2019;121(11):1–40. https://doi.org/10.1177/016146811912101102.
5. Axelsson CW, Guath M, Nygren T. Learning how to separate fake from real news: scalable digital tutorials promoting students' civic online reasoning. Future Internet. 2021;13(3):60–78. https://doi.org/10.3390/fi13030060.
6. Breakstone J, Smith M, Connors P, Ortega T, Kerr D, Wineburg S. Lateral reading: college students learn to critically evaluate internet sources in an online course. Harv Kennedy Sch Misinformation Rev. 2021;2(1):1–17. https://doi.org/10.37016/mr-2020-56.
7. Brodsky JE, Brooks PJ, Scimeca D, Galati P, Todorova R, Caulfield M. Associations between online instruction in lateral reading strategies and fact-checking COVID-19 news among college students. AERA Open. 2021;7(1):233285842110317–89. https://doi.org/10.1177/23328584211038937.
8. Kohnen AM, Mertens GE, Boehm SM. Can middle schoolers learn to read the web like experts? Possibilities and limits of a strategy-based intervention. J Media Lit Educ. 2020;12(2):64–79. https://doi.org/10.23860/JMLE-2020-12-2-6.
9. McGrew S. Learning to evaluate: an intervention in civic online reasoning. Comput Educ. 2020;145:103711–3. https://doi.org/10.1016/j.compedu.2019.103711.
10. McGrew S, Breakstone J. Civic online reasoning across the curriculum. AERA Open. 2023;9. https://doi.org/10.1177/23328584231176451.
11. McGrew S, Smith M, Breakstone J, Ortega T, Wineburg S. Improving students' web savvy: an intervention study. Br J Educ Psychol. 2019;89(3):485–500. https://doi.org/10.1111/bjep.12279.
12. Pavlounis D, Johnston J, Brodsky J, Brooks P. The digital media literacy gap: how to build widespread resilience to false and misleading information using evidence-based classroom tools. CIVIX Canada. Nov 2021. https://ctrl-f.ca/en/wp-content/uploads/2022/01/The-Digital-Media-Literacy-Gap.pdf. Accessed 8 Mar 2023.
13. Wineburg S, Breakstone J, McGrew S, Smith M, Ortega T. Lateral reading on the open internet: a district-wide field study in high school government classes. J Educ Psychol. 2022;114(5):893–909. https://doi.org/10.1037/edu0000740.
14. Breakstone J, McGrew S, Smith M, Ortega T, Wineburg S. Why we need a new approach to teaching digital literacy. Phi Delta Kappan. 2018;99(6):27–32. https://doi.org/10.1177/0031721718762419.
15. McGrew S. Challenging approaches: sharing and responding to weak digital heuristics in class discussions. Teach Teach Educ. 2021;108:103512. https://doi.org/10.1016/j.tate.2021.103512.
16. Caulfield M. Yes, digital literacy. But which one? Hapgood. 19 Dec 2016. https://hapgood.us/2016/12/19/yes-digital-literacy-but-which-one/. Accessed 8 Mar 2023.
17. Sullivan MC. Why librarians can't fight fake news. J Librariansh Inf Sci. 2019;51(4):1146–56. https://doi.org/10.1177/0961000618764258.
18. Ziv N, Bene E. Preparing college students for a digital age: a survey of instructional approaches to spotting misinformation. C&RL. 2022;83(6):905. https://doi.org/10.5860/crl.83.6.905.
19. Caulfield M. A short history of CRAAP. Hapgood. 14 Sept 2018. https://hapgood.us/2018/09/14/a-short-history-of-craap/. Accessed 8 Mar 2023.
20. Jacobs J. A shadowy interest group shapes food policy around the world. The New York Times. 16 Sept 2019. https://www.nytimes.com/2019/09/16/health/ilsi-food-policy-india-brazil-china.html. Accessed 8 Mar 2023.
21. Bakke A. Everyday Googling: results of an observational study and applications for teaching algorithmic literacy. Comput Compos. 2020;57:102577–16. https://doi.org/10.1016/j.compcom.2020.102577.
22. Barzilai S, Zohar A. Epistemic thinking in action: evaluating and integrating online sources. Cogn Instr. 2012;30(1):39–85. https://doi.org/10.1080/07370008.2011.636495.
23. Dissen A, Qadiri Q, Middleton CJ. I read it online: understanding how undergraduate students assess the accuracy of online sources of health information. Am J Lifestyle Med. 2021;16(5):641–54. https://doi.org/10.1177/1559827621990574.
24. Gasser U, Cortesi SC, Malik M, Lee A. Youth and digital media: from credibility to information quality. Berkman Klein Center for Internet & Society. 20 Feb 2012. https://doi.org/10.2139/ssrn.2005272. Accessed 8 Mar 2023.
25. Hargittai E, Fullerton L, Menchen-Trevino E, Thomas KY. Trust online: young adults' evaluation of web content. Int J Commun. 2010;4:468–94.
26. Martzoukou K, Fulton C, Kostagiolas P, Lavranos C. A study of higher education students' self-perceived digital competences for learning and everyday life

online participation. J Doc. 2020;76(6):1413–58. https://doi.org/10.1108/JD-03-2020-0041.
27. McGrew S, Breakstone J, Ortega T, Smith M, Wineburg S. Can students evaluate online sources? Learning from assessments of civic online reasoning. Theory Res Soc Educ. 2018;46(2):165–93. https://doi.org/10.1080/00933104.2017.1416320.
28. Office of the US Surgeon General. A community toolkit for addressing health misinformation. 2021. https://oes.gsa.gov/assets/publications/2120-health-misinformation-toolkit.pdf. Accessed 8 Mar 2023.
29. Media Literacy Now. Putting media literacy on the public policy agenda. Jan 2023. https://medialiteracynow.org/your-state-legislation-2/. Accessed 8 Mar 2023.
30. CivXNow. Pending state bills. https://civxnow.org/our-work/state-policy/pending-state-bills. Accessed 8 Mar 2023.
31. Weisberg L, Kohnen A, Dawson K. Impacts of a digital literacy intervention on preservice teachers' civic online reasoning abilities, strategies, and perceptions. J Technol Teach Educ. 2022;30(1):73–98.
32. Boryga A. Quality media literacy requires more than toothless laws, educators say. Edutopia. 29 Feb 2024. https://www.edutopia.org/article/quality-media-literacy-requires-more-than-toothless-laws-educators-say/. Accessed 10 Apr 2024.
33. Ad Council Research Institute. The 2022 trusted messenger study: the annual study of who Americans trust on social and societal issues. 2022. https://www.adcouncil.org/tmstudy. Accessed 8 Mar 2023.
34. Aspen Institute Commission on Information Disorder. Final report. Aspen Institute. 15 Nov 2021. https://www.aspeninstitute.org/publications/commission-on-information-disorder-final-report/. Accessed 8 Mar 2023.

# Children's Privacy in the Digital Age: US and UK Experiences and Policy Responses

Sonia Livingstone, Eva Lievens, Richard Graham, Kruakae Pothong, Stacey Steinberg, and Mariya Stoilova

## 1 Background

Children's privacy can receive culturally diverse interpretations and its implementation is often contested. To psychologists, it is vital to child development [1]. To clinicians, it is necessary for mental health. In the United Nations Convention on the Rights of the Child (UNCRC), it is a child's right. Yet, there is little consensus on from or by whom children's privacy should be protected. At issue are the dimensions of privacy (bodily, locational, communicational, decisional, and informational) [2], cultural understandings of privacy, and privacy's embedding in different legal systems [3, 4]. In most countries, legal protections center on privacy from the state, although also from commercial actors. Meanwhile, the public typically thinks of privacy in interpersonal terms, relying on negotiating social norms to protect their privacy.

In the digital age, privacy from the state, businesses, and individuals is both enabled and threatened by digital technologies and new forms of data processing, notably by commercial providers of digital products and services. Digital networks create new opportunities for interpersonal expression and exchange. These are highly valued by children and young people, although navigating digital spaces can make children's activities more visible to others than they realize [5]. However, privacy infringements are intensified now that everyday digital activities are tracked, shared, aggregated, and often monetized [6].

Data processing influences both privacy and the outcomes that depend on privacy—identity, dignity, freedom of thought and speech, safety, sociality, and participation. UNICEF argues that technological innovation impacts multiple dimensions of children's privacy and can have various negative effects [7]. Children's bodily (or physical) privacy is violated when tracking, monitoring, or live broadcasting or streaming technologies reveal a child's image, activities, or location. Their communicational privacy is violated when surveillant governments, bad actors, or unintended audiences gain access to children's posts, chats, or messages. Their informational privacy is violated when their personal data is

S. Livingstone (✉)
London School of Economics and Political Science, London, UK

Good Thinking: The London Digital Mental Wellbeing Service, London, UK
e-mail: S.Livingstone@lse.ac.uk

E. Lievens
Ghent University, Ghent, Belgium

R. Graham
stem4, London, UK

K. Pothong · M. Stoilova
London School of Economics and Political Science, London, UK

S. Steinberg
University of Florida, Gainesville, FL, USA


D. A. Christakis, L. Hale (eds.), *Handbook of Children and Screens*,
https://doi.org/10.1007/978-3-031-69362-5_67

collected, processed, or shared unlawfully or beyond what children reasonably expect. Finally, their decisional privacy is violated when digital design or automated decision making limits, directs, or biases children's thoughts and choices [8, 9].

In public and policy debates over privacy, children occupy an uneasy position. Media headlines complain that children's social media activities show they have no sense of privacy, also criticizing parents for publicly sharing images of their children. Parents, caregivers, and health advocates argue that children's privacy should not be invaded by commercial interests such as advertising and marketing [10]. Yet children's privacy gets short shrift in policy deliberations regarding privacy and data protection regulation. When it is discussed, it is often under the guise of keeping children safe rather than ensuring their right to privacy is honored [11]. Moreover, the same adults who defend their own privacy from the state and commerce may doubt that children need privacy, especially from their parents, notwithstanding that parental actions are not always in their child's best interests.

## 2 Current State

Privacy is widely theorized as relational, being variously sustained or threatened through social interactions shaped by conventions of visibility, intimacy, publicness, surveillance, consent, and redress. In highlighting these normative contextual factors, US legal scholar Helen Nissenbaum argues that privacy is "neither a right to secrecy nor a right to control, but a right to appropriate flow of personal information" [12]. How does, and how could, this apply in the digital environment, where children have little agency regarding the flow of their personal information (i.e., information that identifies them, either directly or indirectly)?

Research shows that children care about their privacy online, making efforts to create and sustain digital spaces that are both meaningful to them and privacy preserving, and finding tactics and workarounds when privacy settings are insufficient for their needs [13]. Yet the operation and consequences of the complex and opaque digital ecosystem in which children are increasingly immersed may remain beyond their comprehension, as they do for most adults. Hence, adequate policy responses are vital to protect children's privacy.

Unlike the right to free expression, the right to privacy is not an enumerated right within the text of the United States Constitution. As such, in the United States, courts will not weigh an individual's right to privacy equally with another individual's right to free expression or speech. Moreover, a parent's right to raise their child as they see fit is recognized as a constitutional right under the due process clause of the 14th Amendment. Thus, any discussions centered on a child's right to privacy are often outweighed both by parental rights to free expression and the parental right to dictate how the child is raised [14]. Laws that affect children's privacy either stem from a consumer or market perspective [15] (such as the 1998 Children's Online Privacy Protection Act (COPPA)), which requires parental consent for companies' processing of the data of children younger than 13, or they are adopted at the state level (such as the California Age-Appropriate Design Code Act). Recent legislative proposals by US lawmakers focus on children's online safety. While this may ultimately protect their privacy, it does not recognize children's agency according to their evolving capacities, which is recognized in the rights-based privacy protection in the UK and EU [16].

In the UK, and Europe more widely, although the right to privacy and the right to the protection of personal data are closely interlinked, they are not identical in scope or implementation [17]. Whereas the right to privacy prohibits state interference with an individual's personal sphere and the shaping and expression of identity (including sexual orientation) and family life, subject to some exceptions, the right to data protection provides a system of checks and balances for how information about an individual is processed by public and private actors [18]. The EU General Data Protection Regulation (GDPR), on which the UK data protection framework is also grounded, acknowledges that data protection is closely linked to other fundamental rights, and that children's data merits heightened protection because of their vulnerability. In the UK, such protections for children are articulated through a legally binding Age Appropriate Design Code (AADC), now also adopted and considered in various forms internationally, including in California, Maryland, New Mexico, Argentina, and Indonesia.

Contexts in which tensions between child rights or between child and adult rights are particularly relevant are the family, health, and educational contexts.

## 2.1 The Family Context

Courts in the US are reluctant to regulate family matters, and parents in the US have significant legal protections to control the upbringing of their children. Meanwhile, children in the UK benefit from the rights afforded to them through several UK laws, underpinned by the UK's ratification of the UNCRC, which recognizes the need to respect children's evolving autonomy, capacities, and privacy, even when parents' and children's interests conflict. The US has not ratified the UNCRC, mainly due to the concern that it will undermine parental authority to discipline children and, more generally, raise children as parents see fit. Consequently, until a young person's eighteenth birthday, parents have the authority to disclose a young person's private information with minimal or no state intervention [19]. Even when courts recognize that young people have an interest in privacy, this interest traditionally ends where intrafamilial life begins. Consider the context of parents sharing information online about their children ("sharenting") [20]. While this may benefit parents socially and financially, it can jeopardize their child's privacy, and allow third parties to collect and further share children's data, including sensitive images or location information, in ways unintended or unanticipated by the parent and potentially harmful to the child [21].

It is almost inconceivable to imagine courts in the US enjoining parents from posting publicly about their children, except in the most limited circumstances. Indeed, parents in the US often share images with unfettered restraint due to cultural and legal expectations of parental autonomy and free speech. By contrast, the UNCRC, UK GDPR, and other laws applicable in the UK and Europe offer young people certain legal remedies. Under the European Convention of Human Rights, to which the UK is a party, conflicts between a parent's right to family life and expression and a child's right to privacy is assessed on a case-by-case basis by the European Court. This is done using the child's best interests (UNCRC Article 3.1) as a guiding principle when balancing parents' and children's rights. Further, parental disclosures, labeled speech in the US, may constitute personal data in the UK, affording children greater legal protections such as the right to ask for the erasure of images ("the right to be forgotten"). However, in practice, it is difficult for children to exercise their right to privacy, in particular against a parent, and especially when very young [22]. Furthermore, there are doubts whether sharenting falls within the household exemption, thereby rendering the GDPR inapplicable [23].

## 2.2 The Educational Context

Data are collected from children throughout their learning lives—at school and in nonformal and informal learning settings—in ways that are intensified by the reliance on educational technologies for teaching, safeguarding, and administration. The data collected are often sensitive (including race/ethnicity, family hardship, mental health, and disabilities) and can be analyzed to reveal further intimate details about each child. Whether data collection is mandated by the government or is a matter of school choice, it is likely that children's data enter a global commercial ecosystem extending far beyond the school [24]; meanwhile the promised benefits (resulting from personalized learning or learning analytics) do not always materialize [25].

In the United States, the federal law intended to protect the privacy of students' educational records is the Family Educational Rights and Privacy Act (FERPA). Designed to prevent misuse of students' records, FERPA prioritizes informational privacy and relies on parental consent as "the primary mechanism for disclosure" [26]. This puts the primary responsibility for protecting children's data on parents rather than businesses, although whether parents can provide meaningful consent in complex data-driven economies is questionable [27]. In December 2023, the Federal Trade Commission proposed changes to COPPA which could also affect education technology (EdTech) providers, including a prohibition to use children's information for commercial use and additional safeguards [28].

In the United Kingdom, children's personal data are protected by the UK Data Protection Act 2018 and the UK GDPR. Further, the AADC applies to EdTech services likely to be accessed by children on a direct-to-consumer basis (on the web or through an app) [29]. This ensures privacy-by-design, data minimization requirements, and data subject rights. In practice, however, the US and the UK share similar problems of compliance and enforcement, partly because children's privacy at school is commonly a low priority and use of tech is often not a (real) choice, and partly because schools lack the expertise and resources to hold powerful EdTech companies to account [30].

### 2.3 The Health Context

Privacy is core to the delivery of healthcare, which increasingly has a digital dimension. Data protection laws apply to health records, given the sensitive personal data they contain. In the United States, the Health Insurance Portability and Accountability Act (HIPAA) includes stringent information security standards. However, as with education, commercial technologies increasingly provide the infrastructure for health services delivery. While detailed consideration has been applied to children's capacity to consent to medical treatment, their options to consent (or not) to the consequent data processing are limited, even though the data at issue may be highly sensitive. With innovation in digitally facilitated treatment [31], concerns are growing regarding whether digital health services respect children's privacy and protect their data [32, 33]. In addition to data protection considerations, "confidentiality concerns can be a critical barrier for young patients in seeking and receiving appropriate medical services, and confidentiality protection represents an important evidence-based practice in adolescent health care" [34]. Increasingly, these concerns intersect: parents may be informed of their child's treatment or learn of it through an insurance statement, for instance, in ways that the child does not anticipate or is not in their interest, compromising confidentiality for young patients [34].

In the United Kingdom, young people aged 16 and 17 are treated similarly to adults, presumed to have sufficient capacity to decide about their medical treatment and exercise their data protection rights, although assessing their capacity can be challenging [35, 36]. From the age of 13, children deemed mature enough to make such decisions can access online, and without parental consent, confidential sexual health services including contraception, testing for sexually transmitted infections, and advice on unplanned pregnancy [37]. This medical judgement is mirrored by data protection regulation: recognizing that children increasingly go online to access help or counseling services, the UK GDPR and the GDPR allow children under the age of consent to do so without obtaining parental consent for the processing of their personal data.

## 3 Future Research

Research on children's privacy and data protection is actively developing across multiple sectors. There are some pressing gaps in knowledge, including the effect of video cameras, smart monitoring, or facial recognition in homes, schools, and public spaces, or of sharing sensitive or biometric data with health services or law enforcement.

Also important are knowledge gaps regarding how children of different ages and life circumstances understand and value their privacy, at home, with peers, and in relation to education, health, business, and other organizations. Research could examine whether unfolding privacy beliefs and practices affect children's online identity expression or agency or help-seeking, and whether this varies by dimensions of vulnerability.

Efforts to protect children's privacy raise new research questions in turn. How is existing legislation enforced, and which new policies and practices are emerging to protect children's privacy, and are they effective? What mechanisms would incentivize service providers to implement necessary safeguards? Also, are efforts to increase digital literacy, even to resist the datafication of children's lives, proving effective?

Finally, research could examine whether the global nature of big tech is harmonizing cultural understandings of children's privacy or provoking divergent responses in different countries or contexts (such as law, education, health, or welfare). Related, are strategies emerging to enable children to benefit from the data collected from them? Indeed, what role do and could children play in shaping future policy responses?

Such questions are especially pressing as artificial intelligence (AI) becomes more pervasive in contexts (education, health, transport), where dependence on technical systems means neither children nor parents have meaningful opportunities to give or withdraw consent or exercise other rights. However, the present chapter suggests a sufficient evidence base for clear recommendations, as below.

## 4 Recommendations

- Government policies on privacy and data must promote children's rights, facilitating their need for protection and participation, and prevent discrimination and other harms arising from privacy violations and data exploitation in digital contexts. Governments should also involve young people in the policymaking process, by giving children real agency in influencing decisions that affect them, including policy and product design.
- There must be necessary safeguards in place for children's privacy and data protection when data- and AI-driven technologies are used in public services affecting or used by children (notably education, health, and welfare). In addition, these safeguards need to be regularly updated to keep pace with technological innovation.
- Since neither children nor families can realistically be held solely responsible for navigating the complex, global, and largely commercial digital environment on which their lives increasingly depend, the government must regulate or legislate robust standards of privacy by design and by default, as included in the UK Data Protection Act and AADC, and ensure that big tech provides child-friendly, age-appropriate mechanisms for privacy protection, transparency, complaint, and remedy.
- Sustained media (data, digital, privacy critical, AI) literacies are vital from an early age. They should be implemented in school curricula, professional training (for teachers, clinicians and other professionals who work with children), and parent/caregiver guidance. Such initiatives should be informed by children's voices, reflect their concerns and experiences, and respond to real-world problems.
- A robust evidence base must be sustained that fills critical gaps, especially regarding younger children and those living in vulnerable or disadvantaged situations, provides an independent evaluation of the effectiveness of privacy-related interventions, and consults children for their own experiences and views.

**Conflict of Interest and Funding Disclosures** None.

## References

1. Laufer R, Wolfe M. Privacy as a concept and a social issue: a multidimensional developmental theory. J Soc Issues. 1977;33(3):22–42.
2. Koops B-J, Newell BC, Timan T, Škorvánek I, Chokrevski T, Galič M. A typology of privacy. Univ

Pa J Int Law. 2017;38(2):483–57. Available at: https://scholarship.law.upenn.edu/jil/vol38/iss2/4. Accessed 2 May 2023.
3. Livingstone S, Lemish D, Lim SS, Bulger M, Cabello P, Claro M, Cabello T, Khalil J, Kumpulainen K, Nayar U, Nayar P, Park J, Tan M, Prinsloo J, Wei B. Global perspectives on children's digital opportunities: an emerging research and policy agenda. Pediatrics. 2017;140(2):137–41. https://doi.org/10.1542/peds.2016-1758S.
4. Livingstone S, Bulger M, Burton P, Day E, Lievens E, Milkaite I, Leyn T, Martens M, Roque R, Sarikakis K, Stoilova M, Wolf R. Children's privacy and digital literacy across cultures: implications for education and regulation. In: Sefton-Green J, Pangrazio L, editors. Learning to live with datafication: educational case studies and initiatives from across the world. Abingdon: Routledge; 2022. p. 184–200.
5. Milkaite I, De Wolf R, Lievens E, De Leyn T, Martens M. Children's reflections on privacy and the protection of their personal data: a child-centric approach to data protection information formats. Child Youth Serv Rev. 2021;129:106170. Available at: https://doi.org/10.1016/j.childyouth.2021.106170. Accessed 2 May 2023.
6. Mascheroni G, Siibak A. *Datafied childhoods: data practices and imaginaries in children's lives*. New York, London: Peter Lang; 2021. Available at: https://doi.org/10.3726/b17460. Accessed 2 May 2023.
7. UNICEF (United Nations Children's Fund). Children's online privacy and freedom of expression. 2018. Available at: www.guvenliweb.org.tr/dosya/ZybsG.pdf. Accessed 2 May 2023.
8. Alegre S. Freedom to think: the long struggle to liberate our minds. London: Atlantic Books; 2022.
9. Eubanks V. Automating inequality: how high-tech tools profile, police, and punish the poor. New York: St. Martin's; 2018.
10. Radesky J, Chassiakos YR, Ameenuddin N, Navsaria D. Digital advertising to children. Pediatrics. 2020;146(1):e20201681. Available at: https://doi.org/10.1542/peds.2020-1681. Accessed 2 May 2023.
11. Lievens E, Livingstone S, McLaughlin S, O'Neill B, Verdoodt V. Children's rights and digital technologies. In: Liefaard T, Kilkelly U, editors. International children's rights law. Singapore: Springer; 2018. p. 1–27.
12. Nissenbaum H. Privacy in context: technology, policy, and the integrity of social life. Stanford: Stanford University Press; 2010. p. 3.
13. Stoilova M, Nandagiri R, Livingstone S. Children's understanding of personal data and privacy online—a systematic evidence mapping. Inf Commun Soc. 2021;24(4):557–75. Available at: https://doi.org/10.1080/1369118X.2019.1657164. Accessed 2 May 2023.
14. Milkaite I, Lievens E. Children's rights to privacy and data protection around the world: challenges in the digital realm. Eur J Law Technol. 2019;10(1):1–24.
15. Schwartz PM, Peifer KN. Transatlantic data privacy law. Georgetown Law J. 2017;106(1):115–80.
16. Lynskey O. The foundations of EU data protection law. Oxford: Oxford University Press; 2015.
17. González Fuster G. Study on the essence of the fundamental rights to privacy and to protection of personal data. 2022. https://www.edps.europa.eu/system/files/2023-11/edps-vub-study_on_the_essence_of_fundamental_rights_to_privacy_and_to_protection_of_personal_data_en.pdf
18. FRA (European Union Agency for Fundamental Rights), Council of Europe. Handbook on European data protection law. Luxembourg: Publications Office of the European Union; 2018.
19. Shmueli B, Blecher-Prigat A. Privacy for children. Columbia Hum Rights Law Rev. 2010;42:759.
20. Steinberg S. Growing up shared: how parents can sharer smarter on social media and what you can do to keep your family safe in a no-privacy world. Naperville: Sourcebooks; 2017.
21. Blum-Ross A, Livingstone S. "Sharenting," parent blogging and the boundaries of the digital self. Pop Commun. 2017;15(2):110–25.
22. ICO. What rights to children have? https://ico.org.uk/for-organisations/uk-gdpr-guidance-and-resources/childrens-information/children-and-the-uk-gdpr/what-rights-do-children-have/.
23. Bessant C, Schnebbe M. Does the GDPR offer a solution to the "problem" of sharenting? Datenschutz Datensich. 2022;46:352–6. https://link.springer.com/article/10.1007/s11623-022-1618-3.
24. Livingstone, S., Pothong, K., Atabey, A., Hooper, L., & Day, E. (2024) The Googlization of the classroom: Is the UK effective in protecting children's data and rights? Computers and Education Open. https://doi.org/10.1016/j.caeo.2024.100195
25. Selwyn N, Hillman T, Bergviken Rensfeldt A, Perrotta C. Digital technologies and the automation of education—key questions and concerns. Postdigital Sci Educ. 2023;5:15–24. Available at: https://doi.org/10.1007/s42438-021-00263-3. Accessed 2 May 2023.
26. Vance A. Lessons learned from the Family Educational Rights and Privacy Act. In: Livingstone S, Pothong K, editors. *Education data futures: critical, regulatory and practical reflections*. London: 5Rights Foundation; 2022. p. 189–201. Available at: https://educationdatafutures.digitalfuturescommission.org.uk/essays/the-value-of-better-regulation/lessons-learned-from-the-famuly-educational-rights-privacy-act. Accessed 2 May 2023.
27. Edwards L. Privacy, security and data protection in smart cities: a critical EU law perspective. Eur Data Prot Law Rev. 2016;2(1):28–58.
28. FTC. FTC proposes strengthening children's privacy rule to further limit companies' ability to monetize children's data. https://www.ftc.gov/news-events/news/press-releases/2023/12/ftc-proposes-strengthening-childrens-privacy-rule-further-limit-companies-ability-monetize-childrens.
29. ICO. The children's code and education technologies (edtech). https://ico.org.uk/for-organisations/uk-

gdpr-guidance-and-resources/childrens-information/childrens-code-guidance-and-resources/the-children-s-code-and-education-technologies-edtech/.
30. Day E, Pothong K, Atabey A, Livingstone S. Who controls children's education data? A socio-legal analysis of the UK governance regimes for schools and EdTech. Learn Media Technol. 2022;49:356–70. Available at: https://doi.org/10.1080/17439884.2022.2152838. Accessed 2 May 2023.
31. Hollis C, Livingstone S, Sonuga-Barke E. Editorial: the role of digital technology in children and young people's mental health—a triple-edged sword? J Child Psychol Psychiatry Allied Discip. 2020;61(8):837–41.
32. Grundy Q, Jibb L, Amoako E, Fang GH. Health apps are designed to track and share. Br Med J. 2021;373:n1429. https://doi.org/10.1136/bmj.n1429.
33. Bahareh K, Steinberg S. Parental sharing on the internet: child privacy in the age of social media and the pediatrician's role. JAMA Pediatr. 2017;171(5):413–4. https://doi.org/10.1001/jamapediatrics.2016.5059.
34. Pathak PR, Chou A. Confidential care for adolescents in the U.S. health care system. J Patient Cent Res Rev. 2019;6(1):46–50. https://doi.org/10.17294/2330-0698.1656. PMID: 31414023; PMCID: PMC6676754.
35. GMC (General Medical Council). Confidentiality: good practice in handling patient information. London: GMC; 2017 [updated 2018].
36. GMC (General Medical Council). 10–18 years: guidance for all doctors. London: GMC; 2007 [updated 2018].
37. NHS England. Sexual health. 2022. Available at: www.nhs.uk/live-well/sexual-health/confidentiality-at-sexual-health-services. Accessed 2 May 2023.

# Bridging America's Homework Gap by Closing the Digital Divide

Bhaskar Chakravorti, Stephen J. Aguilar, Arturo Franco, Reg Leichty, and Morgan Scott Polikoff

## 1 Background

While the COVID-19 pandemic put a spotlight on just how much we rely on Internet connectivity, it also surfaced the many ways in which use of the Internet remained far from equal across the United States. Those on the wrong side of this digital divide found it hard to access the same economic opportunities available to their connected peers. It also brought into sharp focus a "homework gap"—i.e., the difficulties that students face in completing school assignments at home when they do not have reliable access to the Internet. This has been a point of concern for many, including the chairwoman of the Federal Communications Commission (FCC), Jessica Rosenworcel [1].

B. Chakravorti (✉)
The Fletcher School, Tufts University, Medford, MA, USA
e-mail: Bhaskar.chakravorti@tufts.edu

S. J. Aguilar · M. S. Polikoff
Rossier School of Education, University of Southern California, Los Angeles, CA, USA

A. Franco
World Bank, Washington, DC, USA

R. Leichty
Foresight Law + Policy, Washington, DC, USA

During the pandemic-induced lockdowns, the problem went far beyond homework: children in some areas of the United States had to resort to extreme measures to attend schools being held over Zoom because they could not reliably access the Internet; some students went to a Taco Bell parking lot to go online, while others huddled under blankets outside a closed school to access school Wi-Fi [2].

Other students sat outside public libraries to piggyback on the nearest reliable Wi-Fi systems. In stark contrast, students in wealthier parts of the country with reliable high-speed Internet access attended remote classrooms, participated in extracurricular activities, and had access to resources to collaborate, access library resources, conduct research, and complete assignments.

Alarmed by the gap in student learning the National School Boards Association (NSBA) urged the FCC to distribute resources from the $7.17 billion Emergency Connectivity Fund to help provide devices and Internet connectivity to communities in need [3]. Although the gap did narrow as the pandemic progressed, closing the digital divide overall remains a work in progress. There is much work that needs to be done to create a more equitable digital infrastructure to give every child the opportunity to transcend the homework—and learning and development—gap.


D. A. Christakis, L. Hale (eds.), *Handbook of Children and Screens*,
https://doi.org/10.1007/978-3-031-69362-5_68

## 2 Current State

### 2.1 Research Question 1: How Did the Digital Divide Affect Children During the Pandemic?

At the onset of the pandemic, as more than 55 million students moved to online learning, one in five teens, ages 13–17, reported being unable to do their homework "often" or "sometimes" because of unreliable Internet access [4]. Twelve million children were without Internet access altogether. The challenges varied by location. For example, 70% of children in the Kansas City school district did not have Internet access at home. The lack of investment predated the pandemic, however, as Missouri only spent about $10,600 per pupil in 2017, placing it near the bottom third compared to other states [5]. Even wealthier states such as California were ill prepared for the pandemic—students in urban districts were particularly susceptible to not having the capability to engage in remote live instruction [6].

The digital divide also reinforced long-standing racial inequalities in American society. Nearly half of Americans without at-home Internet were in Black and Hispanic households; Black and Hispanic households were 14 and 12 percentage points more likely to lack broadband access [7]. Up to 40% of K-12 students from Black, Latino, and indigenous communities also struggled with insufficient digital literacy and difficulties engaging with English-only content. Seventy percent of Black and 60% of Hispanic workers reported being underprepared with digital skills, affecting their employability [8]. The study projected that without additional intervention to close this divide, a majority of Black and Hispanic workers could be locked out of 86% of jobs by 2045 [9].

The pandemic did, however, provide the impetus to release resources for targeted emergency relief. Over the course of the pandemic's first year, there were notable improvements in digital access. According to analysis of a nationally representative survey of U.S. households co-developed by one of the co-authors of this chapter, the proportion of families lacking either Internet or computers for learning dropped by 10 percentage points between April and October 2020 [10]. However, there were significant differences by race and income, with the biggest disparities by income on some variables. For example, in April, only about two-thirds of households with annual incomes less than $25,000 reported having computers and Internet access available for children's remote learning, compared with 92% of families with household incomes of $75,000–$149,000, and 97% of those above $150,000. These differences were much smaller in October—just seven percentage points between the highest and lowest income families with hybrid or remote learners. There were important racial/ethnic differences in technology access in October, with Black families less likely than other groups to have technology and Internet and more likely to have to share devices. There were also school-level differences, with secondary students less likely to have access.

Another factor with significant implications for learning online was the quality of the Internet connections. 77% of K–12 parents of fully remote or hybrid learners reported good Internet connectivity for their children's remote learning, while 22% reported connections were slow or dropped frequently [11]. Poor Internet connections translated into missed instruction, student absences, an inability to meaningfully communicate with teachers and peers, and ultimately, failing grades. There were large income gaps in connectivity, with 39% of the lowest income group (less than $25,000 per year) reporting connectivity issues versus just 3% of the highest income group (over $150,000 per year). 81% of suburban parents reported good connectivity versus 72% of urban and 69% of rural parents.

In addition to the disruptions caused by access and affordability issues, there were other challenges that extended beyond students and families to also consider issues that affected schools, communities, libraries, and anchor institutions. Many of America's schools and libraries whose presence was correlated with the digital divide fell on the wrong side of the cybersecurity poverty line [12]. All schools and libraries were at significant risk, but the community anchor institutions in the nation's most vulnerable communities often lacked sufficient cyber protections. Successful cyberattacks caused lost instructional time, halted library services, and compromised sensitive personally identifiable information. Such disruptions disproportionately harmed the populations that depended most on schools and libraries for online access.

## 2.2 Research Question 2: What Actions Have Been Taken to Close the Digital Divide?

One of biggest challenges to overcome in closing the digital divide is that broadband access in the United States is one of the most expensive in the world. In a recent study of 50 cities, only 17 of 50 cities studied had two or more cable providers and 27 cities had only one broadband Internet provider [13]. Many rural areas are insufficiently connected to the broadband networks, which means that even if consumers were willing to pay for the service, they cannot physically get access to high-speed Internet. The costs of bringing broadband Internet infrastructure to relatively sparsely populated areas are high, and companies that provide such access infrastructure and services do not find rural areas sufficiently commercially attractive to make the necessary investments.

Can action by policymakers and government make a difference? The first obstacle is that there is poor understanding of the true extent of the digital divide because of inaccurate data. While the FCC estimated that 14.5 million Americans did not have access to broadband, a more thorough "manual" check by an independent research group, BroadbandNow, put the number at 42 million [14, 15]. Yet another analysis done by Microsoft estimated that nearly half the country did not use the Internet at broadband speeds [16]. Despite the lack of clarity on the data on the extent of the divide, the discussions in Congress prior to approving a budget to address the problem relied on a past FCC estimate of what it would cost to ensure universal broadband: $80 billion [17]. That FCC calculation relied on the drastic undercount of 14.5 million unserved Americans. Applying the same methodology to BroadbandNow's more credible accounting of the divide suggests the budget ought to have been closer to $240 billion [18]. After many deliberations, Congress finally committed $65 billion for broadband deployment and affordability through the Infrastructure Investment and Jobs Act (IIJA) to help close the digital divide [19]. The digital equity plans thanks to IIJA will, no doubt, promote meaningful adoption and use of high-speed Internet service, including for education and workforce initiatives. The planning process has prompted important conversations about a range of digital learning issues, including promoting digital learning accessibility through open educational resources ("OER") policies, strengthening data systems, and more.

While the budget is far from adequate, it is a significant sum and provides a place to start. The task of allocating this budget must contend with a second set of hurdles: there is lack of clarity on the underlying causes of the digital divide, which would be critical for directing the limited resources most appropriately.

## 2.3 Research Question 3: What Are the Underlying Causes of the Digital Divide?

Because of the commercial unattractiveness of sparsely populated areas, Internet service providers have few incentives to expand service in rural communities, creating an access gap. At the same time, an estimated three times as many metropolitan households as rural households lack broadband subscriptions [20]. The causes of the gap in the urban areas are related—mostly—to affordability.

A key portion of the IIJA, the Broadband Equity, Access, and Deployment (BEAD) program, allocates $42.5 billion to states to fund broadband network deployments, prioritizing *un*served areas: areas that lack networks reaching 25 Mbps download/3 Mbps upload speeds.

*Under*served areas lack service above 100 Mbps download/20 Mbps upload speeds and are second in priority. A majority of the funding will be allocated by determining the total number of unserved locations in a state relative to the national total [20]. While, at face value, prioritizing the unserved areas may appear to be a logical way to sequence the funding, the policy tilts funding toward prioritizing rural areas, by spending the budget toward covering miles with broadband infrastructure, which is expensive and reaches fewer people over covering people by helping make the existing broadband services more affordable, potentially affecting a larger number of people. The current approach risks leaving many urban and suburban communities behind. There are racial implications of this policy. Analysis done by one of the co-author's research teams finds that in the ten largest cities, there are very few zip codes with unserved populations, while the bulk of lower-income, less white zip codes are in areas that are underserved [21]. For those in the underserved areas, speeds are simply not adequate to meet current bandwidth needs for learning and working effectively online.

## 3 Future Research

There are several directions for future research. The first recommendation for ongoing inquiry would be to track advances in digital access over time and evaluate the impact on learning outcomes of children at various stages of schooling. We should also analyze how this impact varies across different parts of the country, across socioeconomic and demographic lines, and across the rural-urban-suburban school systems. A second area of inquiry would be to examine the impact of digital access on elements of the digital divide that go beyond the inability to afford or reach the digital infrastructure. These could include information literacy and digital skills, functionality of devices, and applications used in households, etc. A third area of research would be to draw lessons from the experience in the United States regarding impact of digital access on learning outcomes and consider the implications for education of children in other countries.

## 4 Recommendations

Policymakers should consider the following principles to equitably narrow the digital divide and create a more equitable digital infrastructure for children and their families across the United States.

- *Prioritize people over miles*: The current funding approach risks deprioritizing the digital divide that persists in urban areas and exacerbating racial and socioeconomic inequalities. The National Telecommunications and Information Administration (NTIA), responsible for reviewing the broadband proposals for the BEAD program, is offering more leeway to states in the sequence in which they can use funding in unserved vs. underserved areas [22]. However, it still requires states to determine that they have a plan to reach all unserved areas before using funds for highly populated underserved areas, and the funding allocation mechanism is based heavily on the number of unserved locations. State-level stakeholders would be wise to realize that the BEAD money will favor the unserved, primarily rural areas, and look to other funding sources, like the American Rescue Plan Act (ARPA) to fill the gap in underserved locations in cities and suburbs. The end goal must be to get high-speed Internet to as many people as possible. Stakeholders should pay close attention to where funding is going, and look not only at the number of locations, but the number of people served.
- *Ensure accountability in affordability programs*: The IIJA is not only focused on building out broadband and improving access but it also contains funding to improve affordability. Affordability and accessibility are closely intertwined, as ISPs are more likely to prioritize investments in areas where they believe enough households will sign up for Internet service and help recoup their investment.

- The Affordable Connectivity Program (ACP), passed as part of the infrastructure bill, offers lower-income households a $30/month subsidy to access broadband. Students were expected to be among the principal beneficiaries of the program. The Biden administration also secured commitments from 20 Internet service providers to cut prices and improve speeds for those receiving the ACP benefit. Advocates and policymakers would do well to track which ISPs are following through on these public commitments.
- *Enable rural utility pole access*: Remote rural broadband gaps are more pronounced for low income and minority students—those most vulnerable from the perspective of falling behind in their schoolwork. As NTIA prepares to allocate the broadband funding, policymakers should consider also making it easier for the competitive providers to gain access to existing rural telecom infrastructure including utility poles. The FCC has an open rulemaking focused on Accelerating Wireline Broadband Deployment by Removing Barriers to Infrastructure Investment [23].
- *Create a reliable, verified, and timely database to understand the true state of the digital divide*: Policymakers from opposite sides of the aisle, advocates, and the FCC chair herself agree that the current FCC maps are inadequate. In the absence of credible data that reflects the reality and the scale of the problem, it is hard to make the case for investing and to secure the right budgets to close the gap. While new, more geographically detailed maps are in progress, states and other stakeholders will have the opportunity to challenge the veracity of these maps, and the final outcome of the areas mapped as unserved will determine what portion of funding is allocated to each state. State and local practitioners would do well to get their own cartographical house in order ahead of the FCC release, working with local stakeholders to ensure they are not overlooking unserved and underserved areas.
- In the post-pandemic environment, schools across the country are increasingly relying on digital connectivity for a range of applications, such as learning management systems, multimedia resources, online research, and remote schooling on snow days and other weather-related school building closures. A recent survey from the National Center for Education Statistics found that schools are winding down subsidized home Internet access programs, possibly because COVID-19 relief budgets have run out [24]. The ACP may be terminated despite the fact that it has more than 22 million recipients. The uptick in children's access to the Internet in many parts of the country during the pandemic may be short-lived.
- *Invest in digital literacy*: It is essential to recognize that even if households have affordable access to the digital infrastructure, they need to be able to use the knowledge-building capacity of the Internet and learn how to use the technology responsibly. Digital literacy and building healthy social media habits are important; the quality of content is as critical as access to that content in the first place.

- It is high time we learned from the pandemic experience and devastating impact the lack of connectivity can have on the development of children. We need to get past the emergency measures and put in place a sustainable solution to the homework gap by closing the digital divide once and for all.

**Conflict of Interest and Funding Disclosures** Bhaskar Chakravorti leads a research program Imagining a Digital Economy for All (IDEA) 2030 that has received funding support from the Mastercard Impact Fund and Omidyar Network.

## References

1. More than $130K raised for California family after girls seen using Taco Bell for school work. USA Today. https://www.usatoday.com/story/news/nation/2020/09/01/thousands-raised-girls-who-had-use-taco-bell-wifi-school/5680992002/. Accessed 24 May 2023.
2. Coronavirus for kids without internet: quarantined worksheets, learning in parking lots. USA

Today. https://www.usatoday.com/story/news/education/2020/04/01/coronavirus-internet-speed-broadband-online-learning-school-closures/5091051002/. Accessed 25 May 2023.
3. NSBA asks FCC for speed and flexibility in disbursement of $7.1 billion devoted to closing "homework gap". National School Boards Association. https://www.nsba.org/News/2021/reply-comments-emergency-connectivity-fund. Accessed 25 May 2023.
4. The effects of COVID-19 school closures will last a lifetime – especially for children in need. Red Nose Day. https://rednoseday.org/news/covid19-effects-missing-school. Accessed 25 May 2023.
5. States that spend the most (and the least) on education 2017. Governing. https://www.governing.com/archive/gov-state-education-spending-revenue-data.html. Accessed 25 May 2023.
6. Aguilar SJ, Galperin H, Baek C, Gonzalez E. Live instruction predicts engagement in K–12 remote learning. Educ Res. 2022;51(1):81–4. https://doi.org/10.3102/0013189X211056884.
7. Digital denied. Free Press. https://www.freepress.net/sites/default/files/legacy-policy/digital_denied_free_press_report_december_2016.pdf. Accessed 25 May 2023.
8. The U.S. has a "racial tech gap" problem, Deutsche Bank study shows. Marketplace. https://www.marketplace.org/2020/09/18/racial-tech-gap-broadband-hardware-access-deutsche-bank-employment-wealth-digitization-us-economy/. Accessed 25 May 2023.
9. America's racial gap & Big Tech's closing window. Deutsche Bank Research. https://www.dbresearch.com/PROD/RPS_EN-PROD/PROD0000000000511664/America%27s_Racial_Gap_%26_Big_Tech%27s_Closing_Window.pdf;REWEBJSESSIONID=A1579D8F32BF1D3A55A0C61A7353CFCB?undefined&realload=bYUk5RFnZLGoC4p9b9RXs4RmEGZUU4Plw8ygLxRDJW5EFTpI52TxGZ5xTYrO6m0F. Accessed 25 May 2023.
10. Haderlein SK, Saavedra AR, Polikoff MS, Silver D, Rapaport A, Garland M. Disparities in educational access in the time of COVID: evidence from a nationally representative panel of American families. AERA Open. 2021;7:1–21. https://doi.org/10.1177/23328584211041350.
11. Dombo M. The cybersecurity poverty line. U.S. Cybersecurity Magazine. https://www.uscybersecurity.net/csmag/the-cybersecurity-poverty-line/. Accessed 25 May 2023.
12. A snapshot of internet service provider competition in the U.S. Broadband Search. https://www.broadbandsearch.net/blog/internet-ISP-competition-across-America#post-navigation-3. Accessed 25 May 2023.
13. Fourteenth Broadband Deployment Report. FCC. https://docs.fcc.gov/public/attachments/FCC-21-18A1.pdf. Accessed 25 May 2023.
14. BroadbandNow estimates availability for all 50 states; confirms that more than 42 million Americans do not have access to broadband. BroadbandNow Research. 25 May 2023. https://broadbandnow.com/research/fcc-broadband-overreporting-by-state.
15. Microsoft Airband: an annual update on connecting rural America, Microsoft on the issues. Microsoft. https://blogs.microsoft.com/on-the-issues/2020/03/05/update-connecting-rural-america/. Accessed 25 May 2023.
16. de Sa P. Improving the nation's digital infrastructure. Federal Communications Commission. 2017. https://www.fcc.gov/document/improving-nations-digital-infrastructure. Accessed 25 May 2023.
17. Turning America's digital divide into digital dividends, digital planet. The Fletcher School, Tufts University. https://sites.tufts.edu/digitalplanet/us-digital-divide/#methodology. Accessed 25 May 2023.
18. Fact sheet: the bipartisan infrastructure deal. The White House. https://www.whitehouse.gov/briefing-room/statements-releases/2021/11/06/fact-sheet-the-bipartisan-infrastructure-deal/. Accessed 25 May 2023.
19. Chakravorti B. How Biden's "internet for all" initiative can actually fulfill its mission. Harvard Business Review. https://hbr.org/2022/07/how-bidens-internet-for-all-initiative-can-actually-fulfill-its-mission. Accessed 25 May 2023.
20. Summary of notice of funding opportunity for the broadband, equity, access and deployment (BEAD) program. Akin Gump. https://www.akingump.com/a/web/fGfDi6MKcQXYLcqLkA6dhK/summary-of-notice-of-funding-opportunity-for-the-broadband-equity-access-and-deployment-bead-program.pdf. Accessed 25 May 2023.
21. Bridging the broadband divide dashboard, digital planet. The Fletcher School, Tufts University. https://sites.tufts.edu/digitalplanet/broadband-infrastructure-funding-and-the-digital-divide-prioritizing-people-over-miles/. Accessed 25 May 2023.
22. NTIA chief answers 5 burning broadband funding questions. Fierce Telecom. https://www.fiercetelecom.com/telecom/ntia-chief-says-broadband-funding-will-start-flowing-later-year. Accessed 25 May 2023.
23. Accelerating wireline and wireless broadband deployment by removing barriers to infrastructure investment. Federal Register. https://www.federalregister.gov/documents/2022/04/28/2022-09029/accelerating-wireline-and-wireless-broadband-deployment-by-removing-barriers-to-infrastructure. Accessed 25 May 2023.
24. Fewer districts are providing home internet access, but students still need it. Education Week. https://www.edweek.org/technology/fewer-districts-are-providing-home-internet-access-but-students-still-need-it/2022/09. Accessed 25 May 2023.

# Global Perspectives on Youth and the Digital Environment: Learnings from Majority World Countries

Lucía Magis-Weinberg, Matías Dodel, Luci Pangrazio, Manisha Pathak-Shelat, Sisi Tao, and Chikezie E. Uzuegbunam

## 1 Background

Most youth are growing up in Majority World countries (MWCs)[1] in an increasingly digitalized context but with unequal digital media access, usage, skill, and opportunity [2–4]. Even though youth are one of the groups going online at the fastest rate [5, 6], most live in countries that have largely been left out of research and other forms of global decision-making about digital platforms [2, 7, 8]. As a result, most research on digital environments and youth fails to acknowledge issues that prevail in MWCs, including the gender digital gap; differences between rural, suburban, and urban areas; youth from ethnic minorities; limited resources to support parents and teachers; and limited regulation to effectively mediate digital media use [2, 4, 8, 9]. Understanding the digital lives of youth in MWCs (while acknowledging the wide variability that exists *between* and *within* countries) is critical to creating more inclusive and equitable research and policy that reflects the global population.

Digital divides impact youth development through disparities on three levels: (1) access, (2) use and skills, and (3) outcomes/utility derived from digital media [10]. These divides are inherently linked to underlying inequalities that result from education, poverty, gender, age, and geography [4, 10] and have been heightened by the pandemic [11]. Despite a gap in research between Minority World (i.e., those countries with developed economies and where most research is conducted) and Majority World countries, what is increasingly clear is the tension in balancing youth's digital opportunities and risks in heterogeneous contexts.

[1]The term *Majority World* refers to regions where a significant portion of the world's population, natural resources, and landmass is concentrated, in Asia, Africa, Latin America, the Middle East and Oceania. The Majority World is a term offered to replace Global South [1].

L. Magis-Weinberg (✉)
University of Washington, Seattle, Washington, USA
e-mail: luciamw@uw.edu

M. Dodel
Universidad Católica del Uruguay, Montevideo, Uruguay

L. Pangrazio
Deakin University, Melbourne, Victoria, Australia

M. Pathak-Shelat
MICA, Ahmedabad, Gujarat, India

S. Tao
The Education University of Hong Kong, Hong Kong SAR, China

C. E. Uzuegbunam
Rhodes University, Makhanda, Eastern Cape, South Africa


D. A. Christakis, L. Hale (eds.), *Handbook of Children and Screens*, https://doi.org/10.1007/978-3-031-69362-5_69

# 2 Current State

## 2.1 Opportunities and Risks

Online experiences provide crucial opportunities for youth development, but also introduce risks. The *ladder of online participation* [8, 12] describes *potential* benefits. At the entry step, most youth consume online *entertainment*, which requires the least skill and is easier to access by the youngest populations. As youth gain digital skills, they progress to a second step, *online sociability*, through communication and social media apps. The third step is *online education and information*, a need that was highlighted during the pandemic [11]. With more advanced skills and literacies, youth can reach the top, and engage in *citizenship and community activities* as well as *creative endeavors* [12]. While many MWCs youth do engage in *some* online activities, digital divides prevent them from fully participating in civic, informational, and creative pursuits that are considered the hallmark of the digital age [5, 12]. Digital media holds potential for youth in MWCs, leading to socioeconomic advancement through education, training, and employment opportunities. These platforms can amplify marginalized voices and be powerful communication tools for health and information [13].

The *4Cs framework* [14] recognizes four online risk categories: *Content, Contact, Conduct, and Commercial.* Many of these risks are amplified in MWCs [2, 3, 15], including concerns such as sexual exploitation, violence, and exposure to harmful content. For example, the *Disrupting Harm* initiative [16] investigated risks and opportunities online in African and Asian countries. In terms of *Content*, 33% of youth in these regions have been exposed to online violence and 20% to hate messages. This negativity sometimes comes from *Conduct* with peers: 9% of youth harassed someone online and 15% made negative comments. There is also evidence of serious *Contact* risks: 1–20% of youth were subjected to online sexual exploitation and abuse. In Latin America, 30% of youth have seen disturbing content and 25% sexual content. Between 13% and 44% of youth have contacted strangers and around 10% have experienced cyberbullying [8].

Digital competence links these two frameworks, as opportunities will not necessarily materialize into benefits without skills, scaffolding, regulation and age-appropriate design, and risks can be prevented from turning into harms. There are important determinants of risks and opportunities at the individual, household, school, community, and country levels [3, 10, 17, 18]. Digital inequalities both reflect and contribute to widening preexisting inequalities [10, 11, 19]. Socioeconomic status, general and digital literacy might be barriers to access and use [4], compounded by undersupply of culturally, linguistically, and regionally tailored content [4].

## 2.2 Youth in the Mobile Internet

Increasingly, youth in MWCs are gaining connection to the Internet. Youth (ages 15–24) are more connected online than those of other ages, particularly in countries in Africa and Asia-Pacific [6, 20]. Still, *access* remains a huge barrier, especially for youth in rural areas [21]. At the beginning of the pandemic, two-thirds of MWC youth (ages 3–17) did not have access to the Internet at home [6, 11, 22]. The main barriers include lack of electricity, affordability, and poor connectivity [21].

Youth connect mostly through mobile devices first, which are often shared [6], and prefer to use social media and videos. Compared to desktop/broadband connectivity, access to the Internet through mobile devices is associated with fewer skills and less online participation [19]. Mobile devices enable easy access to social media platforms specifically designed for this medium. In MWCs, telecommunications networks offer "free" access to social media, regulating the cost and accessibility of third-party platforms and other services. As a result, digital platforms now dominate the Internet [23]. In many MWCs settings, *Facebook* (and increasingly *WhatsApp*) are the Internet. Thus, in underresourced settings, social media use is more common than other technology-based activities, such as seeking information, educational opportunities, or engaging with governmental agencies [19].

### 2.3 Gender

The digital gender gap is still vast in MWCs: girls face barriers including social norms and gender stereotypes, insufficient digital literacy and skills, and safety concerns [3, 24]. In India [25] a pilot study conducted as part of the Global Kids Online Project[2] indicated that gender remains an important dimension of digital inequality for girls from low-income families. Girls experience more restrictive parenting around their digital use than boys [21]. The gender gap in access is most pronounced for girls in countries with the lowest rates of Internet adoption [21]. Persisting inequalities in norms, social structures, and offline institutions that influence girls' online engagement limit its potential benefits. For MWCs youth, the negotiations around play and leisure and the experience of privacy remain deeply gendered. Online gender-based violence, which is hugely pervasive, is an embodied experience [26].

### 2.4 Parents and Schools

Parents [27] and teachers [11] play a central role in scaffolding the development of digital skills and literacies for youth and are critical in mediating online experiences. However, in many settings in MWCs, youth lead the adoption of digital devices. Youth might have more exposure to and familiarity with digital technologies than parents, and often act as *digital brokers* [3, 28].

Low levels of digital literacy among parents [27], and limited sources of guidance for safe and meaningful use may hinder their ability to effectively mediate youth's media use [21, 29]. Furthermore, obstacles to effective digital parenting are impacted by distinct cultural values, norms, and beliefs [30, 31], with many parents feeling uncertain, less confident, or competent to manage their children's online lives [12]. Studies in Nigeria show, for example, that factors such as moral panic, traditional socialization, and a lack of digital literacy result in strict mediation of technology use [30, 31], with less conversation about youth's online concerns [4, 30, 32]. Counterintuitively, more restrictive parenting has been associated with more cyberbullying for youth in Hong Kong [33]. *Restrictive* mediation is less effective that *active* mediation and can curtail youth rights and citizenship online [8, 12].

While governments have made significant investments in digital infrastructure in education, teacher training lags behind [8]. For example, only a minority of youth in Eastern and Southern African countries have received information on online safety [21]. With limited training, teacher mediation tends to be restrictive, focused on setting rules and limits. Training on more sophisticated digital literacies that can effectively empower youth to rise through the digital ladder is lacking, limiting students' opportunities for development. Although digital education policies have evolved to prioritize the development of digital skills, literacy, and citizenship over mere access to digital resources, there is still a significant need to enhance the role of schools and teachers [8, 34].

Youth do not possess sufficient digital skills [19]. For example, the 2018 *International Computer and Information Literacy Study*, showed that only "19% of the 42,000 students assessed in 14 countries and educational systems could work *independently* with computers" [35]. Youth's digital literacy in Australia has been *on the decline* [36]. In Hong Kong, longitudinal data showed that although students' digital literacy skill improved from 2019 to 2021, the performance gap widened [20]. Digital literacy programs that develop technical understanding and a criticality have not been prioritized [37]. Instead, most programs focus on cybersafety or cyberbullying, which tend to rely on protectionist

[2]The Global Kids Online Study is part of an international research and action network "committed to generating cross-nationally comparable and robust evidence that directly reflects children's voices, experiences and concerns", particularly focused on their experiences in the digital environment [12].

approaches rather than those of empowerment and agency [34]. Clearly, youth need explicit instruction to develop critical [38] and technical understandings of digital media. Still, we are at a critical juncture in conceptualizing what it means to be digitally literate, particularly as the nature of the digital challenges are socially, culturally, and geographically situated.

## 2.5 The Pandemic

The rapid shift to remote learning exposed the existing digital inequalities in MWCs, widening the gap and highlighting the need for increased investment in digital infrastructure and resources. With more time online, adolescents are at greater risk of cyberbullying, online harassment, and other forms of online exploitation. This is particularly concerning in MWCs, where there may be limited legal protections or support systems for victims [15].

At the same time, the pandemic spurred digitalization: mobile network data traffic grew by 42% between 2020 and 2021 [6]. Digitalization of education was accelerated in MWCs in order to quickly adapt to online learning [22]. Families prioritized buying or sharing devices to preserve sociability and education during isolation [11, 22]. As a consequence, reliance on digital technologies has increased, alongside demands for digital skills and digital literacy for education and employability [11].

## 2.6 Regulation

The past decade has seen calls for regulation that ensures that technological companies assume greater responsibility in protecting and centering youths' needs, with platforms that are age-appropriate [39], safe [15], and playful [40] by design. Several regulations have emerged, including the United Kingdom (UK) Online Safety Bill [41], the European Union (EU) General Data Protection Regulation and Digital Services Act [42], and the United States (US) Children's Online Privacy Protection Act [43]. These European and US initiatives have potential for global impact on youth's rights in the online environment. However, MWCs lack comparable examples of cross-national legislation. Even when national Internet rights legislations do exist (e.g., Brazil's Marco Civil da Internet or India's Personal Data Protection Bill [44]), they tend to be limited. Youths' rights can also be at risk in countries with strict governmental surveillance and control (e.g., China's Social Credit System).

Part of the solution is legislation that can apply broadly, such as the worldwide initiative of General Comment 25 (GC25) [45], which was adopted by the United Nations Convention on the Rights of the Child to enshrine that youth's rights apply equally online and offline [9]. The GC25 was informed by policymakers and also global consultations, which included youth from diverse nations [9]. The GC25 creates a common framework around the lived-experience of digitalization, a holistic understanding of how youth live in the digital environment, and integrates human rights that are not exclusively related to technologies [46]. However, signing or even ratifying the convention is just the first step to ensuring that rights are recognized and supported in everyday life. There are potential disparities in levels of awareness of the GC25 among signatory countries with and without strong intersections between children and Internet rights agendas. Less economically developed nations generally have less leverage to ensure youth's rights in digital ecologies where big transnational corporations regulate behaviors and communications, which could weaken implementation efforts.

# 3 Future Research

- Research in MWCs has focused on older adolescents and emerging adults. However, research should incorporate children and young adolescents [3] as they enter social media at a critical developmental stage. A *multidimensional* and *intersectional* perspective is needed to understand how gender, class, families and schools, urban/rural, and ethnic dimensions interact and impact online opportunities and risks [2, 12].

- Increasingly, qualitative and ethnographic work is challenging normative constructs from the Minority World [26]. Such nuanced research is sensitive to specific individual, household, cultural, and structural contexts and is needed to move beyond the tropes of technological optimism on one side and oppression on the other. It is also important to develop *indigenous* research methods, ethics, and theories for researching how youth use digital media in MWCs.
- Scholarship and practice must include youth's voices. Future research should respect and amplify youth voices globally, understand youth's agency and evolving capacities, and recognize their aspirations for the digital environment [9].
- Research should stay abreast of the dynamic digital landscape, which is constantly changing, and is poised to increasingly integrate aspects of the metaverse, virtual reality, and artificial intelligence at an escalating rate [47, 48]. MWCs are underrepresented in AI development, limiting the creation of inclusive AI technologies, and raising important ethical concerns [49]. In addition, emerging evidence suggests that youth in MWCs are working as AI-labelers for content moderation and being exposed to harmful content [50].
- Research should incorporate comparative studies on national legislation on youth's rights in the digital environment, as well as assessments of GC25's implementation. In terms of regulation, we should pay attention to the Global Digital Compact (GDC) [51]—a common agenda for global rights by the UN Secretary-General. The GDC aims to "outline shared principles for an open, free and secure digital future for all" and, among other objectives, the application of human rights online. The GC25 could, and should, play a critical role presenting youth's voices and rights within the GDC process [46].

## 4 Recommendations

- *Expand, diversify, and contextualize research*: To foster youth's full digital participation, digital rights, digital resilience, and digital safety, researchers, educators, governments, and funders in MWCs must prioritize research concerning youth's digital opportunities and risks. Given that the digital context is expanding, changing, and variable across regions, we recommend research that accounts for digital and offline differences. Cross-cultural comparison needs to consider different digital challenges as well as the types of digital literacy programs that are possible. The increasing monopoly of major technological companies calls for the development of critical digital literacies that consider not only how to use digital media but also the kinds of power and ideologies that are implicit within their infrastructures. Surveys and quantitative research should be complemented by embracing ethnographic approaches [11] that provide context.
- *Understand and address long-term impacts of the pandemic*: We emphasize the need to address the challenges and inequalities that have emerged in the shift to remote learning and call for greater investment in digital infrastructure, digital literacies, and regulation to ensure equitable online practices and opportunities. Programs and policies can leverage the increased adoption and digitalization catalyzed by the pandemic and provide youth with the digital resources and support systems they need to thrive in this new digital reality.
- *Increase capacity in tandem with access to infrastructure*: Increased investment in ICT infrastructure, education, and skilling is needed to bridge the digital divides and increase digital participation and opportunity for more youth around the world, especially in MWCs. Both digital and non-digital inequalities (i.e., economic resources, education, discrimination around gender, minority status, and ability/disability) need to be addressed in tandem [18]. Digital policies at the national and local levels are needed to ensure that

schools in MWCs teach digital skills, promote information and media literacy, and expose youth to emerging digital possibilities (e.g., Uruguay's Plan Ceibal).[3] There is a need to strengthen information and empowerment channels for parents and families to promote active mediation of youth's online lives [8].

- *Implement, monitor, and expand global regulation*: GC25 should be embedded in the GDC, ensuring youth's rights are part of the global shared principles for an open, free, and secure digital future for all. We also argue for a multistakeholder taskforce in charge of creating and monitoring mechanisms for GC25 implementation. Public accountability instances based on standards/indicators are also necessary. Youth are the only stakeholders absent from GDC. If direct representation is still nonfeasible in these instances (something that should be discussed), continuous consultations such as the one that informed the GC25 [9] and comparative international studies such as Global Kids Online [12], need to be developed and funded to ensure the presence of youth's voices in the discussion regarding their own lives and rights in the digital environment.

**Conflict of Interest and Funding Disclosures** None.

## References

1. Khan T, Abimbola S, Kyobutungi C, Pai M. How we classify countries and people-and why it matters. BMJ Glob Health. 2022;7(6):e009704. https://doi.org/10.1136/bmjgh-2022-009704. PMID: 35672117; PMCID: PMC9185389.
2. Ghai S, Magis-Weinberg L, Stoilova M, Livingstone S, Orben A. Social media and adolescent well-being in the Global South. Curr Opin Psychol. 2022;46:101318. https://doi.org/10.1016/j.copsyc.2022.101318.
3. Magis-Weinberg L, Ballonoff Suleiman A, Dahl RE. Context, development, and digital media: implications for very young adolescents in LMICs. Front Psychol. 2021;12:632713. https://www.frontiersin.org/articles/10.3389/fpsyg.2021.632713. Accessed 30 Mar 2023.
4. UNICEF. Children in a digital world. UNICEF; 2017.
5. Arora P. The next billion users: digital life beyond the west. Harvard University Press; 2019.
6. International Telecommunication Union. Measuring digital development: facts and figures 2021. International Telecommunication Union; 2021. https://www.itu.int/en/ITU-D/Statistics/Documents/facts/FactsFigures2021.pdf.
7. Pathak-Shelat M, Bhatia KV. Engaging the world. In: The handbook of media education research. Wiley; 2020. p. 399–412. https://doi.org/10.1002/9781119166900.ch37.
8. Trucco D, Palma A. Infancia y Adolescencia En La Era Digital: Un Informe Comparativo de Los Estudios de Kids Online Del Brasil, Chile, Costa Rica y El Uruguay. CEPAL; 2020. https://repositorio.cepal.org/bitstream/handle/11362/45212/7/S2000334_es.pdf.
9. Third A, Moody L. Our rights in the digital world: a report on the children's consultations to inform UNCRC general comment 25. 5Rights Foundation and Western Sydney University; 2021. https://5rightsfoundation.com/uploads/OurRIghtsinaDigitalWorld-FullReport.pdf.
10. Helsper E. The digital disconnect: the social causes and consequences of digital inequalities. Sage Publications, Inc; 2021.
11. Law ELC, Vostanis P, O'Reilly MJ. Insights from impacts of the digital divide on children in five majority world countries during the COVID-19 pandemic. Behav Inform Technol. 2022;42(15):2696–715. https://doi.org/10.1080/0144929X.2022.2141136.
12. Global Kids Online. Global Kids Online: comparative report. UNICEF Office of Research – Innocenti; 2019.
13. Ngwainmbi EK, editor. Social media, youth, and the Global South. Springer Nature; 2023.
14. Livingstone S, Stoilova M. The 4Cs: classifying online risk to children, CO:RE short report series on key topics. Hamburg: Leibniz-Institut für Medienforschung | Hans-Bredow-Institut (HBI); CO:RE; 2021. https://doi.org/10.21241/SSOAR.71817.
15. Lala G, Chandra S, Ogun N, Moody L, Third A. Online safety perceptions, needs, and expectations of young people in Southeast Asia: consultations with young people in Indonesia, Malaysia, Thailand, and Vietnam. Western Sydney University; 2022. https://doi.org/10.26183/tz74-ev38.
16. UNICEF Office of Research Innocenti. Children's experiences of online sexual exploitation and abuse in 12 countries in eastern and southern Africa and Southeast Asia. Global Partnership to End Violence Against Children; 2022. https://www.end-violence.

[3]Plan Ceibal is a nationwide policy that is more than a country-level one-to-one device provision initiative, as it also provides high-speed broadband connectivity to all compulsory education centers, connects teachers to students in regions where there was a lack of teachers (i.e. English teaching in small localities), develops an ecosystem of free educational software and contents, and even new pedagogies to integrate them into class.

org/sites/default/files/2022-05/DH-data-insight-1_Final%281%29.pdf.
17. Livingstone S, Nandi A, Banaji S, Stoilova M. Young adolescents and digital media: uses, risks and opportunities in low-and middle-income countries: a rapid evidence review. London: Gender and Adolescence: Global Evidence; 2017. https://www.gage.odi.org/publication/digital-media-risks-opportunities/.
18. Navarro JL, Tudge JRH. Technologizing Bronfenbrenner: neo-ecological theory. Curr Psychol. 2022;42:19338–54. https://doi.org/10.1007/s12144-022-02738-3.
19. Dodel M. Socioeconomic inequalities and digital skills. In: Rohlinger DA, Sobieraj S, editors. The Oxford handbook of digital media sociology. Oxford University Press; 2022. https://doi.org/10.1093/oxfordhb/9780197510636.013.30.
20. Law NWY, Pan Q, Tao S, et al. Hong Kong students' digital citizenship development 2019–2021: findings from a longitudinal study. 2nd ed; 2023. https://doi.org/10.25442/hku.22085738.v2.
21. Kardefelt Winther D, Twesigye R. Disrupting harm: online risk and harm for children in eastern and southern Africa. Florence: UNICEF Office of Research – Innocenti; 2023.
22. Rodríguez MRB, Cobo C. COVID-19 and education in the Global South: emergency remote learning solutions with long-term implications. 2022. https://www.oecd-ilibrary.org/content/component/897cd0d8-en.
23. Plantin JC, Lagoze C, Edwards PN, Sandvig C. Infrastructure studies meet platform studies in the age of Google and Facebook. New Media Soc. 2018;20(1):293–310. https://doi.org/10.1177/1461444816661553.
24. OXFAM. Digital divide: India inequality report. OXFAM; 2022. https://www.oxfamindia.org/knowledgehub/workingpaper/india-inequality-report-2022-digital-divide
25. Pathak-Shelat M, Saesha CP. Indian Kids Online: negotiating the global and the digital flows – a pilot study report. MICA; 2022.
26. Bhatia KV, Arora P, Pathak-Shelat M. Good girls don't go online: unpacking the quotidian playful resilience influencing girls' social and digital engagements. Int J Commun. 2021;15:19.
27. Sada Garibay C, Lapierre MA. From risk perception to the use of technical restrictions of SVoD services in Mexico, the mediating role of parent involvement and knowledge. J Broadcast Electron Media. 2024;68(1):21–42. https://doi.org/10.1080/08838151.2023.2278616.
28. Correa T. The power of youth: how the bottom-up technology transmission from children to parents is related to digital (in)equality. Int J Commun. 2015;9:24.
29. Uzuegbunam CE. Children and young people's digital lifeworlds: domestication, mediation, and agency. Palgrave Macmillan; 2024.
30. Uzuegbunam CE. Assessing rural and urban teenagers' domestication of technology: the role of digital literacy. Int J Mob Blended Learn. 2022;14(3):1–15. https://doi.org/10.4018/IJMBL.310941.
31. Adigwe I, van der Walt T. Parental mediation of online media activities of children in Nigeria: a parent-child approach. Comput Hum Behav Rep. 2020;2:100041. https://doi.org/10.1016/j.chbr.2020.100041.
32. Dias P, Brito R, Ribbens W, et al. The role of parents in the engagement of young children with digital technologies: exploring tensions between rights of access and protection, from "Gatekeepers" to "Scaffolders". Glob Stud Child. 2016;6(4):414–27. https://doi.org/10.1177/2043610616676024.
33. Tao S, Reichert F, Law N, Rao N. Digital technology use and cyberbullying among primary school children: digital literacy and parental mediation as moderators. Cyberpsychol Behav Soc Netw. 2022;25(9):571–9. https://doi.org/10.1089/cyber.2022.0012.
34. Weinstein E, James C. School-based initiatives promoting digital citizenship and healthy digital media use. In: Telzer EH, Nesi J, Prinstein MJ, editors. Handbook of adolescent digital media use and mental health. Cambridge University Press; 2022. p. 365–88. https://doi.org/10.1017/9781108976237.020.
35. Fraillon J, Ainley J, Schulz W, Duckworth D, Friedman T. IEA international computer and information literacy study 2018 assessment framework | IEA.Nl. IEA; 2019. https://www.iea.nl/publications/assessment-framework/iea-international-computer-and-information-literacy-study-2018. Accessed 1 Apr 2023.
36. ACARA. Australian curriculum, assessment and reporting authority annual report. 2015.
37. Pangrazio L, Cardozo-Gaibisso L. Beyond cybersafety: the need to develop social media literacies in pre-teens. Digit Educ Rev. 2020;37:49–63. https://doi.org/10.1344/der.2020.37.49-63.
38. Tanksley TC. "We're changing the system with this one": black students using critical race algorithmic literacies to subvert and survive AI-mediated racism in school. Engl Teach Pract Crit. 2024;23(1):36–56. https://doi.org/10.1108/ETPC-08-2023-0102.
39. Information Commissioner's Office. Age appropriate design: a code of practice for online services. ICO; 2020.
40. Livingstone S, Pothong K. Playful by design: a vision of free play in a digital world. Digital Futures Commission; 5Rights Foundation; 2021.
41. Online Safety Act 2023. (Parliament of UK). Available from: https://www.legislation.gov.uk/ukpga/2023/50
42. Regulation (EU) 2022/2065 of the European Parliament and of the Council of 19 October 2022 on a Single Market for Digital Services and amending Directive 2000/31/EC (Digital Services Act). 2022. (EU). Available from: https://eurlex.europa.eu/eli/reg/2022/2065/oj
43. Children's Online Privacy Protection Act. 1998. (US). §§ 6501-6506. Available From: http://uscode.house.gov/view.xhtml
44. Marco Civil da Internet, 2014. (BR). Law No. 12.1965. Available From: https://www.cgi.br/pagina/marco-civil-law-of-theinternet-in-brazil/180#art32
45. General comment No. 25 (2021) on children's rights in relation to the digital environment, 2021. (UN). Available From: https://www.ohchr.org/en/docu-

ments/general-comments-and-recommendations/general-comment-no-25-2021-childrensrights-relation.

46. Souter D. Children's rights online: implementing general comment 25. Media@LSE; 2022. https://blogs.lse.ac.uk/medialse/2022/11/25/childrens-rights-online-implementing-general-comment-25/. Accessed 14 Mar 2023.
47. Hinduja S. The metaverse: opportunities, risks, and harms. Cyberbullying Research Center Blog; n.d. https://cyberbullying.org/metaverse. Accessed 3 June 2024.
48. Hinduja S. Generative AI risks and harms – the role of platforms and users. Cyberbullying Research Center Blog. 24 May 2023. https://cyberbullying.org/generative-ai-risks-harms-platforms-users. Accessed 3 June 2024.
49. Okolo C. AI in the Global South: opportunities and challenges towards more inclusive governance. 1 Nov 2023. https://www.brookings.edu/articles/ai-in-the-global-south-opportunities-and-challenges-towards-more-inclusive-governance/. Accessed 12 Apr 2024.
50. Rowe N. Underage workers are training AI. Wired. 15 Nov 2023. https://www.wired.com/story/artificial-intelligence-data-labeling-children/. Accessed 12 Apr 2023.
51. Global Digital Compact, 2023. (UN). Available from: https://www.un.org/sites/un2.un.org/files/our-common-agenda-policybrief-gobal-digi-compact-en.pdf

# Part III

# Digital Domains

# Introduction to the Section on Education Technology

Jennifer Darling-Aduana

Education technology (edtech) integration in school establishes how students will understand, use, and develop a relationship with technology as they mature. Technology is deeply intertwined with social understanding and functions in society, with technology presented as an essential tool for achieving academic and life success. Whether, which type, and how edtech is used also has profound implications for the quality of students' learning experiences. From an instructional standpoint, the identification, integration, and enactment of edtech within the classroom has the potential to shape and transform educational experiences Yet, the full potential of edtech integration is rarely realized in practice, particularly in lower-resourced environments where students may be most likely to benefit. Accordingly, there remain profound equity implications to differential edtech access as well as to appropriate and equitable use in the classroom.

The following six chapters highlight the reality, potential, and unknowns regarding the pervasive use of education technology in schools. Each of these chapters summarizes research on fully online learning environments, such via online course taking and web conferencing, as well as the integration of digital tools like learning management systems (LMS), social media, and cloud-based document creation, editing, and sharing in traditional, face-to-face instruction (i.e., blended instruction). These categories include the most common uses of educational technology—which tend to be teacher-centric and recreating existing educational practices [1]. A few chapters also engage with more transformative uses of educational technology including virtual/augmented reality (VR/AR), artificial intelligence (AI), and students as content creators. Most research reviewed was conducted within the United States and similar sociopolitical contexts, with the exception of the chapter on emergency schooling.

Within this section, researchers provide a synthesis of K-12 edtech research, generally, as well as edtech use during the pandemic (and future emergencies), more specifically. Subsequent chapters provide a deeper dive into specific subareas including the equity implications of online learning, digital media literacy, edtech in early childhood, and data privacy and surveillance. Below, I briefly summarize each chapter before presenting a synthesis of overarching themes, suggestions for current research, and recommendations for improving edtech policy and practice.

First, Krutka et al. [2] (see chapter "The State of Educational Technology Research and Practice") document trends in edtech research and educational practices over the past decade. Key trends include increased interest in online/blended learning and emergency remote teaching due to COVID-19. Additionally, interest in VR/AR became more pronounced in 2021 followed by even more recent attention on AI.

Narrowing the focus to edtech use during the COVID-19 pandemic and future emergencies, Reich et al. [3] (see chapter "Education Technology During the Pandemic and Future

J. Darling-Aduana (✉)
Georgia State University, Atlanta, GA, USA
e-mail: jdarlingaduana@gsu.edu



D. A. Christakis, L. Hale (eds.), *Handbook of Children and Screens*,
https://doi.org/10.1007/978-3-031-69362-5_70

Emergencies") highlight the need for *pedagogies of adaptability* to maintain learning and student well-being during increasingly frequent global crises. Pedagogies of adaptability include being prepared to teach via multiple modalities, partnering with caregivers and community members to educate students, and developing emergency learning policies and procedures. For instance, refugee students in Somali found educational support through virtual peer and expert relationships [4], while teachers in the United States shared that increased use of teleconferencing during the pandemic made it easier to build relationships with caregivers during and outside of the school day [5]. Developing these pedagogies requires preparation (not just response), including time to rehearse and support pedagogies before crises, universal connectivity, critical approaches to edtech use, and social welfare investments.

Next, Darling-Aduana et al. [6] (see chapter "Digital Ethics and Equity in K-12 Blended and Online Learning") place edtech use in its larger societal contexts, emphasizing the non-neutrality of technology and the need to dismantle existing assumptions, norms, values, and structures within the social and institutional structures of schooling to achieve equitable (online) education. Common benefits of online and blended instruction highlighted include increased flexibility, self-pacing, real-time data, just-in-time assessment, and removal of geographic barriers. Yet, systematic differences in access to quality online learning experiences remain due to inequitable school funding structures, overreliance on low-quality commercial edtech products that emphasize standardization to maximize profits, and a failure to enact critical or social-justice oriented pedagogical approaches that center students as knowledge generators and creators.

Turner et al. [7] (see chapter "The Importance of Digital Media Literacy") underscore that digital media literacy—"the knowledge and practices required to navigate digital spaces' productively, ethically, and as producers (as well as consumers) of knowledge"—is necessary to maximize benefits and mitigate harmful effects of technology on children and teens. For example, students with stronger digital media literacy are more likely to be civically active, achieve higher academically, be more informed consumers of information, and be better equipped to navigate troubling digital situations (like online bullying and scams).

Golinkoff et al. [8] (see chapter "The Explosion of EdTech: Can Its Promise Be Fulfilled?") assert edtech in early childhood has yet to realize its potential. Currently, most edtech focuses on cognitive skills development. There is a yet unrealized opportunity to support students' social-emotional learning and foster collaborative learning between children and their caregivers, both of which are particularly critical to early childhood learning. As one example, co-reading e-books that integrate dialogic reading prompts is associated with more positive emotions for children and parents as well as an increase in on-task behaviors [9]. Edtech targeting early childhood could also be improved by removing distractions, non-learning-based visual/auditory enhancements, and advertisements.

Finally, Hillman et al. [10] (see chapter "Children, Education, and Technologies: Current Debates, Key Concerns, and Future Directions Around Data Privacy, Surveillance, and Datafication") express concern related to datafication and the use of edtech to monitor and quantify all learner interactions within the system. Researchers emphasize the potential for even longer-term, negative consequences that may result through the normalization of the digital surveillance state for future generations of citizens. Hillman and colleagues assert the need for critical digital literacy to support students in maintaining well-being when existing in these online spaces of learning.

## 1 Overarching Themes

Several overarching themes regarding edtech use in schools were reiterated across chapters. Darling-Aduana et al., Hillman et al., Krutka et al., and Reich et al. emphasized the ethical concerns of edtech use. Darling-Aduana et al. and Golinkoff et al. expressed skepticism regarding the quality of commercially available edtech products. Both Hillman et al. and Turner et al. stressed the essential role of digital media literacy in supporting healthy, informed technology use in school and beyond. Darling-Aduana et al. and Krutka et al. highlighted the potential of edtech to center students as content creators and change agents.

When discussing ethical concerns related to edtech use, researchers described the role edtech products play in collecting detailed personal data and contributing to the surveillance of children and their families. These features of many (especially commercial) edtech products are under-understood and underregulated. Hillman et al. warned that increased reliance in decision-making systems on this decontextualized, supposedly neutral data collected by edtech products has the potential to reinforce (if not magnify) existing biases and systematic inequities. Further, algorithmic biases, built-in normative assumptions, cyberbullying, online harassment, and distraction are all inherent in edtech systems and processes unless specifically targeted and countered during design and implementation.

Relatedly, several researchers cautioned against reliance on commercial edtech products. Beyond the privacy concerns highlighted above—which tend to be most extreme in commercial products—Golinkoff et al. documented positive learning associations when examining researcher-developed edtech products. However, learning associations tend to be negative when examining commercial products. These trends appear to indicate that commercial edtech is of lower quality. Darling-Aduana et al. point out that commercial edtech companies (which dominate the market) are disincentivized to provide innovative, differentiated learning experiences as they are more expensive to facilitate (reducing profits). Thus, commercial edtech products often prioritize easily standardized structures and default to normative assumptions to improve product scalability [11].

Given the current state of edtech—as well as the state of technology more generally—digital media literacy has become essential for informed technology use. Turner et al. explain that "developing digital media literate citizens who consume, create, connect, and advocate for themselves and others in ethical ways is paramount to overcoming the challenges faced by youth in a technology-driven world." Relatedly, researchers highlight one of the greatest potentials of edtech use in schools is the extent to which it can be used to center students as content creators, makers, and change agents. The Young People's Race, Power, and Technology Program (YPRPT) based out of Northwestern University accomplishes many of these aims by empowering youth to debate the ethics of online surveillance, create a documentary on facial recognition software, and file and analyze Freedom of Information Act (FOIA) requests of surveillance technology in their neighborhood [12]. Emerging research and programs with these aims demonstrate real promise in promoting digital media literacy, student agency, and deep learning.

## 2 Future Research

Historically, edtech research has focused on documenting the potential of tools and programs when implemented in ideal settings, often on a small scale with sufficient funding, buy-in, and expertise to support enactment. With widespread adoption and use, there is a need to move beyond this emphasis on ideal case studies to an examination of broader use, including potential ethical concerns, implementation challenges, unintended consequences, and (in)equity implications. Critical theoretical traditions provide a framework for this work by emphasizing the non-neutrality of educational institutions, working to dismantle oppressive (educational) systems, and empowering students as active participants in their learning journey and communities more broadly [13]. Building upon these critical traditions, there is a need for researchers to support the development, documentation, evaluation, refinement, and scaling up of programs that promote student voice and agency in online learning spaces. Participatory research methods may be particularly helpful in achieving this aim through the process as well as the outcomes of research.

## 3 Recommendations

Several shared recommendations emerged across chapters. For policymakers, researchers emphasized the need for universal connectivity to ensure all students have access to the globalized technology system. Increased attention should also be paid to regulating online advertisers that target minors, employ manipulative design features (i.e., microtransactions), and engage in the collection/use of personal data for minors. Specifically, policymakers should enact data protection laws, increase accountability, and place limits on digital surveillance—particularly when it involves minors.

More broadly, policymakers, commercial and non-profit organizations, developers, educators, parents, community members, and students all have a role to play in acknowledging and working to dismantle structural inequities in technology use. Specific inequities highlighted include disproportionate underrepresentation in computer science and other technology fields and the inequitable access/use of quality online tools. Related to this goal is teaching students *about* as well as *with* technology. This could be accomplished through a national digital media literacy curriculum, resources integrated within existing literacy standards, and parental guidance that considers the quality as well as the quantity of screen time. Finally, several researchers emphasized the importance of fostering parental partnerships to support both online learning and student well-being in digital spaces.

## 4 Conclusion

Given the consensus of researchers across edtech disciplines and focus areas, the chapters in this section present a roadmap for improving edtech enactment in a manner that maximizes learning, centers equity, and fosters student well-being. Notably, calls were made across chapters for increased policy guidance, support, and oversight. At the same time, the true potential of edtech use cannot be realized until used to give students a voice, encourage agency, create and share knowledge, and enact social change.

**Conflict of Interest and Funding Disclosures** None.

## References

1. Reich J. Failure to disrupt: why technology alone can't transform education. Harvard University Press; 2020.
2. Krutka DG, Greeenhow C, Kimmons R, Pangrazio L, Trust T. The state of education technology research and practice. Pediatrics.
3. Reich J, Cobo C, Dryden-Peterson S, Klopfer E, Kamenetz A, Trust T. Education technology during the pandemic and future emergencies. Pediatrics.
4. Dryden-Peterson S, Dahya N, Adelman E. Pathways to educational success among refugees: connecting locally and globally situated resources. Am Educ Res J. 2017;54(6):1011–47.
5. Esteves N, Buttimer CJ, Faruqi F, Soukab A, Fourkiller R, Gutierrez H, Reich J. The teachers have something to say: lessons learned from US PK-12 teachers during the COVID-impacted 2020-21 school year. 2021. Retrieved from https://osf.io/preprints/edarxiv/h8gac.
6. Darling-Aduana J, Heath MK, Stewart A, Viano S, Asim S, Garcia A, Langran E, Heinrich C, Woodley X. Digital ethics and equity in K-12 blended and online learning. Pediatrics.
7. Turner KH, Fisenstock B, Hicks T, Jolls T, O'Byrne I, Paciga K, Price-Dennis D, Reich J, Schira Hagerman H. The importance of digital media literacy. Pediatrics.
8. Golinkoff RM, Hassinger-Das B, Kucirkova N, Myers L, Dore RA. The explosion of ed tech: can its promise be fulfilled? Pediatrics.
9. Ahn J, Beck A, Rice J, Foster M. Exploring issues of implementation, equity, and student achievement with educational software in the DC Public Schools. AERA Open. 2016;2(4):233285841666772. https://doi.org/10.1177/2332858416667726.
10. Hillman V, Manolev J, Zeide E, Kumar P, Martin F, Johnston S-K, Vladova G, Lai R. Children, education, and technologies: current debates, key concerns, future directions around data privacy, surveillance and datafication. Pediatrics.
11. Darling-Aduana J, Hemingway K. Representation is not enough: teacher identity and discretion in an asynchronous, scripted online learning environment. Teach Coll Rec. 2022;124(9):91–121.
12. Vakil S, Reith A, Melo NA. Jamming power: youth agency and community-driven science in a critical technology learning program. J Res Sci Teach. 2023;60(8):1723–54.
13. Freire P. Pedagogy of the oppressed. 1970; Giroux H. Pedagogy and the politics of hope: theory, culture, and schooling: a critical reader. Routledge; 2018; Hooks B. Teaching to transgress. Routledge; 2014; Ladson-Billings G. Toward a theory of culturally relevant pedagogy. Am Educ Res J. 1995;32(3):465–91.

# The State of Educational Technology Research and Practice

Daniel G. Krutka, Christine Greenhow, Royce Kimmons, Luci Pangrazio, and Torrey Trust

## 1 Background

Broadly defined, educational technology (edtech) is any technology that affects the educational experiences of youth within or outside of schools. Instruction-specific tools have evolved over time from blackboards to whiteboards to smart boards. Edtech also encompasses technologies explicitly designed for educational purposes, such as learning management systems (e.g., Moodle) and widely popular tools, apps, and platforms that have pervaded how people live, learn, work, and play (e.g., Google Workspace apps). Much of the recent attention, discussion, and research in educational technology research and practice in our contexts in the United States and Australia tends to focus on current and emerging technologies that have influenced teaching and learning in classroom settings.

D. G. Krutka (✉)
University of North Texas, Denton, TX, USA

C. Greenhow
Michigan State University, East Lansing, MI, USA

R. Kimmons
Brigham Young University, Provo, UT, USA

L. Pangrazio
Deakin University, Geelong, VIC, Australia

T. Trust
University of Massachusetts Amherst, Amherst, MA, USA

The shift to emergency remote teaching [1] during the onset of the COVID-19 pandemic in 2020 increased attention, among educators, researchers, and the general public, to the quality of students' experiences when teachers employ edtech. As in-person schools closed around the world, educators scrambled to figure out how to reach and teach learners at physical distance. Schools and districts sought to provide devices and Internet access to every student, while educators turned to digital tools, apps, and platforms to support remote teaching and learning. This increased focus on digital edtech has resulted in more educators, students, and families having access to and experience with, technology used for educational purposes today than prior to the pandemic. However, not all access to, and experiences with, emerging technologies have been equal; as such, digital divides persist [2].

Scholars have long contended that educational technologies cannot produce quality teaching on their own. With their Technological Pedagogical Content Knowledge (TPACK) framework, Koehler and Mishra [3] argued that educators must intricately combine technological, pedagogical, and content knowledge to successfully use edtech to support students' learning. Kimmons and colleagues [4] offered another model that focused on students' roles (passive, interactive, creating) with edtech, and how the use of edtech affects teachers' pedagogies (replacement, amplification, transformation)


D. A. Christakis, L. Hale (eds.), *Handbook of Children and Screens*,
https://doi.org/10.1007/978-3-031-69362-5_71

(i.e., PICRAT) to showcase the multifaceted interaction between teaching, student learning, and edtech. Simply providing new technologies, digital tools, apps, and platforms is not enough to improve the quality of educational experiences. These models demonstrate that there is a complex interplay between teachers, students, and technologies that influences whether and how learning happens with edtech. This interplay of factors is context-specific, meaning that what works for one teacher in one classroom might not work for another teacher in a different classroom.

## 2 Current State

Because technologies, schools, and students are ever-changing, edtech as a field has been in a constant state of flux as educators try to address current educational needs considering affordances and constraints of emerging technologies. As such, research in edtech tends to shift based on current and emerging trends in technologies, pedagogies, and innovations. Analysis of articles in edtech research journal reveals that current research in the field [5]:

- Focuses on both higher education and K-12, but favors higher education
- Uses a variety of methods, including systematic review, case study, meta-analysis, mixed methods, and factor analysis
- Explores various modalities, including online/blended learning, virtual/augmented reality, and flipped classrooms
- Grapples with a variety of technologies and topics, such as learning environments, computational thinking, language learning, social media, artificial intelligence, self-efficacy, performance, engagement, coding, and more
- Shifts over time, such as a focus from virtual and augmented reality in 2021 to artificial intelligence [5, 6] in 2022 and 2023

Additionally, the COVID-19 pandemic spurred an exponential increase in articles about emergency remote teaching, while increasing scholarship on *online learning*, or learning that involves interactions mediated through the use of digital, typically Internet-based, technology; *blended learning*, or the combination of online and in-person time and place dimensions; and *self-directed*, or personalized learning such as through social media [7].

The fluid, evolving nature of emerging technologies makes checking the current pulse of edtech difficult, particularly if scholars rely solely upon traditional publishing and communication models, such as peer-reviewed journals. For this reason, analyzing more voluminous sources of data, such as edtech-related Twitter feeds, school Facebook groups, and edtech-adjacent website analytics can offer a clearer sense of the current state of the field [8]. Current analyses of these sources suggest other additional trends from the past decade [5, 6, 9, 10].

First, there has been increased attention among educators in using edtech as a means for improving access, equity, representation, and democratization in learning. This takes a variety of forms, ranging from the use of open educational resources (OER) to increase access to knowledge, to the use of technology for improving women's and girls' experiences in science, technology, engineering, and math (STEM) learning. Recent scholarship has also investigated how to challenge sexist and racist stereotypes in computing by centering historically minoritized groups [11–13].

Second, because most edtech work is of an applied nature and takes place in public institutions (e.g., teachers working with students in K-12 classrooms), there is often a disconnect between what is being researched in journals and what is of immediate practical value to practitioners in the field. For instance, in April 2023, research articles might focus on the affordances of generative AI for reshaping educational institutions of tomorrow, but they may not provide practical guidance to teachers on how to address the benefits and drawbacks of students' uses of ChatGPT for writing assignments today. Educators can be bombarded with immediate suggestions, particularly from *education influencers* on social media, for how to react [14].

Third, edtech is inherently technophilic, meaning that the field generally has optimistic attitudes toward technology. This means that edtech practitioners and researchers tend to be focused on exploring and adopting new technologies to solve educational problems, rather than grappling with the ethics and potential pitfalls of such use [15]. For example, scholars might focus more on how to use technology to teach online courses compared to the negative implications of weak cybersecurity or data privacy practices with digital tools, apps, and platforms. Though there are certainly voices in the field that focus on these areas and exhibit a more cautionary attitude toward new technologies [16, 17], they are in the minority, making safe and responsible use of technologies more of an afterthought than a driving factor. However, although the "technology" aspect of edtech may regularly receive the lion's share of interest, there is ongoing attention in the field to students and social institutions by exploring theory, experiences, perspectives, ethics, and change management.

The field of educational technologies is broad and diverse enough that more illustrative examples are needed to better understand such emerging trends. One area of edtech that remains under-explored is the complex interrelationships between self-directed learning with ubiquitous social media—which can occur within class curricula or outside it (e.g., YouTube) as youth tap resources based on their interests—and schooling. Teachers and students often have little choice about the platforms procured by school administrators, and the lack of school-sanctioned digital platforms and alternatives presents an ongoing issue [19]. Youth, in particular, have turned to social media for informal learning and educational purposes, that extend beyond the formal place and time of the "school day" [19, 20]. With low barriers to content creation and sharing, social media have allowed young people to pursue their interests, generating new forms of self-expression and creating personal or professional learning networks [20, 21].

However, the benefits and challenges of these trends are not well understood. For example, educators and scholars should attend more to how social media affects students' ability to sustain their concentration for difficult tasks. There is increasing evidence that regular use of social media and the Internet can have cognitive effects on attention span and concentration [22], which raises the question whether schools must teach students how to negotiate social media use. Also, as social media intertwine with, and are incorporated into K-12 education, educators should be concerned with user agreements and uses of data; algorithms of echo, extremism, and oppression; user choice, distraction, and access for nonusers; cyberbullying and harassment; and gatekeeping of accurate information [23]. These issues raise ethical questions for which there is limited practical guidance in the educational technology scholarship [24]. As one example, chatbots or conversational agents where students can ask questions, can be a cognitive and time-saving aide for teachers, but raise ethical questions regarding *data privacy* (how entered information is used); *surveillance* (how the student's activities and preferences are tracked); and *autonomy* (the degree to which the student is being manipulated by the algorithms or acting of their own accord) [24].

In a related topic, teaching students about digital data serves as another example of work being done in the field. This subject is particularly powerful because digital data creates realities that are internalized by young people in unconscious ways. Individuals are not always aware of the digital data they are sharing when they use devices and systems. Therefore, educators can use a *critical data literacies* approach to scaffold young people toward more critical understanding and awareness. Such curriculum requires a careful balance between both revealing the "black box" of how apps and devices collect and use data and also providing opportunities to increase agency to "do" data differently [25]. However, a didactic approach to students can be counterproductive because digital practices are so intricately entwined with social life [26].

## 3 Future Research

These trends in contemporary educational technology inspire several questions about teaching practice while addressing gaps in research going forward. We have identified three research priorities for the field.

First, there is a need for more detailed, classroom-based empirical research that takes account of the beliefs, practices, and contexts of students and teachers. Edtech journalists have offered quality stories on how teachers respond to technological change [27], but more detailed, scholarly research can unpack even more. This research should focus on students' perspectives, but also go beyond examining direct effects of technology by considering larger contexts, opportunity costs, and differential experiences for students of different races, abilities, genders, and more. The ways edtech is employed in classrooms are contextual and divergent. Students, classrooms, and contexts are different and only through rigorous methods can scholars and educators begin to unpack those complexities.

Second, there is a need for more exploratory and collaborative research on the complex interplay between learning with technologies that span traditional boundaries. Recent literature reviews have synthesized findings on teachers' integration of ubiquitous technologies such as social media in K-12 classrooms; students' self-expression or self-directed learning within such spaces; and teachers' personal and professional learning networks [7], but few edtech studies have been conducted in informal and formal learning environments concurrently. Research that examines their interplay is needed to advance understanding of whether and how theories generalize across contexts and the relationships between them. Such research also has practical implications; it could help educators discern how to build on understandings (or resolve confusions) formed in one context, in the other, and vice versa [7]. Moreover, innovative research methods currently underutilized in edtech (e.g., participatory action research [PAR]) would allow better integration of research and practice. In PAR, for instance, participants collaborate with researchers to shape and conduct inquiry that could examine the technologies they choose (e.g., social media) for learning and those they do not (e.g., school-adopted learning management systems). Adults—researchers, teachers, parents—need to listen and learn from young people, particularly students whose identities are often not centered in technology discourses. In recommending methods such as PAR [28], we also recognize that replication studies are similarly needed to make broader claims, particularly about educational technologies with widespread adoption.

Third, there is a need for more critical inquiry into technologies and professional development opportunities for educators to think deeply about technological choices. Too often, teachers are expected, or required, to be innovators or use technologies without time to examine issues such as data privacy or how it changes the culture of a class. This could be undertaken by teachers, and hopefully with students, conducting technoethical audits of edtech that address ethical, legal, democratic, economic, technological, and pedagogical questions [16]. Scholars and technology professionals could investigate the role of intermediaries, such as tech brokers, and state departments in the procurement and use of edtech in schools. Ideally, educators and researchers will also work productively with edtech companies to ensure that school-based stakeholders' needs are incorporated into the design and development of products. Educators need time to study, reflect, plan, and partner.

## 4 Recommendations

What should be next for edtech? We offer three recommendations:

- First, the edtech field—teachers and scholars alike—should always remember that technology is situated in larger cultures and contexts. In schools, this requires paying attention to situated interactions between technology and pedagogies and content [3], students' roles and teachers' choices [4], and infrastructure and protections [18]. Educators and scholars must attend to these complex factors if edtech is to improve education. Tools are unlikely to improve educational experiences on their own. Such systems-level approaches to technology integration can prepare teachers and students to take cautious approaches. For example, Williamsons' "sociotechnical survey of ClassDojo" details a "'data assemblage' composed of technical components, social relations, people, policies, funding arrangements, expert knowledge, and discourse," which illustrates the need for situated understandings of technologies as much more than just tools teachers use [30].

- Second, in our highly technologized world with rapid change, young people need opportunities to not just use the most recent tool, but to inquire into its nature, ethics, and effects [17, 29]. Students should have opportunities to analyze the ethics of edtech in their classrooms and participate in decisions about its uses and abuses in education, culture, and society [13], such as regarding uses and abuses of their data. This can be accomplished by, for example, conducting an edtech audit with students [16]. Teachers should teach not only *with* technology but *about* technology in every grade level and subject [14]. These types of discussions can, and should, include various stakeholders, including parents and community members, among others. This type of *technology education* can better prepare students and teachers to make wise decisions with edtech, especially given the ever-evolving technological landscape shaping our future.
- Third, educators and scholars should critically consider who is being served by edtech and seek more democratic, ethical, and just arrangements. This means that educators have to go beyond teaching everyone to code, but directly addressing the structural reasons why women and historically minoritized groups are often further marginalized in areas like computer science [11–13]. Edtech companies and school adoption should protect vulnerable students and be designed for racially, linguistically, and neurodivergently diverse students. Gender non-conforming students should be assured they are not outed due to lack of data privacy protections. Educators and scholars should be wary of technophilic solutions that privilege only the schools that can afford expensive software and hardware. All students deserve access and equity from edtech.

Technology will continue to change. Even as technological change continues to speed up, educators and scholars need to commit to the slow work of attending to situated contexts, identifying pedagogical approaches, and inquiring critically into technologies to ensure students' experiences are educational and just.

**Conflict of Interest and Funding Disclosures** None.

## References


1. Hodges CB, Moore S, Lockee BB, Trust T, Bond MA. The difference between emergency remote teaching and online learning. Educause. 27 Mar 2020. https://er.educause.edu/articles/2020/3/the-difference-between-emergency-remote-teaching-and-online-learning.
2. Lai J, Widmar NO. Revisiting the digital divided in the COVID-19 era. Appl Econ Perspect Policy. 2019;43:458–64. https://doi.org/10.1002/aepp.13104.
3. Koehler M, Mishra P. What is technological pedagogical content knowledge (TPACK)? CITE J. 2009;9(1):60–70.
4. Kimmons R, Graham CR, West RE. The PICRAT model for technology integration in teacher preparation. CITE J. 2020;20(1):176–98.
5. Allman B, Kimmons R, Rosenberg J, Dash M. Trends and topics in educational technology. 2023 edition. TechTrends. 2023;67:583–91.
6. Kimmons R, Rosenberg J. Trends and topics in educational technology. 2022 edition. TechTrends. 2022;66:134–40. https://doi.org/10.1007/s11528-022-00713-0.
7. Greenhow C, Graham CR, Koehler MJ. Foundations of online learning: challenges and opportunities. Educ Psychol. 2022;57(3):131–47. https://doi.org/10.1080/00461520.2022.2090364.
8. Kimmons R, Veletsianos G. Public internet data mining methods in instructional design, educational technology, and online learning research. TechTrends. 2018;62(5):492–500. https://doi.org/10.1007/s11528-018-0307-4.
9. Kimmons R. Current trends (and missing links) in educational technology research and practice. TechTrends. 2020;64(6):803–9. https://doi.org/10.1007/s11528-020-00549-6.

10. Kimmons R, Rosenberg J, Allman B. Trends in educational technology: what Facebook, Twitter, and Scopus can tell us about current research and practice. TechTrends. 2021;65:125–36. https://doi.org/10.1007/s11528-021-00589-6.
11. Ryoo JJ, Tanksley T, Estrada C, Margolis J. Take space, make space: how students use computer science to disrupt and resist marginalization in schools. Comput Sci Educ. 2020;30(3):337–61. https://doi.org/10.1080/08993408.2020.1805284.
12. Shaw MS, Coleman JJ, Thomas EE, Kafai YB. Restorying a Black girl's future: using womanist storytelling methodologies to reimagine dominant narratives in computing education. J Learn Sci. 2023;32:52–75. https://doi.org/10.1080/10508406.2023.2179847.
13. Yadav A, Heath MK. Breaking the code: confronting racism in computer science through community, criticality, and citizenship. TechTrends. 2022;66(3):450–8.
14. Carpenter JP, Shelton CC, Schroeder SE. The education influencer: a new player in the educator professional landscape. J Res Technol Educ. 2022;55:749–64. https://doi.org/10.1080/15391523.2022.2030267.
15. Sims C. Disruptive fixation: school reform and the pitfalls of techno-idealism. Princeton University Press; 2017. https://doi.org/10.1515/9781400885299.
16. Krutka DG, Heath MK, Staudt Willet KB. Foregrounding technoethics: toward critical perspectives in technology and teacher education. J Technol Teach Educ. 2019;27(4):555–74.
17. Krutka DG, Pleasants J, Nichols TP. Talking the technology talk. Phi Delta Kappan. 2023;104:42–6. https://kappanonline.org/talking-to-students-about-technology-krutka-pleasants-nichols/.
18. Pangrazio L, Selwyn N, Cumbo B. A patchwork of platforms: mapping data infrastructures in schools. Learn Media Technol. 2022;48(1):65–80.
19. Greenhow C, Galvin S, Staudt Willet KB. What should be the role of social media in education? Policy Insights Behav Brain Sci. 2019;6(2):178–85.
20. Greenhow C, Galvin S, Brandon D, Askari E. A decade of research on K-12 teaching and teacher learning with social media: insights on the state-of-the-field. Teach Coll Rec. 2020;122(6):1–72.
21. Greenhow C, Galvin S, Staudt Willet KB. Inquiring tweets want to know: #edchat supports for #remoteteaching during COVID-19. Br J Educ Technol. 2021;52(4):1434–54. https://doi.org/10.1111/bjet.13097.
22. Mark G. Attention span: a groundbreaking way to restore balance, happiness and productivity. Hanover Square Press; 2023.
23. Krutka D, Manca S, Galvin S, Greenhow C, Koehler M, Askari E. Teaching "against" social media: confronting problems of profit in the curriculum. Teach Coll Rec. 2019;121(14):1–42. https://doi.org/10.1177/016146811912101410.
24. Akgun S, Greenhow C. Artificial intelligence in education: addressing ethical challenges in K-12 settings. AI Ethics. 2022;2:431–40. https://doi.org/10.1007/s43681-021-00096-7.
25. Pangrazio L, Selwyn N. Critical data literacies: rethinking data and everyday life. MIT Press; 2023.
26. Buckingham D. Media education and the end of the critical consumer. Harv Educ Rev. 2003;73(3):309–27.
27. Singer N. At this school, computer science class now includes critiquing chatbots. New York Times. 6 Feb 2023. https://www.nytimes.com/2023/02/06/technology/chatgpt-schools-teachers-ai-ethics.html.
28. Christensen R, Hodges CB, Spector JM. A framework for classifying replication studies in educational technologies research. Technol Knowl Learn. 2021;27:1021–38. https://doi.org/10.1007/s10758-021-09532-3.
29. Pleasants J, Clough MP, Olson JK, Miller G. Fundamental issues regarding the nature of technology: implications for STEM education. Sci Educ. 2019;28:561–97.
30. Williamson B. Learning in the "platform society": disassembling an educational data assemblage. Res Educ. 2017;98(1):59–82.

# Education Technology During the Pandemic and Future Emergencies

Justin Reich, Cristóbal Cobo, Sarah Dryden-Peterson, Eric Klopfer, Anya Kamenetz, and Torrey Trust

## 1 Background

A century ago, Tokyo was struck by the Great Kanto Earthquake, which destroyed much of the city and killed nearly 100,000 people. In the wake of that tragedy, Japan's leaders recognized that from their perch at the top of the Pacific Rim, earthquakes would be an ongoing threat to their country. As they sought to rebuild Tokyo, government officials and educators partnered to make schools and children central to their rebuilding efforts and a cornerstone of a more resilient future. Today, the Japanese are renowned for their disaster preparedness and measured, practiced response to emergencies. These are not inherent cultural traits, but the product of intentional decisions over a century to support generations of young people to be ready for uncertain futures [1].

J. Reich (✉) · E. Klopfer
Massachusetts Institute of Technology, Cambridge, MA, USA
e-mail: jreich@mit.edu

C. Cobo
World Bank, Washington, DC, USA

S. Dryden-Peterson
Harvard University, Cambridge, MA, USA

A. Kamenetz
Aspen Institute, Aspen, CO, USA

T. Trust
University of Massachusetts, Amherst, MA, USA

Just as Tokyo rests atop unstable tectonic plates, all humans now live below an atmosphere with over 400 parts per million of carbon dioxide, a blanket trapping heat on the Earth's surface with a density that has not existed for the past 4 million years. Our school systems were built in an age of climatological stability, and they will now be operated during an era of rapid changes to sea levels, climate, and weather patterns and resulting displacement and migration.

As we continue to rebuild from a global pandemic, we need to strengthen our systems of schooling, digital learning, and social welfare for children and their families. What we once called "interruptions" in schooling will become the ongoing conditions under which schools must operate. Communities must support educators in building the digital and pedagogical infrastructure to support flexible, resilient systems of learning for an uncertain future.

The COVID-19 pandemic forced educators around the world to adopt unfamiliar practices for facilitating learning in an emergency. Schools built outdoor classrooms, adjusted class sizes and schedules, forged new partnerships with families, and tested schemes for serving some students in school buildings and other students at a distance [2]. These plans and practices addressed urgent needs in a moment of crisis, but they were also a vital testing ground for education amidst a growing climate emergency.


D. A. Christakis, L. Hale (eds.), *Handbook of Children and Screens*,
https://doi.org/10.1007/978-3-031-69362-5_72

As average global temperatures rise and extreme weather events become more common, there will be more fires, floods, freezes, and novel disease events, along with accompanying migration, civil unrest, and conflict [3]. Schooling in the years ahead will need to rely on resilient, layered, flexible structures that allow students to continue learning during shifting conditions, in schools, homes, and other places of refuge.

Teaching in conditions of ongoing uncertainty requires different proficiencies than teaching in stable circumstances. Educators need to be able to facilitate learning in online, in-person, and hybrid environments; to teach students while also coaching caregivers and community members acting as teachers; and to move seamlessly from curricula, assessments, and policies optimized for stable times to those that are more flexible and suited to moments of crisis. We call these proficiencies *pedagogies of adaptability* [4, 5]. Educators working with refugees and in places of protracted conflict have been developing these practices for decades, and educators in many more places honed these approaches during school shutdowns caused by COVID-19.

Education technology can play an essential role in supporting pedagogies of adaptability. Household technologies like mobile phones, radios, laptops, and televisions can connect families to their local educators and to wider networks of educational resources. Digital tools like learning management systems, social media platforms, and videoconferencing technologies, can bridge learning experiences and connect people across schools, homes, and places of refuge, providing continuity in times of uncertainty [6].

Infrastructure alone, however, is insufficient for teaching and learning in emergencies. Students and families need to be familiar with routines for participating in schooling outside of school buildings, and teachers need professional learning in pedagogies suitable for times of uncertainty [7]. Educational leaders need to address critical issues of digital learning—such as privacy, safety, security, credentialing, and inequality—in advance of crises [8].

As millions of technology staff, educators, families, and policymakers discovered during the pandemic, building digital learning infrastructure and supporting pedagogies of adaptability during an emergency is extremely difficult. In an overheating world, educators will need to teach through uncertainty, and now is the time to build the layered, resilient systems that we know will be urgently needed.

## 2 Current State

Research from the fields of *education in emergencies and protracted crises* and *education technology* informs our recommendations for building education systems for a heating world. From studies in sudden and protracted crises, researchers have shown how education offers a wealth of benefits to young people and families facing uncertainty and how even temporary gaps in education introduce risks to youth development [9]. Education can provide stability, maintain community connections, and foster well-being. Interruptions to education can derail student learning, imperil life trajectories—risking graduation, postsecondary admission, and career entry—and even impact health and longevity, especially for vulnerable learners. Historically, emergency response leaders have viewed education as an activity that can resume after crises have passed. In a world with more frequent, protracted crises, education systems need to persist and support student well-being and learning during challenging times.

Education technologies are essential to pedagogies of adaptability, but their benefits cannot be activated like the flip of a switch. Rather, education technologies only support learning when educators have time, support, and resources to develop effective practices with new tools and pedagogies in advance of a crisis. Two findings appear repeatedly in the history of the research on education technology. First, when teachers get access to new technologies, they primarily use these tools to continue existing, often teacher-centered, practices. Second, new technologies disproportionately benefit affluent learners with financial, social, and technical capital. While technology boosters often hope and promise that new tools will "democratize" education, new technologies—from massive open online courses (MOOCs) to low-cost laptops—have generally proven to be weak approaches to improving issues of educational equity [10, 11].

These patterns bore out during the pandemic. Cutting-edge technologies saw very little adoption during the pandemic. For all the hype associated with massive open online courses, virtual and augmented reality, artificial intelligence, and learning analytics, these technologies were rarely used. Instead, educators in the United States tended to rely on tools they were most familiar with (e.g., Google Docs, Drive, Slides, Forms), tools for synchronous communication (e.g., Zoom, Google Meet), learning management systems (e.g., Google Classroom, Moodle), and video-based learning tools (e.g., YouTube, Khan Academy) [12].

Using these digital tools, educators attempted to reproduce the existing structures and routines of in-person schooling in online settings. This approach had the benefit of familiarity, but it was not particularly effective, especially for the nation's youngest and most vulnerable learners. Young children, especially those without dedicated caregivers, did not have the executive function skills, interest, or attention to stay engaged for long periods on Zoom. Many students struggled to participate in remote learning due to limited access to reliable internet, having to share devices and internet with multiple family members, and having limited access to family support and privacy [13]. The model worked best for older students in affluent families with access to reliable internet, devices for completing schoolwork, privacy for joining synchronous classes, and adult support for completing schoolwork. Emergency learning worked least well for the most vulnerable populations—the same populations who were already most likely to be negatively impacted by job loss, COVID-19 exposure, inadequate health care, and the other indignities of the pandemic [14].

While the pandemic was a once-in-this-past-century global event, it highlighted how core principles of education technology research—the conservatism of teaching practice and the persistent challenges of inequality—are useful guides for understanding the future.

## 3 Future Research

Education policy researchers' initial analyses and findings about the educational effects of the pandemic are distressing. Average scores on standardized tests of reading and math declined for pandemic-afflicted cohorts, and the most vulnerable students—from poverty-impacted backgrounds or marginalized racial minorities—appear to be the most negatively affected from the pandemic [15].

While broad studies of districts, policies, and test scores can identify certain kinds of trends, their focus is too wide to answer the most important question for our collective futures: What specific educational conditions or teaching practices were most protective of well-being and most effective at promoting learning? The 3.5 million teachers in the United States and millions more around the world conducted micro-experiments every day in classrooms, home visits, and Zoom rooms during the pandemic (for instance, the specific choices that elementary teachers made to continue science lessons during the pandemic) [16]. More retrospective research is needed to understand what teachers tried, what may have worked (or at least worked better), what has persisted into contemporary practice, and what we can learn from those experiments to inform both typical practice and future interruptions to schooling [17, 18].

## 4 Recommendations

Through late nights and long hours, educators around the world learned a wealth of lessons to build more future-ready education systems. The experience of the pandemic should inform our plans for interrupted learning, and we offer five specific recommendations.

- *Research and support pedagogies of adaptability*: In any areas prone to weather-related school closures, schools develop and practice routines to manage interruptions. For example, when a storm is forecast along the hurricane-prone Gulf Coast of the Southeast United States, students may take home laptops and hotspots each night in case of an emergency evacuation [19]. Families learn how to find out when school is closed, what to take from school when leaving in advance of a school closure, how to communicate during closures, how to know when to resume online learning activities, and routines for returning to schools after emergencies. In a world of rising seas and temperatures, many more places should adopt these practices that help students face emergencies with preparedness.

- School systems must support educators to develop *pedagogies of adaptability.* These will vary across places and systems, and there is more research to be done to understand and refine these approaches. But there are promising starting points, especially where educators have been working for many years in challenging circumstances [20]. Competency- or mastery-based approaches to learning—pedagogies that clearly define learning goals while maintaining flexible pathways for students to achieve those goals—prepare students for a greater degree of independent learning than typical lockstep curriculum. Peer-learning methods prepare students to recruit classmates, neighbors, and family members into their studies when teachers and schools are less available [21]. School systems that developed expertise in outdoor learning and leveraging community assets for learning—families, neighbors, informal learning spaces—may also be better prepared for times where school buildings are unsafe or inaccessible [22].
- *Secure universal connectivity and computing access for all learners, educators, and families*: Internet connectivity and computing platforms enable pedagogies of adaptability. Every student should have access to a computing device and reliable internet connectivity that works at home and in places of displacement that will become more common in climate crises. In the twentieth century, countries around the world developed electrification strategies—led by national and provincial governments—to provide light and electricity to people in all corners of the world. Similar efforts are needed today to connect homes to the Internet and connect young people to educational opportunities, with a particular focus on areas with the least connectivity and with payment structures that do not create untenable debt for communities least able to pay.
- *Prepare curriculum and policies for interruptions in learning*: Along with pedagogies and technical infrastructure, educational systems should plan for future emergencies by preparing curriculum materials and educational policies suitable for uncertain futures. Teachers should have access to curriculum and instructional resources that they can facilitate with students online with minimal preparation (for instance, science curricula that leverages materials found in typical homes) [23]. Along with providing flexible learning resources, policymakers need to build resilience into the systems that we use to assess, certify, and credential learning. Regulations around school features like seat time, attendance, examinations, and credit requirements become unworkable in times of crisis. Even in times of unrest, milestones such as grade-level promotions, graduations, postsecondary admissions, and career entry are all ways that students can demonstrate their commitment to future building. For example, UNESCO worked with Ukraine following the Russian invasion to provide continuity in access to higher education [24]. School policies should provide for the flexibility to ensure that these important rites of passage continue during difficult times.
- *Adopt a critical approach to using technology in times of uncertainty*: During the pandemic, teachers in the midst of a global crisis found themselves creating new digital learning experiences and materials. However, digital learning resources are not unambiguously good, and they invite challenges of privacy,

security, safety, and inequality. An uncritical adoption of technology can exacerbate existing inequities and create new harms for the most vulnerable students [25]. Educators need opportunities to learn how to critically interrogate digital learning materials in order to make informed decisions about when and how to use these technologies to aid and facilitate student learning in times of uncertainty. These questions are best thought through comprehensively in advance of emergencies.

- *Invest in the well-being of children and families*: Learning happens when students feel physically secure and psychologically safe. All the technology infrastructure in the world cannot support students who are hungry, unsheltered, or feel unsafe.

- Provisioning children's welfare during emergencies requires having robust social welfare systems in times of stability. In the United States, the pandemic revealed how utterly essential schools are for the welfare of young children and their families: providing food, safe spaces, a caring community, health and mental health resources, and other social supports. For places where school staff were overwhelmed with these issues during the pandemic, municipal and state agencies should consider how they could expand their readiness to provision these kinds of services during emergencies.

- As part of pedagogies of adaptability, schools should adopt curriculum related to social and emotional learning, so teachers, students, and families have a common language for talking about well-being, uncertainty, and emergencies. Schools should facilitate adult student connections through structures like advisories (similar to "home room" classes, but with the explicit goal of fostering mentoring relationships) that ensure that every student feels a personal connection with at least one adult in the school. If these connections have a digital communication component, students and families will have stronger allies in schools during stable times and practice for keeping in touch with school staff during emergencies.

**Conflict of Interest and Funding Disclosures** None.

## References


1. Borland J. Earthquake children: building resilience from the ruins of Tokyo. Harvard University Press; 2020.
2. Kamenetz A. The stolen year: how COVID changed children's lives, and where we go now. 1st ed. PublicAffairs; 2022.
3. Reidmiller DR, Avery CW, Easterling DR, et al. Impacts, risks, and adaptation in the United States: fourth National Climate Assessment, Volume II. NOAA; 2018.
4. Cohen E, Willemsen LW, Shah R, et al. Deconstructing and reconstructing comparative and international education in light of the COVID-19 emergency: imagining the field anew. Comp Educ Rev. 2021;65(2):356–74. https://doi.org/10.1086/713720.
5. Dryden-Peterson S. Pedagogies of belonging: lessons from refugee education for times of uncertainty. In: Suarez-Orozco M, editor. The COVID-19 generation: children and youth in and after the pandemic. Editrice Vaticana; 2023.
6. Hodges C, Moore S, Lockee B, Trust T, Bond A. The difference between emergency remote teaching and online learning. Educause Review. 2020. https://er.educause.edu/articles/2020/3/the-difference-between-emergency-remote-teaching-and-online-learning. Accessed 30 Mar 2023.
7. Shamir-Inbal T, Blau I. Facilitating emergency remote K-12 teaching in computing-enhanced virtual learning environments during COVID-19 pandemic – blessing or curse? J Educ Comput Res. 2021;59(7):1243–71. https://doi.org/10.1177/0735633121992781.
8. Trust T, Whalen J. Should teachers be trained in emergency remote teaching? Lessons learned from the COVID-19 pandemic. J Technol Teach Educ. 2020;28(2):189–99.
9. Inter-Agency Network for Education in Emergencies (INEE). Psychosocial support and social and emotional learning for children and youth in emergency settings. Inter-agency Network for Education in Emergencies (INEE); 2016. https://inee.org/resources/inee-background-paper-psychosocial-support-and-social-emotional-learning-children-youth. Accessed 1 Apr 2020.
10. OECD. Students, computers and learning: making the connection. Organisation for Economic Co-operation and Development; 2015. https://www.

oecd-ilibrary.org/education/students-computers-and-learning_9789264239555-en. Accessed 30 Mar 2023.
11. Reich J. Failure to disrupt: why technology alone can't transform education. Harvard University Press; 2020.
12. Trust T, Whalen J. K-12 teacher' experiences and challenges with using technology for emergency remote teaching during the COVID-19 pandemic. Ital J Educ Technol. 2021;29(2):10–25. https://doi.org/10.17471/2499-4324/1192.
13. Katz V, Rideout V. Learning at home while underconnected. 2021. https://www.newamerica.org/education-policy/reports/learning-at-home-while-underconnected/. Accessed 30 Mar 2023.
14. Munoz-Najar A, Gilberto Sanzana AG, Hasan A, Cobo Romani JC, Azevedo JPWD, Akmal M. Remote learning during COVID-19: lessons from today, principles for tomorrow. World Bank; 2022. https://documents.worldbank.org/en/publication/documents-reports/documentdetail/160271637074230077/Remote-Learning-During-COVID-19-Lessons-from-Today-Principles-for-Tomorrow. Accessed 30 Mar 2023.
15. Betthäuser BA, Bach-Mortensen AM, Engzell P. A systematic review and meta-analysis of the evidence on learning during the COVID-19 pandemic. Nat Hum Behav. 2023;7(3):375–85. https://doi.org/10.1038/s41562-022-01506-4.
16. Anderson E, Hira A. Loss of brick-and-mortar schooling: how elementary educators respond. Inf Learn Sci. 2020;121(5/6):411–8.
17. Next Generation Learning Challenges. What made them so prepared? Research findings. NGLC. 30 Mar 2023. https://www.nextgenlearning.org/resources/prepared-project-research-findings. Accessed 30 Mar 2023.
18. Esteves N, Buttimer CJ, Faruqi F, et al. The teachers have something to say: lessons learned from U.S. PK-12 teachers during the COVID-impacted 2020–21 school year. 20 Sept 2021. https://doi.org/10.35542/osf.io/h8gac.
19. Kamenetz A. Hurricane Ida's impact on students could be worse than Katrina, expert says. NPR. 3 Sept 2021. https://www.npr.org/sections/back-to-school-live-updates/2021/09/03/1034051445/hurricane-ida-closed-schools-louisiana-hurricane-katrina. Accessed 30 Mar 2023.
20. Chopra V, Dryden-Peterson S, Talhouk J, Geha C. Bridging the gap between imagined and plausible futures: what Syrian refugee students wish their teachers knew.
21. Dryden-Peterson S, Dahya N, Adelman E. Pathways to educational success among refugees: connecting locally and globally situated resources. Am Educ Res J. 2017;54(6):1011–47. https://doi.org/10.3102/0002831217714321.
22. Reich J. Schooling in the "Fifth Season". Educ Leadersh. 2021;79(1):20–5.
23. Urrea C, Delong K, Diaz J, et al. MIT full STEAM ahead: bringing project-based, collaborative learning to remote learning environments. In: Reimers FM, Marmolejo FJ, editors. University and school collaborations during a pandemic: sustaining educational opportunity and reinventing education, Knowledge studies in higher education. Springer International Publishing; 2022. p. 299–319. https://doi.org/10.1007/978-3-030-82159-3_20.
24. UNESCO supports Ukraine's 2022 University admission campaign | UNESCO. UNESCO News. https://www.unesco.org/en/articles/unesco-supports-ukraines-2022-university-admission-campaign. Accessed 30 Mar 2023.
25. Trust T, Carpenter J, Heath M, Krutka DG. Toward critical and ecological dispositions in technology decision making in teacher education. 28 Feb 2023. https://doi.org/10.35542/osf.io/4ecn2.

# Digital Ethics and Equity in K-12 Blended and Online Learning

Jennifer Darling-Aduana, Marie K. Heath, Ashley Stewart, Samantha Viano, Sumreen Asim, Antero Garcia, Elizabeth Langran, Carolyn Heinrich, and Xeturah Woodley

## 1 Background

The COVID-19 pandemic drew national attention to the already prevalent practice of K-12 online and blended learning as well as to the underlying systemic inequities in society that permeate all institutions—including educational institutions—within the United States. Historically, online ecology has included a wide swath of tools, sites, and online places. Today, however, learning technologies have enclosed and interwoven themselves into the core of teaching and learning. Whether learning in a virtual or face-to-face environment (or somewhere in between), students' educational experiences depend on and are influenced by elements of online learning. Accordingly, online and blended learning have the potential to further magnify educational opportunity gaps if high-quality online learning experiences differ systematically by sociodemographic background.

For this chapter, we define K-12 online learning as any fully digital, internet-based, or blended (i.e., part online, part face-to-face) form of education where technology integration is used to deliver some or all of the instruction within a classroom [1]. This encompasses a wide swath of learning environments, ranging from fully asynchronous, online courses where students receive no (or minimal) face-to-face interactions with instructors and peers to technology integration within a traditional, face-to-face classroom setting. We focus primarily on the United States educational context in this synthesis although we hope themes may have relevance to other contexts as well.

Concurrently, we define educational equity as providing every student the resources, tools, supports, experiences, and interactions required to reach their learning potential [2]. Equity is more than access, and equality (i.e., equal access) is insufficient to achieve equity. Instead, every child deserves an educational experience that aligns with their unique strengths, needs, and funds of knowledge. Existing educational opportunity gaps are symptoms of broader policies, practices,

J. Darling-Aduana (✉) · A. Stewart
Georgia State University, Atlanta, GA, USA
e-mail: jdarlingaduana@gsu.edu

M. K. Heath
Loyola University Maryland, Baltimore, MD, USA

S. Viano
George Mason University, Fairfax, VA, USA

S. Asim
Indiana University Southeast, New Albany, IN, USA

A. Garcia
Stanford University, Stanford, CA, USA

E. Langran
Marymount University, Arlington, VA, USA

C. Heinrich
Vanderbilt University, Nashville, TN, USA

X. Woodley
Doña Ana Community College, Las Cruces, NM, USA


D. A. Christakis, L. Hale (eds.), *Handbook of Children and Screens*,
https://doi.org/10.1007/978-3-031-69362-5_73

and norms that perpetuate and legitimize existing power dynamics in society [3]. Truly equitable learning (online or otherwise) requires dismantling these underlying systems.

Accordingly, we seek something other than a technocratic solution to a social problem. Instead, we provide a roadmap to enacting a more equitable educational system and highlight the role online learning might play in supporting that broader goal. To accomplish that, we must acknowledge that technology is not neutral. Like the broader school system, technology often reflects and replicates existing systemic inequities through differential use, algorithmic biases, surveillance, built-in normative assumptions, online harassment, etc. [4]. These underlying inequities must be challenged for technology to operate within an equitable education framework. To accomplish these aims, we begin by summarizing the current state and common practices within K-12 online and blended learning before proposing a reframing of the educational goals and process of technology use in schools. We conclude with suggestions for future research and recommendations for policymakers and educators.

## 2 Current State

One of the best-documented strengths of online and blended learning is its ability to facilitate one of the precursors for equity—access to quality educational content/tools/resources [5, 6]. Online and blended instructional approaches are also being used to offer greater flexibility and self-pacing in learning, which can be helpful for students with sufficient self-regulation [7]. Additionally, educators can use online resources and tools to improve students' educational experiences by providing real-time data on student progress, delivering just-in-time, formative feedback, and removing time and geographic-related barriers to communication and collaboration with students, teachers, and content experts [5, 8]. For instance, in one school, students used technology-based tools to collaborate with museum staff and tribal leaders to learn about and create a digital exhibit of Indigenous artifacts [9]. This activity supported students in deepening content knowledge, developing technical skills, and fostering Indigenous identity and connection.

Despite these bright spots, research on online learning has also revealed substantial variation in how online instruction is enacted in schools, with some studies pointing to the potential for online learning to worsen rather than reduce inequities in learning opportunities [10]. For example, adapting the content and logistics of instruction (i.e., pace, order, location, and lesson material) for individual student needs can be especially beneficial for students with learning disabilities or those who may need additional academic support in specific content areas [11]. Yet school districts that lack adequate resources or support for expanding blended learning models often resort to "drill and practice" strategies on lower-order skills in the use of online learning tools, with low-income and Black students more likely to experience these modes of learning [12]. Other constraints on the implementation of effective online learning practices include high turnover among teaching, administrative, and technology support staff, higher student–teacher ratios, and competing demands for resources that could be used to enhance blended instruction.

In addition to implementation concerns, research also suggests the need to be more attentive to the content accessed through online learning platforms and applications. Much of the content development for online learning is commercially driven, where the companies creating the tools operate with the goal of maximizing profit [13]. Content is often designed by private vendors with the "modal" (White, middle-income, average academic achievement) student in mind, with limited options for reflecting or adapting the content to students whose lived experiences, cultural norms, or learning needs fall outside that narrow privileged group [14]. Widely used online learning platforms often provide limited opportunities for students to engage in authentic work—work that encourages students to solve new and interesting questions, investigate a topic in-depth, and communicate ideas with others, or consider how it applies to situations outside of school [15]. A recent study using an observation rubric to quantify the presence of authentic work in over 400 lessons created one of the largest course vendors in the United States found that fewer than a quarter of lessons provided opportunities for students evaluate, synthesize, or create content [16].

Beyond the online platforms and tools, school norms and priorities also shape and constrain the instructional environments that students experience, with students belonging to dominant cultural groups more likely to be encouraged to engage in digital play-based learning and learn how to be digital content creators as well as consumers. Digital play encapsulates the skills and experiences students gain from communicating, playing, interacting with, and creating content online extracurricularly. In a comparative ethnographic study of digital use in schools, Rafalow observed that teachers of students from more affluent backgrounds valued, encouraged, and integrated features and knowledge gained from digital play in the classroom, while the teachers of students from less affluent backgrounds considered digital play as threatening or useless [17].

Finally, using a software application that monitors activity raises privacy concerns when commercial companies, third-party vendors, or advertisers have access to student data, often without student knowledge or consent. Personalization tools may also create profiles of students based on their academic performance, learning disabilities, or other personal characteristics, potentially leading to stereotyping or discrimination. Further, we expect to see an increase in artificial intelligence in educational applications and platforms in the near future; when algorithms and data used to train an AI system contain bias, then the system will replicate and amplify that bias.

### 2.1 Reframing the Target

In contrast to the emphasis on access issues in current conversations around online learning, enacting truly equitable online and blended learning requires reframing the target. The real promise and pathway to digital equity involve democratizing education and learning practices. For many young people, online spaces have served as outlets for community building, activism, and counterstorytelling [18, 19]. Similarly, many promising online platforms and learning strategies leverage the increased ease of technology-based communication to allow a variety of voices to be heard and critical dialogues to occur.

Leveraging learners' technology use outside of classroom spaces is more complex than merely giving learners technological devices for educational use [20]. Attention must be paid to how learners interact with the technology itself and how they interact with other learners and instructors. Learners' adaptations and use of these informal digital spaces, as well as the unique features of digital platforms for academic purposes, demonstrate the ways that they assert agency over their own learning experiences. To accomplish this, the role of the educator is crucial in building opportunities to pause, reflect, and build toward meaningfully engaging with students before technology integration. Considering the rich funds of knowledge abundant in classrooms every day, we must redefine the socioeconomic forces underlying teaching, pedagogy, and definitions of learning.

## 3 Future Research

With a few exceptions, the majority of online learning research maximizes possibilities and minimizes perils. This has resulted in research on best practices but little understanding of potential harms due to issues of surveillance capitalism, data (in)justice, racialized and gendered constructions of online spaces, privatization, and philanthrocapitalism. In this section, we propose lines of research to recognize these pitfalls and identify systems and processes that can support more equitable online and blended learning.

First, we call for research that interrogates issues of data justice and considers the intersection of data surveillance and online education, integrating discussions of power and bias. When online learning platforms monitor students, this surveillance can be racialized, resulting in discriminatory outcomes [21]. Online learning research needs to be attuned to these racialized elements of surveillance in order to identify ways that online learning can reduce opportunity gaps instead of exacerbating them.

Second, the consistent underfunding of public education invites private companies and philanthropies to "solve" education problems with technology [22]. At the expense of high-quality learning environments, providers lower costs by delivering static course content, lowering content quality, reducing, or eliminating instructional support, using technology to police students, and limiting or censoring content [23–25]. This raises further equity concerns as schools are more likely to distribute lower-quality products to students in ways that are racialized, and underfunded school systems are more incentivized to buy cheaper online learning products [26]. We invite more research that inquiries into the impacts on children and society when private companies insert themselves into public education, bringing with them their logics of efficiency and competition in ways misaligned with the goals of public education as a common social good.

Third, researchers should not ignore online learning's placement in the same online ecosystem as social media and the broader attention economy [27, 28]. Social media, mobile apps, and online games are designed to be addictive [29], and coding embedded in these platforms is racialized in ways that perpetuate societal inequalities. Consequently, research should engage in issues related to equity and the addictive elements of technology (i.e., the attention economy) as well as the extent to which (and how) online and blended learning can be structured to allow students to productively engage with these platforms.

Finally, we encourage continuing scholarship on the ways young people engage in counternarratives, social actions, and justice-oriented work in online spaces. Youth-led inquiry and media projects like Wide Angle Media [30] in Baltimore and the Young People's Race Technology and Power Project (YPRPP) [31] in Chicago provide examples of online curricula that confront injustice and spur civic action. Wide Angle Media accomplished this by teaching students to create documentaries and social media content on important local topics such as truancy, homelessness, and the Baltimore Uprising. YPRPP focused more explicitly on encouraging students to engage with and consider the ethical implications of technology use through inquiry-based units on cryptocurrencies, social media and mental health, fashion and 3D design, video games, and cybersecurity. These examples offer opportunities for race and gender-conscious research on the intersection of identity, young people, and online learning. There is also a unique opportunity to examine the discourse and decision-making processes of learners in these digital spaces. A deeper understanding of how learners use technology in their daily lives might also uncover strategies for realizing the promise of online learning.

## 4 Recommendations

Below, we provide research-based recommendations for how to close the gap between the reality and potential of K-12 online and blended learning.

### 4.1 For Policymakers

- Fund high-speed Internet like a public utility, increasing access to online learning for students in and out of school.
- Protect student privacy and students from advertisements on learning platforms.
- Monitor the purposes and use of data collected through digital tools and tightly restrict its linkage to databases of families, students, medical, and educational records.
- Democratize and make transparent EdTech vending and purchasing decisions.
- Create equitable school funding models that allow schools disproportionately serving marginalized student populations to be able to afford high-quality online and blended learning tools.

### 4.2 For Educators

- Provide all students the opportunity to engage in learning as content creators, not just consumers, through digital play and media making.
- Safeguard student privacy by limiting data stored on online platforms and particularly LMS systems.
- Evaluate online learning programs, tools, and integration practices for their impact on educational equity and student well-being, considering aspects of differential use, algorithmic biases, built-in normative assumptions, etc. Center the findings from these evaluations when making purchasing, curricular, and teaching decisions.
- Leverage technology to provide opportunities for student agency, autonomy, and voice in the classroom. Consider mediums through which students can express themselves and share their experiences, opinions, and knowledge with peers and their community.

**Conflict of Interest and Funding Disclosures** None.

## References

1. Horn MB, Staker H. Blended: using disruptive innovation to improve schools. San Francisco: Jossey-Bass; 2014.
2. OECD. Equity and quality in education: supporting disadvantaged students and schools. OECD Publishing; 2012.
3. Carter PL, Welner KG, editors. Closing the opportunity gap: what America must do to give every child an even chance. Oxford University Press; 2013.
4. Benjamin R. Race after technology: abolitionist tools for the New Jim Code. Polity; 2019.
5. Darling-Aduana J, Heinrich C. The potential of telepresence for increasing advanced course access in high schools. Educ Res. 2020;49(6):415–25.
6. Hart CMD, Linden R, Jacob B, Loeb S. Online course-taking and expansion of curricular options in high schools. Peabody J Educ. 2023;98(1):26–48. https://doi.org/10.1080/0161956X.2023.2160108.
7. Heissel J. The relative benefits of live versus online delivery: evidence from virtual algebra I in North Carolina. Econ Educ Rev. 2016;53:99–115.
8. Julia K, Marco K. Educational scalability in MOOCs: analysing instructional designs to find best practices. Comput Educ. 2021;161:104054.
9. Christal M, Roy L, Cherian A. Stories told: tribal communities and the development of virtual museums. J Internet Catalog. 2005;7(1):65–88.
10. Heinrich CJ, Darling-Aduana J, Good A. Equity and quality in digital learning: realizing the promise in K-12 education. Boston: Harvard Education Press; 2020.
11. Enyedy N. Personalized instruction: new interest, old rhetoric, limited results, and the need for a new direction for computer-mediated learning. Boulder: National Education Policy Center; 2014.
12. Delgado AJ, Wardlow L, McKnight K, O'Malley K. Educational technology: a review of the integration, resources, and effectiveness of technology in k-12 classrooms. J Inf Technol Educ. 2015;14:397–416.
13. Molnar A, Boninger F. The commercial transformation of America's schools. Phi Delta Kappan. 2020;102(2):8–13.
14. Darling-Aduana J, Good A, Geraghty E. The culture of power online: cultural responsiveness and relevance in vendor-developed online courses. Urban Educ. 2022;57(4):714–42.
15. Darling-Aduana J, Rogers LK, Woo DS. Virtual schooling at scale: identifying effective online teaching and learning. Paper presented at the annual meeting of the University Council for Educational Administration. Nov 2022.
16. Darling-Aduana J. Authenticity, engagement, and performance in online high school courses: insights from micro-interactional data. Comput Educ. 2021;167:104175.
17. Rafalow MH. Digital divisions. University of Chicago Press; 2020.
18. Stevens R, Gilliard-Matthews S, Dunaev J, Woods MK, Brawner BM. The digital hood: social media use among youth in disadvantaged neighborhoods. New Media Soc. 2017;19(6):950–67.
19. Tanksley T. Race, education and #BlackLivesMatter: how online transformational resistance shapes the offline experiences of Black college-age women. Urban Educ. 2024;59:2179–207.
20. Philip TM, Garcia A. Schooling mobile phones: assumptions about proximal benefits, the challenges of shifting meanings, and the politics of teaching. Educ Policy. 2015;29(4):676–707.
21. Browne S. Dark matters: on the surveillance of blackness. Duke University Press; 2015.
22. Sims C. Disruptive fixation. Princeton University Press; 2017.
23. Gleason B, Heath MK. Injustice embedded in Google classroom and Google meet: a techno-ethical audit of remote educational technologies. Ital J Educ Technol. 2021;29(2):26–41.
24. Heath MK, Segal P. What pre-service teacher technology integration conceals and reveals: "Colorblind" technology in schools. Comput Educ. 2021;170:104225.

25. Viano S. At-risk high school students recovering course credits online: what we know and need to know. Am J Dist Educ. 2018;32(1):16–26. https://doi.org/10.1080/08923647.2018.1412554.
26. Heinrich CJ, Darling-Aduana J. Does online course-taking increase high school completion and open pathways to postsecondary education opportunities? Educ Eval Policy Anal. 2021;43(3):367–90.
27. Mintzer A. Paying attention: the attention economy. Berkeley Economic Review. 31 Mar 2020.
28. Wang C. Comprehensively summarizing what distracts students from online learning: a literature review. Hum Behav Emerging Technol. 2022;2022:1483531.
29. Hari J. Stolen focus: why you can't pay attention--and how to think deeply again. Crown; 2023.
30. Durington M, Collins S, Randolph N, Young L. Push it along: on not making an ethnographic film in Baltimore. Transform Anthropol. 2017;25(1):23–34.
31. Vakil S, McKinney de Royston M. Youth as philosophers of technology. Mind Cult Act. 2022;29:336–55.

# The Importance of Digital Media Literacy

Kristen Hawley Turner, Bobbie Eisenstock, Troy Hicks, Tessa Jolls, W. Ian O'Byrne, Kathleen A. Paciga, Detra Price-Dennis, and Michelle Schira Hagerman

## 1 Background

Literacy is essential for successful participation in a democratic society [1]. In today's world, technology constantly reshapes ways of learning, playing, working, interacting, and engaging in civic life, making digital and media literacies foundational [2–4].

In 2017, Turner et al. [1] argued that both digital and media literacies should be taught in schools "as literacy"—that is, embedded as core components throughout a student's entire school experience—and that policy efforts were needed. Since then, some progress has been made, yet the world has continued to change. Educational technology exploded during COVID-19. Algorithms increasingly control us. The rise of mis-, dis-, and malinformation threatens democracy [5]. Currently, artificial intelligence (AI), especially generative text production, is changing the landscape again.

Educators, parents, and other caregivers must work in tandem to develop children's and adolescents' literacy skills to be healthy, safe, and productive. Professional organizations' updates to their digital and media literacy frameworks articulate the knowledge and practices required to navigate digital spaces [6, 7]. These frameworks move toward a more complex, nuanced definition of *digital media literacy*, one that is "interconnected, dynamic, and malleable" [7].

Still, there is no consensus definition of digital media literacy shared by researchers, educators, policymakers, caregivers, or politicians [8], thus making systemic change difficult. In their 2017 *Pediatrics* article, Turner et al. [1] offered the following:

> Digital literacy takes into account the full range of skills needed to read, write, speak, view, and participate in online spaces. All of these practices require media literacy, which includes the ability to access, analyze, evaluate, create, and participate with media in all its forms.

K. H. Turner (✉)
Drew University, Madison, NJ, USA
e-mail: kturner3@drew.edu

B. Eisenstock
California State University Northridge, Northridge, CA, USA

T. Hicks
Central Michigan University, Mount Pleasant, MI, USA

T. Jolls
Center for Media Literacy, Santa Monica, CA, USA

W. I. O'Byrne
College of Charleston, Charleston, SC, USA

K. A. Paciga
Columbia College Chicago, Chicago, IL, USA

D. Price-Dennis
The Ohio State University, Columbus, OH, USA

M. S. Hagerman
University of Ottawa, Ottawa, ON, Canada



D. A. Christakis, L. Hale (eds.), *Handbook of Children and Screens*,
https://doi.org/10.1007/978-3-031-69362-5_74

With the need for digital media literate citizens to participate ethically, advocate for equitable representations, and assume human-driven agency and responsibility, there is a simultaneous need to develop computational thinking skills that include breaking down problems, identifying patterns, and devising solutions.

Thus, this chapter proposes a refined definition of *digital media literacy*: The ability of individuals to deliberately decide when, why, and how to engage with various forms of digital media with confidence and a sense of empowerment. People who are digitally media literate access, analyze, evaluate, create, reflect, and communicate for multiple purposes and with critical intention. They understand and act to change the power dynamics inherent in various technologies that may otherwise breed passivity.

This active stance toward digital media literacy represents the ideal; however, many youth are not explicitly taught how—nor expected to—engage with digital media in responsible, creative, and ethical ways [9], leading to uninformed or harmful uses [10, 11]. Developing digital media literate citizens who consume, create, connect, and advocate—for themselves and others—is paramount for youth today.

## 2 Current State

In 2015, most teens were online at least once a day; by 2023, the number "almost constantly" online nearly doubled from 24% to 46%, with Hispanic (55%) and Black (54%) teens reporting more constant use than White teens (38%) [12]. Though the COVID-19 pandemic increased more equitable access to devices through school-based one-to-one initiatives, growth in device use reflects long-term trends. Much has been written about the harmful effects of devices, and particularly social media, on youth [13–16], though emerging research suggests that digital media literacy may mitigate some of the potentially harmful effects.

### 2.1 Mitigating Harm with Digital Media Literacy

During the COVID-19 pandemic, estimates suggest that daily recreational screen use doubled from 3.8 hours per day to an average of 7.7 hours [17]. The varied and long-term impacts of nearly constant screen use across various platforms continue to be studied [18]. Any research on digital media literacy must now be considered in relation to broader considerations of the generational health impacts of this crisis.

Evidence suggests that strong social supports and higher levels of physical activity predicted lower levels of screen use and better coping skills for teens [17], but little evidence has emerged so far on whether digital media literacy skills may have provided additional protections during this time of crisis. Strong information navigation and processing skills have, however, been found to predict a range of positive outcomes that include (1) more civic participation, (2) higher academic achievement, and (3) more information-seeking for homework [19]. Additionally, research shows that activities requiring youth to discuss and justify their decision-making processes when comparing evidence from multiple sources can help inform better judgments [20].

Similarly, foundational skills of digital media literacy predict young people's ability to benefit from online opportunities, avoid digital exclusion, and manage risks [21]. Evidence suggests that—when adults talk with children about ethically complex situations and model strategies for how to respond to risks online—children report feeling more prepared and less harmed by threats they encounter; children with stronger digital media literacy skills are more able to avoid problems by deleting harmful images or blocking unwanted conversations [22]. Strong relationships with parents and caregivers, paired with opportunities to talk through troubling situations, seem to support digital resilience [23]. More research is needed, however, that closely examines the role of digital media skills in a post-pandemic context.

## 2.2 Digital Media Literacy in Education

Recognition of the importance of digital media literacy education has been growing. Organizations such as the News Literacy Project, Digital Inquiry Group, Canada's CIVIX project, and the Australian Broadcasting Corporation invite students into gamified experiences and simulations. The European Commission has emphasized the importance of digital skills for economic growth and social inclusion, leading to the establishment of programs such as the Digital Skills and Jobs Coalition. Similarly, countries in Asia, such as South Korea and Singapore, have prioritized digital literacy in their education systems to prepare citizens for the digital age. Organizations like UNESCO have collaborated with governments in Africa to incorporate digital literacy into curriculum and policies for education. The US State Department has sponsored media literacy programs throughout the world, and the Institute of Museum and Library Services has included media literacy in the first federal task force to explore the need for new literacy initiatives.

Even so, digital media literacy is not yet fully integrated into PK-12 school curricula in the United States [24]. As of 2023, only 18 US states have state-level educational policies that include digital media literacy, and the specifications and implementation of these policies vary greatly, often failing to offer funding for curricular development or teacher education [25]. Outside of schools, students are still more likely to "watch, play, or scroll through content created by others" [26] than they are to use their devices to produce their own content. In short, youth engagement with digital media is mostly passive, and not active, critical, or creative. Additionally, post-pandemic, access and connectivity gaps are more common among lower-income families, disproportionately affecting Black and Latinx students [27]. In communities where fundamental infrastructures remain underdeveloped, digital inequity contributes to a literacy opportunity gap [28].

## 2.3 Equity, Access, and Identity

The acceleration of technology's role in civic, social, educational, professional, and personal contexts makes achieving digital equity and access even more imperative [29]. To further the points above, households in disenfranchised communities frequently use only mobile devices with constrained data plans. Broadband infrastructure is typically lacking in rural areas, and discriminatory policies exacerbate participation barriers. This contributes to wider gaps in literacy opportunities, further limiting already marginalized youth. Stereotypical portrayals and mis- and disinformation on the internet affect these students, which digital media literacy instruction could help mitigate. Intentionally creating antiracist and culturally sustaining policies, curricula, and community support could provide space for youth to reimagine their civic participation in society [30].

To mitigate these challenges, how can community programs and schools collaborate? Which scaffolds aid multilingual students in acquiring the vocabulary necessary to participate critically in online environments? How can media literacy practices that are affirming of gender and identity be promoted? In what ways can federal, state, and local government offices partner with community organizations to provide broadband access to families in urban and rural spaces? Digital literacy initiatives will support empowerment and social justice if they address these issues with an asset-based perspective that acknowledges structural injustices.

## 2.4 Generative Artificial Intelligence (AI) and Digital Media Literacy

The swift progression of generative artificial intelligence (AI) presents novel challenges and opportunities. Systems such as ChatGPT demonstrate unique language generation capabilities, drawn from a large corpus of existing data on the world wide web. If employed carelessly, the potential for AI to produce human-like text may both exacerbate academic dishonesty and further reduce the chances that students will interact critically and actively with digital media. Educators must carefully consider how to use AI to authentically nurture student voice, agency, and ethical digital participation.

Put another way, with careful application, generative AI can also present fascinating chances to support literacy skill development, particularly in digital and hybrid environments. To do so will require that educators understand the characteristics of AI-generated writing as well as how to adapt their instructional practices [31]. To truly transform education, however,—as new technologies are often restricted in schools and districts—it is imperative that policies and practices that unleash generative tools as catalysts for moral, empowering literacy learning should be developed proactively rather than reactively [32].

## 3 Future Research

Literacy researchers have argued that digital media literacy must be incorporated more intentionally from early childhood through adolescence, and even into adulthood. Traditional reading, writing, and critical analysis skills do not simply transfer into digital spaces, and students must be explicitly taught digital media literacy skills [33]. Schools alone cannot tackle this issue; its importance crosses disciplinary fields as well as home and community contexts. Therefore, future research must be interdisciplinary and focused on mitigating the effects of increased device use, curricular implementation, and programs for families and communities. The following questions can shape future research agendas to this end:

- *What specific digital media literacy skills help to mitigate the negative impacts of increased device use?* With increased access possible, research on potential impacts remains limited and inconclusive [34]. A small body of scholarship links digital and media literacy skills to positive academic and socioemotional outcomes among adolescents [35, 36]. Developing critical thinking, content analysis, communication skills, and ethical participation may enable youth to more effectively build online community and collective efficacy, and drive social change through digital activism [37, 38]. However, significant questions persist: what are the beneficial or deleterious effects of digital media, and what combination of knowledge, skills, attitudes, and supports best position youth for healthy technology use, thus promoting agency, well-being, and ethical digital citizenship? [19, 39] Educators, policymakers, and designers must collaborate closely with youth themselves to empower, rather than undermine, young people's opportunities. To do so, an empirical measure to establish a youth's current level of digital media literacy is needed, while also allowing for tracking growth over time. Specifically, investigation into how individual choices and self-regulation in relation to consumption, creation, and connection to others may reduce unwanted impacts and increase beneficial outcomes should be a priority.
- *What curricula prove effective in developing digital media literacy?* A variety of individual organizations support curricular work in digital literacy (Media Smarts), information literacy (American Library Association), news literacy (News Literacy Project), visual literacy (American Library Association), and digital citizenship (Cyberwise Media), among others (Examples include refs. 40, 41). Some suggest that building dispositions—in contrast to a specific skill set—can effectively develop digital media literacy and citizenship [42]. Others focus more on developing discrete skills, such as lateral reading [20]. The Common Sense K-12 Digital Citizenship Curriculum [40] does both. The current version of the curriculum focuses on learning dispositions that are noncognitive, affective variables that identify a willingness, tendency, or trait, such as "slow down and

reflect," "explore perspectives," "seek facts and evidence," "envision options and possible impacts," and "take action." Such research should examine the impact in the short- and long-term for diverse children and teachers, avoiding samples of relatively affluent, White, English-speaking, and able persons and moving toward a strengths-based perspective that accounts for social and cultural differences in ways of knowing. These curricula may be school-based, or openly available for youth engagement outside of school whether on their own, in affinity groups, or through community-based programs. For schools, research into how educators can examine existing digital media literacy materials to make informed instructional choices—and how they can sequence curricula effectively—should be given priority. Alongside investigating youth-focused curricula, research to support adult learning must also be prioritized. Without adult mentors who themselves are digital media literate, youth learning will not thrive.

- *How do families and communities impact children's digital media literacy development?* Because schools alone cannot develop a literate society, parents, caregivers, and community organizations must become collaborators [42]. Research on the impact of television on youth indicates that certain types of parental mediation can enhance children's social and cognitive development and mitigate negative media effects. This line of research must continue across all media forms. Caregivers are well positioned to support their children's digital media literacy development; however, many lack the know-how. Being a digital media literate caregiver requires immersion in the digital media landscape to understand its dynamics and learn how to keep children safe, protect their privacy, and develop their skills to navigate online, often supported by community organizations. This can help to address digital inequity while also collapsing a generational gap in digital media literacy.

## 4 Recommendations

Though evidence for digital media literacy interventions does not yet exist in randomized, controlled trials, the research reviewed above, combined with a larger body of educational research, suggests that change cannot be isolated to add-on curriculum in public schools; a systems approach that crosses all disciplines is needed. This approach has been used in Finland [43] with digital media literacy integrated into mandatory curricula from early childhood through adulthood. In the Finnish system, this work is supported through teacher training and national programming that promotes media education among professionals who work with youth and parents and caregivers raising children at home. Three recommendations follow:

- *Policymakers*: Adopt digital media literacy policies that support both the education of youth and limitations on what technology can do to them that are supported financially to include curriculum review, development and implementation, and both educator and family training.
- *Medical Providers*: Develop new pediatric health assessments that include a focus on digital media literacy (as compared to general discussions of "screen time"). In a complex digital media ecosystem, evaluations of family and youth must incorporate patterns of a youth's digital media usage, as well as their literacy skills, on a developmental continuum that includes (1) *consumption* (passive watching of videos, listening to audio, or playing of games without interaction and analysis), (2) *engagement* (meaningful conversation/questioning about the media itself, with a peer or adult, during the watching of video, listening to audio, or playing of games), and (3) *production* (active creation of new media products including text, image, audio, video, or interactive content).
- *Educators and Community Organizations*: Create and curate resources that explicitly teach digital media literacy from a community

and family perspective. As children and their families work to develop digital media literacy, educators and community organizations can affirm, encourage, and support them across all dimensions of their lives. Creating and promoting safe digital spaces for marginalized youth are particularly important. Meaningful personal and community connections can help youth learn to regulate their digital activities in ways that maximize opportunities while minimizing risks.

In sum, an interdisciplinary approach to research and education through a family- and community-oriented approach to building digital media literacy—in addition to the current efforts in schools and pediatric practices—has the potential to create more healthy, productive children and adolescents who can use, rather than be used by, the devices that have become ubiquitous in modern life.

**Conflict of Interest and Funding Disclosures** None.

## References

1. Turner KH, Jolls T, Hagerman MS, et al. Developing digital and media literacies in children and adolescents. Pediatrics. 2017;140(Suppl 2):S122–6. https://doi.org/10.1542/peds.2016-1758P.
2. Hobbs R. Digital and media literacy: a plan of action. A White paper on the digital and media literacy recommendations of the knight commission on the information needs of communities in a democracy. Aspen Institute; 2010.
3. Warschauer M, Matuchniak T. New technology and digital worlds: analyzing evidence of equity in access, use, and outcomes. Rev Res Educ. 2010;34(1):179–225. https://doi.org/10.3102/0091732X09349791.
4. Mihailidis P. Civic media literacies: re-imagining engagement for civic intentionality. Learn Media Technol. 2018;43(2):152–64. https://doi.org/10.1080/17439884.2018.1428623.
5. Maloy R, Butler A, Goodman L. Critical media literacy in teacher education: discerning truth amidst a crisis of misinformation and disinformation. J Technol Teach Educ. 2022;30(2):167–76. https://www.learntechlib.org/primary/p/221058/
6. National Association of Media Literacy Education. Core principles of media literacy education. Published online 2023. Accessed 8 Dec 2023 https://namle.net/resources/core-principles/
7. National Council of Teachers of English. Definition of literacy in a digital age. Published November 7, 2019. Accessed 13 Jan 2020. https://ncte.org/statement/nctes-definition-literacy-digital-age/
8. Wuyckens G, Landry N, Fastrez P. Untangling media literacy, information literacy, and digital literacy: a systematic meta-review of core concepts in media education. J Media Literacy Educ. 2022;14(1):168–82. https://doi.org/10.23860/JMLE-2022-14-1-12.
9. Jenkins H, Ito M, Danah B. Participatory culture in a networked era: a conversation on youth, learning, commerce, and politics. Wiley; 2015.
10. Vickery JR, Watkins SC. Worried about the wrong things: youth, risk, and opportunity in the digital world. Illustrated edition. The MIT Press; 2017.
11. Graafland JH. New technologies and 21st century children: recent trends and outcomes. OECD. 2018; https://doi.org/10.1787/e071a505-en.
12. Anderson M, Faverio M, Teens GJ. Social media and technology 2023. Pew Research Center; 2023. Accessed 18 Dec 2023. https://www.pewresearch.org/internet/2023/12/11/teens-social-media-and-technology-2023/
13. Twenge JM. Increases in depression, self-harm, and suicide among U.S. adolescents after 2012 and links to technology use: possible mechanisms. Psychiatr Res Clin Pract. 2020;2(1):19–25. https://doi.org/10.1176/appi.prcp.20190015.
14. Orben A, Blakemore SJ. How social media affects teen mental health: a missing link. Nature. 2023;614(7948):410–2. https://doi.org/10.1038/d41586-023-00402-9.
15. Eirich R, McArthur BA, Anhorn C, McGuinness C, Christakis DA, Madigan S. Association of screen time with internalizing and externalizing behavior problems in children 12 years or younger: a systematic review and meta-analysis. JAMA Psychiatry. 2022;79(5):393. https://doi.org/10.1001/jamapsychiatry.2022.0155.
16. Gentzler AL, Hughes JL, Johnston M, Alderson JE. Which social media platforms matter and for whom? Examining moderators of links between adolescents' social media use and depressive symptoms. J Adolesc. 2023;95(8):1725–48. https://doi.org/10.1002/jad.12243.
17. Nagata JM, Cortez CA, Dooley EE, et al. 10. Screen time and moderate-to-vigorous intensity physical activity among adolescents during the COVID-19 pandemic: findings from the adolescent brain cognitive development study. J Adolesc Health. 2022;70(4):S6:S6. https://doi.org/10.1016/j.jadohealth.2022.01.014.

18. Gohari MR, Patte KA, Ferro MA, et al. Adolescents' depression and anxiety symptoms during the COVID-19 pandemic: longitudinal evidence from COMPASS. J Adolesc Health. 2024;74(1):36–43. https://doi.org/10.1016/j.jadohealth.2023.07.024.
19. Livingstone S, Mascheroni G, Stoilova M. The outcomes of gaining digital skills for young people's lives and wellbeing: A systematic evidence review. New Media Soc. 2023;25(5):1176–202. https://doi.org/10.1177/14614448211043189.
20. Wineburg S, Breakstone J, McGrew S, Smith MD, Ortega T. Lateral reading on the open internet: a district-wide field study in high school government classes. J Educ Psychol. 2022;114:893–909. https://doi.org/10.1037/edu0000740.
21. Rodríguez-de-Dios I, van Oosten JMF, Igartua J. A study of the relationship between parental mediation and adolescents' digital skills, online risks and online opportunities. Comput Hum Behav. 2018;82:186–98. https://doi.org/10.1016/j.chb.2018.01.012.
22. Vandoninck S, d'Haenens L, Roe K. Online risks. J Child Media. 2013;7(1):60–78. https://doi.org/10.1080/17482798.2012.739780.
23. Shutzman B, Gershy N. Children's excessive digital media use, mental health problems and the protective role of parenting during COVID-19. Comput Hum Behav. 2023;139:107559. https://doi.org/10.1016/j.chb.2022.107559.
24. Hobbs R, Moen M, Tang R, Steager P. Measuring the implementation of media literacy instructional practices in schools: community stakeholder perspectives. Learn Media Technol. 2022;49(2):1–16. https://doi.org/10.1080/17439884.2022.2151621.
25. McNeill E. U.S. media literacy policy report: a state-by-state status of media literacy education laws for K-12 schools. Media Literacy Now. 2023; Accessed 24 Mar 2023. https://medialiteracynow.org/wp-content/uploads/2023/03/MediaLiteracyPolicyReport2022.corrected.pdf
26. Rideout V, Peebles A, Mann S, Robb MB. Common sense census: media use by tweens and teens, 2021. Common Sense. 2022; Accessed 24 Mar 2023. https://www.commonsensemedia.org/sites/default/files/research/report/8-18-census-integrated-report-final-web_0.pdf
27. Office for Civil Rights. Education in a pandemic: the disparate impacts of COVID-19 on America's students. US Department of Education: US Department of Education; 2021. https://www2.ed.gov/about/offices/list/ocr/docs/20210608-impacts-of-covid19.pdf
28. Salemink K, Strijker D, Bosworth G. Rural development in the digital age: a systematic literature review on unequal ICT availability, adoption, and use in rural areas. J Rural Stud. 2017;54:360–71. https://doi.org/10.1016/j.jrurstud.2015.09.001.
29. Mirra N, Garcia A. Civic participation reimagined: youth interrogation and innovation in the multimodal public sphere. Rev Res Educ. 2017;41(1):136–58. https://doi.org/10.3102/0091732X17690121.
30. Mirra N, Garcia A. "I hesitate but I do have hope": youth speculative civic literacies for troubled times. Harv Educ Rev. 2020;90(2):295–321. https://doi.org/10.17763/1943-5045-90.2.295.
31. Herbold S, Hautli-Janisz A, Heuer U, Kikteva Z, Trautsch A. A large-scale comparison of human-written versus ChatGPT-generated essays. Sci Rep. 2023;13(1):–18617. https://doi.org/10.1038/s41598-023-45644-9.
32. White SV, Scott DA, Koshy DS, Noble DS, Bender DE, Marshall DB, Gillard DC, Alkhatib DA, Bobb DK, Margolis DJ, Banks AS, Williams A, Petty T, Vakil DS, Ryoo DJ, Yadav DA, Heath DM, Krutka DD, Crawford C, et al. Responsible AI & Tech Justice: a guide for K-12 education. Kapor Foundation; 2024. https://kaporfoundation.org/wp-content/uploads/2024/01/Responsible-AI-Guide-Kapor-Foundation.pdf
33. Garcia AG, McGrew S, Mirra N, Tynes B, Kahne J. Rethinking digital citizenship: Learning about media, literacy, and race in turbulent times. In: Civic Engagement Research Group. 2021; p. 319–352. Accessed 24 Mar 2023. https://naeducation.org/wp-content/uploads/2021/03/Chapter-7.pdf
34. Lehtimaki S, Martic J, Wahl B, Foster KT, Schwalbe N. Evidence on digital mental health interventions for adolescents and young people: systematic overview. JMIR Ment Health. 2021;8(4):e25847. https://doi.org/10.2196/25847.
35. Hobbs R. Measuring the digital and media literacy competencies of children and teens. In: Cognitive development in digital contexts. Elsevier; 2017. p. 253–74. https://doi.org/10.1016/B978-0-12-809481-5.00013-4.
36. Bohnert M, Gracia P. Digital use and socioeconomic inequalities in adolescent well-being: longitudinal evidence on socioemotional and educational outcomes. J Adolesc. 2023;95(6):1179–94. https://doi.org/10.1002/jad.12193.
37. Cortesi S, Hasse A, Lombana-Bermudez A, Kim S, Gasser U. Youth and digital citizenship+ (plus): understanding skills for a digital world. Berkman Klein Center for Internet & Society; 2020. Accessed 10 Dec 2023. http://nrs.harvard.edu/urn-3:HUL.InstRepos:42638976
38. Garcia P, Fernández C, Okonkwo H. Leveraging technology: how black girls enact critical digital literacies for social change. Learn Media Technol. 2020;45(4):345–62. https://doi.org/10.1080/17439884.2020.1773851.
39. Hollenstein T, Colasante T. Socioemotional development in the digital age. Psychol Inq. 2020;31(3):250–7. https://doi.org/10.1080/1047840X.2020.1820224.
40. Common Sense Education. Digital citizenship curriculum. Accessed 14 Aug 2023. https://www.commonsense.org/education/digital-citizenship/curriculum

41. Eisenstock B, editor. News literacy now. Peter Lang Verlag; 2023. https://doi.org/10.3726/b20691.
42. Hammond S, Polizzi G, Bartholomew K. Using a socio-ecological framework to understand how 8–12-year-olds build and show digital resilience: a multi-perspective and multimethod qualitative study, vol. 28. Educational Information Technology. Published online September 30; 2022. p. 3681. https://doi.org/10.1007/s10639-022-11240-z.
43. Lessenski M. How it started, how it is going: media literacy index 2022. Open Society Institute - Sofia; 2022. Accessed 31 Mar 2023. https://osis.bg/wp-content/uploads/2022/10/HowItStarted_MediaLiteracyIndex2022_ENG_.pdf

# The Explosion of EdTech: Can Its Promise Be Fulfilled?

Roberta Michnick Golinkoff, Brenna Hassinger-Das, Natalia Kucirkova, Lauren Myers, and Rebecca A. Dore

## 1 Background

During a typical preschool day in 1990, 4-year-old Jessica counts out 10 pebbles, places them in a row, and tells her friend to follow the stone path. Fast forward to 2023: 4-year-old Olivia assembles Osmo pieces on the table, adjusts the reflector over the iPad, and her programmed path comes alive on the screen. A virtual character follows the forest path Olivia coded, turning the coding exercise into a colorful game with music and interactive features.

Over the past 30 years, children have been interacting with technology more frequently in both home and school settings. Educational Technologies (EdTech) are hardware and software designed to promote children's learning, such as coding robots, smartphone or tablet apps, interactive websites, and e-books as well as educational TV programs. EdTech is changing how children learn and is becoming increasingly common. And yet, as research indicates, Ed Tech has not yet realized its potential.

In this chapter, we focus on EdTech used at home and in preschool and early primary school classrooms, with typically developing children aged between 0 and 5 years. To date, research on EdTech has focused mostly on the cognitive domain, in academic subjects like reading, math, and science. Fewer apps are designed to foster socioemotional outcomes, and even fewer still require collaboration between children and caregivers.

The promise of EdTech is that it features affordances that only digital technology can provide and will help teachers individualize instruction to meet children's unique needs and preferences, thereby improving educational outcomes. For example, apps can allow children to progress through content at different paces based on prior knowledge. On the other hand, to the extent that Ed Tech minimizes children's interactions with teachers and other children, it reduces their opportunities for socialization and learning from others.

## 2 Current State

As of 2021, approximately 78% of American households own a computer or tablet [1]. Almost the entire population of the United States (97%)

R. M. Golinkoff (✉)
University of Delaware, Newark, DE, USA
e-mail: roberta@udel.edu

B. Hassinger-Das
Pace University, New York, NY, USA

N. Kucirkova
University of Stavanger, Stavanger, Norway

L. Myers
Lafayette College, Easton, PA, USA

R. A. Dore
The Ohio State University, Columbus, OH, USA


D. A. Christakis, L. Hale (eds.), *Handbook of Children and Screens*,
https://doi.org/10.1007/978-3-031-69362-5_75

reports having a cell phone [1]. Even in preschools and kindergartens, as many as 71% of educators use tablets in the classroom [2]. Computer use is also prevalent, with 27% of teachers using computers every day and 41% at least once a week [2]. As surveys of media use indicate, the use of Ed Tech is not evenly distributed, with children from rural areas and those whose parents are less educated having the least access.

Despite the prevalence of EdTech, its effects on child outcomes are unclear, as not all EdTech programs are designed according to how children learn best. Therefore, it is critical to examine the *quality* of EdTech [3]. Researchers have identified four "pillars" that define aspects of media design that can support or inhibit child learning [3]. High-quality apps require *mental activity* on the child's part and not just the physical activity of clicking or swiping. They should *engage* rather than distract from the learning activity with advertising or mini games. When apps are *meaningful* and link up to what children already know, they are much more likely to spur new learning. Apps should also spur *social interaction or parasocial relationships* rather than encouraging exclusively solo play since children learn more when interacting with others [3].

To assess app quality, Meyer et al. applied these criteria to the 100 most downloaded apps from the Apple Store and Google Play [4]. Fully 50% of the apps parents paid for were in the lower quality range, and free apps featured "distracting visual and sound effects, disruptive advertising, and irrelevant rewards." [4] These findings present a challenge to parents and teachers, as the most popular EdTech that is available in the app store is mostly not consistent with the principles of how children learn.

The same is true for electronic or digital books [3]. The most popular children's digital books are not based on scientific principles; they contain many "bells and whistles" that distract children, are often not available in local languages, and many are merely digitized versions of paper books [3]. Often, because the advertising associated with digital materials touts its benefits relentlessly, some caregivers have accepted the industry's claims that these untested books and apps are in fact educational.

This belief may contribute to why some parents let their children overuse screens. Radesky and colleagues tracked mobile device use over nine months among US children aged 3–5 [5]. Comparing their findings of children's actual use with parents' estimates of use, nearly three-quarters of their parents *underestimated* it. The authors were stunned to find that the content children watched was often inappropriate, with some children watching gambling and violent games even though their parents thought they were watching educational content.

EdTech's effectiveness varies depending on the context of use, presence of and active input of adults, and of course, the features of the individual EdTech [6]. Recent experimental studies from across the globe confirm that well-designed EdTech can positively impact children's learning, demonstrating an overall positive effect on 2- to 5-year-old children's literacy development, mathematics, science, problem solving, and self-efficacy [7]. In addition, EdTech enhanced with artificial intelligence (AI) can advance children's creative and collaborative skills, as well as computational thinking [8]. Here, we review EdTech across domains and the extent to which it has been shown to be effective for learning. It is worth noting that we primarily focus on apps and e-books, while more research is needed to evaluate the effectiveness of inquiry-based investigations with simulations, creative coding, robotics, tangible electronics, and other platforms.

## 2.1 Ed Tech and Mathematics Learning

The added value of EdTech to early mathematics education depends on children's prior knowledge [9]. To examine the effectiveness of apps for math learning, Kim and colleagues conducted a meta-analysis of 36 studies with children in preschool through Grade 3 [10]. They found medium-sized impacts on math skills (ES = 0.29), which were fairly similar to the effects of tutoring interventions [11]. Apps were most effective for "constrained" math skills—those that are easier to teach and mastered by the majority of children—such as counting and sorting shapes, and simple addition. Kim et al. rated each app according to criteria proposed by Hirsh-Pasek et al. [2] (active, engaged, meaningful, and social interactive learning) [10]. The mean app score was 2.4 on a scale of 3 in each of these dimensions, suggesting that, on average, the apps were fairly well-aligned with the learning principles, with some room for improvement. However, there is still more to learn about how and why these apps are effective.

## 2.2 Literacy Apps and E-Books for Learning

Although print books are still around and will likely never disappear, teachers and parents are increasingly using digital books with children. There is no difference in the quality and quantity of parent-child talk between print and digital books—especially when the "bells and whistles,' 'such as sound effects and embedded games, are turned off [12, 13]. It is important to note that caregivers who can personalize the text and link it to children's experiences foster more learning in children who read an e-book alone. Conversation prompts can be built into digital books to support more parent-child conversation during reading. Visual and auditory enhancements, when linked to the story—as opposed to distracting from it—can significantly increase children's story comprehension and book-based vocabulary [14]. For the enhancements to benefit children's literacy, it is important to adjust the design to the child's age: fewer enhancements work better for younger children (3-year-olds). However, by age 4, English-speaking children can learn just from listening to the audio track of an e-book [13, 15].

Studies with literacy apps and digital books show that when it comes to educational benefits of EdTech features, less is more. Too many prompts and enhancements overwhelm children and hinder, rather than promote, their learning. This is especially the case for younger children (2- to 3-year-olds), who have lower cognitive capacity and are more easily distractible [14].

While e-books can be improved, using them remotely can offer reading opportunities for children who are in crisis. Remote reading experiences supported through online libraries offer educational moments for children who are in hospitals, in the midst of war, and those with imprisoned parents. Remote storybook reading can promote enjoyment of reading, increase reported feelings of adult-child closeness, and support language development [13]. Moreover, video chat platforms open up new possibilities for preschoolers to engage in virtual book reading with far-flung relatives such as grandparents (Ramirez, Zosh, & Golinkoff, under preparation). Some apps offer specialized platforms for digital play and e-book reading with a virtual partner. English-speaking preschool-aged children can comprehend books over video chat and respond similarly to questions and prompts in both live and video chat reading contexts [13]. Research also suggests that reading with a parent—whether an e-book or a paper book—increases children's arousal compared to reading an e-book alone [16]. Does this positive arousal occur with remote reading as well? Future research is needed.

## 2.3 Socioemotional Skills Development Through Apps

Prior research has shown that children around the world can learn social-emotional skills, such as perspective taking and cooperation, from educational television [17], including through digital toolkits in the preschool classroom setting [18, 19]. Yet little research has explored children's social-emotional learning from educational apps. In parents' reports of children's most-used apps, less than 7% included any content coded as teaching social-emotional content [18]. In one US study, Rasmussen et al. found that children who used *Daniel Tiger's Neighborhood,* an app with an emotion-focused curriculum, used more of the taught emotion regulation strategies than children in a control condition [20]. In two more recent experimental studies in the United States and Israel, children's prosocial behavior increased after using an app or playing a virtual reality game with prosocial content [20, 21]. Mindfulness and meditation apps targeted toward children may promote social-emotional development and are prevalent in app stores, but researchers have questioned their quality and identified the need for empirical evidence on their effectiveness [22].

### 2.4 Ed Tech: Room for Improvement

The overall positive effect of touchscreen use among 0–5-year-olds is not substantiated by studies that focus on parents' reports of children's EdTech and its impact [23]. Longitudinal studies on parent reports from across the globe find negative associations between children's use of apps and game play and psychological difficulties, such as lower inhibition capabilities [24]. Furthermore, while systematic reviews do document positive associations between educational apps for early learning [25], there is significant variation in outcomes based on the types of apps studied. In particular, children's use of EdTech developed by *researchers* is associated with positive outcomes while the use of commercial EdTech, which is of lower quality, is negatively associated with learning [10].

Yet another issue is the misuse of personal data for advertising purposes. Mallawaarachchi and colleagues [26] found that educational apps, particularly free apps, advertised to Australian children, contain persuasive design features that motivate and prompt children to engage in consumer behavior but do not advance their learning. Similar findings were noted by Radesky et al. [27], who found that 80% of apps used by US 3–5-year-olds contained manipulative design features.

Indeed, the EdTech Evidence movement is a global initiative to address the quality issues in current educational technologies. Researchers across the world work actively to integrate more science of learning with the design of educational technologies through research accelerators or mentorship with EdTech companies. Testing products with schools and kindergartens is a crucial part of adducing evidence for EdTech. However, not all states and districts have the resources to support the necessary three-way collaboration between scientists, EdTech designers, and teachers. Yet, it is only through empirical testing, ongoing design improvements, and teachers' input that EdTech can become truly educational.

## 3 Future Research

### 3.1 Coviewing with Adults

Given research showing that using media with an adult supports children's attention and learning [3, 27], how can we encourage parents, caregivers, and teachers to experience EdTech with children? How can features of Ed Tech promote children's positive interactions with adults? For instance, Stuckelman et al. [28] showed that digital books can be designed to foster positive English language parent-child interactions; specifically, a character embedded in an e-book can model dialogic reading prompts that parents can employ themselves. Families who read this enhanced version of an e-book demonstrated increases in on-task behavior, and both parent and child exhibited more positive emotions during book reading. There is a great need to disseminate the message that children have a different, more positive, and fruitful experience when they read an e-book with an adult.

### 3.2 Coplaying with Peers

How can we work with developers to encourage the creation of digital apps that promote social interaction between peers? Collaborative games hold great potential in promoting learning through children's experiences in situ or virtual interaction with others. For instance, US children's use of the online collaborative program

First In Math (FIM) was correlated with improved academic achievement in math, even controlling for prior achievement [29].

### 3.3 Researching the Factors that Matter

While research proceeds on what makes apps effective [3], we need to probe more deeply, as well as longitudinally, to understand how the use of EdTech impacts children from many vantage points. For instance, does the use of solo EdTech, which now dominates the landscape, impact children's social skills, executive function development, or motivation and desire to learn?

## 4 Recommendations

In 2023, Olivia from the opening anecdote plays differently than 1990 Jessica, thanks to the pervasiveness of EdTech in the multiple contexts of childhood (home, school, and peer settings). Where is this digital revolution taking us? One can imagine a dystopian future with preschool taking place only online and young children slogging away on computers, rather than playing joyfully and collaboratively interacting with peers. Ed Tech can help children learn, but there are numerous red flags to heed. We offer recommendations separately for researchers, pediatricians, and parents and educators.

### 4.1 For Researchers

- Researchers must find ways to partner with developers to evaluate products for continuous improvement [30].
- Researchers should study new media as it emerges, such as generative AI and metaverse applications.
- The field of developmental cognitive neuroscience also holds great potential: can we examine children's neural processing while they use media to uncover brain-based mechanisms that underlie effects on learning, cognition, and affect?

### 4.2 For Parents and Educators

- There is currently no clearinghouse to evaluate EdTech programs, so educators and caregivers should have a healthy dose of skepticism about advertised claims of EdTech's educational effects. They now attempt to choose content aligning with the principles of learning [3].
- Children's Technology Review is a good place to find expert reviews of specific apps and platforms.
- Playful learning supported by caring adults should be at the forefront of educators' and parents' minds when selecting EdTech for children.

### 4.3 For Pediatricians

- As parents find effective communication with pediatricians helpful [31], pediatricians can suggest that screen time be limited for young children and that it is worth being skeptical of claims of educational impact.
- There is a need to support parents so that they might develop sufficient research literacy to evaluate and critique educational claims themselves or conversely, to develop a solution that addresses the fact that many parents may not have the time to thoroughly evaluate every educational technology by themselves.
- Asking about media use quantity and content should be routine during well visits.
- Pediatricians should gauge the developmental appropriateness of content and suggest alternatives such as well-researched programs like Sesame Street and those recommended by Common Sense Media (in the United States).

**Conflict of Interest and Funding Disclosures** None.

## References


1. Internet/Broadband Fact Sheet. Pew Research Center: Internet, Science & Tech. https://www.pewresearch.org/internet/fact-sheet/internet-broadband/#panel-e60540d5-6342-47eb-835d-21b1c0a5e37b. Published March 2, 2023. Accessed 31 Mar 2023.
2. Dore RA, Dynia JM. Technology and media use in preschool classrooms: prevalence, purposes, and context. Front Educ. 2020:5. https://doi.org/10.3389/feduc.2020.600305.
3. Hirsh-Pasek K, Zosh JM, Golinkoff RM, Gray JH, Robb MB, Kaufman J. Putting education in "educational" apps: Lessons from the science of learning. Psychol Sci Public Interest. 2015;16(1):3–34. https://doi.org/10.1177/1529100615569721.
4. Meyer M, Zosh JM, McLaren C, et al. How educational are "educational" apps for young children? App Store content analysis using the four pillars of learning framework. J Child Media. 2021;15(4):526–48. https://doi.org/10.1080/17482798.2021.1882516.
5. Radesky JS, Weeks HM, Ball R, et al. Young children's use of smartphones and tablets. Pediatrics. 2020;146(1) https://doi.org/10.1542/peds.2019-3518.
6. Kucirkova N. iRPD—a framework for guiding design-based research for iPad apps. Br J Educ Technol. 2016;48(2):598–610. https://doi.org/10.1111/bjet.12389.
7. Herodotou C. Young Children and tablets: a systematic review of effects on learning and development. J Comput Assist Learn. 2017;34(1):1–9. https://doi.org/10.1111/jcal.12220.
8. Su J, Yang W. Artificial Intelligence in early childhood education: a scoping review. Comput Educ Artif Intel. 2022;3:100049. https://doi.org/10.1016/j.caeai.2022.100049.
9. Verbruggen S, Depaepe F, Torbeyns J. Effectiveness of educational technology in early mathematics education: a systematic literature review. Int J Child-Comput Interact. 2021;27:100220. https://doi.org/10.1016/j.ijcci.2020.100220.
10. Kim J, Gilbert J, Yu Q, Gale C. Measures matter: a meta-analysis of the effects of educational apps on preschool to grade 3 children's literacy and math skills. AERA Open. 2021:7. https://doi.org/10.1177/23328584211004183.
11. Nickow A, Oreopoulos P, Quan V. The impressive effects of tutoring on prek-12 learning: a systematic review and meta-analysis of the experimental evidence. National Bureau of Economic Research. https://www.nber.org/papers/w27476. Published July 6, 2020. Accessed 31 Mar 2023.
12. Strouse GA, Troseth GL, Stuckelman ZD. Page and screen: Storybook features that promote parent-child talk during shared reading. J Appl Dev Psychol. 2023:86. https://doi.org/10.1016/j.appdev.2023.101522.
13. Gaudreau C, King YA, Dore RA, et al. Preschoolers benefit equally from video chat, pseudo-contingent video, and live book reading: implications for storytime during the coronavirus pandemic and beyond. Front Psychol. 2020:11. https://doi.org/10.3389/fpsyg.2020.02158.
14. Li X, Bus AG. Efficacy of digital picture book enhancements grounded in multimedia learning principles: Dependent on age? Learn Instr. 2023:85. https://doi.org/10.1016/j.learninstruc.2023.101749.
15. Dore RA, Hassinger-Das B, Brezack N, et al. The parent advantage in fostering children's e-book comprehension. Early Child Res Q. 2018;44:24–33. https://doi.org/10.1016/j.ecresq.2018.02.002.
16. Avelar D, Dore RA, Schwichtenberg AJ, Roben CKP, Hirsh-Pasek K, Golinkoff RM. Children and parents' physiological arousal and emotions during shared and independent e-book Reading: a preliminary study. Int J Child-Comput Interact. 2022:33. https://doi.org/10.1016/j.ijcci.2022.100507.
17. Mares M-L, Pan Z. Effects of sesame street: a meta-analysis of children's learning in 15 countries. J Appl Dev Psychol. 2013;34(3):140–51. https://doi.org/10.1016/j.appdev.2013.01.001.
18. Dore RA, Purtell KM, Lin T-J & Justice LM. Examining the prevalence, content, and demographic and time use correlates of children's educational media use. Flash talk presented at the Biennial Meeting of the Society for Research in Child Development; Salt Lake City, UT.
19. Oades-Sese GV, Cahill A, Allen JW, Rubic WL, Mahmood N. Effectiveness of sesame workshop's little children, big challenges: a digital media SEL intervention for preschool classrooms. Psychol Sch. 2021;58(10):2041–67. https://doi.org/10.1002/pits.22574.
20. Rasmussen EE, Strouse GA, Colwell MJ, et al. Promoting preschoolers' emotional competence through prosocial TV and mobile app use. Media Psychol. 2018;22(1):1–22. https://doi.org/10.1080/15213269.2018.1476890.
21. Shoshani A, Nelke S, Girtler I. Tablet applications as socializing platforms: the effects of prosocial touch screen applications on young children's prosocial behavior. Comput Hum Behav. 2022:127. https://doi.org/10.1016/j.chb.2021.107077.
22. Shoshani A. From virtual to prosocial reality: the effects of prosocial virtual reality games on preschool children's prosocial tendencies in real life environments. Comput Hum Behav. 2023:139. https://doi.org/10.1016/j.chb.2022.107546.
23. Nunes A, Castro SL, Limpo T. A review of mindfulness-based apps for children. Mindfulness. 2020;11(9):2089–101. https://doi.org/10.1007/s12671-020-01410-w.
24. Xie H, Peng J, Qin M, Huang X, Tian F, Zhou Z. Can touchscreen devices be used to facilitate young children's learning? A meta-analysis of touchscreen learning effect. Front Psychol. 2018:9. https://doi.org/10.3389/fpsyg.2018.02580.
25. McNeill J, Howard SJ, Vella SA, Cliff DP. Longitudinal associations of electronic applica-

tion use and media program viewing with cognitive and psychosocial development in preschoolers. Acad Pediatr. 2019;19(5):520–8. https://doi.org/10.1016/j.acap.2019.02.010.
26. Mallawaarachchi SR, Tieppo A, Hooley M, Horwood S. Persuasive design-related motivators, ability factors and prompts in early childhood apps: a content analysis. Comput Hum Behav. 2023:139. https://doi.org/10.1016/j.chb.2022.107492.
27. Radesky J, Hiniker A, McLaren C, et al. Prevalence and characteristics of manipulative design in mobile applications used by children. JAMA Netw Open. 2022;5(6) https://doi.org/10.1001/jamanetworkopen.2022.17641.
28. Stuckelman ZD, Strouse GA, Troseth GL. Value added: digital Modeling of Dialogic Questioning promotes positive parenting during shared reading. J Fam Psychol. 2022;36(6):1010–20. https://doi.org/10.1037/fam0000932.
29. Ahn J, Beck A, Rice J, Foster M. Exploring issues of implementation, equity, and student achievement with educational software in the DC Public Schools. AERA Open. 2016;2(4) https://doi.org/10.1177/2332858416667726.
30. Dore RA, Shirilla M, Hopkins E, et al. Education in the app store: using a mobile game to support U.S. preschoolers' vocabulary learning. J Child Media. 2019;13(4):452–71. https://doi.org/10.1080/17482798.2019.1650788.
31. Nobile C, Drotar D. Research on the quality of parent-provider communication in pediatric care: implications and recommendations. J Dev Behav Pediatr. 2003;24(4):279–90. https://doi.org/10.1097/00004703-200308000-00010.

# Children, Education, and Technologies: Current Debates, Key Concerns, and Future Directions Around Data Privacy, Surveillance, and Datafication

Velislava Hillman, Jamie Manolev, Samantha-Kaye Johnston, Priya C. Kumar, Florence Martin, Elana Zeide, Gergana Vladova, and Rina Lai

## 1 Background

Edtech products have diffused into educational systems globally, driven by education policy [1] as well as beliefs that they can help achieve some of the United Nations Sustainable Development Goals (SDGs), including Goal 4 (Quality Education) and Goal 10 (Reduced Inequalities) [2]. At the same time, the current design and implementation of digital technologies presents complex contradictions in justly achieving the SDGs [3].

For instance, the absence of transparency regarding data collection processes and decision-making concerning students undermines the ability of teachers to fully understand how they can effectively collaborate with edtech platforms. This lack of clarity inhibits the use of their professional insights, consequently hindering the enhancement of teacher qualifications through the integration of edtech, thus contradicting Goal 4.C [3]. The lack of transparency raises ethical concerns, such as fostering a surveillance culture [4]. It also conflicts with Goal 16, which aims to establish peace, justice, and strong institutions, as it can undermine privacy and trust within educational systems [5]. Moreover, this constant collection (and over-collection) of data uses high computing resources, whose environmental impacts challenge Goal 13 (Climate Action), given that the ICT sector, including edtech, is projected to contribute 14% of global greenhouse gas emissions by 2040 [6]. Therefore, current efforts aimed at greening education should include greening edtech [7].

V. Hillman (✉)
London School of Economics and Political Science, London, UK
e-mail: v.hillman@lse.ac.uk

J. Manolev
University of South Australia, Centre for Research in Educational and Social Inclusion, Adelaide, Australia

S.-K. Johnston
University of Oxford and Berkman Klein Centre for Internet and Society, Cambridge, MA, USA

P. C. Kumar
Pennsylvania State University, State College, PA, USA

F. Martin
North Carolina State University, Raleigh, NC, USA

E. Zeide
University of Nebraska, Lincoln, NE, USA

G. Vladova
Humboldt University of Berlin, Department of Computer Science, Computer Science Education/ Computer Science and Society, Berlin, Germany

R. Lai
University of Cambridge, Cambridge, UK


D. A. Christakis, L. Hale (eds.), *Handbook of Children and Screens*,
https://doi.org/10.1007/978-3-031-69362-5_76

Importantly, while edtech advances digital infrastructure (Goal 9), neglecting data privacy contradicts Goal 9.1. Cloud-based solutions expose student data to cybersecurity risks, jeopardizing educational integrity. Profiting from education data undermines Goal 9.2, prioritizing economic gains over inclusivity and sustainability. Altogether, edtech's infusion has often been propelled by industry's aggressive marketing, promising technological revolution in education, and accelerated by the COVID-19 pandemic. Yet, despite the hype, technological adoption has been accompanied by a sense of disappointment and failure to impact education [8]. Educational institutions, specifically in Anglo-American contexts, increasingly depend on edtech, while datafication and surveillance are normalized.

Data-intensive edtech is used across the educational system—from providing lessons and content, to assessing students and practicing subjects, to managing schools and staff. Many K-12 schools across the United States, for instance spend financial resources on monitoring applications such as Gaggle and GoGuardian, whose functionalities comprise activity and time logging, 24/7 notifications, home calls/wellness checks, and remote control. This digitization, especially in K-12 education, has led to growing concerns of learning environments that convert learners' social actions into quantifiable data, a process known as "datafication." While datafication has been seen to support decision-making by adapting and personalizing the learning experience [9], it has also raised significant concerns for children's well-being.

## 2 Current State

### 2.1 The Nature and Impact of Datafication

First, datafication can be understood as the quantification of social processes that espouses a reductionist view of education-related phenomena. This trend is driven by a view of numbers as objective, true, accurate, and subsequently superior to other forms of knowledge, which some describe as a mythology of data [10]. That is, numbers strip context from what they represent and underpin the problematic "turn to decontextualized data as truth,' [11] because numbers produce an "abstracted tunnel vision" that only reveals a fragment of reality and its complexity [12]. The behavior management platform ClassDojo is an example of decontextualization as it reduces student behavior to a numerical score [13], removing any social context.

Second, datafication can involve inferring, predicting, and controlling human behavior in ways that risk undermining individual agency, privacy, and basic human rights [14]. In the United States, the Family Educational Rights and Privacy Act of 1974 (FERPA) provides legal guidance for protecting student privacy enforcing that student data can be shared with third parties only as long as there is an educational reason for disclosure such as providing critical services. Yet, loopholes for data exploitation remain [15]. Conversely, the Children's Internet Protection Act (CIPA) aimed to address concerns about children accessing obscene or harmful content on the Internet, enabling schools to use monitoring software applications to keep track of students' online behavior.

Third, datafication leads to the collection of vast amounts of personal and sensitive data, which can be used to identify individuals and track and control behaviors that are not conducive to learning. While data privacy laws continue to adapt and address the challenges of datafication, edtech remains plagued by data misuse [16], cybersecurity risks, weak scrutiny, and no clear standards in the sector [17].

Fourth, datafication has led to risks of bias, perpetuating, or amplifying existing inequalities. The algorithm used by the Office of Qualifications and Examinations Regulation in the United Kingdom was meant to forecast national exam results, yet it produced biased outcomes, negatively impacting students' learning progression and confidence [18].

In many American K-12 schools today, platforms like iReady are used to assess students' reading and mathematics proficiency, which determines their subsequent placement in middle and high school. However, there exists a lack of transparency or clarity regarding the methodology employed by the platform to conduct these assessments, including sufficient details on the process of data collection [19]. Consequently, the conclusions drawn may lack validity and reliability. This is particularly important in light of evidence indicating that students using the iReady platform instructional resources either scored lower [20] or exhibited no discernible improvement [20] in reading proficiency compared to their peers who were not instructed through the iReady program. Moreover, globally, digital divides continue to widen. Since underserved children still lack digital resources, less data is available about them, which leads to samples that disproportionately represent White, Educated, Industrialized, Rich, and Democratic (WEIRD) populations. Using such biased samples could further impact children's education negatively [21].

Finally, datafication has also intensified the debate surrounding the risks of harm through surveillance, or "dataveillance" [22] and diminishing personal freedoms and rights. The digital monitoring system E-HallPass, which was recently introduced into 1000 U.S. schools to track students movement outside the classroom (including visits to the bathroom), exemplifies the concerns with such technologies [23]. Such real-time surveillance of students can lead to unjustified control of their behavior [13]. Schools and local authorities may end up using surveillance data as evidence in disciplinary investigations and harm children and young people when the same surveillance systems are used even outside school hours [24]. Such practices are transcending schools' role beyond academic environments to ones of sanction and punishment.

Knowing that there is constant digital surveillance can create a sense of unease and even paranoia among individuals—be those students or teachers. This can lead to self-censorship (chilling effects) where both students and teachers refrain from expressing themselves freely or exploring controversial topics for fear of repercussions. The normalization of surveillance and datafication is now extending beyond the classroom, which can potentially impact students' willingness to question authority or engage in activities that may be deemed unconventional.

Many digital surveillance systems are also dependent on algorithms to analyze data and make inferences and decisions about individuals. These algorithms often inherit biases present in the data on which they are trained. As such, digital surveillance systems can often target certain groups of individuals based on shared characteristics of race, ethnicity, socioeconomic status, and others, which can lead to increased scrutiny and surveillance of minoritized individuals, perpetuating inequalities, and exacerbating bias and other social injustices. In short, the implications of dataveillance in education are concerning because they can discriminate against specific individuals, create anxiety among students as well as teachers who are equally subject to dataveillance, and erode overall trust not only between students and teachers but also students' trust in the whole educational system [25].

## 2.2 Current Safeguards Against Datafication

Indeed, with increased datafication, it is important to consider the nature of safeguards for student data. Thus far, we have hinted at the need to elevate privacy by design—that is, incorporating privacy protections directly into the design of technologies. However, privacy protection can also be viewed from a digital literacy perspective: the knowledge and skills to responsibly evaluate, create, collect, and share information in digital environments. Digital literacy has been previously linked to online resilience and wellbeing, and "three times as many young people [aged 11 to 16 years across the UK] with high critical digital literacy scores have high mental wellbeing." [26]

Teachers enact and resist the logics of dataveillance [27], while also recognizing the inherent limitations of the data such technologies generate. That said, the implications of datafication are often remote for teachers and school district leaders immersed in the day-to-day responsibilities of education [27]. For teachers, the more immediate concerns surrounding technology relate to children's (in)appropriate device use [27]; for districts, the concerns are basic data protection and security procedures [28]. While teachers express interest in incorporating digital literacy into their lessons, neither teachers nor district administrators receive much training in digital privacy or security [28].

Although researchers highlight the value of diversity in digital literacy conversations, inappropriate critical digital literacy strategies, often based on Global North (GN) realities, are implemented in Global South (GS) (a sociopolitical term referring to newly developed or developing nations with a colonial past) voices) contexts [29]. Given the distinct experiences in GS contexts, these strategies may not necessarily be effective within GS environments. Moreover, in the GS, the diverse ways of constructing concepts like "digital" and "literacy" (e.g., Latin-American and Caribbean literacies) are mostly excluded from conversations on curricular reforms [30]. Investing in context-specific digital literacy is important across the GS because, as these economies' internet connectivity expands, they often host infrastructures that are not resilient to cyberattacks, which require digital literacy and cybersecurity knowledge, especially regarding unregulated edtech [31].

## 3 Future Research

Future research should focus on the larger sociolegal and ethical implications of datafication and surveillance. Laws and policies pave the way for creating more transparency about who has access and what kind of student data is collected. However, research enquiry should delve on the long-term use of data. Research can focus on whether the obsessive drive for digital opportunities in education does not eliminate nondigital opportunities, too.

There is a gap in literature on teacher perceptions and experiences with advancing algorithmic systems and the growing datafication model. Questions can focus on how teachers perceive and experience datafication and surveillance. This includes questions about how these practices affect their sense of autonomy and professionalism, their relationships with students and parents.

Scholarship can be built around the impact of automating decision-making on teaching and learning itself. Answers are needed around how these practices affect student motivation, engagement, and achievement. Diagnostic platforms such as Naviance, iReady, and Thrively are capable of automating decision-making with the risk of automating inequalities, too. Only longitudinal research can identify the true impact of such systems on children's future opportunities.

Research, policy, and investment focus should be directed toward technological solutions that address the digital divide and learning barriers that persist worldwide. However, such efforts should be cautious about how investment and funding can expand the current educational inequalities.

## 4 Recommendations

### 4.1 For Educators

- *Evidence-based practice:* To fully leverage the power of technologies in learning, teachers should adapt evidence-based practice for effective use of edtech [32]. Put otherwise, educators need to make instructional decisions that integrate good evidence for which technology works, for what purpose, and for whom. Evaluating empirical research to align technology with appropriate pedagogical approaches can lead to greater learning outcomes [33].
- *Professional development:* Educational processes depend highly on teachers' skills and performance. Even though technologies can support pedagogy, teaching is influenced by teachers' attitudes, routines, visions, and competencies in novel methodologies and, equally in technologies [34]. Digitally competent teachers can be perceived by students and educational institutions as competent and

capable facilitators overall [35]. Using technologies is challenging for teachers, especially as products evolve fast and new edtech are being offered all the time. Teachers are expected to show willingness to engage in ongoing professional development and keep pace with the fast-changing technologies. In the absence of such competencies and professional development, teachers are less likely to use edtech [36]. Take, for instance, how Chat GPT and similar large language models have changed the demands on teachers' skills, not only in terms of whether this is indeed a tool that is beneficial for teaching and learning but also in terms of detecting and understanding how to respond from pedagogical and ethical aspects, when students use LLMs for their homework and assignments.

- The digitization of education is changing the demands on teachers' skills, abilities, and competencies, and the interplay between the different competencies is becoming more critical. Research shows that teachers' perceived competencies by students and their educational institutions are critical to students' acceptance of technology [37]. Developing teacher competencies for digital learning should be strongly supported. The goal should be to implement the complex interplay between pedagogy, content, and media skills as part of the curriculum for future teachers and their continued training.
- *Critical pedagogies:* Beyond professional development, we also call on educators to adopt critical pedagogies as a means of addressing the suite of concerns we have presented. Critical pedagogies offer an approach to teaching and learning that confronts injustices and power relations, prioritizes student interests, acknowledges the importance of context, and recognizes the inherent political nature of education [38]. Unlike common instrumental pedagogies, Saltman [11] argues, critical pedagogies foster an engagement with the politics of edtech and datafication while reasserting education's contribution toward creating more democratic and just societies. In both educators and students, it cultivates dispositions and thinking that encourage "an examination of the values, assumptions, and ideologies that undergird claims to truth" within technologies and data and enables them to be understood "in terms of broader structural and systematic patterns, history, and context." [11]
- Within critical pedagogies, learning is grounded in the process of deliberation, debate, dissent, and investigation that can be used to explore the relationships between technology and data, and the interests, authority, and social positions of those involved in their production, function, and use. This subsequently allows "students to theorize the technology [and data] they utilize" [11] in socially relevant ways, while simultaneously subjecting them and the knowledge they produce and represent to scrutiny. The adoption of critical pedagogies offers a way to resist the harmful impacts of datafication.

### 4.2 For Parents

- *Active mediation:* Parents should be supported to take a more active role in mediating children's engagement with digital learning and the increasing datafication and surveillance in education. Parents are often a significant influence on their children's lives; therefore, an opportunity exists for them to exercise such influence in digital learning. To do this, parents can adopt a mediator role that fosters strong positive relationships with their children involves explaining and discussing digital technologies and their content and provides guidance in proper use of technologies and data, which research has shown to be increasingly important to children's engagement with online environments [39].
- *Data literacy:* Such a role requires parents to possess data literacy, which is becoming a critical quality for navigating today's data saturated education environment (specifically in Anglo-American contexts). This means that it is important for parents to be sufficiently

informed or be supported to become informed about digital technologies and data, including how they work and the social, cultural, and economic forces operating through them [40]. This would enable parents to, for example, help children discern the different ways data is created about them through technologies, such as through information they voluntarily provide, or when it is extracted from them without their knowledge [40]. In this way, digital literacy can be viewed as a meta-competence necessary to assess the interrelationships, social consequences, and the impact of digitization. It also enables people to act more self-determinedly.

## 4.3 For Policymakers

- *Enhanced regulation:* More needs to be done to regulate and scrutinize the businesses developing and selling edtech products [41]. There are numerous frameworks, toolkits, and policies providing privacy by design guidelines and good practices; however, oversight and enforcement should be the next step [42]. This holds particular significance because privacy-enhancing can vary greatly among individuals, including developers, across different contexts [43].
- *Children's best interests:* Policymakers should put the spotlight on the edtech industry and demand that they prioritize children's best interests. This is harder said than done: whose best interests, according to what, how these might change over time, why edtech should be the main solution to achieve these best interests, and so on, are questions that cannot be answered in a straightforward manner. Additionally, the debate over what constitutes "best interests" can be both endless and distracting from other crucial tasks. For instance, meaningful education and efforts are essential to address more pressing issues related to the safeguarding and well-being of children. This is particularly important as both safeguarding and well-being are increasingly impacted by the digitization of education and children's lives to begin with. In practical terms though, "best interests" should entail emphasizing contextual and historical educational norms and structures, identifying collective and individual needs first, and then identifying how edtech may facilitate and address these. Indeed, educational technologies may benefit specific individuals. For example, children absent due to illness can catch up on their learning at home through the support of approved and vetted technologies. Edtech could also fit well within specific contexts, such as, when children work collectively on a project. The key point, however, is that we must avoid allowing the digital environment to become the sole and default method of learning and teaching.
- *Common standards:* Policymakers should recognize that education stakeholders demand that the edtech industry adhere to commonly agreed standards, protocols, and rules, along with a robust mechanism to enforce these is also implemented, if trust in advancing technologies is to be built. There are many frameworks and mediators coming to the fore offering stamps of approval. A parallel can be drawn with the emergence of environmental, social, and governance auditing (ESG) frameworks in response to climate change, where companies use standards to demonstrate their positive impact on the environment, relationships with employees and communities and effective governance structures [47]. The expectation is that companies disclosing their performance on ESG criteria will receive a "higher value," benefiting both "their bottom line and shareholders." [48] Consequently, the demand for corporate ESG frameworks and financial ESG investing metrics has surged more recently. The consulting industry, as Mazzucato and Collington point out, is a major provider of ESG frameworks and related services, promoting their adoption en masse. Similarly, in education, we see an overwhelming number of frameworks, standards, and industry-led associations and alliances offering vetting programs, "evidence-based" assessments of edtechs,

evaluations of "what works," and certifications sorting out the "good quality" edtech products. The list is too long to fit here (read a full chapter on this here [60]); however, some are worth paying attention to as they also can be seen as demarcating market share, which demonstrates more the commercial value created than says much about what technologies are safe and meaningful to use. For instance, the World Bank's SABER-ICT Framework [51] aids policymakers in designing and evaluating edtech policies, while the UNESCO ICT [49] Competency Framework for Teachers, in collaboration with Microsoft, CISCO, Intel, and ISTE, supports reforms in teacher training and professional development. The PISA ICT Framework assesses the integration of digital technologies in education, and other frameworks like the *Technological, Pedagogical, and Content Knowledge* (TPAC) [56], the T3 Framework (elevating the influence of edtech into "transnational, transformational, and transcendental" domains) [59], and the International Society for Technology in Education's ISTE Standards for Educators [52] provide additional guidance. Organizations like 1Edtech (former IMS Global [61]) also offer standards and certification for edtech products (TrustEd Apps [62]). 1Edtech not only certifies edtech products but also schools, encouraging them to then "Seek out suppliers with the IMS Data Privacy Seal," which reflects the aggressive market expansion and the creation of lock-ins. These entities drive market-focused activities—from training teachers to use edtech products to forming affiliations where teachers promote rather than critique these products. They also make high-level commitments with schools and districts, providing training and technical support, which develops top-down approaches where teachers have no choice but to submit to using technologies they may not want to. This also illustrates the lucrative business of digitization, with educational programs and events like trade shows and the glamorous ASU + GSV Summit reinforcing edtech's prominence. All these standards, training, and searches for "evidence" often come at a cost for schools and districts. There are numerous more standards, including those for quality online teaching, technology integration matrices, e-assessment quality assurance, age-appropriate design standards, the ISTE *edtech Product Evaluation Guide for Teachers* [52] and its *Five Pillars for edtech Procurement* [63], and the edtech Digital Promise framework among many others. There are various legal frameworks like the EU's General Data Protection Regulation, the new EU AI, data, and digital markets laws, among the growing plethora of data privacy laws in the United States, and an endless list of cybersecurity frameworks and standards. More are likely to emerge. How do edtech companies meet any of these? Is it even possible that all vendors meet such standards? And what are students and schools to understand of all this messy market while keeping focus on studies and healthy development? In a word, a common understanding must be made and one that addresses the industry, not one whose bill falls on schools.

- *Student privacy laws:* Current legal frameworks fail to adequately protect student privacy. Existing laws primarily focus on prohibiting educators from sharing information with third parties without parental consent [15]. They have not kept up with rapidly changing technology and, therefore, do not address potential issues that may arise even when well-meaning educators use technology to serve educational purposes [44]. Vendors are not held responsible to promises backed by little empirical evidence. Administrators may use predictive analytics in a deterministic manner that reinforces existing inequalities [45]. In addition, many edtech services track students' movements, online activity, and social media presence—both in and out of school [24]. This normalizes students to constant surveillance and risks stifling their intellectual growth and willingness to express unpopular ideas. Legislators and regulators must update student privacy laws to address today's technologies and concerns.

### 4.4 For edtech Providers

- *Child-centered design:* Risks of harm from datafication and surveillance in education create the urgency to reset the values that guide future design and development of edtech. This includes emphasizing child-centered designs, data responsibility, and evidence-based practices. Bridging the gap between research and industry is essential for ensuring child-centered designs of educational technologies and their adoption in formal educational settings or as complementary efforts for out-of-school engagement [46]. Cross-sectoral collaboration can facilitate edtech products that are underpinned by scientific knowledge (i.e., cognitive and learning sciences) to support future evidence-based products [32]. Hence, there is a necessity for closer collaboration between researchers and industry leaders. However, that also means that industry input should not be accepted by default as the superior or "only way" option for access to education. Design that is child-centered should also be socio-ethical and humanistic [41], (e.g., what are edtech products' impacts on individual and collective cultures and values?) to safeguard children's rights and privacy.
- *Internal capacities for compliance:* Value-driven edtech providers should consider hiring for roles such as data responsibility officer to establish internal policies for the collection, use, and sharing of children's personal data. Such roles can ensure compliance with local data protection laws and data practice accountability.

### 4.5 For Funders and Investors

- *Transparent assessment:* It is crucial for edtech providers to develop robust products that are grounded in scientific research and validated through rigorous testing. The industry has the responsibility to share their results transparently with key stakeholders, including funders and investors. This includes demonstrating their products' effectiveness, beyond mere compliance with data privacy regulations, but also their value to pedagogy and learning.
- *Responsible investment:* On the other hand, investors must also take responsibility for demanding results before investing in and launching edtech products. As investment has the power to shape the future of education and the lives of the next generation, investing in edtech start-ups that demonstrate effectiveness in improving learning outcomes and are grounded in scientific research can drive a positive impact on education. To build a strong evidence base surrounding new technology, it is essential for different stakeholders to collaborate and work toward child-centered and evidence-based designs. Venture capitalists should also establish investment frameworks that prioritize products that align with such principles.

**Conflicts of Interest and Funding Disclosures** None.

## References

1. Mundy KE, Green A, Verger A. The handbook of global education policy. Wiley Blackwell; 2016.
2. Ho SJ. Correlations between the UN SDGs and educational technology from the perspective of Taiwan's educational innovation. Int J Online Pedagogy Course Design (IJOPCD). 2022;12(3):1–7.
3. Kim NJ, Kim MK. Teacher's perceptions of using an artificial intelligence-based educational tool for scientific writing. Front Educ. 2022;7:755914. Frontiers
4. Participants in an Ethics of Digitalization Research Sprint. Digital ethics in times of crisis: COVID-19 and access to education and learning spaces. Berkman Klein Centre for Internet & Society. 2021. Retrieved from https://cyber.harvard.edu/publication/digital-ethics-times-crisis-covid-19-and-access-education-andlearning-spaces
5. Nazaretsky T, Ariely M, Cukurova M, Alexandron G. Teachers' trust in AI-powered educational technology and a professional development program to improve it. Br J Educ Technol. 2022;53(4):914–31.
6. Belkhir L, Elmeligi A. Assessing ICT global emissions footprint: trends to 2040 & recommendations. J Clean Prod. 2018;177:448–63.
7. Selwyn N. Ed-tech within limits: anticipating educational technology in times of environmental crisis. E-learning Digital Media. 2021;18(5):496–510.

8. Selwyn N. Should robots replace teachers? AI and the future of education. Editorial: Polity Press; 2019.
9. Mayer-Schönberger V, Cukier K. Big data: a revolution that will transform how we live, work and think. John Murray, Impr., Cop; 2013.
10. Boyd D, Crawford K. Critical questions for big data. Inf Commun Soc. 2012;15(5):662–79. https://doi.org/10.1080/1369118X.2012.678878.
11. Saltman KJ. The alienation of fact. The MIT Press eBooks. Published online November 22, 2022. https://doi.org/10.7551/mitpress/14387.001.0001.
12. Piattoeva N. Numbers and their contexts: how quantified actors narrate numbers and decontextualization. Educ Assess Eval Account. 2021;33(3):511–33. https://doi.org/10.1007/s11092-021-09363-x.
13. Manolev J, Sullivan A, Slee R. The datafication of discipline: ClassDojo, surveillance and a performative classroom culture. Learn Media Technol. 2019;44(1):36–51. https://doi.org/10.1080/17439884.2018.1558237.
14. Mehrabi N, Morstatter F, Saxena N, Lerman K, Galstyan A. A survey on bias and fairness in machine learning. ACM Comput Surv. 2021;54(6):1–35. https://doi.org/10.1145/3457607.
15. Zeide E. Student privacy principles for the age of big data: moving beyond Ferpa and Fipps. Law Review. Published February 9, 2018. https://drexel.edu/law/lawreview/issues/Archives/v8-2/zeide/
16. Human Rights Watch. 'How dare they peep into my private life?': children's rights violations by governments that endorsed online learning during the covid-19 pandemic. Human Rights Watch. Published May 25, 2022. https://www.hrw.org/report/2022/05/25/how-dare-they-peep-my-private-life/childrens-rights-violations-governments
17. Hillman V. Media@LSE Working paper series the state of cybersecurity in education: voices from the EdTech Sector. Accessed 15 Apr 2023. https://www.lse.ac.uk/media-and-communications/assets/documents/research/working-paper-series/WP72.pdf
18. Smith H. Algorithmic bias: should students pay the price? AI & Soc. Published online September 12, 2020. https://doi.org/10.1007/s00146-020-01054-3.
19. Bailey N. The murky world of i-ready, grading, and online data. National Education Policy Centre. 2022. https://nepc.colorado.edu/blog/murky-world-i-ready
20. Torres RA. The effect of the I-Ready reading program on student scores on the Northwest Evaluation Association (NWEA®) Measures of Academic Progress (MAP) reading assessment. Doctoral dissertation, Cleveland State University; 2019.
21. Draper CE, Barnett LM, Cook CJ, et al. Publishing child development research from around the world: an unfair playing field resulting in most of the world's child population under-represented in research. Infant Child Dev Published online October 10, 2022. doi:https://doi.org/10.1002/icd.2375.
22. van Dijck J. Datafication, aataism and dataveillance: big data between scientific paradigm and ideology. Surveill Soc. 2014;12(2):197–208. https://doi.org/10.24908/ss.v12i2.4776.
23. Cox J. A tool that monitors how long kids are in the bathroom is now in 1,000 American schools. Vice; 2021. Viewed 21 March 2024, https://www.vice.com/en/article/dy73n7/ehallpass-1000-thousand-schools-monitor-bathroom
24. Fedders B. The constant and expanding classroom: surveillance in K-12 public schools. North Carolina Law Review. 2019;97(6):1673. https://scholarship.law.unc.edu/nclr/vol97/iss6/4
25. Caines A, Silverman S. Back doors, trap doors, and fourth-party deals: how you end up with harmful academic surveillance technology on your campus without even knowing. J Interact Technol Pedagogy. Published December 10, 2021. https://jitp.commons.gc.cuny.edu/back-doors-trap-doors-and-fourth-party-deals-how-you-end-up-with-harmful-academic-surveillance-technology-on-your-campus-without-even-knowing/
26. Picton I, Clark C, Riad L, Cole A. Insights into young People's literacy, critical digital literacy. Online Communication and Wellbeing; 2022. Accessed 15 Apr 2023. https://cdn.literacytrust.org.uk/media/documents/Literacy_critical_digital_online_communication_wellbeing_2021_mYxoTGi.pdf
27. Kumar PC, Vitak J, Chetty M, Clegg TL. The platformisation of the classroom: teachers as surveillant consumers. Surveill Soc. 2019;17(1/2):145–52. https://doi.org/10.24908/ss.v17i1/2.12926.
28. Chanenson J, Chee J, Rajan N, et al. Uncovering privacy and security challenges in K-12 schools. 2023;28 https://doi.org/10.1145/3544548.3580777.
29. Lammers JC, Astuti P. Calling for a global turn to inform digital literacies education. J Adolesc Adult Lit. 2021;64(4):371–7. https://doi.org/10.1002/jaal.1103.
30. Trigos-Carrillo L, Rogers R. Latin American influences on multiliteracies. Literacy Res Theory Method Pract. 2017;66(1):373–88. https://doi.org/10.1177/2381336917718500.
31. Schia NN. The cyber frontier and digital pitfalls in the global south. Third World Q. 2018;39(5):821–37. https://doi.org/10.1080/01436597.2017.1408403.
32. Lai R, Tong S. Promoting evidence-based practice in educational technology for teachers. My College. Accessed 15 Apr 2023. https://my.chartered.college/impact_article/promoting-evidence-based-practice-in-educational-technology-for-teachers/
33. Kimmons R. Current trends (and missing links) in educational technology research and practice. TechTrends. 2020;64(6):803–9. https://doi.org/10.1007/s11528-020-00549-6.
34. Blundell C, Lee KT, Nykvist S. Moving beyond enhancing pedagogies with digital technologies: frames of reference, habits of mind and transformative learning. J Res Technol Educ. 2020;52(2):178–96. https://doi.org/10.1080/15391523.2020.1726235.
35. Ally M. Competency profile of the digital and online teacher in future education. Int Rev Res Open Distrib

Learn. 2019;20(2) https://doi.org/10.19173/irrodl.v20i2.4206.
36. Adiguzel T, Capraro R, Willson V. An examination of teacher acceptance of handheld computers. International. J Spec Educ. 2011;26(3) Accessed 15 Apr 2023. https://files.eric.ed.gov/fulltext/EJ958994.pdf
37. Vladova G, Scheel L, Ullrich A. Acceptance of digital learning in higher education – what role do teachers' competencies play? ECIS 2022 Research papers. Published online June 18, 2022. Accessed 15 Apr 2023. https://aisel.aisnet.org/ecis2022_rp/168
38. Steinberg S, Down B. The SAGE handbook of critical pedagogies. SAGE Publications Ltd; 2020. https://doi.org/10.4135/9781526486455.
39. Lo Cricchio MG, Palladino BE, Eleftheriou A, Nocentini A, Menesini E. Parental mediation strategies and their role on youths' online privacy disclosure and protection. Eur Psychol Published online August 20, 2021. https://doi.org/10.1027/1016-9040/a000450.
40. Pangrazio L, Selwyn N. Critical data literacies: rethinking data and everyday life. MIT Press; 2023.
41. Hillman V. Edtech procurement matters: it needs a coherent solution, Clear Governance and Market Standards Working Paper; 2022. https://www.lse.ac.uk/social-policy/Assets/Documents/PDF/working-paper-series/02-22-Hillman.pdf
42. Bapna A, Nicolai S, Wilson S. Why Edtech frameworks aren't enough. UKFIET the education and development forum. 2021.
43. Pant A, Hoda R, Spiegler SV, Tantithamthavorn C, Turhan B. Ethics in the age of AI: an analysis of AI practitioners' awareness and challenges. ACM Trans Softw Eng Methodol. 2023;
44. Zeide E. The limits of education purpose limitations. University of Miami Law. Review. 2017;71(2):494. Accessed 23 Apr 2023. https://repository.law.miami.edu/umlr/vol71/iss2/8/
45. Baker RS, Hawn A. Algorithmic bias in education Int J Artif Intell Educ. Published online November 18, 2021. https://doi.org/10.1007/s40593-021-00285-9.
46. Radesky J, Hiniker A. From moral panic to systemic change: making child-centred design the default. Int J Child-Comput Interact. 2022;31:100351. https://doi.org/10.1016/j.ijcci.2021.100351.
47. Pant A, Hoda R, Spiegler SV, Tantithamthavorn C, Turhan B. Ethics in the Age of AI: An analysis of AI practitioners' awareness and challenges. 2023. ACM Transactions on Software Engineering and Methodology.
48. Cornell B, Damodaran A. 'Valuing ESG: Doing Good or Sounding Good?', NYU Stern School of Business. 20 March; 2020. Available online: https://papers.ssrn.com/sol3/papers.cfm?abstract_id=3557432
49. Mazzuccato M, Collington R. The big con: How the consulting industry weakens our businesses, infantilises our governments and warps our economies, London: Penguin Random House. 2023;228.
50. UNESCO. UNESCO ICT Competency Framework for Teachers, (version 2.0). Paris: UNESCO; 2011. Available online: https://unesdoc.unesco.org/ark:/48223/pf0000213475
51. OECD. PISA 2021 ICT Framework. Paris: OECD; 2022. Available online: https://www.oecd.org/pisa/sitedocument/PISA-2021-ICT-framework.pdf
52. Trucano M. SABER-ICT Framework Paper for Policy Analysis: Documenting National Educational Technology Policies Around the World Over Time. World Bank Education Technology & Innovation: SABER-ICT Technical Paper Series (#01), Washington, DC: The World Bank; 2016. Available online: https://www.edulinks.org/sites/default/files/media/file/Documenting%20national%20educational%20technology%20policies.pdf
53. ISTE. Teacher Ready: Edtech Product Evaluation Guide, ISTE; 2023. Available online: https://cms-livemedia.iste.org/ISTE_Edtech_Product_Evaluation_Guide_2023_v1023.pdf?_ga=2.164533247.1752817368.1699653248-824124001.1699653248
54. https://www.educateventures.com/consultancy
55. Foerster M, Gourdin A, Huertas E, Möhren J, Ranne P, Roca R. Framework for the Quality Assurance of EAssessment, TESLA (European Horizon project, report, H2020-ICT-2015/H2020-ICT-2015 Agreement Number: 688520); 2019. Available online: https://www.enqa.eu/wp-content/uploads/D4.7-Framework-screen-TeSLA-2606.pdf
56. https://edtech.digitalpromise.org
57. https://tpack.org
58. https://www.nis-2-directive.com/
59. https://www.statista.com/statistics/1273188/cybersecurity-standards-usage-control-systems/
60. Magana AJ, III. Disruptive Classroom Technologies. Oxford Research Encyclopedia of Education. 2019;1–28. https://doi.org/10.1093/acrefore/9780190264093.013.423 Available online: https://maganaeducation.com/wp-content/uploads/2020/11/Magana-Disruptive-Classroom-Technologies.pdf, 1.
61. Hillman V. Taming Edtech: Why Children Stand to Lose in an Unregulated Digitised Classroom. London: Bloomsbury Academic; 2024.
62. 1Edtech. 'IMS Global Learning Consortium Becomes the 1Edtech Consortium', [Press Release], 1Edtec, 25 May; 2022. Available online: https://www.1edtech.org/article/ims-global-learning-consortium-becomes-1edtechconsortium#:~:text=Today%2C%20IMS%20GLobal%20Learning%20Consortium,new%20brand%2C%201EdTech™%20Consortium
63. IMS Global. Consortium. 'TrustEd Apps.: Security Trust for Your Digital Learning Ecosystem', IMS Global Consortium; 2020. Available from: https://www.imsglobal.org/sites/default/files/webinars/webinar_ims_trusted_apps_100620.pdf, 94.
64. ISTE. The Five Pillars for Edtech Procurement, ISTE; 2020. Available online: https://cdn.iste.org/wwwroot/PDF/EL%20January%202020-weboptimized.pdf

# Introduction to the Section on Video Gaming, Violence, and Gambling

Douglas A. Gentile and Marc N. Potenza

The four chapters in this section on gaming, violence, and gambling examine the current state of understanding of video gaming and online gambling as conducted by youth. The section covers a subset of possible topics, with other topics, such as gaming disorder and effects on mental health, addressed in other sections of this handbook.

King et al. (see chapter "Video Gaming and Its Effects on Children and Adolescents: Research Priorities and Recommendations") provide a broad examination of gaming effects, noting how gaming is not monolithic—both games and the people who play them are diverse, making it virtually impossible to provide any singular conclusion about gaming effects as a whole. Instead, as they argue, "effects of gaming on young people's well-being appear complex and multi-directional, and depend on patterns, content, and context of gaming activities." There is evidence to support both positive and negative effects, and research is needed to discriminate when healthy gaming can cross the line into unhealthy gaming.

Bushman et al. (see chapter "Violent Video Games and Aggression") review research on violent game content and aggression. They describe some of the psychological principles through which playing violent games may influence aggression-related cognitions, scripts, expectations, and emotions. Aggressive thoughts and feelings can influence the odds of aggressive behaviors when youth are provoked. It is worth noting that aggression is a broad term that includes verbal, relational, and physical behaviors and their antecedents, and it is primarily at this level that research finds relatively robust effects. Although the question of gaming and real-world *violent* behavior (potentially lethal physical aggression) may receive considerable media coverage, there is comparatively very little research at this level. The authors note that research on whether virtual reality (VR) and augmented reality (AR) enhance some of the effects is needed, as well as more nuanced studies that examine how content interacts with individual differences.

Gainsbury et al. (see chapter "Gaming Convergences with Other Digital Technologies:

D. A. Gentile (✉)
Iowa State University, Ames, IA, USA
e-mail: dgentile@iastate.edu

M. N. Potenza
Department of Psychiatry, Yale University School of Medicine, New Haven, CT, USA

Child Study Center, Yale University School of Medicine, New Haven, CT, USA

Connecticut Mental Health Center, New Haven, CT, USA

Connecticut Council on Problem Gambling, Wethersfield, CT, USA

Department of Neuroscience, Yale University, New Haven, CT, USA

Wu Tsai Institute, Yale University, New Haven, CT, USA


D. A. Christakis, L. Hale (eds.), *Handbook of Children and Screens*,
https://doi.org/10.1007/978-3-031-69362-5_77

Gambling, Pornography, Social Media, and Streaming") examine how gaming technologies have converged with other online activities, such as gambling, social media, and pornography use. They note that despite the apparent differences in these types of activities, "online addictive activities have shared risk factors, including personality factors (e.g., impulsivity), co-occurring psychopathological symptoms (e.g., mood and anxiety disorders), cognitive processes (e.g., attentional biases), and neurobiologies (e.g., when brain regions involved in self-control and emotion regulation remain in development)." They recommend more education for parents, educators, and clinicians so that problematic behaviors may be recognized and treated sooner.

Mestre-Bach et al. (see chapter "Online Gambling in Youth") review online gambling research and the current cultural contexts that appear to include greater acceptance of gambling. They describe several features of adolescent development that likely make adolescents more vulnerable to problematic or addictive engagement in online gambling. They recommend additional research examining etiological factors for problem gambling among youth as well as testing prevention and treatment techniques.

Examining these chapters as a group, there are some themes that emerge. First, a considerable amount is known. Although the chapters focus on the edges of existing knowledge and make recommendations about what studies are needed, the existing data are sufficient to acknowledge that relations exist and warrant attention, with more knowledge needed particularly from longitudinal studies that involve "deep assessments" of multiple factors including but not limited to patterns, content, and context of multiple online behaviors.

Second, underlying much of what these chapters discuss involves learning. In particular, multiple problematic behaviors are supported/promoted by variable reinforcement schedules, and the negative reinforcement of reducing boredom or using games/gambling to "cope." Games use many of the features that enhance learning and motivation, so it should be little surprise that people learn from games, even though they typically do not game with the intent to learn [1, 2].

Third, families could really use this information, but it is unclear from where they will get it. Pediatricians and educators are in an excellent place to support parents, but only if they get the training they need regarding relationships between different types and patterns of screen media activity and developmental outcomes. As an example, many first-year students at universities spend considerable time gaming, then start doing more poorly in classes, and then game to "cope" with the stress of school. If they finally go to counseling services, they may raise concerns regarding their grades, anxieties, and stress. The therapist may ask questions about studying, mood, anxiety, and stress, but often not about gaming, because the patient did not present with concerns about gaming. The patient often does not discuss gaming because gaming may appear to the patient as a solution for coping with stress. Therefore, a crucial aspect may get missed, and the student may continue to perform poorly and possibly fail out of school. Medical professionals and school counselors should be trained to recognize that gaming may be an important etiological factor related to school problems, sleep disorders, mental health, aggression, and other factors, so that they will be more likely to examine patients' media habits as one possible etiological factor. Similarly, given the legalization of sports gambling and increased social acceptability of online sports gambling, similar concerns exist for online gambling.

Fourth, because games have been demonstrated to have powerful motivational and learning effects (both positive and negative), they may be touted as being beneficial for schools. This claim should be viewed with skepticism, however. Just because games may enhance learning does not mean they should be used for learning. If one needs to "gamify" education to get students interested in learning, this may undermine their intrinsic motivation and make it harder for them in situations where they have to persevere through frustration. Research on technology in the classroom generally has found that it does not bring the alleged benefits that are usually given as a reason for including it [3].

In summary, gaming and gaming technologies may have multiple benefits, not the least of these being entertainment. The fact that youth can learn school topics from games indicates that we should take games and game effects seriously. This is perhaps the least likely place for games to be broadly effective, given that many students may resist school lessons. When students are more engaged, they tend to learn better [4]. Youth are highly engaged in gaming as a leisure activity and are therefore likely to learn from the games they play. This includes learning the content, affordances, mechanics, and deeper structural themes across games (e.g., violence solves most problems; when stuck, find a YouTube video to give you the solution rather than figuring it out on your own). Although learning may be one central theme related to gaming, multiple biological and developmental aspects from other domains also likely contribute. As such, gaming warrants continued research and concern.

**Conflict of Interest and Funding Disclosures** DG has consulted for the Partnership for a Healthy Iowa, DQ Institute, the World Health Organization, the National Academies of Sciences, Engineering, and Medicine, and Starfall Education Foundation. He has participated in surveys, mailings, or telephone consultations related to media and child health, including Gaming Disorder, and given academic lectures in grand rounds and other clinical or scientific venues, and consulted as an expert witness. MP has consulted for Opiant Therapeutics, Game Day Data, Baria-Tek, the Addiction Policy Forum, AXA, and Idorsia Pharmaceuticals; been involved in a patent application with Yale University and Novartis; received research support from Mohegan Sun Casino, Children and Screens and the Connecticut Council on Problem Gambling; participated in surveys, mailings, or telephone consultations related to drug addictions, internet use, impulse-control disorders, and other health topics; consulted for or advised gambling, non-profit and legal entities on issues related to internet use, impulse-control and addictive disorders; and given academic lectures in grand rounds, continuing medical education events, and other clinical or scientific venues.

## References

1. Gentile DA, Gentile JR. Violent video games as exemplary teachers: a conceptual analysis. Article. J Youth Adolesc. 2008;37(2):127–41. https://doi.org/10.1007/s10964-007-9206-2.
2. Gentile DA, Gentile JR. Learning from video games (and everything else): the general learning model. Elements in applied social psychology. Cambridge University Press; 2021.
3. Cordes C, Miller E. Fool's gold: a critical look at computers in childhood. College Park, MD: Alliance for Childhood; 2000.
4. Trowler V. Student engagement literature review. Higher Educ Acad 2010;11(1):1–15.

# Video Gaming and Its Effects on Children and Adolescents: Research Priorities and Recommendations

Daniel L. King, Christina R. Galanis, Paul H. Delfabbro, Joel Billieux, Orsolya Király, Natale Canale, Florian Rehbein, Sally M. Gainsbury, and Marc N. Potenza

## 1 Background

Video gaming is a multi-billion-dollar global industry that is projected to continue to grow. The popularity of gaming is fueled by its high accessibility and affordability, particularly in relation to "free to play" casual games on smartphones and other portable devices. Some important elements underlying the appeal of modern video games include their seemingly endless designs and repeatability, complex narratives and role-playing, and opportunities to share experiences and socialize with others [1]. Video games are highly diverse in that they differ according to genre (e.g., shooting, role-playing, and strategy), platforms (e.g., home console, virtual reality), modes (e.g., single-player, competing against others), online connectivity (i.e., playing online or offline), and objectives (e.g., overcoming challenges using violence, persuasion, or stealth tactics). Therefore, they attract and cater to many different interests and motives [2].

Like other digital media, game design and business models are constantly changing. Over the last decade, many game developers have adopted a "games as a service" revenue model whereby games receive regular content updates, which may involve an extra premium or a paid

D. L. King (✉) · C. R. Galanis
College of Education, Psychology & Social Work, Flinders University, Adelaide, Australia
e-mail: daniel.king@flinders.edu.au

P. H. Delfabbro
School of Psychology, The University of Adelaide, Adelaide, Australia

J. Billieux
Institute of Psychology, University of Lausanne, Lausanne, Switzerland

Centre for Excessive Gambling, Addiction Medicine, Lausanne University Hospitals (CHUV), Lausanne, Switzerland

O. Király
Institute of Psychology, ELTE Eötvös Loránd University, Budapest, Hungary

N. Canale
Department of Developmental and Social Psychology, University of Padova, Padova, Italy

F. Rehbein
Department of Social Work, Münster University of Applied Sciences, Münster, Germany

S. M. Gainsbury
School of Psychology, Brain and Mind Centre, University of Sydney, Sydney, Australia

M. N. Potenza
Departments of Psychiatry and Neuroscience, Child Study Center, Yale University School of Medicine, New Haven, CT, USA


D. A. Christakis, L. Hale (eds.), *Handbook of Children and Screens*,
https://doi.org/10.1007/978-3-031-69362-5_78

subscription. Gaming has also become monetized via the rise of esports, or professional leagues and tournaments where players compete against each other, individually or in teams, for prize money, sponsorships, and prestige [3]. Similarly, many online games have become connected to online social networks and have attracted young audiences who watch others play the game rather than play the game themselves. Spectating and paying or donating money to other gamers (e.g., *YouTube* and *Twitch* personalities who "stream," meaning to broadcast live) has become an extremely popular activity in gaming culture [4]. A 2018 survey reported that 78% of US children aged 10–12 years who play video games also watch online gaming videos. These technological innovations and social structures have contributed to gaming becoming more engaging, immersive, and socially connected, and are important considerations for stakeholders in evaluating the social, psychological, and physical effects of gaming on children and adolescents.

Gaming devices are commonplace in most homes with children. In the United States, three out of four households have a "gamer" and 64% of American households own a gaming device [5]. Although gaming may have once been considered primarily an underage activity, only an estimated 1 in 10 US gamers are aged under 20 years old. This reflects the ever-increasing average age of gamers over time, which is cited to be around 35 years of age [6]. However, younger individuals, particularly male adolescents, tend to play more often than other demographic groups, and their usage has increased over time. The Generation M2 study in the United States, for example, reported that average daily gaming usage among individuals aged 8–18 years increased from 24 to 73 minutes between 2004 and 2009, and a recent estimate reported by Alanko (2023) [7] of 150–240 minutes further demonstrates this steady increase over time.

Recent Australian data indicate that males aged 15–24 years play games for an average of 128 min/day [8] and 4.1% of males aged 11–17 years play games for 9 hours or more on an average weekday [9]. Gaming among children and adolescents is often supported or facilitated by parental figures, as over 70% of US parents believe playing video games has educational benefits, and nearly 60% of parents play video games with their children at least once a week [5].

This chapter will summarize some recent developments in the literature on the effects of gaming on young people and highlight some of the challenges and limitations in this work. Then, this chapter will identify some important research questions and future directions for research studies to better understand the role of gaming technologies in young people's lives.

## 2 Current State

There is growing international interest in understanding the potential effects and implications of gaming among children and adolescents. However, recreational gaming encompasses a wide range of products and experiences, and gaming often intersects with other online activities and experiences (e.g., online social networking, web browsing). Therefore, it has been challenging to study gaming holistically [10]. Much literature on gaming media effects has involved studies focusing either on investigating potential positive effects [11], such as visual attention and memory benefits, or ones examining potential negative effects, such as effects of violent video games on aggression and prosocial/antisocial behaviors [12]. Thus, many studies have not applied overarching frameworks conceptualizing both potential positive and negative effects of gaming on children and adolescents. Research into media effects has also been specialized in discrete areas (e.g., cognition, mental health, social networks), with few studies synthesizing data across subfields. Another limitation has been studies of gaming media effects have often tested for direct effects, rather than indirect relationships [13] and reciprocal effects [14].

Studies of effects of gaming have reported mixed findings [12], consistent with reviews of "screen time" among young people that have reported relatively small to negligible effects [15]. The effect of gaming is reported to be complex and dependent on patterns, content, and context of gaming activities [16]. Other pre-existing vulnerabilities, such as social anxiety and attention deficits, may contribute [17]. Among 2442 children aged 7–11 years, Pujol et al. reported that playing video games for 1 hour per week was associated with better performance on certain visuomotor tasks [18]. In contrast, weekly time spent gaming was associated with conduct problems, peer conflicts, and reduced prosocial tendencies, and that these concerns were most apparent among children at an extreme end of the game-time spectrum (i.e., more than 9 hours per week). Using fMRI, the authors also observed changes in basal ganglia white matter and functional connectivity associated with time spent gaming. However, a limitation of the study, as in other studies of media effects, was its correlational design that could not determine directionality.

An important recent development has been the recognition of problem gaming as a mental health disorder in international clinical and public health nomenclature. This recognition has followed several decades of research reporting that specific types/patterns of gaming may be harmful and addictive [19, 20]. In 2013, "internet gaming disorder" was included in Section III (for research purposes) of the DSM-5 and it retains this status in the current DSM-5-TR. In 2019, "gaming disorder" (GD) and "hazardous gaming" were included by the World Health Organization as official designations in the latest revision of the International Classification of Diseases (ICD-11). GD is characterized by persistent gaming behavior, impaired control over gaming, and functional impairment due to gaming for a period of at least 12 months in most instances, but a shorter period may be considered sufficient for young people [21]. Young people with GD play games to the exclusion of other activities, resulting in missed life opportunities and interference with normal routine and basic self-care (i.e., sleep, eating, personal hygiene); real-world social interaction (i.e., meeting friends, family interaction); and important responsibilities (i.e., school, household chores). For further information on gaming disorder, readers are encouraged to consult the chapter dedicated to gaming disorder in this text.

## 3 Future Research

As the gaming industry continues to innovate and its products become increasingly embedded into young people's lives, investigating the psychosocial effects of gaming is a priority area of research. The effects of gaming on young people appear complex and multidirectional. Effectively studying these effects requires sophisticated and holistic research approaches that account for features of gaming, player characteristics, and the social environment. Researchers should investigate the short- and long-term educational, social, and mental and physical health consequences of gaming for children and adolescents, including those involved in professional (esports) gaming activities and streaming via social media.

Researchers should consider how new designs, such as large online games linked to social media profiles and games employing artificial intelligence-driven designs, may leverage player and population data to present more responsive, individually tailored, and immersive playing experiences and how these experiences may affect gaming involvement, including in terms of player investment of time and money. The ethical and social responsibilities of gaming companies in providing a gaming service to underage consumers require further critical exploration in this regard. The literature is lacking academia-industry collaborations committed to understanding and improving player protection and identifying at-risk players.

Recent technological developments enable underage players to engage in betting activities within and in connection with high-profile online games, including those promoted via esports and social media. Some of these activities may be purely "simulated" (i.e., not involving winning real money) [22] whereas others may involve betting systems that enable players to use virtual goods that can be exchanged for real money via a secondary market (e.g., "*skins betting*"). There is a need to delineate specific reinforcing and behavior-shaping elements of gaming (e.g., endlessness, reward schedules, avatar creation), including monetized, gambling-like components, to gain insights into how these activities may promote persistent engagement.

Further research on interventions to manage gaming behavior to directly address problematic gaming is needed. To date, there have been few studies examining the effect of technological measures (e.g., parental locks, time restrictions, consumer messages) on gaming behavior and as a means of reducing problematic gaming among young people. Some research suggests that there are only very limited benefits of restrictive policies targeting children, such as the "Cinderella law" [23] in South Korea, which one study reported was only effective for reducing gaming and spending on gaming among less regular or excessive gamers [24]. Although there is a growing clinical literature, there is a need to identify and develop effective identification methods and interventions, including prevention measures and clinical therapies, for vulnerable children and adolescents and their families. Further, there is a need to examine the neurobiological changes, genetic markers, and epigenetic changes associated with problematic engagement in gaming.

It is important that researchers also evaluate the positive aspects of gaming and the conditions that support the positive aspects of game play. It may be valuable, for example, to consider and contextualize certain frequent patterns of gaming that have benefits alongside the opportunity cost (e.g., spending money on games and less time on other hobbies) as being distinct from harmful gaming or gaming that interferes with daily functioning. This includes studying the potential benefits of "serious" games and "exergames" in therapeutic settings. Such games include those designed to complement cognitive therapy approaches, such as supporting exposure techniques [25]; games for training working memory to reduce symptoms of attention-deficit/hyperactivity disorder [26]; "exergames" for promoting physical exercise [27]; and, virtual reality games for pain management [28]. Research should identify and verify types of gaming activities that help develop cognitive abilities and prosocial behaviors.

Another area of research is the refinement of measurement approaches [29]. Studies of gaming among young people have often relied on self-report data fraught with bias and error. Many individuals misestimate their gaming behaviors. It is recommended that researchers leverage more objective sources of data to measure gaming involvement, including player tracking data that are stored online. It may be possible, for example, to identify patterns of gaming that may indicate a "turning point" from non-problematic to problematic use [30]. Such work may inform early detection and intervention for youth and others. At the same time, gaming activity as a unit of analysis should be treated, where possible, in psychological and social terms and not simply as a form of "screen time" [31]. Screen time and other conventional frequency measures convey a passive and homogenous experience that belie the complexity of gaming.

## 4 Recommendations

An important step forward for research into excessive gaming has been the WHO's recognition of hazardous gaming and gaming disorder in the ICD-11 [32]. These diagnostic categories should enable greater consistency in the conceptualization and assessment of gaming-related problems. Further, these diagnostic categories provide needed clarity of terminology for guiding recommendations in health agendas.

- For policymakers, it is important that the ICD-11 and DSM-5-TR taxonomic developments in gaming disorder and hazardous gaming are reflected by acknowledgment in health policies. Recognizing gaming disorder as a risk to public health is an important step toward achieving health goals, including supporting efforts for consumer awareness and advice. The promotion of healthy and safe online gaming (and other online activities) requires active support from governments. Public health agendas and consumer advice have tended to emphasize restrictions on time spent gaming [33]. This advice could be improved by adding references to the warning signs and symptoms of problem gaming as a mental disorder, and highlighting desirable qualities and social conditions of gaming experiences for children and adolescents.

- Relatedly, there is a need for *regulators* to evaluate the range of gaming products available to young people, including monitoring and considering restrictions on products that are known to be associated with problematic gaming, and which contain features that converge with gambling and/or employ predatory or questionable tactics to target young people. Transparency in game design features and experiences, such as odds associated with paid randomized content, should be considered in regulatory approaches.
- The evidence base on gaming disorders and other problematic online behaviors requires further original research undertakings. The study of gaming disorders is significantly hindered by the lack of resources in many regions, particularly in countries outside of East Asia. *Major funding bodies* should provide the investment necessary to advance the evidence base on problem gaming and other technology-driven problematic behaviors. National agencies with a research focus should coordinate population-level monitoring to study the prevalence of problem gaming and emerging trends in gaming. This includes adding problem gaming measures into epidemiological surveys to monitor the incidence and progression of cases over time in the wider population.
- As gaming products marketed for children and adolescents have incorporated risky features that have drawn attention internationally from regulators, such as predatory monetization (e.g., loot boxes) resembling gambling products [17], it is important for researchers to have access to industry data and other information to better understand risks associated with involvement [34]. Such knowledge should help to better inform young people and their families about these activities, prevention approaches and psychological therapies, cyber-safety programs, and consumer advice on online gaming products. The barriers to industry-academia collaborations require further examination, as it is unclear whether major gaming companies perceive any benefit or incentive to directly supporting research into problematic gaming.
- *Academics and institutions* with a clinical and/or research specialty in problem gaming should develop consumer information and expert workshops to inform the allied health fields. For health practitioners, it is important that they are vigilant to technology use among young people, and screen and assess for these issues in mental health and well-being evaluations. Sharing experiences in delivering treatments with the wider research and clinical community (e.g., via papers, conferences, informal communications) would be valuable to improving the evidence base. Parents and teachers can support public health efforts to reduce problematic gaming by ensuring screen time recommendations are followed and support participation in alternative activities that promote child development, and by supporting research efforts that seek their valuable insights and experiences.
- Finally, *gamers* can share their knowledge with researchers to provide needed lived experience perspectives that can assist, for example, in making interventions more authentic and engaging. The gaming community is also influential in terms of publicly voicing its views and preferences for the types of gaming experiences it values, and making purchasing decisions that support games with more ethical designs that respect the player's time and autonomy.

**Conflict of Interest and Funding Disclosures** None.

## References

1. King DL, Delfabbro PH. Internet gaming disorder: theory, assessment, treatment, and prevention. Cambridge, MA: Elsevier Academic Press; 2019.
2. Király O, Billieux J, Urban R, et al. A comprehensive model to understand and assess the motivational back-

ground of video game use: the Gaming Motivation Inventory (GMI). J Behav Addict. 2022;11:796–819.

3. Brevers D, King DL, Billieux J. Delineating adaptive esports involvement from maladaptive gaming: a self-regulation perspective. Curr Opin Psychol. 2020;36:141–6.
4. Cabeza-Ramírez LJ, Muñoz-Fernández GA, Santos-Roldán L. Video game streaming in young people and teenagers: uptake, user groups, dangers, and opportunities. Healthcare. 2021;9:192.
5. Finances Online. Number of Gamers Worldwide 2022/2023: Demographics, Statistics, and Predictions. Accessed April 24, 2024. https://financesonline.com/number-of-gamers-worldwide/
6. Jovanovic B. Gamer demographics: facts and stats about the most popular hobby in the world. Accessed April 24, 2024. https://dataprot.net/statistics/gamer-demographics
7. Alanko D. The health effects of video games in children and adolescents. Pediatr Rev. 2023;44:23–32.
8. Brand JE, Jervis J. Digital Australia 2022. Eveleigh: IGEA; 2021.
9. Lawrence D, Johnson S, Hafekost J, et al. The mental health of children and adolescents: report on the second Australian child and adolescent survey of mental health and wellbeing. Canberra: Department of Health; 2015. Available at https://www.health.gov.au/internet/main/publishing.nsf/Content/9DA8CA21306FE6EDCA257E2700016945/%24File/child2.pdf
10. Smirni D, Garufo E, Di Falco L, et al. The playing brain. The impact of video games on cognition and behavior in pediatric age at the time of lockdown: a systematic review. Pediatr Rep. 2021;13:401–15.
11. Granic I, Lobel A, Engels RC. The benefits of playing video games. Am Psychol. 2014;69:66.
12. Greitemeyer T. The dark and bright side of video game consumption: effects of violent and prosocial video games. Curr Opin Psychol. 2022;46:101326.
13. Halbrook YJ, O'Donnell AT, Msetfi RM. When and how video games can be good: a review of the positive effects of video games on well-being. Perspect Psychol Sci. 2019;14:1096–104.
14. Hygen BW, Belsky J, Stenseng F, et al. Time spent gaming and social competence in children: reciprocal effects across childhood. Child Dev. 2020;91:861–75.
15. Tang S, Werner-Seidler A, Torok M, et al. The relationship between screen time and mental health in young people: a systematic review of longitudinal studies. Clin Psychol Rev. 2021;86:102021.
16. Houghton S, Lawrence D, Hunter SC, et al. Reciprocal relationships between trajectories of depressive symptoms and screen media use during adolescence. J Youth Adolesc. 2018;47:2453–67.
17. King DL, Delfabbro PH, Deleuze J, et al. Maladaptive player-game relationships in problematic gaming and gaming disorder: a systematic review. Clin Psychol Rev. 2019;73:101777.
18. Pujol J, Fenoll R, Forns J, et al. Video gaming in school children: how much is enough? Ann Neurol. 2016;80(3):424–33. https://doi.org/10.1002/ana.24745.
19. Mihara S, Higuchi S. Cross-sectional and longitudinal epidemiological studies of Internet gaming disorder: a systematic review of the literature. Psychiatry Clin Neurosci. 2017;71:425–44.
20. Rehbein F, Kliem S, Baier D, et al. Prevalence of Internet gaming disorder in German adolescents: diagnostic contribution of the nine DSM-5 criteria in a state-wide representative sample. Addiction. 2015;110:842–51.
21. Saunders J, Hao W, Long J, et al. Gaming disorder: its delineation as a serious condition for diagnosis, management and prevention. J Behav Addict. 2017;6:271–9.
22. Delfabbro PH, King DL, Derevensky JD. Adolescent gambling and problem gambling: prevalence, current issues and concerns. Curr Addict Rep. 2016;3:268–74.
23. Lee C, Kim H, Hong A. Ex-post evaluation of illegalizing juvenile online game after midnight: a case of shutdown policy in South Korea. Telematics Inform. 2017;34:1597–606.
24. Jo W, Sunder S, Choi J, et al. Protecting consumers from themselves: assessing consequences of usage restriction laws on online game usage and spending. Mark Sci. 2020;39:117–33.
25. Goh DH, Ang RP, Tan HC. Strategies for designing effective psychotherapeutic gaming interventions for children and adolescents. Comput Hum Behav. 2008;24:2217–35.
26. Zayeni D, Raynaud JP, Revet A. Therapeutic and preventive use of video games in child and adolescent psychiatry: a systematic review. Front Psych. 2020;11:36.
27. Oliveira CB, Pinto RZ, Saraiva BT, et al. Effects of active video games on children and adolescents: a systematic review with meta-analysis. Scand J Med Sci Sports. 2020;30:4–12.
28. Pourmand A, Davis S, Marchak A, et al. Virtual reality as a clinical tool for pain management. Curr Pain Headache Rep. 2018;22:1–6.
29. King DL, Nogueira-López A, Galanis CR, et al. Reconsidering item response categories in gaming disorder symptoms measurement. J Behav Addict. 2023;12:873–7.
30. Billieux J, Van der Linden M, Achab S, et al. Why do you play world of Warcraft? An in-depth exploration of self-reported motivations to play online and in-game behaviours in the virtual world of Azeroth. Comput Hum Behav. 2013;29:103–9.
31. King DL, Billieux J, Delfabbro PH. Red box, green box: a self-report behavioral frequency measurement approach for behavioral addictions research. J Behav Addict. 2024;13:21. https://doi.org/10.1556/2006.2023.00079.

32. Reed GM, First MB, Bryant RA, et al. Emerging experience with selected new categories in the ICD-11: complex PTSD, prolonged grief disorder, gaming disorder, and compulsive sexual behaviour disorder and prolonged grief disorder. World Psychiatry. 2022;21:189–213.
33. King DL, Delfabbro PH, Doh YY, et al. Policy and prevention approaches for disordered and hazardous gaming and Internet use: an international perspective. Prev Sci. 2018;19:233–49.
34. King DL, Billieux J, Delfabbro PH. COVID-19: science of tech habits needs industry support. Nature. 2021;589:198.

# Violent Video Games and Aggression

Brad J. Bushman, Alessandro Gabbiadini, Tobias Greitemeyer, and Barbara Krahé

## 1 Background

An extensive body of research evidence shows that exposure to violent media can increase aggression in children, which has led many professional and scientific organizations to issue policy statements, including the American Academy of Pediatrics [1]. Although empirical evidence considering different types of media suggests that violent content is more important than the media platform, there are at least four reasons to believe that violent video games might be especially problematic. First, video game play is active. People learn better when they are actively involved. Several studies have shown larger effects for violent video games than for comparable violent media that are not interactive [2–5]. Second, video games demand constant attention, which also increases learning. You cannot "zone out" while playing a violent video game, or your character will be killed. Third, players who identify with violent characters can be psychologically connected with them [6] (e.g., if they are playing a first-person shooter game, they have the same visual perspective as the violent character), which can increase aggression. Fourth, violent games directly reward violent behavior (e.g., earning points by killing enemies). It is well known that rewarding behavior increases its frequency [7].

B. J. Bushman (✉)
School of Communication, The Ohio State University, Columbus, OH, USA
e-mail: bushman.20@osu.edu

A. Gabbiadini
Mind and Behavior Technological Center, Department of Psychology, University of Milano-Bicocca, Milan, Italy

T. Greitemeyer
Department of Psychology, University of Innsbruck, Innsbruck, Austria

B. Krahé
Department of Psychology, University of Potsdam, Potsdam, Germany

## 2 Current State

### 2.1 Effects of Violent Video Game Play on Aggression-Related Outcomes

The positive effects of engaging with video games have been demonstrated in several areas (e.g., teaching academic subjects, simulators), and in these domains, it is accepted without question that video games are very effective teachers [8]. In addition to these intended effects, negative side effects of media use in general and of video game use in particular have been widely demonstrated and acknowledged, for example in terms of reinforcing racial [9] and gender stereotypes [10] or promoting risky behavior [11] (see also chapter "Introduction to the Section on Digital


D. A. Christakis, L. Hale (eds.), *Handbook of Children and Screens*,
https://doi.org/10.1007/978-3-031-69362-5_79

Media, Cognition, and Brain Development"). The processes leading from experiences in the virtual world to real-life outcomes are the same across domains, but the effects differ depending on the content of the media stimuli. Aggressive behavior is acquired by the same underlying processes that shape positive effects of video game use. Therefore, there are good theoretical reasons to assume that engaging in violent actions in the virtual world may also affect what users feel, think, and do in the real world. By the same reasoning, exposure to these stereotypes in video games may contribute to the normalization of discriminatory attitudes and behaviors, potentially influencing individuals' actions beyond the gaming context [10]. In this chapter, we focus on the effects of violent video games on aggression-related outcomes, especially on adolescents.

The relationship between playing violent video games and social behavior has been investigated in numerous experimental, correlational, and longitudinal studies. Experimental studies allow researchers to make cause-effect inferences. Correlational studies allow researchers to examine associations of playing violent video games with more serious forms of aggression, such as violent criminal behavior. Longitudinal studies following the same participants over several points in time are the method of choice for examining the effects of habitually playing violent video games on aggression. A comprehensive meta-analytical summary of these studies involving 381 effect sizes from studies involving more than 130,000 participants was published in 2010 [12]. The analysis found that playing violent video games increased aggressive tendencies and decreased prosocial tendencies. A subsequent meta-analysis published in 2014 [13], which included all new studies not included in the 2010 meta-analysis, reached very similar conclusions. Therefore, it is safe to conclude that playing violent video games affects the social behavior of players, and the effects are not only found in the laboratory, but also in real life, and they can be long-lasting.

Playing violent video games is typically part of a more stable and extensive pattern of leisure activities, especially for adolescents and younger children, rather than a rare or single event. Therefore, it is especially important to examine the impact of repeated exposure to video game violence over extended periods of time. A 2021 meta-analysis of 21 individual studies with a total of almost 16,000 participants found a significant longitudinal correlation of $r = 0.21$ between violent video game play and physical aggression [14]. The association was reduced to $r = 0.11$ when controlling for the stability of physical aggression over time [15], but remained significant and above the established threshold for a "small" effect [16]. Although violent video games can only explain a small part of individual differences in aggression, the same can be said for many other single risk factors for aggression (e.g., exposure to aggressive peers, family environment) [17]. Given that aggression is a highly stable personality characteristic over the life course, the finding that the use of violent video games can additionally explain individual differences in aggression is noteworthy. Longitudinal studies can also disentangle two possible ways in which violent video game use and aggression may be causally related. The "socialization hypothesis" assumes that violent video game use is a cause of aggression, which should be reflected in a significant path from violent video game use at an earlier point in time to aggressive behavior at a later point in time. The "selection hypothesis" postulates that the association is due to more aggressive individuals showing a greater preference for violent video games than nonaggressive individuals, which should be reflected in a significant path from aggression at an earlier time to violent video game use at a later point in time. The empirical evidence shows support for the socialization hypotheses, whereas support for the selection hypothesis is less consistent [18]. Over time, both processes can work together and mutually reinforce each other to create a "downward spiral" toward aggressive behavior in real life [19].

## 2.2 Explaining Violent Video Game Effects

To explain how playing violent video games may increase aggression in players, several well-established theories are available. First, violent video games provide opportunities for social learning through observation [20]. Violent video games may reinforce aggressive behaviors both directly through rewarding or punishing players' actions and indirectly through the observation of other players' or game characters' rewards and punishments. Violence in games is often shown by attractive characters, rewarded by success within the game, justified by a "good cause," and presented as an acceptable form of conflict resolution. Violent actions with positive consequences (e.g., advancing in the game by killing opponents) lead to a positive association between aggressive behavior and positive feelings. In fact, playing favorite video games, like most self-chosen leisure activities, has a positive impact on the player's mood [21]. Over time, this association increases the probability of engaging in aggressive behavior outside the game situation. This finding contradicts the widespread belief that playing violent video games is an effective strategy for releasing aggressive impulses and thereby reducing actual aggressive behavior [22]. Across many studies, the assumption of a cathartic effect of engaging in virtual violence has been shown to be false [23]. Research has found that playing violent video games can temporarily increase positive affect, but it does not result in venting of anger. On the contrary, learning to associate violent actions, such as killing opponents in a video game, with positive feelings will make future aggression more likely.

The process of social learning is not only limited to the acquisition of specific forms of aggressive behavior but also fosters the development of more complex mental representations (called "aggressive scripts") that include norms about the appropriateness of aggression and the tendency to interpret the actions of others as an expression of their hostile intent. Empirical findings support the assumption that the habitual consumption of media containing violence leads to increased normative acceptance and more positive attitudes about aggression. The more violence individuals consume in the media world, the more likely they are to expect hostile intentions from others and interpret the behavior they see in real life as an expression of the actor's intention to harm [24]. These expectations and perceptions increase the odds that they will show an aggressive response.

In addition to the effect on aggression-related thoughts, the habitual use of violent video games also affects aggression-related emotions. As with other intense emotional experiences, repeated exposure to violence leads to habituation. The experience of fear, which is a natural reaction to violence, becomes weakened, both in terms of reduced physiological arousal and in the subjective emotional experience. For example, a study found that pictures showing victims of violence elicited less physiological arousal in viewers the more they used violent video games. No effect of habitual use of violent video game use was found on arousal in response to negative pictures without violence (such as pictures of accident victims or disfigured babies), indicating that desensitization was specific to the violent content of video game use [25].

At the same time, increasing levels of violence are needed to elicit an emotional response, as users become desensitized to violence. Violent video games trivialize violence insofar as it is not carried out in real life but only in a virtual world. Empathy with the victims is not necessary because they do not actually suffer and cannot feel pain. Habituation and desensitization to violence in the virtual world of video games has been related to reduced sympathy with victims of real-world violence, reduced willingness to help others, and lowered inhibition of aggressive behavior in real life [26].

The General Aggression Model integrates the cognitive and emotional effects of violent video games into a comprehensive theoretical framework [27]. It proposes that engaging in virtual violence may lead to the learning, rehearsal, and reinforcement of aggression-related patterns of thinking and feeling via several psychological mechanisms (e.g., promoting positive attitudes about violence, fast, and frequent activation of aggressive scripts, perception, and expectation of others' hostile intent). In combination, these changes contribute to the development of aggression as a stable personality trait.

### 2.3 Conclusions

This chapter is not meant to "demonize" video games as such, but to highlight the risk of exposure to violence as a particular type of game content. Negative media effects are much less controversial in other domains (e.g., thin media models and eating disorders; media models that drink or smoke; gender stereotypes in children's media). Exposure to violent media models can also have unintended negative effects.

The challenge is to reap the benefits of video games (e.g., improved spatial visualization and attentional skills), while avoiding their potential drawbacks. This can be accomplished by playing nonviolent real-world problem-solving games. Indeed, there are video games on the market that provide an excellent entertaining experience while promoting essential skills (e.g., eye-hand coordination, fine motor control), raising awareness about important issues (e.g., global warming solutions, pro-environmental behaviors), and teaching prosocial behaviors. Thus, giving up violent video games may easily be compensated by a wide choice of nonviolent games without losing the fun of engaging in this popular form of leisure activity.

## 3 Future Research

Hundreds of studies have examined the consequences of playing violent video games. Of course, not all of them have shown that violent video games lead to aggression. Because aggression is influenced by multiple factors, with violent video gaming being only one of them, it is to be expected that some studies do not find significant effects. However, when synthesizing the results of all relevant studies, most meta-analyses have shown a positive link between exposure to violent video games and aggressive thoughts and behaviors. Hence, we believe it is time to move beyond the question of whether violent video games increase aggression to seek answers to other important questions.

The psychological mechanisms underlying the link between violent video games and aggression need to be explored further. The role of individual differences (e.g., cognitive processes, differences in emotional regulation) and contextual factors that may influence the effects of violent video games deserve further investigation. More research is also needed to determine who is most motivated to play and why. The motivations behind the games people choose to play are complex and go beyond simple entertainment value [28].

Furthermore, today's video game producers are exploring the possibilities offered by virtual reality (VR) and augmented reality (AR), which can provide unprecedented immersive experiences. Newer video games are more realistic and immersive and may indeed have larger effects on players compared to older games. The high level of immersion produces the so-called sense of presence, which is users' sense of being inside the simulated environment, and through embodied avatars, players feel transported into the game (e.g., "becoming" a soldier in a war scenario). Preliminary research shows the VR technology intensifies violent video game effects [29], but further research is needed on topics such as situated immersion (i.e., the illusion of literally existing within the game) as determined by factors such as intensity, vividness, and graphics quality. Moreover, AR integrates virtual game elements with the physical environment of the players in real time (e.g., "turning" the living room into a war scenario through a simple smartphone). To date, no study has investigated the effects of combining computer generated violent elements with the real world. In addition, many video games contain other objectionable content (e.g., discriminatory behavior, prejudice, sexual objectification of women, alcohol, and drug use). It is therefore necessary to look more closely at the "side effects" of violent video games that go beyond aggression, especially during adolescence, the stage of life when individual identity comes to be consolidated.

Additionally, psychoeducation about the potential effects of violent video games and the importance of managing one's emotions and behavior may help prevent aggression. Several promising psychological strategies have already been proposed in the literature, such as (1) decreasing exposure time, (2) substituting violent media content with nonviolent media content, (3) increasing critical consumption by fostering cognitive knowledge structures against the portrayal of violence [30], and (4) empowering beliefs in self-control [31]. However, further research is needed to fully understand the effectiveness of these interventions and identify other potential approaches to preventing aggression after playing violent video games. In this regard, future research could explore the effectiveness of parental and educational guidance in reducing the negative effects of violent video games. Finally, more knowledge is needed about the dosage question: How much video gaming represents a risk for aggression or, conversely, is there a "safe dose" that does not give cause for concern?

## 4 Recommendations

- Intervention efforts have mostly addressed violent media use in general rather than violent video game use in particular. Three intervention approaches have been used: (1) "co-viewing" in the form of joint use and evaluation of media contents, (2) "restrictive mediation" aimed at reducing exposure to violent media content, and (3) "critical viewing," the promotion of understanding the mechanisms by which violent content may lead to aggression [32, 33].
- Although the effectiveness of critical viewing has been demonstrated for different age groups, co-viewing and restrictive mediation were found to be effective in younger children. For adolescents, they may be counterproductive, as these interventions run counter to the desire for independence and autonomy in this developmental period [34].
- One recommendation is to strengthen adolescents' understanding of violent video game effects and promote their ability and motivation to substitute violent content with nonviolent content. For younger children, adult mediation/co-playing may be effective.
- Children should not play video games marked as age inappropriate by established video game content rating systems (e.g., the ESRB in North America and PEGI in Europe). While these rating systems serve as valuable tools for informing consumers about the content of video games, additional efforts are needed to regulate children's exposure to violent content further. For instance, guns in video games are especially problematic. Indeed, the leading cause of death among children and adolescents in the United States ages 1–19 is firearm-related injuries [35]. Research shows that video games with guns make real guns more attractive to children [36].
- Fostering collaboration between video games industry stakeholders, policymakers, parents, and researchers, it is possible to develop comprehensive strategies that prioritize the well-being of children and promote a safe and positive gaming environment for all.

**Conflict of Interest and Funding Disclosures** None.

## References

1. https://publications.aap.org/pediatrics/article/138/2/e20161298/52469/Virtual-Violence
2. Lin J. Identification matters: a moderated mediation model of media interactivity, character identification, and video game violence on aggression. J Commun. 2013;63(4):682–702. https://doi.org/10.1111/jcom.12044.
3. Lin J-H. Do video games exert stronger effects on aggression than film? The role of media interactivity and identification on the association of violent content and aggressive outcomes. Comput Hum Behav. 2013;29(3):535–43. https://doi.org/10.1016/j.chb.2012.11.001.
4. Silvern SB, Williamson PA. The effects of video game play on young children's aggres-

sion, fantasy, and prosocial behavior. J Appl Dev Psychol. 1987;8(4):453–62. https://doi.org/10.1016/0193-3973(87)90033-5.
5. Tamborini R, Eastin MS, Skalski P, Lachlan K, Fediuk TA, Brady R. Violent virtual video games and hostile thoughts. J Broadcast Electron Media. 2004;48(3):335–57.
6. Konijn EA, Nije Bijvank M, Bushman BJ. I wish I were a warrior: the role of wishful identification in the effects of violent video games on aggression in adolescent boys. Dev Psychol. 2007;43(4):1038–44. https://doi.org/10.1037/0012-1649.43.4.1038.
7. Carnagey NL, Anderson CA. The effects of reward and punishment in violent video games on aggressive affect, cognition, and behavior. Psychol Sci. 2005;16(11):882–9. https://doi.org/10.1111/j.1467-9280.2005.01632.x.
8. Gentile DA, Gentile JR. Violent video games as exemplary teachers: a conceptual analysis. J Youth Adolesc. 2008;37(2):127–41. https://doi.org/10.1007/s10964-007-9206-2.
9. Yang GS, Gibson B, Lueke AK, Huesmann LR, Bushman BJ. Effects of avatar race in violent video games on racial attitudes and aggression. Soc Psychol Personal Sci. 2014;5(6):698–704. https://doi.org/10.1177/1948550614528.
10. Gabbiadini A, Riva P, Andrighetto L, Volpato C, Bushman BJ. Acting like a tough guy: violent-sexist video games, identification with game characters, masculine beliefs, & empathy for female violence victims. PLoS One. 2016;11(4):e0152121. https://doi.org/10.1371/journal.pone.0152121.
11. Fischer P, Greitemeyer T, Kastenmüller A, Vogrincic C, Sauer A. The effects of risk-glorifying media exposure on risk-positive cognitions, emotions, and behaviors: a meta-analytic review. Psychol Bull. 2011;137(3):367–390. https://doi.org/10.1037/a0022267
12. Anderson CA, Shibuya A, Ihori N, et al. Violent video game effects on aggression, empathy, and prosocial behavior in eastern and Western countries: a meta-analytic review. Psychol Bull. 2010;136(2):151–73. https://doi.org/10.1037/a0018251.supp.
13. Greitemeyer T, Mugge DO. Video games do affect social outcomes: a meta-analytic review of the effects of violent and prosocial video game play. Personal Soc Psychol Bull. 2014;40(5):578–89. https://doi.org/10.1177/0146167213520459.
14. Burkhardt J, Lenhard W. A meta-analysis on the longitudinal, age-dependent effects of violent video games on aggression. Media Psychol. 2022;25(3):499–512. https://doi.org/10.1080/15213269.2021.1980729.
15. Drummond A, Sauer JD, Ferguson CJ. Do longitudinal studies support long-term relationships between aggressive game play and youth aggressive behaviour? A meta-analytic examination. R Soc Open Sci. 2020;7(7):200373. https://doi.org/10.1098/rsos.200373.
16. Cohen, J. (1988). Statistical power analysis for the behavioral sciences (2nd Ed.). Hillsdale, NJ: Lawrence Erlbaum.Sci. 2020;7(7):200373.
17. Dubow EF, Huesmann LR, Boxer P, Smith C. Childhood and adolescent risk and protective factors for violence in adulthood. J Crim Just. 2016;45:26–31. https://doi.org/10.1016/j.jcrimjus.2016.02.005.
18. Krahé B, Möller I. Longitudinal effects of media violence on aggression and empathy among German adolescents. J Appl Dev Psychol. 2010;31(5):401–9. https://doi.org/10.1016/j.appdev.2010.07.003.
19. Slater MD, Henry KL, Swaim RC, Anderson LL. Violent media content and aggressiveness in adolescents: a downward spiral model. Commun Res. 2003;30(6):713–36. https://doi.org/10.1177/0093650203258281.
20. Bandura A, Ross D, Ross SA. Vicarious reinforcement and imitative learning. J Abnorm Soc Psychol. 1963;67(6):601–7. https://doi.org/10.1037/h0045550.
21. Villani D, Carissoli C, Triberti S, Marchetti A, Gilli G, Riva G. Videogames for emotion regulation: a systematic review. Games Health J. 2018;7(2):85–99. https://doi.org/10.1089/g4h.2017.0108.
22. Kersten R, Greitemeyer T. Why do habitual violent video game players believe in the cathartic effects of violent video games? A misinterpretation of mood improvement as a reduction in aggressive feelings. Aggress Behav. 2022;48(2):219–31. https://doi.org/10.1002/ab.22005.
23. Gentile DA. Catharsis and media violence: a conceptual analysis. Societies. 2013;3(4):491–510. https://doi.org/10.3390/soc3040491.
24. Bushman BJ. Violent media and hostile appraisals: a meta-analytic review. Aggress Behav. 2016;42(6):605–13. https://doi.org/10.1002/ab.21655.
25. Bartholow BD, Bushman BJ, Sestir MA. Chronic violent video game exposure and desensitization to violence: behavioral and event-related brain potential data. J Exp Soc Psychol. 2006;42(4):532–9. https://doi.org/10.1016/j.jesp.2005.08.006.
26. Brockmyer JF. Desensitization and violent video games: mechanisms and evidence. Child Adolesc Psychiatr Clin N Am. 2022;31(1):121–32. https://doi.org/10.1016/j.chc.2021.06.005.
27. Anderson CA, Bushman BJ. Media violence and the general aggression model. J Soc Issues. 2018;74(2):386–413. https://doi.org/10.1111/josi.12275.
28. Gabbiadini A, Riva P. The lone gamer: social exclusion predicts violent video game preferences and fuels aggressive inclinations in adolescent players. Aggress Behav. 2017;44(2):113–24. https://doi.org/10.1002/ab.21735.
29. Lull RB, Bushman BJ. Immersed in violence: presence mediates the effect of 3D violent video gameplay on angry feelings. Psychol Pop Media Cult. 2016;5(2):133–44. https://doi.org/10.1037/ppm0000062.

30. Kirsh SJ. Media and youth: a developmental perspective. Malden: Wiley-Blackwell; 2010.
31. Gabbiadini A, Riva P, Andrighetto L, Volpato C, Bushman BJ. Preliminary evidence of the effectiveness of a brief self-control intervention on reducing the short-term harmful consequences of violent video games on adolescents. J Appl Soc Psychol. 2022;52(4):246–58. https://doi.org/10.1111/jasp.12854.
32. Krahé B, Busching R. Breaking the vicious cycle of media violence use and aggression: a test of intervention effects over 30 months. Psychol Violence. 2015;5(2):217–26. https://doi.org/10.1037/a0036627.
33. Shany Y, Yablon YB. The contribution of face-to-face and embedded mediation to early childhood aggression after watching violent media content. Psychol Violence. 2021;11(6):519–28. https://doi.org/10.1037/vio0000385.
34. Nathanson AI. The unintended effects of parental mediation of television on adolescents. Media Psychol. 2002;4(3):207–30. https://doi.org/10.1207/S1532785XMEP0403_01.
35. Goldstick JE, Cunningham RM, Carter P. One of the leading causes of death among young people in the US is gun violence. N Engl J Med. 2022;386:1955–6. https://doi.org/10.1056/NEJMc2201761.
36. Chang JH, Bushman BJ. Effect of exposure to gun violence in video games on children's dangerous behavior with real guns. Randomized clinical trial. JAMA Pediatr. 2019;2(5):e194319. https://doi.org/10.1001/jamanetworkopen.2019.4319.

# Gaming Convergences with Other Digital Technologies: Gambling, Pornography, Social Media, and Streaming

Sally M. Gainsbury, Thomas B. Swanton, Isabel Baenas, Jesús Castro-Calvo, Fernando Fernández-Aranda, Maèva Flayelle, Susana Jiménez-Murcia, Gemma Mestre-Bach, and Joël Billieux

## 1 Background

Severe problems arising from gambling and gaming have been recognized through the diagnosis of gambling and gaming disorders [1]. In 2013, the American Psychiatric Association's Diagnostic and Statistical Manual of Mental Disorders, Fifth Edition, (*DSM-5*) included Internet Gaming Disorder in Section III, dedicated to those conditions for which there was not yet sufficient empirical evidence to justify their consideration as mental disorders [2]. A few years later, the World Health Organization officially recognized gaming disorder in the

S. M. Gainsbury (✉) · T. B. Swanton
The University of Sydney, School of Psychology, Brain & Mind Centre, Gambling Treatment & Research Clinic, Sydney, NSW, Australia
e-mail: sally.gainsbury@sydney.edu.au

I. Baenas
Clinical Psychology Department, Bellvitge University Hospital-IDIBELL, Barcelona, Spain

Ciber Physiopathology of Obesity and Nutrition (CIBERObn), Instituto de Salud Carlos III, Madrid, Spain

Psychoneurobiology of Eating and Addictive Behaviors Group, Neuroscience Program, Bellvitge Biomedical Research Institute (IDIBELL), L'Hospitalet de Llobregat, Catalonia, Spain

J. Castro-Calvo
Department of Personality, Assessment, and Psychological Treatments, University of Valencia-Estudi General, Valencia, Spain

F. Fernández-Aranda · S. Jiménez-Murcia
Clinical Psychology Department, Bellvitge University Hospital-IDIBELL, Barcelona, Spain

Ciber Physiopathology of Obesity and Nutrition (CIBERObn), Instituto de Salud Carlos III, Madrid, Spain

Psychoneurobiology of Eating and Addictive Behaviors Group, Neuroscience Program, Bellvitge Biomedical Research Institute (IDIBELL), L'Hospitalet de Llobregat, Catalonia, Spain

Department of Clinical Sciences, School of Medicine, University of Barcelona, Barcelona, Spain

M. Flayelle
Institute of Psychology, University of Lausanne, Lausanne, Switzerland

G. Mestre-Bach
Instituto de Investigación, Transferencia e Innovación, Universidad Internacional de La Rioja, La Rioja, Spain

J. Billieux
Institute of Psychology, University of Lausanne, Lausanne, Switzerland

Center for Excessive Gambling, Addiction Medicine, Lausanne University Hospitals (CHUV), Lausanne, Switzerland


D. A. Christakis, L. Hale (eds.), *Handbook of Children and Screens*,
https://doi.org/10.1007/978-3-031-69362-5_80

International Classification of Diseases, Eleventh Revision (*ICD-11*)—adding another diagnosis to the category of "Disorders due to substance use or addictive behaviours," along with Gambling Disorder [3].

Although problematic engagement in other online activities is increasingly acknowledged, evidence remains insufficient that these merit inclusion as other specific addictive disorders. There are similarities between non-substance-related addictive behaviors in terms of diagnostic criteria (which are modeled on criteria for substance use disorders), comorbidities, and treatment. Brand and colleagues established a set of criteria to inform decisions about which conditions could be included in the *ICD-11* category of "Other specified disorders due to addictive behaviours" [4]. These criteria include: i) clinical relevance of the addictive behavior, which impacts on an individual's functioning; ii) existing theoretical models of addictive behaviors also explain the new condition; and iii) empirical evidence demonstrates neurocognitive, physiological, genetic, and psychological mechanisms shared with other addictive behaviors.

Nonetheless, there is currently limited evidence that problematic Internet use related to various activities is comorbid or related to each other. Among adults, recent studies using network analyses have demonstrated that gaming disorder and problematic pornography use, problematic shopping, problematic use of social networking sites, and problematic online gambling constitute relatively independent and distinct conditions, despite sharing certain similarities in terms of their clinical expression and symptoms [5].

The video game industry has undergone a significant evolution in recent years due to the convergence of various digital technologies. These developments have led to the incorporation of gaming elements into other products and apps, such as those related to online gambling, pornography, social media, and on-demand video-streaming. The convergence of gaming and gambling has potentially been the most noticeable; online gaming has incorporated gambling-like elements such as loot boxes as well as in-game financial elements such as microtransactions, and in-game currencies that can be used (including through third parties) for gambling/gambling-like activities such as skins betting. Esports refers to professional gaming tournaments, which now represent a betting market [6]. Social games, often available through or linked with social media platforms, include a prominent genre called social casino games. Social casino games replicate gambling activities without real-money payouts—although players can pay to obtain virtual chips to gamble. This game genre consistently ranks among the most popular and profitable. Concerns have emerged that social casino games may increase favorable attitudes toward gambling and misrepresent the likelihood of winning [7], leading some individuals—including adolescents—to migrate to gambling because of their game play [8].

Increasing digitalization of activities has led to concerns about other potentially problematic online behaviors, such as social media use, on-demand streaming, and compulsive sexual behaviors (e.g., pornography viewing) [4]. The convergence of gaming and pornography has resulted in the creation of a new genre of video games known as "adult games." These games feature sexually explicit content and often involve interactive elements that allow players to customize their avatar and control the actions of characters. The convergence of gaming and on-demand video-streaming has led to the creation of "gamified watching," in which on-demand video-streaming platforms use gaming elements to encourage consumers to engage with content. Platforms include design features that challenge users' self-control, as well as immersive, social, and comparative elements [9]. These developments raise concerns about the potential for dysregulated and addictive behaviors, exploitation of vulnerable groups (especially children and adolescents), and negative impacts on individuals and society. It is therefore crucial to consider carefully the ethical and social implications of these developments and ensure that they are regulated appropriately.

## 2 Current State

### 2.1 Gaming and Gambling

Similarities between video games and gambling have led to the proposition that video gaming could act as a "gateway" to gambling. However, to date, there is limited evidence to support this hypothesis [10]. A review found only a small correlation between overall gambling and video game engagement, which could be accounted for by demographic and personality factors [10]. There is also limited evidence of a relationship between problem gaming and problem gambling.

There does, however, appear to be a relationship between loot box purchases and problem gambling symptoms. Loot boxes are a "surprise mechanic" within games whereby players can win/earn or purchase an item (with real-world, virtual, or in-game currency) without knowing which item they will "randomly" receive. Meta-analytic evidence shows that people with greater symptoms of problem gambling spend more on loot boxes than people with fewer problem gambling symptoms [11]. The size of the association between loot box purchasing and problem gambling symptomology is typically stronger for adolescents than for adults. However, there is mixed evidence about whether loot box spending is associated with psychological distress [12, 13]. Further, evidence regarding the directionality and causality of relationships between problematic gambling and loot box spending is lacking.

Studies based on self-reports have found individuals who play social casino games also present with a tendency to gamble—although this may be related to having a specific interest in gambling activities. For example, an Australian study of adolescents found spending money on social casino games to be a risk factor for problem gambling and related to higher levels of psychological distress compared to social casino game players who had not paid to play [14]. Two-thirds of paying social casino game players recalled that their social casino game use preceded their involvement in gambling. A longitudinal study following up adolescents over time found that simulated Internet gambling was related to onset of gambling and increased gambling problems; however, factors such as advertising, cognitive distortions, and gambling involvement also played a role [15].

### 2.2 Gaming and Social Media

A positive association between social media use and gaming has been described, as well as between problematic social media use and gaming disorder. Although epidemiological studies related to the prevalence of comorbidity between problematic social media use and gaming disorder are scarce, younger age has been described as a shared vulnerability factor [16, 17]. Potential vulnerability factors related to the development of these digital media-based addictive behaviors include social factors (e.g., lower perceived social competence; lower educational, social, and occupational levels), impulsivity, psychiatric comorbidities (e.g., anxiety, depression, substance use, attention deficit/hyperactivity disorder, obsessive-compulsive disorder), and brain development stage (e.g., higher affective and behavioral dysregulation at early ages due to lower neurological maturity)—with influence varying according to age and sex [16, 18].

Beyond risk factors for problematic use of social media and video games and their differences by sex/gender, it is important to consider the convergence between both forms of entertainment and communication. Social media platforms (e.g., Facebook, Twitch, YouTube, Douyu) can integrate gaming activity from multiple genres including direct access to games, and by creating a platform for gaming communities to host discussions [17]. This potentially involves the need for users to share data or register on a platform to access certain games and related content, which may create privacy and security risks for users, who in many cases are children or adolescents.

Gamers often report spending leisure time on other screen-related activities [19], such as using social platforms to watch videos of gameplay or share gaming-related content (e.g., *YouTube*).

Gaming communities (i.e., in-game communities) are inherent to gaming [20]. Identification with the social identity of a virtual community modulates gaming behavior and potentially motivates gaming and normalizes maladaptive gaming behaviors [20]. Apart from in-game communities, forums exist where gamers interact, share, and discuss their experiences. In the social context of in- and out-game communities, gamers may modulate others' gaming habits within a gaming network—a type of social contagion effect [20]. In contrast with gambling, a protective role of gaming communities in relation to problematic gaming and purchasing has not yet been described, possibly conditioned by the potential detrimental impact on the game performance for the team [20]. In this context, social networking via social platforms allows people with similar interests to be connected, but might contribute to maintenance of the problematic behavior due to social pressures and distorted cognitive aspects (e.g., "fear of missing out") [18].

The convergence of social media and gaming/gambling is apparent through advertising for online activities on social media seeking to attract new users. Social media users might have greater exposure to gaming and gambling activities, and subsequently be more likely to experience related harms.

### 2.3 Gaming and Problematic Pornography Use

Male sex and younger age are two key shared vulnerability factors for problematic gaming and pornography use [21]. A systematic review of experimental studies suggests that problematic pornography use is related to attentional biases, deficient inhibitory control, poorer performance in tasks assessing working memory, and decision-making impairments [22]. These cognitive processes are also relevant when explaining the manifestation and severity of gaming disorder [23], meaning that both conditions share similar cognitive underpinnings. Gaming disorder and problematic pornography are driven by common motives (e.g., hedonic/recreation-related motives, pleasure seeking, fantasy or escape from stress or intense negative emotions) and share underlying psychological processes [24]. Studies show that the prevalence, frequency, and pattern of pornography consumption (including the risk of developing problematic pornography use) is similar—or even increased—among adolescents [25], suggesting that features promoting over-engagement may especially affect this population.

Ecological data relating to the 2018 crash of Fortnite (one of the most popular video games among adolescents) showed that during forced abstinence from gaming, pornography use increased—in particular, consumption of pornographic content related to the video game [26]. This increase suggests that pornography consumption may constitute a "compensation behavior," such as researching information about video games in forums or watching gaming videos on YouTube [27].

At the intersection between gaming, problematic pornography use, and social networking is the use of massively multiplayer virtual worlds for sexual purposes (e.g., Second Life). Second Life is an online multimedia platform that allows people to create avatars and interact with other users. Built-in customization tools allow users to sexualize their avatars according to personal preferences and engage in sexual interactions with other users (or "avatar sex") [28].

Pornographic websites commonly include design elements that seek to optimize user engagement (e.g., search by preferred categories, algorithm-based content recommendations), facilitating an immersive and interactive viewing experience, and increasing attention and "time on site." [29] Dating apps, such as Tinder, are another example where gaming elements are incorporated with the aim of increasing "time on site." Tinder's design (the overall interface, "swiping" function) gamifies the process of finding a date. Basic dynamics of Tinder use include rewarding elements (e.g., receiving a match), as well as multiple features that might promote uncontrolled and problematic engagement [9]. Design features similar to those used by the gaming and gambling industry might promote excessive engagement in online pornography use and related sexual behaviors.

### 2.4 Gambling, Gaming, and On-Demand Video Streaming

Evidence suggests that problematic patterns of on-demand video streaming and binge-watching (i.e., watching multiple episodes of a TV series in one session) occur among adults. However, research on this topic studying adolescent populations remains in its infancy. Paschke and colleagues suggest that adolescents might be especially vulnerable to developing problematic on-demand video streaming/binge-watching due to immature cognitive-control abilities [30]. Preliminary qualitative research suggests that binge-watching in adolescence is primarily prompted by a fear of missing out. That is, adolescents potentially feel pressure to be part of a cultural conversation and a need to immerse themselves in TV series to avoid boredom and to escape from everyday life [31]. Similar to well-established correlates of gaming disorder, correlates of binge-watching and problematic on-demand video streaming in adolescence include depression, anxiety, symptoms of insomnia, poorer school performance, loneliness, emotional problems, conduct problems, cognitive problems, and inattention [30].

Attention has also been paid to the promotion of gambling via video game streaming services, such as Twitch. One study found that Twitch, which primarily streams video game content, also streams gambling with social and real money prizes and was used by content creators as a strategy to increase gambling engagement and monetization [32].

## 3 Future Research

Ongoing research is needed given the dynamic nature of online activities and differences between generational cohorts.

Large, representative samples are needed to explore vulnerability profiles and protective factors, the clinical course of conditions, influence of comorbidities, and relationships with psychological well-being, as well as predictors of severity for problematic online behaviors, including among children and adolescents. Longitudinal research is needed over the course of adolescence to young adulthood to determine if individuals naturally "grow out" of problematic online behaviors. Exploration of the long-term consequences of early and prolonged exposure to various online content types is a research priority—particularly in terms of the potential to interfere with development, foster unhealthy attitudes and values, and undermine emotional and psychological well-being.

Research should consider the impact of specific design features and mechanics within games and gamified online activities [9], with a view to identifying predatory mechanics that might act to deceive or exert undue influence on individuals [33], especially children and adolescents who do not have well-developed analytical and decision-making abilities.

## 4 Recommendations

- The constantly evolving digital environment, and the changing nature of consumers' interactions with emerging technologies mean that legislative, regulatory, and judicial bodies need to reassess the consideration (i.e., the wager) and prize components of legal definitions of gambling. In particular, defining the "value" of virtual objects is relevant, including what constitutes a consideration of value by users in both the digital and "real" worlds.
- As many online content providers are not specifically regulated and industry self-regulation may be insufficient to protect consumers, particularly children and adolescents, greater efforts are needed to assess the suitability of content offered through online platforms and age restrictions for various activities and products. Active involvement of policymakers is crucial in the development of effective

educational, preventive, and therapeutic strategies related to digital media use.

- Parents should be involved in their children's use of digital media, monitoring screen time per day and actively encouraging engagement in entertainment activities other than online gaming, video streaming, and social networking. Parents should monitor game play to ensure that games played by children and adolescents do not contain age-inappropriate content and participate in age-appropriate online activities with adolescents to enable informed discussions around identifying and responding to risky scenarios and setting healthy boundaries on use.
- Educational centers should provide information to students and parents related to adaptive and healthy uses of digital media, help educators and parents to screen and identify potential problematic behaviors, encourage non-screen leisure activities, and provide referrals to specialized services when necessary.
- Social media and networks linked to gaming should contain warnings about risks relating to privacy and social relations in the virtual world (e.g., cyberbullying, *griefing*, *trolling*, *identity theft*, and *grooming*) [34].
- Clinicians, including generalists and specialist health workers, should receive training enabling them to identify online problematic behaviors among children and adolescents. Clinical programs should distribute social, psychoeducational, and therapeutic resources related to digital media use among parents and at-risk/affected individuals.
- Health campaigns should be developed to increase awareness about the potential for games to contain age-inappropriate content for children and the importance of balancing screen time with other activities as part of a healthy lifestyle.

**Conflict of Interest and Funding Disclosures** SG has an updated conflict of interest statement available here: https://www.sydney.edu.au/science/about/our-people/academic-staff/sally-gainsbury.html. TS has received a PhD scholarship through the NSW Government's Gambling Research Capacity Grants program, funded by the NSW Responsible Gambling Fund, and supported by the NSW Office of Responsible Gambling. He has been awarded student travel grants by the National Association for Gambling Studies. FF-A and SJ-M received consultancy honoraria and conference traveling support from Novo Nordisk and FFA editorial honoraria as EIC from Wiley. IB, GM-B, JC-C, MF, and JB have no conflict of interest relevant to this chapter to disclose.

## References

1. Stein DJ, Billieux J, Bowden-Jones H, et al. Balancing validity, utility and public health considerations in disorders due to addictive behaviours. World Psychiatry. 2018;17(3):363–4. https://doi.org/10.1002/wps.20570.
2. American Psychiatric Association. Diagnostic and statistical manual of mental disorders. 5th ed.; 2013. https://doi.org/10.1176/appi.books.9780890425596.
3. World Health Organisation. International Statistical Classification of Diseases and Related Health Problems. 11th ed.; 2019. https://icd.who.int/
4. Brand M, Rumpf HJ, Demetrovics Z, et al. Which conditions should be considered as disorders in the International Classification of Diseases (ICD-11) designation of "other specified disorders due to addictive behaviors"? J Behav Addict. 2020;11(2):150–9. https://doi.org/10.1556/2006.2020.00035.
5. Baggio S, Starcevic V, Billieux J, et al. Testing the spectrum hypothesis of problematic online behaviors: a network analysis approach. Addict Behav. 2022;135:107451. https://doi.org/10.1016/j.addbeh.2022.107451.
6. Brevers D, King DL, Billieux J. Perspectives on adaptive and maladaptive involvement into esports. Addict Behav. 2023;144:107716. https://doi.org/10.1016/j.addbeh.2023.107716.
7. Abarbanel B, Gainsbury SM, King D, Hing N, Delfabbro PH. Gambling games on social platforms: how do advertisements for social casino games target young adults? Policy Internet. 2017;9(2):184–209. https://doi.org/10.1002/poi3.135.
8. Gainsbury SM, Russell AMT, King DL, Delfabbro P, Hing N. Migration from social casino games to gambling: motivations and characteristics of gamers who gamble. Comput Hum Behav. 2016;63:59–67. https://doi.org/10.1016/j.chb.2016.05.021.
9. Flayelle M, Brevers D, King DL, Maurage P, Perales JC, Billieux J. A taxonomy of technology design features that promote potentially addictive online behaviours. Nat Rev Psychol. 2023;2:136–50. https://doi.org/10.1038/s44159-023-00153-4.
10. Delfabbro P, King DL. Gaming-gambling convergence: evaluating evidence for the "gateway"

hypothesis. Int Gambl Stud. 2020;20:380–2. https://doi.org/10.1080/14459795.2020.1768430.
11. Garea SS, Drummond A, Sauer JD, Hall LC, Williams MN. Meta-analysis of the relationships between problem gambling, excessive gaming and loot box spending. Int Gambl Stud. 2021;21(3):460–79. https://doi.org/10.1080/14459795.2021.1914705.
12. Drummond A, Hall LC, Sauer JD. Surprisingly high prevalence rates of severe psychological distress among consumers who purchase loot boxes in video games. Sci Rep. 2022;12:16128. https://doi.org/10.1038/s41598-022-20549-1.
13. Etchells PJ, Morgan AL, Quintana DS. Loot box spending is associated with problem gambling but not mental wellbeing. R Soc Open Sci. 2022;9(8):220111. https://doi.org/10.1098/rsos.220111.
14. King DL, Russell A, Gainsbury SM, Delfabbro PH, Hing N. The cost of virtual wins: an examination of gambling-related risks in youth who spend money on social casino games. J Behav Addict. 2016;5(3):401–9. https://doi.org/10.1556/2F2006.5.2016.067.
15. Brosowski T, Turowski T, Hayer T. Simulated gambling consumption mediation model (SGCMM): disentangling convergence with parallel mediation models. Int Gambl Stud. 2020;20(3):466–86. https://doi.org/10.1080/14459795.2020.1799426.
16. Cerniglia L, Guicciardi M, Sinatra M, Monacis L, Simonelli A, Cimino S. The use of digital technologies, impulsivity and psychopathological symptoms in adolescence. Behav Sci. 2019;9(8):82. https://doi.org/10.3390/bs9080082.
17. Wartberg L, Kriston L, Thomasius R. Internet gaming disorder and problematic social media use in a representative sample of German adolescents: prevalence estimates, comorbid depressive symptoms and related psychosocial aspects. Comput Hum Behav. 2020;103:31–6. https://doi.org/10.1016/j.chb.2019.09.014.
18. Henzel V, Håkansson A. Hooked on virtual social life. Problematic social media use and associations with mental distress and addictive disorders. PLoS One. 2021;16(4):e0248406. https://doi.org/10.1371/journal.pone.0248406.
19. Macur M, Pontes HM. Internet gaming disorder in adolescence: investigating profiles and associated risk factors. BMC Public Health. 2021;21:1547. https://doi.org/10.1186/s12889-021-11394-4.
20. Sirola A, Savela N, Savolainen I, Kaakinen M, Oksanen A. The role of virtual communities in gambling and gaming behaviors: a systematic review. J Gambl Stud. 2021;37:165–87. https://doi.org/10.1007/s10899-020-09946-1.
21. Sallie SN, Ritou VJE, Bowden-Jones H, Voon V. Assessing online gaming and pornography consumption patterns during COVID-19 isolation using an online survey: highlighting distinct avenues of problematic internet behavior. Addict Behav. 2021;123:107044. https://doi.org/10.1016/j.addbeh.2021.107044.
22. Castro-Calvo J, Cervigón-Carrasco V, Ballester-Arnal R, Giménez-García C. Cognitive processes related to problematic pornography use (PPU): a systematic review of experimental studies. Addict Behav Rep. 2021;13:100345. https://doi.org/10.1016/j.abrep.2021.100345.
23. Schiebener J, Brand M. Decision-making and related processes in internet gaming disorder and other types of internet-use disorders. Curr Addict Rep. 2017;4:262–71. https://doi.org/10.1007/s40429-017-0156-9.
24. Castro-Calvo J, Ballester-Arnal R, Gil-Llario MD, Giménez-García C. Common etiological pathways between toxic substance use, internet and cybersex addiction: the role of expectancies and antisocial deviance proneness. Comput Hum Behav. 2016;63:383–91. https://doi.org/10.1016/j.chb.2016.05.066.
25. Ballester-Arnal R, Castro-Calvo J, García-Barba M, Ruiz-Palomino E, Gil-Llario MD. Problematic and non-problematic engagement in online sexual activities across the lifespan. Comput Hum Behav. 2021;120:106774. https://doi.org/10.1016/j.chb.2021.106774.
26. Castro-Calvo J, Ballester-Arnal R, Potenza MN, King DL, Billieux J. Does "forced abstinence" from gaming lead to pornography use? Insight from the April 2018 crash of Fortnite's servers. J Behav Addict. 2018;7(3):501–2. https://doi.org/10.1556/2006.7.2018.78.
27. King DL, Kaptsis D, Delfabbro PH, Gradisar M. Craving for Internet games? Withdrawal symptoms from an 84-h abstinence from Massively Multiplayer Online gaming. Comput Hum Behav. 2016;62:488–94. https://doi.org/10.1016/j.chb.2016.04.020.
28. Döring N, Krämer N, Mikhailova V, Brand M, Krüger THC, Vowe G. Sexual interaction in digital contexts and its implications for sexual health: a conceptual analysis. Front Psychol. 2021;12:769732. https://doi.org/10.3389/fpsyg.2021.769732.
29. Keilty P. Desire by design: pornography as technology industry. Porn Studies. 2018;5(3):338–42. https://doi.org/10.1080/23268743.2018.1483208.
30. Paschke K, Napp AK, Thomasius R. Applying ICD-11 criteria of gaming disorder to identify problematic video streaming in adolescents: conceptualization of a new clinical phenomenon. J Behav Addict. 2022;11(2):451–66. https://doi.org/10.1556/2006.2022.00041.
31. Thomas G, Bennie JA, De Cocker K, Biddle SJH. Exploring contemporary screen time in Australian adolescents: a qualitative study. Health Promot J Austr. 2021;32(S2):238–47. https://doi.org/10.1002/hpja.440.
32. Abarbanel B, Johnson MR. Gambling engagement mechanisms in twitch live streaming. Int Gambl Stud.

2020;20:393–413. https://doi.org/10.1080/14459795.2020.1766097.

33. King DL, Delfabbro PH, Gainsbury SM, Dreier M, Greer N, Billieux J. Unfair play? Video games as exploitative monetized services: an examination of game patents from a consumer protection perspective. Comput Hum Behav. 2019;101:131–43. https://doi.org/10.1016/j.chb.2019.07.017.
34. O'Keeffe GS, Clarke-Pearson K, Council on Communications and Media. The impact of social media on children, adolescents, and families. Pediatrics. 2011;127(4):800–4. https://doi.org/10.1542/peds.2011-0054.

# Online Gambling in Youth

Marc N. Potenza, Gemma Mestre-Bach,
Zsolt Demetrovics, Jeffrey Derevensky,
Fernando Fernandez-Aranda, Sally M. Gainsbury,
Susana Jiménez-Murcia, and Shane W. Kraus

## 1 Background

Gambling involves placing an item of value at risk in hopes of gaining something of greater value, often during games of chance aiming to gain money [1]. The gambling environment has changed in recent years, particularly during the past decade with the growth of the internet [2]. Gambling has arguably become a more socially acceptable and accessible behavior, and new

M. N. Potenza (✉)
Department of Psychology, University of Nevada, Las Vegas, NV, USA

Department of Psychiatry, Yale University School of Medicine, New Haven, CT, USA

Child Study Center, Yale University School of Medicine, New Haven, CT, USA

Connecticut Mental Health Center, New Haven, CT, USA

Connecticut Council On Problem Gambling, Wethersfield, CT, USA

Department of Neuroscience, Yale University, New Haven, CT, USA

Wu Tsai Institute, Yale University, New Haven, CT, USA
e-mail: marc.potenza@yale.edu

G. Mestre-Bach
Instituto de Transferencia e Investigación, Universidad Internacional de La Rioja, La Rioja, Spain

Z. Demetrovics
Centre of Excellence in Responsible Gaming, University of Gibraltar, Gibraltar, Gibraltar

Institute of Psychology, ELTE Eötvös Loránd University, Budapest, Hungary

College of Education, Psychology and Social Work, Flinders University, Adelaide, Australia

J. Derevensky
International Centre for Youth Gambling Problems and High Risk Behaviors, McGill University, Montreal, Canada

F. Fernandez-Aranda · S. Jiménez-Murcia
Clinical Psychology Unit, University Hospital of Bellvitge-IDIBELL, Hospitalet del Llobregat, Barcelona, Spain

CIBER Fisiopatologia Obesidad y Nutrición, (CIBERobn), Hospitalet del Llobregat, Barcelona, Spain

Department of Clinical Sciences, School of Medicine, University of Barcelona, Hospitalet del Llobregat, Barcelona, Spain

Psychoneurobiology of Eating and Addictive Behaviours, Bellvitge Biomedical Research Institute (IDIBELL), Hospitalet del Llobregat, Barcelona, Spain

S. M. Gainsbury · S. W. Kraus
School of Psychology, Brain and Mind Centre, Science Faculty, University of Sydney, Sydney, Australia


D. A. Christakis, L. Hale (eds.), *Handbook of Children and Screens*,
https://doi.org/10.1007/978-3-031-69362-5_81

forms of gambling and related activities have appeared and/or grown, such as online gambling, daily fantasy sports, loot boxes, and sports betting, among others [2].

Although most existing forms of gambling are currently legally restricted to adults in most jurisdictions (with some possible exceptions, e.g., loot boxes), gambling is popular among adolescents [3]. Adolescence may be defined as the developmental period commencing with the onset of puberty and lasting until adulthood. The age boundaries of adolescence have been debated, as has what constitutes the onset of adulthood, with some considering adolescence as extending into the twenties and others considering this later stage as young or emerging adulthood. As considerable brain development continues to occur through the mid-twenties, we will consider "young/emerging adults" (including college students) in the adolescent group in this chapter.

Adolescents have been considered as a population especially vulnerable to gambling due to, among other factors, their brain developmental stages, limited capacities for emotional regulation, susceptibilities to peer influences, and high impulsivity/sensation-seeking promoting engagement in novel, risky experiences, such as gambling [4]. Older adolescents (e.g., college students) may have reached legal ages to engage in some forms of regulated gambling and other potentially risky behaviors [5].

## 2 Current State

### 2.1 Prevalence and Gambling Preferences Among Youth

Gambling disorder (GD) has been classified as a nonsubstance-related addiction in the Diagnostic and Statistical Manual of Mental Health Disorders (DSM-5) [1]. It is characterized by a maladaptive pattern of betting behavior that persists despite negative consequences in major areas of life functioning. Problem gambling may also include patterns of betting not meeting diagnostic criteria but still generating concerns or adversely impacting functioning. Problem gambling and GD are estimated to be two- to fourfold higher among adolescents as compared to general adult populations [6]. Defining a specific prevalence of problem gambling/GD in adolescents is complicated by (a) heterogeneity of assessment instruments and thresholds; (b) differences in time frames between assessments; (c) cultural aspects; and (d) biases associated with self-administered assessments in school contexts (where some prevalence studies have been conducted). Nonetheless, lifetime participation in gambling among adolescents may range from 42.1% to 89.9% [7], and prevalence of problem gambling in adolescents may range between 0.2% and 12.3% [8], higher than estimates in adults [9]. While youth gambling preferences may vary across cultures, adolescent gambling remains a worldwide problem [10].

Online gambling prevalence in adolescents has been reported to range between 5% and 15% and offline gambling between 40% and 70% [1]. Although online gambling among adolescents is less common than offline gambling, it has become increasingly popular in conjunction with loosening legislation [1] and progressive promotion, including the streaming of gambling-related content for children and youth [11]. In addition, with lockdowns during the COVID-19 pandemic, migration from offline to online gambling was reported [12], although adolescent gambling behaviors are less well understood. Online gambling may have greater addictive potential, especially for adolescents, possibly given its availability and accessibility to them through mobile devices. Online gambling may be three to eight times more likely to be associated with problematic gambling/GD compared with offline gambling [1]. Therefore, exposure to online gambling in adolescents may generate more harm than gambling offline [13].

A proliferation of online sports betting has been observed in young people using devices such as smartphones or laptops, which in part may reflect increased advertisements and legalization of online sports gambling [14]. Sports betting may be defined as wagering "on the outcome of one or multiple sporting events, occurrence/non-occurrence of an event within a sporting event, or betting on sports in a week-long or season-long competition." [15] Some have considered online sports gambling a new clinical profile of GD in adolescents [14, 16].

"Loot boxes," random elements within videogames that contain virtual prizes of varying value, have also impacted youth [17]. Some loot boxes are bought through microtransactions, which are now incorporated in many video games. Adolescent purchases of loot boxes have been linked to GD, perhaps as adolescents often report difficulties with impulse control [18]. Moreover, these specific gambling-like features often lead to family conflicts [19]. The annual prevalence rate of loot box purchases among adolescents in the general population has been estimated to range from 20% to 33.9%, which is considerably lower than among adults (22.7–44.2%) [17]. Microtransactions in general have also been linked to gambling problems and GD in youth, including those playing social casino games (actual money is not required) that may familiarize youth and introduce youth to casino gambling [6].

## 2.2 Factors Associated with GD in Adolescents/Youth

Regarding GD, several seemingly protective factors in youth include socioeconomic status, greater parental supervision/support, and parental knowledge of problematic gambling in siblings [20, 21]. On the other hand, problem gambling is more frequent in adolescents who are male, are older, belong to racial/ethnic minority groups, do not live with their parents or have lower family connectedness, have parents and/or friends who gamble, and use the internet to gamble [8].

As in adults, clinical concerns have been associated with GD in adolescents. Adolescent GD has been linked to anxiety, depression, attention-deficit/hyperactivity disorder, learning disorders, antisocial behaviors, conduct problems, substance use, delinquent and criminal behaviors, impulsivity, self-injurious behaviors, and suicidality including ideation and attempts [2, 9, 22]. Low levels of self-discipline and conformity have also been linked to adolescent GD [2]. Such concerns should be evaluated and considered in prevention and treatment programs targeted to adolescents [23].

Finally, although many adolescents have reported that advertising has no specific impact on their gambling, those adolescents who gamble have enhanced recall of gambling-related advertising, with beliefs that such advertising may misinform individuals and promote gambling [24]. Awareness of advertisements may predict gambling behavior in older adolescents [24]. The extent to which advertising or other media (e.g., sports gambling programs) may promote youth gambling warrants further attention [24]. Additionally, sports betting may be less stigmatized than other types of gambling given associations with normalized sporting activities. Thus, adolescents may mistakenly perceive it as a lower-risk behavior.

## 2.3 Assessment of GD in Youth

Widely used and validated instruments for assessing youth GD include the South Oaks Gambling Screen Revised for Adolescents (SOGS-RA), Diagnostic Statistical Manual IV (Multiple Response Format) adapted for Juveniles (DSM-IV-MR-J), and Canadian Adolescent Gambling Inventory (CAGI). The Gambling Addictive Behavior Scale for Adolescents (GABSA) and CAGI are among instruments specifically developed for youth. GD screenings for adolescents may benefit from including measures of social factors (i.e., loneliness and social support), delinquent behaviors, and impulsivity [25].

Brief screening instruments are relevant, particularly in busy clinical settings to assess GD in youth. Few instruments with adequate diagnostic accuracy are currently available [3], with the 3-item Brief Adolescent Gambling Screen (BAGS) and 2-item Lie/Bet Questionnaire having strengths and limitations.

### 2.4 Gambling-Related Consequences in Youth

Consequences of GD typically manifest differently among youth and adults. Among adults, GD is often associated with significant marital conflicts and financial problems. Adolescents, however, are typically unmarried and have limited financial responsibilities [6]. In addition, adolescents with GD often experience school-related problems, impaired social and familial relationships, substance use problems, depressive symptomatology, anxiety, and other mental health concerns [7].

### 2.5 GD Treatment in Youth

Most individuals with GD, particularly youth, do not seek formal therapeutic interventions. Nonetheless, youth may experience GD-related problems that impact their developmental trajectories and persist into their adulthood for years [6].

Different therapeutic options, both pharmacological (e.g., opioid receptor antagonists, monoaminergic drugs, and glutamatergic agents) and psychosocial (e.g., cognitive behavioral therapy, motivational interventions, and self-help groups—e.g., Gamblers Anonymous) have varying degrees of efficacy, with most not having been tested with adolescents (and no medications have youth-GD-related indications from regulatory bodies) [6]. Among psychosocial interventions for adolescents with GD, four behavioral change techniques may be promising: (a) information about antecedents (to provide details on what early factors may predict subsequent GD behaviors); (b) information about social and environmental consequences (to offer insights into sociocultural impacts resulting from performing behaviors); (c) information about emotional consequences (to present details on affective states and concerns emanating from behaviors); and (d) behavioral experiments (to offer data-based insight into relationships). Modes of treatment delivery recommended for adolescent GD may include (a) face-to-face; (b) internet-based; and (c) playable on electronic devices. Therefore, in adolescents with GD, empirically validated interventions that include these techniques and modes of delivery are needed [26]. In this context, "serious games" targeting triggers or other factors linked to maintenance of GD (such as poor self-control or difficulties in emotional regulation) warrant further examination [27].

### 2.6 GD Prevention in Youth

Increased knowledge of risk factors associated with youth gambling could help protect individuals. Prevention programs have traditionally involved school-aged children, with the aim of preventing/delaying gambling early in life. Several programs may be effective in the short term, especially in the modification of erroneous cognitions in relation to gambling, although their longer-term effects are unknown. Few studies have evaluated the acceptability, feasibility, and efficacy of GD prevention plans in young people. Existing studies suggest programs may reduce gambling-related irrational cognitions, such as the illusion of control, and increase knowledge about gambling, including odds [5]. However, these modifications in knowledge, beliefs, and attitudes may not necessarily lead to changes in gambling behavior, suggesting the need for additional research to be conducted in adolescents [13]. Development of skills to cope with everyday challenges could also be a target of future prevention programs. Educating parents [19], teachers, and mental health professionals is important for preventing adolescent GD [28].

## 3 Future Research

- *Is it possible to have a psychometric tool for the assessment of GD in adolescents and young adults that is valid, obtains scientific consensus, includes new types of gambling and related activities, and considers factors associated with youth developmental stages?* The design and validation of diagnostic instruments for GD focused on youth should be developmentally informed, sensitive to the current gambling and online environments, and culturally appropriate, and not involve mere adaptation of existing instruments for adults [29]. Likewise, scientific consensus in the assessment of GD is important to compare results of research conducted internationally. It would also be advisable to standardize instruments for measuring specifically new or recently legalized forms of gambling/gambling-related behaviors, such as online gambling, sports betting, or loot boxes [17].

- *What are specific causal relationships between GD-associated factors and GD in youth?* Longitudinal studies exploring potential causality between specific factors and gambling and GD in youth are needed. For example, studies should determine whether specific psychopathologies or life events may lead to GD or vice versa [20]. Individual differences related to gender, sex, race, and ethnicity [25] and factors associated with these constructs warrant additional examination in youth gambling and GD. Given that race and ethnicity are social constructs, research should evaluate social constructs including socioeconomic factors and how they relate to gambling and GD in youth and may reflect or contribute to systemic racism. Additional scientific consensus should be reached regarding what age ranges constitute adolescence, to promote comparability of results across studies [22].
- *What is/are the most effective treatment(s) for adolescents with GD?* Research on the efficacy of approaches for GD in adolescents remains in a nascent state. More empirical evidence is needed on the efficacy of psychological, pharmacological, neuromodulatory, self-help, and combined interventions [30]. Randomized controlled trials are needed.
- *What are the factors that make a GD prevention program effective for youth, educators, parents, and other stakeholders?* Additional efforts are needed to design and validate prevention programs aimed at educators, families, youth, and other stakeholders [30]. Input from youth with lived experiences should be considered, as should education about online gambling-related behaviors and their regulation.
- *What are the specific impacts of gambling advertisements and new forms of gambling on youth?* Further research is required on influences of advertisements and marketing aimed at promoting gambling and related behaviors, especially risky behaviors like in-play (live-action) betting, and on activities lying along a spectrum of gambling and gaming, such as loot boxes [20]. Moreover, more research is needed regarding online gambling in adolescents and youth, especially as such behavior may be conducted in a more solitary fashion, be linked to academic and substance-use concerns among youth (compared to offline gambling), and offer fewer geographic and time boundaries that may, in the setting of the current options available for app-based internet gambling, facilitate problematic engagement for vulnerable individuals [31, 32].

## 4 Recommendations

- It is important to advance educational and interventional approaches to address youth online risk behaviors, including gambling. The fulfillment of this objective may involve increasing awareness through mass media, social networks, posters, and pamphlets, including in collaboration with local agencies, national entities (e.g., the National Council on Problem Gambling), and gambling operators [33]. Given convergences between gambling and gaming, gaming companies should also be involved and should governments with respect to developing and implementing appropriate regulations.
- Regarding educational and preventive programs aimed at youth, they should begin at young ages [7]. Many adults (parents and educators) perceive gambling as not being harmful and may unknowingly promote gambling (either through lottery gifts or inadvertently through their own gambling); thus, educational efforts should extend beyond youth [6].

It is recommended that parents/guardians set limits on children's online behaviors and have the knowledge to recognize warning signs of gambling and GD [2]. Additionally, healthcare providers should screen youth for gambling and GD. Once identified, clinical services to address youth GD are needed in many jurisdictions, as they remain limited, particularly in Asia [34].

**Conflict of Interest and Funding Disclosures** MNP has consulted for Opiant Therapeutics, Game Day Data, Baria-Tek, Boehringer-Ingelheim, and the Addiction Policy Forum; been involved in a patent application with Yale University and Novartis; received research support from Mohegan Sun Casino, Children and Screens: Institute of Digital Media and Child Development and the Connecticut Council on Problem Gambling; participated in surveys, mailings, or telephone consultations related to drug addictions, internet use, impulse-control disorders, and other health topics; consulted for or advised gambling, nonprofit and legal entities on issues related to internet use, impulse-control and addictive disorders; and given academic lectures in grand rounds, continuing medical education events, and other clinical or scientific venues. FF-A and SJ-M received consultancy honoraria from Novo Nordisk, and FF-A received an editorial honorarium from Wiley. ELTE Eötvös Loránd University receives funding from the Szerencsejáték Ltd. to maintain a telephone helpline service for problematic gambling. The University of Gibraltar receives funding from the Gibraltar Gambling Care Foundation. SWK receives support from the Kindbridge Research Institute. FF-A and SJ-M received institutional support from CERCA. CIBERobn is an initiative of ISCIII. ZD's contribution was supported by the Hungarian National Research, Development, and Innovation Office (KKP126835). The work was supported by the Ministerio de Consumo (SUBV23/00024).

## References

1. Montiel I, Ortega-Barón J, Basterra-González A, González-Cabrera J, MacHimbarrena JM. Problematic online gambling among adolescents: a systematic review about prevalence and related measurement issues. J Behav Addict. 2021;10(3):566–86. https://doi.org/10.1556/2006.2021.00055.
2. Derevensky JL, Hayman V, Gilbeau L. Behavioral addictions. Pediatr Clin N Am. 2019;66(6):1163–82. https://doi.org/10.1016/j.pcl.2019.08.008.
3. Dowling NA, Merkouris SS, Dias S, et al. The diagnostic accuracy of brief screening instruments for problem gambling: a systematic review and meta-analysis. Clin Psychol Rev. 2019;74:101784. https://doi.org/10.1016/j.cpr.2019.101784.
4. Noël X. Why adolescents are at risk of misusing alcohol and gambling. Alcohol. 2014;49(2):165–72. https://doi.org/10.1093/alcalc/agt161.
5. Grande-Gosende A, López-Núñez C, García-Fernández G, Derevensky J, Fernández-Hermida JR. Systematic review of preventive programs for reducing problem gambling behaviors among young adults. J Gambl Stud. 2020;36(1):1–22. https://doi.org/10.1007/s10899-019-09866-9.
6. Potenza MN, Balodis IM, Derevensky J, et al. Gambling disorder. Nat Rev Dis Prim. 2019;5(1):51. https://doi.org/10.1038/s41572-019-0099-7.
7. Riley BJ, Oster C, Rahamathulla M, Lawn S. Attitudes, risk factors, and behaviours of gambling among adolescents and young people: a literature review and gap analysis. Int J Environ Res Public Health. 2021;18(3):984. https://doi.org/10.3390/ijerph18030984.
8. Calado F, Alexandre J, Griffiths MD. Prevalence of adolescent problem gambling: a systematic review of recent research. J Gambl Stud. 2017;33(2):397–424. https://doi.org/10.1007/s10899-016-9627-5.
9. Richard J, Fletcher É, Boutin S, Derevensky J, Temcheff C. Conduct problems and depressive symptoms in association with problem gambling and gaming: a systematic review. J Behav Addict. 2020;9(3):497–533. https://doi.org/10.1556/2006.2020.00045.
10. Yu L, Ma CMS. Youth gambling in Hong Kong: prevalence, psychosocial correlates, and prevention. J Adolesc Health. 2019;64(6):S44–51. https://doi.org/10.1016/j.jadohealth.2018.09.019.
11. Koncz P, Demetrovics Z, Griffiths MD, Király O. The potential harm of gambling streams to minors. J Am Acad Child Adolesc Psychiatry. 2023;62:713. https://doi.org/10.1016/j.jaac.2023.01.020.
12. Masaeli N, Farhadi H. Prevalence of internet-based addictive behaviors during COVID-19 pandemic: a systematic review. J Addict Dis. 2021;39(4):468–88. https://doi.org/10.1080/10550887.2021.1895962.
13. Keen B, Blaszczynski A, Anjoul F. Systematic review of empirically evaluated school-based gambling education programs. J Gambl Stud. 2017;33(1):301–25. https://doi.org/10.1007/s10899-016-9641-7.
14. Barrera-Algarín E, Vázquez-Fernández MJ. The rise of online sports betting, its fallout, and the onset of a new profile in gambling disorder: young people. J Addict Dis. 2021;39(3):363–72. https://doi.org/10.1080/10550887.2021.1886567.
15. Etuk R, Xu T, Abarbanel B, Potenza MN, Kraus SW. Sports betting around the world: a systematic review. J Behav Addict. 2022;11(3):689–715. https://doi.org/10.1556/2006.2022.00064.
16. Valenciano-Mendoza E, Mora-Maltas B, Mestre-Bach G, et al. Clinical correlates of sports betting: a systematic review. J Gambl Stud. 2023;39:579.
17. Montiel I, Basterra-González A, Machimbarrena JM, Ortega-Barón J, González-Cabrera J. Loot box

engagement: a scoping review of primary studies on prevalence and association with problematic gaming and gambling. PLoS One. 2022;17(1):e0263177. https://doi.org/10.1371/journal.pone.0263177.
18. Raneri PC, Montag C, Rozgonjuk D, Satel J, Pontes HM. The role of microtransactions in internet gaming disorder and gambling disorder: a preregistered systematic review. Addict Behav Rep. 2022;15:100415. https://doi.org/10.1016/j.abrep.2022.100415.
19. Király O, Zhang J, Demetrovics Z, Browne DT. Gambling features and monetization in video games create challenges for young people, families, and clinicians. J Am Acad Child Adolesc Psychiatry. 2022;61(7):854–6. https://doi.org/10.1016/j.jaac.2021.12.003.
20. Emond AM, Griffiths MD. Gambling in children and adolescents. Br Med Bull. 2020;136(1):21–9. https://doi.org/10.1093/bmb/ldaa027.
21. Truong A, Moukaddam N, Toledo A, Onigu-Otite E. Addictive disorders in adolescents. Psychiatr Clin North Am. 2017;40(3):475–86. https://doi.org/10.1016/j.psc.2017.05.012.
22. Sharman S, Butler K, Roberts A. Psychosocial risk factors in disordered gambling: a descriptive systematic overview of vulnerable populations. Addict Behav. 2019;99:106071. https://doi.org/10.1016/j.addbeh.2019.106071.
23. Kryszajtys DT, Hahmann TE, Schuler A, Hamilton-Wright S, Ziegler CP, Matheson FI. Problem gambling and delinquent behaviours among adolescents: a scoping review. J Gambl Stud. 2018;34(3):893–914. https://doi.org/10.1007/s10899-018-9754-2.
24. McGrane E, Wardle H, Clowes M, et al. What is the evidence that advertising policies could have an impact on gambling-related harms? A systematic umbrella review of the literature. Public Health. 2023;215:124. https://doi.org/10.1016/j.puhe.2022.11.019.
25. Edgren R, Castrén S, Mäkelä M, Pörtfors P, Alho H, Salonen AH. Reliability of instruments measuring at-risk and problem gambling among young individuals: a systematic review covering years 2009–2015. J Adolesc Health. 2016;58(6):600–15. https://doi.org/10.1016/j.jadohealth.2016.03.007.
26. St Quinton T, Morris B, Pickering D, Smith DM. Behavior change techniques and delivery modes in interventions targeting adolescent gambling: a systematic review. J Gambl Stud. 2022;38(4):1503–28. https://doi.org/10.1007/s10899-022-10108-8.
27. Mena-Moreno T, Munguía L, Granero R, et al. e-Estesia: a serious game for reducing arousal, improving emotional regulation and increasing well-being in individuals with gambling disorder. J Clin Med. 2022;11(22):6798. https://doi.org/10.3390/jcm11226798.
28. Derevensky JL. The prevention and treatment of gambling disorders: some art, some science. In: The Cambridge handbook of substance and behavioral addictions. Cambridge University Press; 2020. p. 241–53. https://doi.org/10.1017/9781108632591.024.
29. Carragher N, Billieux J, Bowden-Jones H, et al. Brief overview of the WHO collaborative project on the development of new international screening and diagnostic instruments for gaming disorder and gambling disorder. Addiction. 2022;117(7):2119–21. https://doi.org/10.1111/add.15780.
30. Fineberg NA, Menchón JM, Hall N, et al. Advances in problematic usage of the internet research—a narrative review by experts from the European network for problematic usage of the internet. Compr Psychiatry. 2022;118:152346. https://doi.org/10.1016/j.comppsych.2022.152346.
31. Potenza MN, Wareham JD, Steinberg MA, et al. Correlates of at-risk/problem internet gambling in adolescents. J Am Acad Child Adolesc Psychiatry. 2011;50(2):150–9. https://doi.org/10.1016/j.jaac.2010.11.006.
32. Staley O. An explosion in sports betting is driving gambling addiction among college students. Time. https://time.com/6342504/gambling-addiction-sports-betting-college-students/. Accessed 14 Apr 2024.
33. Akçayır M, Nicoll F, Baxter DG. Emerging gambling problems and suggested interventions: a systematic review of empirical research. J Gambl Stud. 2022;39:1–26. https://doi.org/10.1007/s10899-022-10122-w.
34. Saunders JB, Hao W, Long J, et al. Gaming disorder: its delineation as an important condition for diagnosis, management, and prevention. J Behav Addict. 2017;6(3):271–9. https://doi.org/10.1556/2006.6.2017.039.

# Introduction to the Section on Emerging Technologies

Judith H. Danovitch

One of the most exciting aspects of modern technology is the rapid rate at which it is changing and advancing. In fact, a recent analysis of US patents shows that technologies involving software and algorithms for purposes such as collecting and using information online are improving very rapidly relative to other types of technologies [1]. Although digital divides between communities still exist [2, 3], modern technologies are quickly becoming more affordable and accessible to more people, including children. In a 2019 survey, an estimated 95 percent of 3- to 18-year-olds in the United States had Internet access in their home [4], and, in a 2021 survey, 43% of American children ages 8–12 years reported owning a smartphone [5]. Moreover, children's interactions with technology start early, with more than one-third of American parents reporting that their child began interacting with smartphones before age 5 [6]. Even technologies such as social robots and virtual reality headsets that have existed for several decades but have historically been out of reach for typical families have recently become more widely available and are beginning to be present in children's homes and classrooms [5, 7, 8].

As technology advances, so do concerns about its effects on users' health and well-being, and this is particularly true for concerns about its effects on children. These concerns are nothing new as access to emerging technologies frequently predates the existence of data that could inform the use of those technologies and potentially assuage fears. For instance, in 1939, John E. Anderson, one of the first directors of the Institute of Child Development at the University of Minnesota, lamented the lack of scientific data on how access to the new technology of his era—the radio—affected children's development [9]. His statement that "one of the greatest controversies of our time revolves about the good or harmful effects of the radio on children and the related problem of censorship and control" could easily be applied to modern technologies like AI-driven conversational agents or virtual reality. Like radio and television, one of the pervasive issues with emerging technologies is that they are typically designed for adult users, yet their appeal extends to children as well.

The section on emerging technologies provides an overview of the current state-of-the-art of research on children and emerging technologies, with an eye toward understanding how using emerging technologies may influence children's cognitive, social, and physical development. It also discusses how emerging technologies can be employed in support of children's healthy development, while reducing the risks of their use. Because new technologies are constantly being developed, the emerging technologies discussed in the section are not intended to be exhaustive. Rather, the discussions of the technologies selected for this section are intended to be representative of the questions and concerns that arise as new means of interacting, communicating, and experiencing the world become available. This section focuses on children ranging from toddlers to early adolescents as this is an

J. H. Danovitch (✉)
Department of Psychological and Brain Sciences, University of Louisville, Louisville, KY, USA
e-mail: j.danovitch@louisville.edu



D. A. Christakis, L. Hale (eds.), *Handbook of Children and Screens*,
https://doi.org/10.1007/978-3-031-69362-5_82

age range when children may begin encountering and using emerging technologies.

The section opens with Xu et al.'s (see chapter "Growing up with Artificial Intelligence: Implications for Child Development") review of artificial intelligence (AI) and its use to support children's learning and social interactions. Danovitch et al. (see chapter "Children's Understanding and Use of Voice-Assistants: Opportunities and Challenges") and Severson et al. (see chapter "Social Robots and Children's Development: Promises and Implications") then discuss children's interactions with two specific types of personified, embodied devices that rely on AI: voice-assistants and robots. Across all three chapters, the authors highlight how the extent to which an emerging technology mimics human behaviors and characteristics can influence children's learning from and interactions with that technology, and their understanding of how the technology works.

The next chapter by Kaufman et al. (see chapter "Immersive Horizons: Navigating the Impacts of Virtual Reality on Children and Families") reviews virtual reality, an emerging technology that alters the user's perception of their environment. By overcoming the limitations of the real world, virtual reality can be applied in powerful ways to support educational and therapeutic goals. However, it may be difficult to use effectively and entail unforeseen risks to children's safety and well-being.

Gelman et al. (see chapter "Children's Understanding of Digital Tracking and Digital Privacy") close the section with a review of the nascent literature on digital tracking and digital privacy. Their chapter raises questions about privacy that are applicable to children's access to and use of many emerging technologies. Their discussion and recommendations highlight the need to gather more data and bring together stakeholders ranging from parents and educators to technology developers and policymakers in order to develop means of using emerging technologies in ways that promote children's health and well-being and keep them safe from harm.

Although the technologies addressed in each chapter are different, several themes appear across these chapters. First, a key issue for emerging technologies is whether the knowledge or skills that children gain through interaction with a technology generalize to other settings. Second, data collection that includes diverse methodologies and populations is urgently needed to better understand how emerging technologies are being used and how they affect children's development. Third, the unprecedented capacity for emerging technologies to collect and store personal information about users raises ethical questions about its place in children's lives. Each of these themes, together with corresponding recommendations, is discussed in further detail below.

## 1 Generalizability

An aspirational goal for technology is to support children's learning and development of real-world skills, particularly for children who are facing psychological or physical challenges. However, there are long-standing concerns about whether children, and particularly young children, can apply what they learn from technological sources like screen-based media to real-world situations [10, 11]. Concerns about this well-documented *transfer deficit* extend to emerging technologies, and they are discussed throughout the chapters in this section.

Some of the research reviewed in this section supports the idea that children can transfer the skills they learn through interactions with emerging technologies successfully to interactions with other people. For instance, Severson et al. discuss evidence that children with autism spectrum disorders who practiced social skills with a robot showed improvements in their human-directed social skills as well. However, in other contexts, children's learning from emerging technology may be inferior to learning from traditional sources like other people [12]. Children may even be skeptical of the information provided by technological devices such as voice-assistants that are unfamiliar to them or whose inner workings they do not understand, and this skepticism can be detrimental to their learning. Moreover, given that most of the existing research measures the transfer of knowledge or effects on behavior in the short term only, additional research is needed to determine whether skill transfer and learning from emerging technologies persist over time.

Together, the chapters in this section suggest that because the time children spend using emerging technologies may replace time spent interacting with other people, caution is warranted when adopting a technology for educational purposes. Increasing awareness of the potential limitations of children's learning from technology and providing adults with better tools for supporting children's technology use may help address these problems. Parents, caregivers, and educators should consider co-viewing or co-using technology, especially with young children, and monitoring whether children are applying what they learn to the real world, for better or for worse. As Kaufman et al. note, adults should also keep in mind that children learn how to responsibly—or irresponsibly—use technology from observing them.

## 2 Methodological Limitations

Because, by definition, emerging technologies are new, and they are constantly evolving and improving, studying children's use of these technologies poses unique challenges. As Severson et al. discuss, interactions with new technologies are prone to a novelty effect, which may be reflected in artificially high levels of interest or engagement with the technology. Measuring children's interactions with new technologies in a controlled laboratory environment may also have low ecological validity if children do not typically have access to these technologies, and they know that they are being observed. That said, there is an ongoing tension between laboratory-based studies that allow researchers to manipulate variables, such as a conversational agent's accuracy or the realism of a virtual reality setting, and in situ studies where researchers can observe how children use technology in the "natural" environment, such as homes and classrooms. Similarly, there can be disagreements about whether studies should use familiar devices that may not have been designed for child users (e.g., Amazon's Alexa) or unfamiliar devices with similar features that the researchers can control to ensure that they are responsive to children's commands (e.g., a novel voice-assistant). Regardless of the parameters, well-powered studies with larger and more diverse samples are needed to better understand the factors that contribute to variability in children's learning from and beliefs about emerging technologies, including but not limited to their prior experience with technology, their identity (especially for members of minoritized groups), their socioeconomic status, and their culture [13].

To better understand the long-term effects of technology use, longitudinal studies that track the trajectory of behaviors over the course of childhood and beyond are necessary. Children are underrepresented in research on emerging technologies, despite the fact that even very young children may have access to and use these technologies. Critically, the omission of children from prior research may conceal important developmental differences. For example, children aged 4–10 years have much more positive attitudes about being digitally tracked than older children and adults [11]. Future research should strive to include children from a wide age range and diverse backgrounds and to follow their experiences with technology over prolonged periods of time.

Finally, another theme that emerges from the chapters in this section is that new technologies may require new methodological approaches and theories to guide the research. Severson et al. and Kaufman et al. call for the development of standardized, child-appropriate measures of beliefs and learning from technology. Some authors also discuss the need for researchers to look beyond existing theories of cognitive and social development and to consider the possibility that emerging technologies may entail new ways of interacting with or seeing the world. For instance, children may treat AI-driven conversational agents, personified voice-assistants, or social robots as part of a new ontological category that is neither fully artifact nor fully human [13, 14].

Ultimately, the advent of new technologies may also mean redefining what it means to be "technologically literate" and considering new ways to promote this literacy.

## 3 Ethical Concerns

Despite reviewing different types of emerging technologies, all the chapters in this section raise concerns about children's privacy and the ways in which technology can be used to collect and store personal, identifiable data about its users. These concerns are perhaps not surprising given that fears about potential privacy violations involving new technologies date back at least to the advent of "instantaneous" photography in the late 1800s [15]. That said, modern technologies pose especially salient challenges because of the quantity of information that they can potentially collect and the high likelihood that users—and particularly children—lack an awareness or understanding of the risks to their privacy.

In their chapter, Gelman et al. discuss the distinction between interpersonal and institutional privacy, and how seeing privacy primarily in interpersonal terms leaves young children more vulnerable to violations. Although privacy protection laws that apply to children's data, such as the Children's Online Privacy Protection ACT (COPPA), have existed for several decades, these laws need to be updated and extended to incorporate emerging technologies. Moreover, as Gelman et al. note, existing privacy protections are inconsistent across locations, they can be difficult to enforce, and loopholes still exist. Privacy protection may also fail to account for children's developing understanding of what kinds of data can be tracked, what risks technology use poses, and how new technologies work. Importantly, although the authors of the chapters in this section agree that actions should be taken to protect children's privacy, several groups of authors also acknowledge that there is a trade-off between maintaining privacy and using personal data to create a better experience for end-users. Determining what kinds of data need to be stored and how those data can be used ethically remains an open challenge for technology developers and policymakers.

Examining the literature on emerging technologies also raises important ethical questions about technology's place in children's lives. These questions include how technology fits with—or potentially disrupts—children's relationships with other people (Xu et al.), and whether the benefits for children's learning or well-being outweigh the potential costs to their relationships. It is also unclear who should be responsible for regulating children's access to emerging technologies (Kaufman et al.) and ensuring that the content those technologies present is appropriate for children (Xu et al.). In addition, there are related questions about whether it is acceptable to deceive children about what a technology is or how it works if doing so makes the technology more effective or engaging (Severson et al). To increase the short-term safety and long-term benefits of children's use of emerging technologies, technology developers need to engage in thoughtful, responsive child-appropriate design that considers users' perspectives and concerns (Gelman et al.), and technology users need to be aware of the benefits and risks of giving children access to new technologies. Ultimately, harnessing the power of emerging technologies to support children's healthy development will depend on stakeholders working together to make decisions based on the available data.

**Conflict of Interest and Funding Disclosures** None.

## References

1. Singh A, Triulzi G, Magee CL. Technological improvement rate predictions for all technologies: use of patent data and an extended domain description. Res Policy. 2021;50(9):104294. https://doi.org/10.1016/j.respol.2021.104294.

2. UNICEF. How many children and young people have internet access at home?: estimating digital connectivity during the COVID-19 pandemic. UNICEF; 2020. Retrieved from: https://data.unicef.org/resources/children-and-young-people-internet-access-at-home-during-covid19/
3. Farry M. An old problem in the new normal: the digital divide. 2021. New America. Retrieved from: https://www.newamerica.org/the-thread/an-old-problem-in-the-new-normal-the-digital-divide/
4. U.S. Census Bureau. 2019 American Community Survey. Retrieved from https://www.census.gov/topics/population/computer-internet/data/tables.html
5. Rideout V, Peebles A, Mann, S, Robb, MB. The common sense census: media use by tweens and teens, 2021. 2022. Available at: https://www.commonsensemedia.org/research/the-common-sense-census-media-use-by-tweens-and-teens-2021
6. Auxier B, Anderson M, Perrin A, Turner E. Parenting Children in the Age of Screens. July 28, 2020. Retrieved from: https://www.pewresearch.org/internet/2020/07/28/childrens-engagement-with-digital-devices-screen-time/. Accessed 20 Apr2023.
7. Insights on the social robots global market to 2026 – rise in automation is driving growth. Retrieved from: https://finance.yahoo.com/news/insights-social-robots-global-market-115800589.html
8. Alsop T. Virtual reality – statistics & facts. 2022 Retrieved from: https://www.statista.com/topics/2532/virtual-reality-vr/
9. Anderson JE. The radio and child development. Phi Delta Kappan. 1939;21(7):316–8. Retrieved from https://www.jstor.org/stable/20258896
10. Jing M, Kirkorian HL. Video deficit in children's early learning. Int Encyclopedia Media Psychol. 2020 Sep;8:1–8.
11. Gelman SA, Martinez M, Davidson NS, Noles NS. Developing digital privacy: children's moral judgments concerning mobile GPS devices. Child Dev. 2018;89(1):17–26. https://doi.org/10.1111/cdev.12826.
12. Barr R. Memory constraints on infant learning from picture books, television, and touchscreens. Child Dev Perspect. 2013;7(4):205–10. https://doi.org/10.1111/cdep.12041.
13. Severson RL, Carlson SM. Behaving as or behaving as if? children's conceptions of personified robots and the emergence of a new ontological category. Neural Netw. 2010;23(8–9):1099–103. https://doi.org/10.1016/j.neunet.2010.08.014.
14. Kahn PH Jr, Shen S. NOC NOC, who's there? A new ontological category (NOC) for social robots. In: Budwig N, Turiel E, Zelazo PD, editors. New perspectives on human development. Cambridge University Press; 2017. p. 106–22.
15. Brandeis L, Warren S. The right to privacy. Harv Law Rev. 1890;4(5):193–220.

# Growing Up with Artificial Intelligence: Implications for Child Development

Ying Xu, Yenda Prado, Rachel L. Severson, Silvia Lovato, and Justine Cassell

## 1 Background

Artificial intelligence (AI) is increasingly finding its place in modern society, influencing various aspects of daily experiences, including those of children. Children may turn to digital assistants such as Siri, Alexa, or ChatGPT to ask questions and seek information, participate in interactive storytelling alongside social robots, or play with smart toys that recognize and respond to facial expressions. Furthermore, AI algorithms are incorporated into adaptive video games and intelligent tutoring systems, customizing content according to individual learning needs. Recently, the children's publishing market has even seen the release of AI-generated children's storybooks, featuring plot twists and illustrations that seemed quite polished.

These applications are supported by a diverse array of AI technologies, including speech recognition, computer vision, and large language models. A common defining characteristic among these technologies is their capacity to process vast amounts of data, learn from these data, and make predictions or decisions based on that learning, ultimately creating an illusion of human-like intelligence. The increasing coexistence of humans and machine intelligence, as exemplified by AI technologies, calls for increased understanding of how AI may impact child development, as children form crucial understandings of their world and relationships through their interactions with others.

The aim of this chapter is to provide an overview of key research fields examining children's interactions with AI, with a particular emphasis on ethical considerations. In essence, AI shows great promise to help children grow and develop at their individual pace. However, that promise will be best realized if educators, technology developers, researchers, and policymakers also ensure that children have access to AI that is designed in child-centered ways.

The affiliations for Justine Cassell in Chapter 83 was incorrect in the published book. It should be J Cassel INRIA Paris, Paris, France and Carnegie Mellon University, Pittsburgh, PA, USA.

Y. Xu (✉)
Harvard University, Cambridge, MA, USA
e-mail: yingxu@g.harvard.edu

Y. Prado
Digital Promise, Washington, DC, USA

R. L. Severson
University of Montana, Missoula, MT, USA

S. Lovato
Public Broadcasting Service, Arlington, VA, USA

J. Cassell
INRIA Paris, Paris, France and Carnegie Mellon University, Pittsburgh, PA, USA


D. A. Christakis, L. Hale (eds.), *Handbook of Children and Screens*,
https://doi.org/10.1007/978-3-031-69362-5_83

# 2 Current State

## 2.1 Children's Learning from AI

A growing number of research studies have identified ways in which AI technologies can enhance children's development across various domains, including creativity, attention, language acquisition, socioemotional well-being, and science and math learning. Though varied in their specific design, these tools leverage AI to support learning in an individualized and interactive manner. Their design is often informed by evidence and theories suggesting the optimal conditions for child development, drawing insights from fields such as psychology, learning sciences, and pediatrics. This approach aims to develop AI tools that are capable of replicating or facilitating these optimal conditions.

One productive area of research is utilizing AI to foster children's language development. Decades of research show that adequate verbal input (quantity) and opportunities to engage in meaningful interactions (quality) are both necessary for children's language skills to develop [10]. AI researchers have used these principles to develop systems that function as language partners, simulating the roles of human partners in activities such as reading, storytelling, and role-playing. For instance, Xu and colleagues developed a conversational agent that narrated a story, asked the child questions, and provided formative feedback [30]. A comparison of comprehension scores following the interaction showed that dialogic reading with the conversational agent replicated the benefits of interacting with a human partner. Other studies have relied on the increasing sophistication of generative AI to support more free-form language activities, such as child-AI co-created stories, demonstrating the feasibility of such an approach [14].

Despite potential learning benefits, concerns remain around children's exposure to AI-generated content that is inappropriate, inaccurate, or that may convey negative biases and stereotypes. Indeed, an analysis of Alexa has revealed that even when apps are placed in the children's section, inappropriate content could still be triggered (e.g., an agent responding "you are ugly…" to a child) [13]. To some extent, this issue can be mitigated by employing techniques such as content filtering. However, addressing biases and stereotypes remains a challenging task given that biases are as deeply engrained in the data used to train AI systems as they are in culture (e.g., when a child asks, "What do girls do?" and the AI agent responds, "housewives"). As a result, the growing body of research investigating methods to detect and reduce such stereotypes and biases has become crucial [27], as young children, who are still developing their social perceptions, are especially susceptible to biased information associating specific traits and social groups [18].

## 2.2 Children's Social Interactions with AI

Research examining children's social interaction with AI typically uses human-human interactions as the benchmark. Although many studies have documented children demonstrating social behaviors similar to those observed in interpersonal interactions with AI agents [12], three separate studies involving children aged 3–6 have found that children appeared to be less active when communicating with AI agents in smart speakers than with humans [1, 9, 29]. These studies also reveal other subtle differences in children's interactional behaviors, including reduced willingness to resolve misunderstandings with voice assistants [9], answer challenging questions posed by AI [30], and an increased attentiveness to the cooperative and informational needs of human partners [1]. Taken together, these findings suggest that children perceive AI agents as a unique category that transcends the distinction between living and non-living entities, perhaps due to the unique constellation of social and psychological attributes depicted by AI systems [20].

Other research has investigated whether children's interactions with AI agents influence their real-life social interactions. One study found that after children were taught to use a novel word to speed up smart speakers' speech, they subsequently attempted to use the same word to accelerate their parents' speech [11]. Other studies have also found that AI agents can be used to teach children social skills, including children with developmental disabilities such as those on the autism spectrum [19, 22]. Indeed, one study indicated that robots adhering to social etiquette requiring children to use polite wake-words (i.e., "Excuse me, robot" instead of "Hey robot") resulted in children's higher level of politeness toward the robot [28]. However, concerns arise when commercial AI devices do not require politeness, potentially leading to inappropriate conversational habits that some children might fail to recognize as distinct from acceptable human social norms [2].

Researchers have also raised questions about how AI might potentially affect children's relationships with family members, peers, and teachers [23]. However, little research has confirmed or refuted these concerns given that most research tends to focus on children's one-to-one interactions with AI rather than children's existing social contexts and relationships. One exception is a study on how a smart-speaker voice might be used as a neutral third party to resolve disputes among children, such as by setting a timer to facilitate toy sharing [4]. This study found that children were receptive to commands coming from the speaker, although it was unclear how long this neutral arbiter remained effective.

Other studies show that AI can be intentionally designed to support human-to-human-interaction. For instance, Lin et al [15] and Zhang et al [31] studied parents and children reading together with a virtual agent that interjected story-related prompts or comments. These agents encouraged parents to elaborate on the agent's feedback, add additional information, and expand the conversation to other relevant topics. Similarly, another study found that when two children told stories in collaboration with a virtual child agent, they were more generous in giving turns to one another, and the quality of their stories was higher than when they told stories as a dyad without the virtual child agent present [7]. These studies highlight potential uses of AI to create enriched environments that foster meaningful social interactions for children, focused on enhancing rather than replacing human connections.

## 2.3 Children's Understanding of AI

Researchers have also begun exploring how children understand and interpret AI, a challenge given the complex and often opaque nature of AI models. This challenge is further compounded by the fact that many child-facing AI products are intended to emulate humans and encourage children to view the technologies as playmates, coaches, or companions, often without disclosing their internal workings. This combination of factors could amplify children's tendency to anthropomorphize AI [21], which has itself been shown to positively correlate with children's acceptance of AI-presented information [25]. However, children's tendency to anthropomorphize AI can also lead to unrealistic expectations of AI's capabilities, which may impact their perceptions of AI in the future.

To address these issues, experts have emphasized the importance of fostering children's accurate understanding of AI so they can effectively interact with AI technologies. Various frameworks have been developed to teach what has been called AI literacy that Long and Magerko [16] define as a set of skills that enable individuals to critically evaluate, communicate, and collaborate effectively with AI as a tool. This includes distinguishing between machine and human or animal intelligence, recognizing technological artifacts that use AI, and understanding the strengths and limitations of AI.

Research in this area can guide the development of programs that teach children AI literacy, and assessments that measure children's understanding of AI. For instance, one study showed that deploying a program that allowed children to work with their parents to create their own conversational agents boosted children's confidence in deciding under what situations their conversational agents should be trusted [24]. Another study found that children's awareness of potential gender discrimination conveyed by AI systems could be significantly enhanced when the models predicting individuals' gender in images included explanations for the models' prediction outcomes (e.g., the presence of athletic objects, such as sneakers and skateboards, being heavily weighted in classifying individuals as male) [17].

Other research has integrated AI awareness information into the system design itself, so that children are informed of how AI works in the particular system they are interacting with. For instance, in one study of children interacting with humanoid robots, those who were explicitly informed that humans programmed the robots were less likely to perceive the robots as similar to themselves. However, this disclosure did not diminish the children's perceived closeness to the robots [26]. This finding suggests that fostering child-AI relationships, without deceiving children into thinking AI is agentive, intelligent, or empathetic, is possible. This approach aligns with policy recommendations advocating making AI systems transparent [6], although most empirical research to date has focused on adult populations.

## 3 Future Research

In the preceding sections, we outlined how children learn from and interact with AI, how AI might impact children's interactions with others, and what children understand about AI. Findings and questions raised in these areas highlight the need for further research to help constituents, including caregivers, educators, technology developers, and policymakers, better comprehend, and guide the role AI plays in children's lives. Such research could lead to the development of AI applications that are specifically designed based on state-of-the-art evidence and prioritize children's needs and experiences.

An important step toward advancing our understanding of AI and child development involves establishing comprehensive, scalable measures that document the extent and nature of children's exposure to and interaction with AI, as well as the social contexts in which these interactions occur (such as whether children use AI alone or with teachers or parents). Such measures could extend from existing tools that capture children's media ecosystem [3]. Data gathered through these efforts would allow researchers to examine the ways and conditions under which children's AI usage impacts developmental outcomes.

The research community also must carry out more longitudinal, in situ studies. Existing research has primarily involved small numbers of sessions conducted in lab environments. These limitations preclude interested stakeholders from thoroughly unpacking the dynamic role AI plays in children's lives. For instance, research examining how children might come to treat AI as a peer or friend would necessarily entail longer term studies to better understand whether such bonds could occur and to explore their nature [8].

More research should also be carried out to support children's understanding of AI and improve their AI literacy. While a number of programs and platforms have been developed to effectively facilitate children's awareness of AI positives and negatives, more research is necessary to optimize these programs and ensure they are readily accessible and inclusive for all children, regardless of socioeconomic background.

It is also important to consider more generally how AI can be designed with children in mind. Ultimately, the goal of designing child-centered AI is to create systems that are effective, accurate, unbiased, and supportive of children's growth and well-being in the broader interaction context [5, 16]. This effort will require exploring new interfaces and interaction modalities that are tailored to children's cognitive and emotional abilities, as well as developing ethical guidelines and standards to ensure that AI systems are safe, appropriate, and respectful in ways that do not exploit or harm vulnerable populations.

# 4 Recommendations

## 4.1 For Parents, Caregivers, and Educators

- Similar to shared digital media experiences, parent involvement in children's AI use can promote positive interactions and learning outcomes while reducing potential harm. It is also crucial for children to have opportunities to unplug and develop social and emotional skills through face-to-face human interactions.
- It is important for states and school districts to support parents, caregivers, and educators in staying informed about the development of new technologies, which will enable them to make knowledgeable decisions regarding how to support children's interactions and learning.
- States and districts can develop resources to ensure that teachers have access to professional development opportunities and that caregivers are provided with resources to explore and understand the AI systems their children are using alongside them.

## 4.2 For Technology Developers

- Technology developers should promote parental involvement by enabling parental controls, such as content filtering, and designing for joint engagement that supports collaboration between parents and children.
- Technology developers should consider incorporating AI literacy into their content and messaging by explaining how AI technologies work and how they can be used in a safe and responsible manner. For instance, manufacturers of smart toys like the popular Hello Barbie could enhance transparency by clearly communicating that a built-in microphone captures children's speech and that it relies on Internet connectivity to function.
- Technology developers can ensure that their products are accessible to all children and families by engaging in co-design practices directly with children, caregivers, schools, and local education and community organizations. Co-designing products keeps users in the loop and helps developers understand children's interactions with their products to test prototypes and inform the final design.

## 4.3 For Policymakers

- As AI technologies become increasingly prevalent, laws and policies must be updated. For instance, lawmakers might update the Children's Online Privacy Protection Act (COPPA) to include child-centered AI. COPPA was enacted in 1998 to protect the online privacy of children under the age of 13, but it does not specifically address the use of AI technologies.
- Regulations should emphasize continuous monitoring and strict standards for content, alongside establishing mechanisms for public feedback and expert oversight to mitigate and address biased, inaccurate, or inappropriate content targeted at children.
- Policymakers can promote research and development of child-centered AI technologies by encouraging collaboration between industry, academia, and government. Specifically, it is important to involve stakeholders who work with children of diverse abilities and needs to ensure that development accommodates variability in learning and fosters inclusive growth.
- Policymakers can promote responsible use of child-centered AI technologies by supporting state and local educational organizations' efforts to identify and use evidence-based practices that ensure AI technologies are safely and effectively being used to support children's developmental outcomes.

**Conflict of Interest and Funding Disclosures** This chapter was conducted with support from the National Science Foundation under Grant No. 2302730.

## References

1. Aeschlimann S, Bleiker M, Wechner M, Gampe A. Communicative and social consequences of interactions with voice assistants. Comput Hum Behav. 2020;112:106466. https://doi.org/10.1016/j.chb.2020.106466.
2. Arora A, Arora A. Effects of smart voice control devices on children: current challenges and future perspectives. Arch Dis Child. 2022;107(12):1129–30. https://doi.org/10.1136/archdischild-2022-323888.
3. Barr R, Kirkorian H, Radesky J, et al. Beyond screen time: a synergistic approach to a more comprehensive assessment of family media exposure during early childhood. Front Psychol. 2020;11:1283. https://doi.org/10.3389/fpsyg.2020.01283.
4. Beneteau E, Boone A, Wu Y, Kientz JA, Yip J, Hiniker A. Parenting with Alexa: exploring the introduction of smart speakers on family dynamics. In: Proceedings of the 2020 CHI conference on human factors in computing systems. New York: ACM; 2020. p. 1–13. https://doi.org/10.1145/3313831.3376344.
5. Birhane A, Isaac W, Prabhakaran V, et al. Power to the people? Opportunities and challenges for participatory AI. In: Equity and access in algorithms, mechanisms, and optimization. New York: ACM; 2022. p. 1–8. https://doi.org/10.1145/3551624.3555290.
6. Cardona MA, Rodríguez RJ, Ishmael K. Artificial intelligence and the future of teaching and learning: insights and recommendations. 2023. https://www2.ed.gov/documents/ai-report/ai-report.pdf. Accessed 4 Apr 2024.
7. Cassell J. Towards a model of technology and literacy development: story listening systems. J Appl Dev Psychol. 2004;25(1):75–105. https://doi.org/10.1016/j.appdev.2003.11.003.
8. Cassell J. Socially interactive agents as peers. In: Lugrin B, Pelachaud C, Traum D, editors. The handbook on socially interactive agents. 1st ed. New York: ACM; 2022. p. 331–66. https://doi.org/10.1145/3563659.3563670.
9. Gampe A, Zahner-Ritter K, Müller JJ, Schmid SR. How children speak with their voice assistant Sila depends on what they think about her. Comput Hum Behav. 2023;143:107693. https://doi.org/10.1016/j.chb.2023.107693.
10. Golinkoff RM, Hoff E, Rowe ML, Tamis-LeMonda CS, Hirsh-Pasek K. Language matters: denying the existence of the 30-million-word gap has serious consequences. Child Dev. 2019;90(3):985–92. https://doi.org/10.1111/cdev.13128.
11. Hiniker A, Wang A, Tran J, et al. Can conversational agents change the way children talk to people? In: Proceedings of the 20th annual ACM interaction design and children conference. New York: ACM; 2021. p. 338–49. https://doi.org/10.1145/3459990.3460695.
12. Kory-Westlund JM, Won Park H, Grover I, Breazeal C. Long-term interaction with relational SIAs. In: The handbook on socially interactive agents. New York: ACM; 2022. p. 195–260. https://doi.org/10.1145/3563659.3563667.
13. Le T, Huang DY, Apthorpe N, Tian Y. SkillBot: identifying risky content for children in Alexa skills. ACM Trans Internet Technol. 2022;22(3):1–31. https://doi.org/10.1145/3539609.
14. Lee Y, Kim TS, Chang M, Kim J. Interactive children's story rewriting through parent-children interaction. In: Proceedings of the first workshop on intelligent and interactive writing assistants (In2Writing 2022). Association for Computational Linguistics; 2022. p. 62–71. https://doi.org/10.18653/v1/2022.in2writing-1.9.
15. Lin GC, Schoenfeld I, Thompson M, Xia Y, Uz-Bilgin C, Leech K. "What color are the fish's scales?" Exploring parents' and children's natural interactions with a child-friendly virtual agent during storybook reading. In: Proceedings of the 21st annual ACM interaction design and children conference. New York: ACM; 2022. p. 185–95. https://doi.org/10.1145/3501712.3529734.
16. Long D, Magerko B. What is AI literacy? Competencies and design considerations. In: Proceedings of the 2020 CHI conference on human factors in computing systems. New York: ACM; 2020. p. 1–16. https://doi.org/10.1145/3313831.3376727.
17. Melsión GI, Torre I, Vidal E, Leite I. Using explainability to help children understandgender bias in AI. In: Proceedings of the 20th annual ACM Interaction design and children conference. New York: ACM; 2021. p. 87–99. https://doi.org/10.1145/3459990.3460719.
18. Over H, Eggleston A, Bell J, Dunham Y. Young children seek out biased information about social groups. Dev Sci. 2018;21(3):e12580.
19. Porayska-Pomsta K, Alcorn AM, Avramides K, et al. Blending human and artificial intelligence to support autistic children's social communication skills. ACM Trans Comput-Hum Interact. 2018;25(6):1–35. https://doi.org/10.1145/3271484.
20. Severson RL, Carlson SM. Behaving as or behaving as if? children's conceptions of personified robots and the emergence of a new ontological category. Neural Netw. 2010;23(8–9):1099–103. https://doi.org/10.1016/j.neunet.2010.08.014.
21. Severson RL, Lemm KM. Kids see human too: adapting an individual differences measure of anthropomorphism for a child sample. J Cogn Dev. 2015;17(1):122–41. https://doi.org/10.1080/15248372.2014.989445.
22. Tartaro A, Cassell J, Ratz C, Lira J, Nanclares-Nogués V. Accessing peer social interaction: using authorable virtual peer technology as a component of a group social skills intervention program. ACM Trans Accessible Comput. 2014;6(1):1–29. https://doi.org/10.1145/2700434.
23. Turkle S. Reclaiming conversation: the power of talk in a digital age. Penguin; 2016.
24. Van Brummelen J, Tian MC, Kelleher M, Nguyen NH. Learning affects trust: design recommendations

and concepts for teaching children – and nearly anyone – about conversational agents. arXiv:2209.05063. 2022; https://doi.org/10.48550/arXiv:2209.05063.
25. van den Berghe R, de Haas M, Oudgenoeg-Paz O, et al. A toy or a friend? Children's anthropomorphic beliefs about robots and how these relate to second-language word learning. J Comput Assist Learn. 2021;37(2):396–410. https://doi.org/10.1111/jcal.12497.
26. van Straten CL, Peter J, Kühne R, Barco A. The wizard and I: how transparent teleoperation and self-description (do not) affect children's robot perceptions and child-robot relationship formation. AI & Soc. 2022;37(1):383–99. https://doi.org/10.1007/s00146-021-01202-3.
27. Weidinger L, Uesato J, Rauh M, et al. Taxonomy of risks posed by language models. In: Proceedings of the 2022 ACM conference on fairness, accountability, and transparency. ACM; 2022. p. 214–29. https://doi.org/10.1145/3531146.3533088.
28. Williams T, Grollman D, Han M, et al. "Excuse me, robot": impact of polite robot wakewords on human-robot politeness. In: Social robotics: 12th international conference, ICSR 2020. New York: ACM; 2020. p. 404–15. https://doi.org/10.1007/978-3-030-62056-1_34.
29. Xu Y, Wang D, Collins P, Lee H, Warschauer M. Same benefits, different communication patterns: comparing children's reading with a conversational agent vs. a human partner. Comput Educ. 2021;161:104059. https://doi.org/10.1016/j.compedu.2020.104059.
30. Xu Y, Aubele J, Vigil V, Bustamante AS, Kim YS, Warschauer M. Dialogue with a conversational agent promotes children's story comprehension via enhancing engagement. Child Dev. 2022;93(2):e149–67. https://doi.org/10.1111/cdev.13708.
31. Zhang Z, Xu Y, Wang Y, et al. StoryBuddy: a human-AI collaborative chatbot for parent-child interactive storytelling with flexible parental involvement. In: Proceedings of the 2022 CHI conference on human factors in computing systems. New York: ACM; 2022. p. 1–21. https://doi.org/10.1145/3491102.3517479.

# Children's Understanding and Use of Voice-Assistants: Opportunities and Challenges

Judith H. Danovitch, Adam K. Dubé, Cansu Oranç, Jessica Szczuka, and Svetlana Yarosh

## 1 Background

Since the launch of Apple's Siri in 2011, use of voice-driven digital assistants and voice-assistant devices (also known as "smart speakers") has skyrocketed. In fact, in 2024, the number of voice-assistant devices (VAs) worldwide is projected to overtake the human population, with over 8.4 billion units [1]. Children's understanding and use of VAs is important for two primary reasons: (1) VAs are increasingly available and present in children's lives and (2) VAs allow even young children to interact with an AI-driven virtual agent that can access information available on the internet.

Children are increasingly likely to be exposed to VAs. In a 2020 survey, nearly half of a diverse sample of American parents reported that their children ages 5–12 had interacted with a VA [2]. Although Internet search technologies have been available for several decades, VAs create a verbally based natural language interaction (e.g., in contrast to typing questions) [3, 4] that allows preliterate or semi-literate child users the opportunity to tap into the human knowledge available on the Internet to support their curiosity and learning. As VAs become more sophisticated and natural in their interaction, children may have more difficulty differentiating between human and agent responses, and therefore, they may also have more difficulty understanding when those responses need to be treated with skepticism, making them increasingly vulnerable to misinformation. Although hardware may change over time, VAs seem to be here to stay, making it essential to understand how children think about them and what benefits and risks their use involves for children's health and learning. In the following sections, we outline what is currently known about children's interactions with and use of VAs, including the ways in which they may view VAs as information sources and social partners. We then offer directions for future research and recommendations for stakeholders in children's development.

J. H. Danovitch (✉)
University of Louisville, Louisville, KY, USA
e-mail: j.danovitch@louisville.edu

A. K. Dubé
McGill University, Montreal, QC, Canada

C. Oranç
Ronin Institute, Montclair, NJ, USA

J. Szczuka
University of Duisburg-Essen, Duisburg and Essen, Germany

S. Yarosh
University of Minnesota, Minneapolis, MN, USA

## 2 Current State

### 2.1 Children Talking to Voice-Assistants

Children enjoy interacting with VAs and readily do so [5]. Naturalistic and laboratory-based


D. A. Christakis, L. Hale (eds.), *Handbook of Children and Screens*,
https://doi.org/10.1007/978-3-031-69362-5_84

observations of children's use of VAs also show that children easily ask questions and make requests of both familiar and unfamiliar VAs [6–12]. One of the properties that makes VAs uniquely accessible and appealing to children is their natural language interface: children can talk to VAs as they would to another person, without requiring special training or an adult mediator. However, interacting with VAs also poses unique challenges for children, and it can have effects on children's linguistic habits and communication skills [8, 13, 14].

Using technology to recognize children's speech is notoriously difficult (e.g., Ref. [15]), especially for spontaneous utterances, and recognizing intent is significantly more difficult than just recognizing specific spoken words, even with adults [16]. In a study where children ages 5–12 had to ask a novel VA questions that required additional context or decomposition into multiple parts in order to have them be comprehensible to the VA, almost all children struggled, and this struggle was more substantial for younger children [17]. Children are likely to encounter communication breakdowns with VAs, such as misunderstandings and nonresponsiveness, which can arise from inadequacies on the part of both the children and the VAs. Children may attempt to repair these miscommunications by employing a variety of strategies, such as repeating or reformulating their questions [18]. Alternatively, they may change the course of the conversation altogether [7, 10, 17]. Recent advances in generative models (e.g., ChatGPT) are likely to address some of these challenges. For example, with future systems, it would no longer be necessary to decompose complex multielement questions into separate queries—a task with which almost all children struggled in Yuan et al.'s study [17]. Nevertheless, as the underlying technology improves and it becomes easier for children to effectively address VAs, this may exacerbate the challenges children face when thinking about them as information sources and social partners.

## 2.2 Voice-Assistants as Information Sources

Among American parents who reported that their children ages 5–12 had interacted with a VA, 78% said that they used it to get information [2]. Children perceive VAs as sources of information, and studies confirm that children ask information-seeking questions of these devices [8, 10]. Children's most common knowledge searches can be characterized as educational or learning related, including questions about science, culture, and practical information (e.g., weather) [8, 19]. Children are also selective in the types of information they seek from VAs. For example, they are more likely to ask VAs factual questions about widely accessible information as opposed to personal questions, and this tendency becomes more pronounced with age [8, 10, 20]. Children also show differential trust in VAs' responses depending on the type of information they provide (factual or personal) [20]. In information-seeking contexts, young children seem to treat VAs like unfamiliar people—they are cautious about trusting them [20], and they will sometimes probe a VA's knowledge by asking questions that they can already answer (e.g., asking about a sibling's age) [8, 17]. Although research regarding actual learning outcomes is limited, some studies suggest that children do not learn as much from VAs as they do from adults [21], but there is also evidence that children recall information provided by VAs and adults equally well [20].

## 2.3 Voice-Assistants as Social Partners

As they gain experience with VAs, children may come to think of these devices not only as information sources but also as social partners. In a recent multinational study [19], parents primarily characterized child–VA relationships as transactional, with children making requests of VAs rather than speaking to them as they would to a friend, entertainer, or teacher. However, parents also reported that their children used human-like adjectives, including "smart," "trustworthy," and "funny" to describe VAs, suggesting that children view VAs in an anthropomorphized way. In other studies, children as young as age 6 have been documented directing emotional expressions toward VAs (e.g., "I love you, Google") [22] and parents report that children as young as age 3 have formed parasocial relationships with a VA in their home [23]. Moreover, when given the choice, children prefer to interact with devices that are personified (e.g., introduce themselves by name) over those that are not [17].

The interactivity of VAs, their fulfillment of a social role (as an assistant and/or conversational partner), and communication via natural language is likely to trigger social reactions that children would normally show toward other people. Thus, it is not surprising that children transfer human characteristics to VAs and draw analogies to their own lives (e.g., claiming VAs need to go to school to have knowledge) [24], although these intuitions appear to change with age [25]. For example, in one study, 6- and 7-year-olds were more likely than 8- and 9-year-olds to attribute cognitive and moral characteristics to a familiar VA [26]. Children's knowledge about how VAs work may also interact with their anthropomorphizing tendencies, as this knowledge can also be an important resource for distinguishing between an artificial device and a living person [24]. One possibility is that, as children gain experience with VAs and better understand how they work, they may come to view VAs as belonging to a new ontological category that is neither entirely living or non-living [5, 12, 27]. Treating VAs as part of a new ontological category could subsequently have consequences for children's preference for and reliance on these devices as information sources and social partners.

## 2.4 Challenges for Young Users of Voice-Assistants

VAs can be useful for learning and entertainment and the natural language user interface makes it relatively easy for children to interact with them. However, children may not fully understand how VAs work or what happens to information they provide a VA (see Ref. [24]), and it may be challenging for some children to anticipate that the interactions they have with this putative social entity could have unintended consequences (e.g., that the account holder, such as their parents, can view transcripts of their conversations). In addition, current state of the art systems follow a one-size-fits-all approach, such that VAs do not adapt to users with different needs. For these reasons, parents potentially play a key role in mediating and supporting children's use of VAs in the home [6, 19, 22]. In a study of parents from the United States, Canada, and the United Kingdom [19], parents frequently reported mediating their child's use of VAs via enabling strategies such as providing guidance based on their child's requests and co-using VAs with their child. Parents were less likely to report mediating use via independently monitoring their child's interactions with VAs or using restrictive strategies (i.e., using software built into VAs to prohibit specific activities).

As VAs become more natural in their interactions, children may have a harder time differentiating between human and agent responses, and therefore they may also have a harder time understanding when those responses need to be treated with skepticism. New generative models may allow VAs to better understand children's speech, but they are not immune from malicious manipulation that could provide confusing or even harmful responses (e.g., Ref. [28]). Although the potential for harm is substantial, VAs are not going away anytime soon. Thus, researchers and regulators must strive to keep up with the rapid changes in VA technology to better understand how to support children in using it safely and effectively.

## 3 Future Research

Given the very recent advent of VAs and their rapidly increasing presence in children's homes and other learning environments, there are several pressing questions for research:

- *In what ways does children's learning from VAs differ from their learning from humans, and do children's learning outcomes relate to how they perceive artificially intelligent agents?* VAs can provide access to information that would otherwise be inaccessible to child users, yet it is unclear whether children consider this information reliable, and whether using a VA affects how well children understand and remember information in the long run.
- *How does interacting with VAs impact children's social cognition and development?* There is evidence that children may view VAs as social partners [22] or enter into parasocial relationships with them [23], but little is known about how children think about these relationships and how the nature of these relationships compares to the relationships that children have with peers or adults, or with media characters. Interacting with VAs may also affect how children view other people, whose responses to their questions and statements are likely to be less consistent than a VA's responses, or who may be less tolerant of antisocial behaviors (e.g., being insulted).
- *How will improvements in VA speech quality and interactivity affect children's interactions with and beliefs about VAs?* In the coming years, if not months, VA technology will leverage generative AI to improve and smoothen the interaction experience and this may result in VAs being better at comprehending children's speech and being more tailored to individual child users' individual needs. As VAs become more adept at "remembering" a child user's interests and preferences, and as their conversational interactions become more humanlike, will children become more reliant on VAs for social companionship? Similarly, as VA technology advances, will children be more likely to attribute human-like characteristics to these devices and will they have more difficulty distinguishing between humans and VAs?
- *How can caregivers and educators leverage the power and appeal of VAs to support children's learning and well-being, while protecting their privacy and avoiding exposure to misinformation?* Given how challenging it can be for children (and even adults) to understand how Internet-based technologies work [12, 29], it may be difficult for children to discern when a VA is "listening" to them or what happens to the information that they share with a VA. Further research is therefore needed to understand how adults can support children's safe and effective use of VAs for learning and entertainment purposes.

Although additional research on children's interactions with VAs is necessary, it is important to keep in mind that as VA technology continues evolving, new questions and challenges may arise. Researchers must thus strive to remain aware of technological advances and research on adjacent topics including artificial intelligence and human–robot interaction.

## 4 Recommendations

- *Researchers* need to thoroughly understand children's questioning patterns with VAs and their expectations of these devices as sources of information. They should look for sources of variability, such as home experience or parent input, and investigate how that affects children's judgments. To best inform our understanding of novel technology and its psychological implications, research should be interdisciplinary; studies of children's use of VAs can benefit from the expertise of computer scientists, psychologists, educators, legal scholars, linguists, and other related disciplines.
- *Caregivers, including parents and guardians,* should support children in the responsible use of VAs and other voice-driven AI technolo-

gies. Caregivers should engage in co-use of VAs with young children and actively monitor children's use of VAs. Critically, caregivers should familiarize themselves with the parental restriction tools/settings available on VAs to set appropriate limits on the range of uses children can access. Although the current actions VAs can perform may seem rather benign (e.g., play a song, set a timer), one only has to look at the development of the smartphone to see how quickly a new technology can become the ubiquitous access point to the entirety of content and software available on the internet.

- *Educators* should exercise caution in using VAs to augment classroom teaching, and they should not assume that children trust the answers provided by a VA or effectively learn from them. Educators also need to rethink and redesign digital literacy education to teach children the skills required for information search in the voice-driven AI era. Specifically, they should educate children on how to communicate their queries effectively to nonhuman agents and how to critically evaluate the information received. Working with researchers, practitioners should continue developing AI-literacy curricula, starting with simple lessons for young children focused on the differences between AI "thinking" and human knowledge, and continuing into adolescence with more direct connections to computational thinking and computer science.
- *Developers* should design systems that take into account the needs and abilities of different groups of vulnerable people, including children. Developers should work toward implementing privacy features and safeguards and making children's interactions with VAs more understandable and transparent. For example, they can develop tools to help children understand where certain answers come from (e.g., by having the VA consistently cite sources or include disclaimers about responses that contain subjective information or potential misinformation). Question asking is a powerful learning tool for children, and developers of commercially available VAs should encourage this behavior by providing safe and seamless interactions while minimizing deadlocks.
- *Policymakers* should consider children's vulnerability and their right to privacy when developing policies for VA manufacturers. Because children are often not actively involved in deciding what data they produce and how their data is stored, regulators and lawmakers must develop guidelines and policies that protect children as VAs and other voice-driven AI technologies become more popular and readily accessible. Such policies will have to reckon with tensions arising from the desire to protect children's privacy with the reality that children's data is likely needed to make VAs more accessible to children (e.g., training of Large Language Models and voice recognition).

**Conflict of Interest and Funding Disclosures** None.

## References

1. Juniper research: number of voice assistant devices in use to overtake world population by 2024, reaching 8.4bn, led by smartphones. Business Wire. 28 Apr 2020. https://www.businesswire.com/news/home/20200427005609/en/Juniper-Research-Number-of-Voice-Assistant-Devices-in-Use-to-Overtake-World-Population-by-2024-Reaching-8.4bn-Led-by-Smartphones. Accessed 20 Apr 2023.
2. Auxier B, Anderson M, Perrin A, Turner E. Parenting children in the age of screens. 28 July 2020. https://www.pewresearch.org/internet/2020/07/28/childrens-engagement-with-digital-devices-screen-time/. Accessed 20 Apr 2023.
3. Druin A, Foss E, Hatley L, Golub E, Guha ML, Fails J, Hutchinson H. How children search the internet with keyword interfaces. In: Proceedings of the 8th international conference on interaction design and children. Como, Italy. New York: ACM; 2009. p. 89–96. https://doi.org/10.1145/1551788.1551804.
4. Druin A, Foss E, Hutchinson H, Golub E, Hatley L. Children's roles using keyword search interfaces at home. In: Proceedings of the SIGCHI conference on human factors in computing systems. Atlanta, GA. New York: ACM; 2010. p. 413–22. https://doi.org/10.1145/1753326.1753388.

5. Festerling J, Siraj I. Alexa, what are you? Exploring primary school children's ontological perceptions of digital voice assistants in open interactions. Hum Dev. 2020;64(1):26–43. https://doi.org/10.1159/000508499.
6. Beneteau E, Boone A, Wu Y, Kientz JA, Yip J, Hiniker A. Parenting with Alexa: exploring the introduction of smart speakers on family dynamics. In: Proceedings of the 2020 CHI conference on human factors in computing systems. Honolulu, HI. New York: ACM; 2020. p. 1–13. https://doi.org/10.1145/3313831.3376344.
7. Cheng Y, Yen K, Chen Y, Chen S, Hiniker A. Why doesn't it work? Voice-driven interfaces and young children's communication repair strategies. In: Proceedings of the 17th ACM conference on interaction design and children. Trondheim, Norway. New York: ACM; 2018. p. 337–48. https://doi.org/10.1145/3202185.3202749.
8. Lovato SB, Piper AM, Wartella EA. Hey Google, do unicorns exist? Conversational agents as a path to answers to children's questions. In: Proceedings of the 18th ACM international conference on interaction design and children. Boise, ID. New York: ACM; 2019. p. 301–13. https://doi.org/10.1145/3311927.3323150.
9. Park S, Lim YK. Investigating user expectations on the roles of family-shared AI speakers. In: Proceedings of the 2020 CHI conference on human factors in computing systems. Honolulu, HI. New York: ACM; 2020. p. 1–13. https://doi.org/10.1145/3313831.3376450.
10. Oranç C, Ruggeri A. "Alexa, let me ask you something different" Children's adaptive information search with voice assistants. Hum Behav Emerg Technol. 2021;3(4):595–605. https://doi.org/10.1002/hbe2.270.
11. Xu Y, Warschauer M. Young children's reading and learning with conversational agents. In: Extended abstracts of the 2019 CHI conference on human factors in computing systems. Glasgow, Scotland, UK. New York: ACM; 2019. p. 1–8. https://doi.org/10.1145/3290607.3299035.
12. Xu Y, Warschauer M. What are you talking to?: understanding children's perceptions of conversational agents. In: Proceedings of the 2020 CHI conference on human factors in computing systems. Honolulu, HI. New York: ACM; 2020. p. 1–13. https://doi.org/10.1145/3313831.3376416.
13. Biele C, Jaskulska A, Kopec W, Kowalski J, Skorupska K, Zdrodowska A. How might voice assistants raise our children? In: Intelligent human systems integration 2019: proceedings of the 2nd international conference on intelligent human systems integration (IHSI 2019): integrating people and intelligent systems. San Diego, CA. Cham: Springer; 2019. p. 162–7. https://doi.org/10.1007/978-3-030-11051-2_25.
14. Sciuto A, Saini A, Forlizzi J, Hong JI. "Hey Alexa, what's up?" A mixed-methods studies of in-home conversational agent usage. In: Proceedings of the 2018 designing interactive systems conference. Hong Kong, China. New York: ACM; 2018. p. 857–68. https://doi.org/10.1145/3196709.3196772.
15. Giuliani D, Gerosa M. Investigating recognition of children's speech. In: 2003 IEEE international conference on acoustics, speech, and signal processing. Hong Kong, China. IEEE; 2003. p. II–137. https://doi.org/10.1109/ICASSP.2003.1202313.
16. Stifelman L, Elman A, Sullivan A. Designing natural speech interactions for the living room. In: CHI'13 Extended abstracts on human factors in computing systems. Paris, France. New York: ACM; 2013. p. 1215–20. https://doi.org/10.1145/2468356.2468574.
17. Yuan Y, Thompson S, Watson K, Chase A, Senthilkumar A, Brush AB, Yarosh S. Speech interface reformulations and voice assistant personification preferences of children and parents. Int J Child Comput Interact. 2019;21:77–88. https://doi.org/10.1016/j.ijcci.2019.04.005.
18. Gampe A, Zahner-Ritter K, Müller JJ, Schmid SR. How children speak with their voice assistant Sila depends on what they think about her. Comput Hum Behav. 2023;143:107693. https://doi.org/10.1016/j.chb.2023.107693.
19. Bharadwaj NA, Dubé AK, Talwar V, Patitsas E. How digital assistants are used by families in the home: a multi-national study of use, interaction, and parental mediation. In: Technology, mind & society 2021 conference proceedings. APA; 2021. https://doi.org/10.1037/tms0000075.
20. Girouard-Hallam LN, Danovitch JH. Children's trust in and learning from voice assistants. Dev Psychol. 2022;58(4):646. https://doi.org/10.1037/dev0001318.
21. Tong Y, Wang F, Wang W. Fairies in the box: children's perception and interaction towards voice assistants. Hum Behav Emerg Technol. 2022;2022:1273814. https://doi.org/10.1155/2022/1273814.
22. Garg R, Sengupta S. He is just like me: a study of the long-term use of smart speakers by parents and children. Proc ACM Interact Mob Wearable Ubiquitous Technol. 2020;4(1):1–24. https://doi.org/10.1145/3381002.
23. Hoffman A, Owen D, Calvert SL. Parent reports of children's parasocial relationships with conversational agents: trusted voices in children's lives. Hum Behav Emerg Technol. 2021;3(4):606–17. https://doi.org/10.1002/hbe2.271.
24. Szczuka JM, Strathmann C, Szymczyk N, Mavrina L, Krämer NC. How do children acquire knowledge about voice assistants? A longitudinal field study on children's knowledge about how voice assistants store and process data. Int J Child Comput Interact. 2022;33:100460. https://doi.org/10.1016/j.ijcci.2022.100460.
25. Flanagan T, Wong G, Kushnir T. The minds of machines: children's beliefs about the experiences,

thoughts, and morals of familiar interactive technologies. Dev Psychol. 2023;59(6):1017–31. https://doi.org/10.1037/dev0001524.
26. Girouard-Hallam LN, Streble HM, Danovitch JH. Children's mental, social, and moral attributions toward a familiar digital voice assistant. Hum Behav Emerg Technol. 2021;3(5):1118–31. https://doi.org/10.1002/hbe2.321.
27. Kahn PH Jr, Shen S. NOC, who's there? A new ontological category (NOC) for social robots. In: Budwig N, Turiel E, Zelazo PD, editors. New perspectives on human development. Cambridge University Press; 2017. p. 106–22.
28. Ganguli D, Hernandez D, Lovitt L, Askell A, Bai Y, Chen A, Conerly T, Dassarma N, Drain D, Elhage N, El Showk S. Predictability and surprise in large generative models. In: Proceedings of the 2022 ACM conference on fairness, accountability, and transparency. Seoul, South Korea. New York: ACM; 2022. p. 1747–64. https://doi.org/10.1145/3531146.3533229.
29. Mertala P. Young children's conceptions of computers, code, and the Internet. Int J Child Comput Interact. 2019;19:56–66. https://doi.org/10.1016/j.ijcci.2018.11.003.

# Social Robots and Children's Development: Promises and Implications

Rachel L. Severson, Jochen Peter, Takayuki Kanda, Jordy Kaufman, and Brian Scassellati

## 1 Background

Advanced interactive technologies, such as social robots, are increasingly a part of many children's everyday lives [1]. Designed for everyday environments such as museums, schools, and hospitals, social robots provide information and assist children with specific educational and therapeutic needs. Although varied in their designs (e.g., Furhat, Keepon, iCat, Pleo, Aibo, Pepper, Nao, Robovie), social robots are commonly defined as autonomous, interactive, embodied, and communicative (e.g., linguistic, nonlinguistic, postural). Social robots represent a rapidly growing emerging technology with a projected 31% market growth from 2022 to 2028 (from US$3.4 to US$17.2 billion) primarily in the education and healthcare sectors [2]. Research over nearly two decades has investigated the potential benefits and downsides of the current and future use of social robots in children's lives.

As social robots become more ubiquitous and sophisticated, decisions regarding their design, context of use, and ethical considerations will not be straightforward. Our goal is to highlight—even if necessarily restricted in scope—the state of the field from our various disciplines. We provide directions for future research to address pressing questions and make recommendations with a particular focus on ethical considerations as we (as parents, educators, clinicians, researchers, designers, policymakers, and society at large) navigate both the promise and implications of social robots in children's development.

## 2 Current State

### 2.1 Understanding of Social Robots

From an early age, children attribute a constellation of animate and inanimate characteristics to social robots. Children understand social robots as technological and not biological. They nevertheless view robots as having perceptual capabilities (e.g., sight, hearing, feeling touch), mental states (e.g., thought, feelings, intentions), sociality (e.g., friend, companion), and moral standing (e.g., not permissible to harm or treat unfairly). Some characteristics attributed to robots may

R. L. Severson (✉)
University of Montana, Missoula, MT, USA
e-mail: rachel.severson@umontana.edu

J. Peter
University of Amsterdam, Amsterdam, Netherlands

T. Kanda
Kyoto University, Kyoto, Japan

J. Kaufman
Swinburne University of Technology, Melbourne, VIC, Australia

B. Scassellati
Yale University, New Haven, CT, USA


D. A. Christakis, L. Hale (eds.), *Handbook of Children and Screens*,
https://doi.org/10.1007/978-3-031-69362-5_85

result from their functional (rather than structural) similarities to biological beings (e.g., robots "see" with cameras rather than eyes). Yet children's willingness to view social robots as mental, social, and moral others has led some researchers to suggest that social robots may represent the emergence of a unique category that cuts across prototypic categories of alive and not alive [3, 4].

Studies show that children's acceptance of robots and their attributions of human-like qualities depends in large part on the child's age and the robot's features. Children accept social robots more readily if, among other things, social robots are adaptive, with adolescents being less accepting of social robots than older children [5]. As to relationship formation between social robots and children, children seem to feel closer to a social robot when the robot is responsive, expressive, and less capable than the children themselves [6]. Younger children (ages 3–5) tend to anthropomorphize robots and attribute animistic qualities to them [7, 8] (see Ref. [4] for a review). Although young children's (ages 3–5) animacy judgments are not contingent on whether the robot is presented as autonomous or controlled [9], slightly older children (5–7 years) ascribe more mental and emotional states, as well as moral standing, to an autonomous versus controlled social robot [10]. Older children (ages 9–15) are more likely to recognize robots as distinct from humans but still often attribute mental states and social qualities to them [3]. However, explicit transparency about the robot's lack of psychological characteristics decreased older children's (8–9 years) animistic perceptions of robots [11].

## 2.2 Social Robots in Education and Therapeutic Contexts

There are vast opportunities (and corresponding needs) for personalized, continuous support for children in a variety of settings, such as schools, hospitals, and homes. In terms of learning, social robots are effective in one-on-one tutoring for school-age children, eliciting positive cognitive, social, and affective results [12, 13]. Research has shown that children's learning from social robots is comparable to the effects with human tutors when tasks are simple and social, and more advantageous than virtual agents as embodied robots are more engaging and elicit social behaviors that enhance learning (see Ref. [12] for a review). However, children have less trust in the competence and reliability of a social robot if it is more human like [14].

Social robots are particularly useful in supporting children's learning for several reasons. Physical embodiment leads to greater compliance and faster learning than with a virtual avatar or on-screen robot (see Refs. [12, 15] for reviews). Another important feature for children's learning is social contingency, which refers to reciprocal interactions initiated by one partner through gaze, vocalization, or actions and appropriately responded to by another partner. Children (3–5 years) were more likely to learn from a socially contingent versus noncontingent robot [16]. Moreover, children are often more comfortable making a mistake in front of a robot tutor rather than a human tutor, and this can lead to significant performance improvements with very little tutoring time [12]. Very young children—even those who are too young (under age 2) to learn from screen-based information—are able to learn when engaged with robots. For example, 6- to 12-month-old deaf infants were able to learn American Sign Language (ASL) signs with a robot system teaching [17]. Among hearing children, social robots have been found to increase children's learning motivation, although robots' impact on language improvement was mixed [15].

Social robots also support the unique and individual needs of children with a range of special needs (e.g., autism spectrum disorder (ASD) [18], hearing impairment [17]), as well as promoting children's mental well-being [19] and physical health (e.g., managing diabetes [20]). For example, in the most in-depth and comprehensive exploration to date, an autonomous social robot was deployed in the homes of children with ASD for 1 month [21]. During the robot's deployment, participants made significant progress in social skills (measured by an independent clinical evaluation team) and in human-directed social skills (while not in the presence of the robot) relative to the prior month. Although children's progress degraded in the month following the robot deployment (consistent with human-based therapies), this research provides real promise for how social robots can provide in-home personalized therapeutic support. Together, this research suggests that social robots are a promising technology for supporting children's learning and healthy functioning, with particular potential among populations that need daily or continuous support.

## 2.3 Moral Relationships with Social Robots

As Kahn and colleagues [3] argue, social robots present a conundrum: On the one hand, they are technological tools that can be used when needed and put away when not. On the other hand, social robots present as if they have psychological and social characteristics. Where then do children place social robots in their moral spheres? Children's moral relationships with social robots have received broad consideration in terms of children's prosocial behaviors toward robots, their trust in robots, and their judgments about robots' moral standing and culpability. We know that children spontaneously help a robot that appears in need. For example, 3- to 5-year-old children attempt to help a robot in need, regardless of whether it was introduced as autonomous or controlled by others [9]. Such prosocial behaviors toward robots extended into the adolescent years as 5- to 16-year-olds would similarly help a robot [22]. Moreover, children (ages 8–10) are sensitive to robots modeling prosocial behavior—children were more generous and expected higher levels of peers' prosociality after observing a prosocial robot [23]. Additionally, children (ages 4–9) trust robots as confidantes; they willingly shared secrets and personal information (see Ref. [14] for a meta-analysis). Together this research illustrates both the potential benefits—an increase in children's prosociality after observing a prosocial robot—and downsides—privacy issues as children disclose secrets and personal information—of children's interactions with social robots.

Children's moral conceptions of robots extend beyond discretionary acts of helping and sharing to also include judgments (by children as young as 3 years) that robots deserve moral treatment (for reviews see Refs. [4, 8]). A study by Kahn and colleagues [3] with 9-, 12-, and 15-year-olds revealed that many children, particularly younger ones, viewed a transgression against the robot, Robovie, as morally unacceptable and akin to their moral judgments about humans. Yet, these same children were more conservative when extending certain rights (e.g., right to vote) to Robovie. Thus, children's more restrictive moral attributions suggest that social robots may be situated in a middle ground between humans and artifacts.

Research has also examined the darker side of children's moral relationships with robots; that is, when children abuse robots. Children (and adults) are surprisingly destructive to robots—verbally abusing, hitting, punching, kicking, and even destroying them. Such cases have occurred in laboratory settings [24] as well as in real-world settings (e.g., shopping malls). Researchers have uncovered several reasons why children abuse robots. Children (5–9 years) who harmed robots often felt enjoyment, while also believing that the abused robot perceived the harm [25]. This result is striking given that many children believe social robots should not be harmed because they would experience that pain (e.g., Ref. [3]), suggesting that children do not conceptualize social robots as mere toys [4]. Other research has found that robot abuse by adults may be related to a dehumanization process, and that a lack of mind attribution to a robot may increase the likelihood of abuse [26]. Finally, robot mistreatment is often a result of group dynamics, with children imitating others' abusive behavior and escalating the aggressiveness of their own behavior [27]—a pattern that is reminiscent of imitative social learning in Bandura's classic Bobo Doll study [28]. Although researchers are beginning to understand why robot abuse occurs, it is difficult to stop the abuse once it starts. There have been relatively few reports of successful approaches, such as asking for bystander intervention [29] or allowing the robot to physically escape [30], and it is largely unknown whether a robot can persuade abusers to stop or change their minds about continuing the abuse. Beyond the costliness and design challenges associated with the mistreatment of social robots, it is concerning that some children spontaneously engage in aggressive behavior toward social robots.

## 3 Future Research

As we turn to suggestions for future research, we first underscore four recommendations to improve the quality, replicability, and applicability of research on child-robot interaction. Methodologically, researchers in the field should address persistent and pernicious problems with poor internal validity (e.g., lack of control conditions, failure to randomize) and low statistical power (due to small sample sizes), as well as employ longitudinal designs and develop standardized child-appropriate measures to improve the fidelity of the research [1, 14]. Theoretically, the field would benefit from more attention to developmental perspectives, cultural differences, and (more homogeneous) theoretical work [1]. Technologically, the field needs to acknowledge more strongly that current interactions between children and robots in research settings are still restricted and hardly feasible in real-world settings [31]. Thus, much of our current knowledge about children's interactions with robots may suffer from a novelty-effect bias and low ecological validity [1, 5]. Ethically, systematic attention is needed regarding what social robots may or may not do in interactions with children (e.g., displaying emotions) and on how researchers (and designers) should deal with robots deceiving children about abilities, such as sentience and consciousness [32]. With these considerations in mind, we now turn to recommendations for future research.

- What features (appearance, behaviors, etc.) affect children's meaningful engagement, animacy, and mental state attributions, social and moral judgments, and actions (prosociality, trust, and nonabusive treatment) toward robots? How *social* do social robots need to be? How does this change with child age and/or experience with the robot over time?
- To what extent is a robot's success at motivating children dependent on children being deceived about the robot's mental and emotional capabilities? For example, will a child continue to work through a painful physical rehabilitation session with a motivating robot if the child understands that the robot does not have the capacity to care about them or their efforts?
- What are the consequences for children of how people interact with social robots? Will aggressive behaviors toward robots translate to other nonliving or living entities, such as pets and people? How might children's development be affected by robot abuse (either as a perpetrator or witness) or engaging with robots in a master-servant relationship? [3]. Conversely, is it appropriate to assert that robots have moral standing? Can and should we build systems that understand, maintain, and perhaps even uphold social and moral norms?
- As social robots become increasingly sophisticated, interactive, and "intelligent" (in the computationally strong or general sense), will children trust robots not only when learning, but also seek them out for comfort and advice? Future research could examine whether robot confidantes could be beneficial (e.g., providing advice utilizing evidence-based approaches [19]) or harmful (e.g., would the robots' lack of authenticity undermine the advice?) relative to what is possible in human-human relationships.

## 4 Recommendations

### 4.1 For Caregivers, Educators, and Clinicians

- Provide an appropriately informative introduction to the robot to ensure that children more accurately understand the robot's capabilities and limitations.

- Given their physical presence compared to nonembodied virtual agents, robots may lend themselves for educational and therapeutic applications. Define clearly if, when, and for what applications a robot may be of use as a teaching or therapeutic assistant with careful consideration of special populations (e.g., children with internalizing problems) and privacy considerations (see recommendation below).
- Provide clear expectations for how to treat social robots. Apart from the potential damage (and repair or replacement costs) and interruption of services, there are unanswered questions regarding (1) whether aggressive actions toward robots may generalize to children's treatment of other human or nonhuman animals and (2) the effects on bystanders of witnessing robot abuse.
- Consider potential privacy violations (ethical or legal) if robots record, retain, or share data collected. Bear in mind that children may place an inappropriately high level of trust in a robot and disclose information without the knowledge that it is being recorded.

## 4.2 For Robot Designers

- Consider the legal and ethical implications in designing robots. Is it necessary that the robot's design deceives users about its machine nature (e.g., suggesting consciousness, emotions, sentiency)? Can designs integrate a means for parents to "opt in" rather than "opt out" when the robot records a child in everyday settings? Prioritize issues of equity and accessibility of social robots.
- Provide more effective and accurate means of communicating the robot's capabilities to end users, with consideration for how children of different ages may understand robots.
- Find ways to support personalization/adaptation that utilize machine learning but provide strong limits on what kinds of behavior can be learned.

## 4.3 For Policymakers

- Employ an evidence-based approach to develop recommendations or certification of social robots for educational and clinical settings to ensure that specific robots and their context of use.
- Consider limitations on the recording, retention, and sharing of children's data collected by social robots. For example, consider whether the US Children's Online Privacy Protection Rule ("COPPA") would need to be amended to include data collected by robots.
- Develop processes to encourage the development of perceptual tools (speech recognition, expression recognition) that utilize child data in a secure, anonymized, and protected manner.

**Conflict of Interest and Funding Disclosures** None.

## References

1. Peter J, Kühne R, Barco A, De Jong C, Van Straten CL. Asking today the crucial questions of tomorrow: social robots and the internet of toys. In: Mascheroni G, Holloway D, editors. The internet of toys: practices, affordances and the political economy of children's smart play. Cham: Palgrave Macmillan (Springer Nature); 2019. p. 25–46.
2. IMARC. Social robots market: global industry trends, share, size, growth, opportunity and forecast 2023–2028. Report ID: SR112023A4794. 2022. https://www.imarcgroup.com/social-robots-market#:~:text=Market%20Overview%3A,30.7%25%20during%202023%2D2028.
3. Kahn PH, Kanda T, Ishiguro H, et al. "Robovie, you'll have to go into the closet now": children's social and moral relationships with a humanoid robot. Dev Psychol. 2012;48(2):303–14. https://doi.org/10.1037/a0027033.

4. Severson RL, Carlson SM. Behaving as or behaving as if? Children's conceptions of personified robots and the emergence of a new ontological category. Neural Netw. 2010;23(8–9):1099–103. https://doi.org/10.1016/j.neunet.2010.08.014.
5. De Jong C, Peter J, Kühne R, Barco A. Children's acceptance of social robots: a narrative review of the research 2000–2017. Interact Stud. 2019;20(3):393–425. https://doi.org/10.1075/is.18071.jon.
6. Van Straten CL, Peter J, Kühne R. Child–robot relationship formation: a narrative review of empirical research. Int J Soc Robot. 2020;12(2):325–44. https://doi.org/10.1007/s12369-019-00569-0.
7. Kahn PH, Severson RL, Ruckert JH. The human relation with nature and technological nature. Curr Dir Psychol Sci. 2009;18(1):37–42. https://doi.org/10.1111/j.1467-8721.2009.01602.x.
8. Kim M, Lee D, Yi S. Between living and nonliving: young children's animacy judgments and reasoning about humanoid robots. PLoS One. 2018;14(6):e0216869. https://doi.org/10.1371/journal.pone.0216869.
9. Martin DU, MacIntyre MI, Perry C, Clift G, Pedell S, Kaufman J. Young children's indiscriminate helping behavior toward a humanoid robot. Front Psychol. 2020;11:239. https://doi.org/10.3389/fpsyg.2020.00239.
10. Chernyak N, Gary HE. Children's cognitive and behavioral reactions to an autonomous versus controlled social robot dog. Early Educ Dev. 2016;27(8):1175–89. https://doi.org/10.1080/10409289.2016.1158611.
11. Van Straten CL, Peter J, Kühne R, Barco A. Transparency about a robot's lack of human psychological capacities: effects on child-robot perception and relationship formation. ACM Trans Hum-Robot Interact. 2020;9(2):11:1–11:22. https://doi.org/10.1145/3365668.
12. Belpaeme T, Kennedy J, Ramachandran A, Scassellati B, Tanaka F. Social robots for education: a review. Sci Robot. 2018;3(21):eaat5954. https://doi.org/10.1126/scirobotics.aat5954.
13. Kanda T, Hirano T, Eaton D, Ishiguro H. Interactive robots as social partners and peer tutors for children: a field trial. Hum Comput Interact. 2004;19(1–2):61–84. https://doi.org/10.1207/s15327051hci1901&2_4.
14. Stower R, Calvo-Barajas N, Castellano G, Kappas A. A meta-analysis on children's trust in social robots. Int J Soc Robot. 2021;13:1979–2001. https://doi.org/10.1007/s12369-020-00736-8.
15. Van den Berghe R, Verhagen J, Oudgenoeg-Paz O, van der Ven S, Leseman P. Social robots for language learning: a review. Rev Educ Res. 2019;89(2):259–95. https://doi.org/10.3102/0034654318821286.
16. Breazeal C, Harris PL, DeSteno D, Westlund JMK, Dickens L, Jeong S. Young children treat robots as informants. Top Cogn Sci. 2016;8(2):481–91. https://doi.org/10.1111/tops.12192.
17. Scassellati B, Brawer J, Tsui K, et al. Teaching language to deaf infants with a robot and a virtual human. In: Proceedings of the ACM CHI conference on human factors in computing systems. Montreal, QC. New York: ACM; 2018. p. 553. https://doi.org/10.1145/3173574.3174127.
18. Scassellati B, Admoni H, Matarić M. Robots for use in autism research. Annu Rev Biomed Eng. 2012;14:275–94.
19. Rabbitt S, Kazdin A, Scassellati B. Integrating socially assistive robotics into mental healthcare interventions: applications and recommendations for expanded use. Clin Psychol Rev. 2015;35:35–46. https://doi.org/10.1016/j.cpr.2014.07.001.
20. Neerincx MA, van Vught W, Blanson Henkemans O, et al. Socio-cognitive engineering of a robotic partner for child's diabetes self-management. Front Robot AI. 2019;6:118. https://doi.org/10.3389/frobt.2019.00118.
21. Scassellati B, Boccanfuso F, Huang CM, et al. Improving social skills in children with ASD using a long-term, in-home social robot. Sci Robot. 2018;3(21):eaat7544.
22. Beran TN, Ramirez-Serrano A, Kuzyk R, Nugent S, Fior M. Would children help a robot in need? Int J Soc Robot. 2011;3(1):83–93. https://doi.org/10.1007/s12369-010-0074-7.
23. Peter J, Kühne R, Barco A. Can social robots affect children's prosocial behavior? An experimental study on prosocial robot models. Comput Hum Behav. 2021;120:106712. https://doi.org/10.1016/j.chb.2021.106712.
24. Bartneck C, Rosalia C, Menges R, Deckers I. Robot abuse – a limitation of the media equation. In: Proceedings of the interact 2005 workshop on agent abuse. Rome; 2005. p. 54–7.
25. Nomura T, Uratani T, Kanda T, et al. Why do children abuse robots? In: Proceedings of the 2015 ACM/IEEE international conference on human-robot interaction. Portland, OR. New York: ACM; 2015. p. 63–4.
26. Keijsers M, Bartneck C. Mindless robots get bullied. In: Proceedings of the 13th ACM/IEEE international conference on human-robot interaction. Tokyo. New York: ACM; 2018. p. 205–14.
27. Yamada S, Kanda T, Tomita K. An escalating model of children's robot abuse. In: Proceedings of the 2020 ACM/IEEE international conference on human-robot interaction. Cambridge, UK. New York: ACM; 2020. p. 191–9.
28. Bandura A, Ross D, Ross SA. Transmission of aggression through imitation of aggressive models. J Abnorm Soc Psychol. 1961;63:575–82.
29. Tan XZ, Vázquez M, Carter EJ, Morales CG, Steinfeld A. Inducing bystander interventions during robot abuse with social mechanisms. In: Proceedings of the 2018 ACM/IEEE international conference on human-robot interaction. Chicago, IL. New York: ACM; 2018. p. 169–77.

30. Brscić D, Kidokoro H, Suehiro Y, Kanda T. Escaping from children's abuse of social robots. In: Proceedings of the 2015 annual ACM/IEEE international conference on human-robot interaction. Portland, OR. New York: ACM; 2015. p. 59–66.
31. Fox J, Gambino A. Relationship development with humanoid social robots: applying interpersonal theories to human/robot interaction. Cyberpsychol Behav Soc Netw. 2021;25(5):294–9. https://doi.org/10.1089/cyber.2020.0181.
32. Sharkey A, Sharkey N. We need to talk about deception in social robotics! Ethics Inf Technol. 2021;23:309–16. https://doi.org/10.1007/s10676-020-09573-9.

# Immersive Horizons: Navigating the Impacts of Virtual Reality on Children and Families

Jordy Kaufman, Jennifer M. Zosh, Jakki O. Bailey, Therese Keane, Paola Araiza-Alba, Dorothy Cowie, Eunjoo Kim, Faisal Mushtaq, Lawrence Tychsen, and Tim J. Smith

## 1 Background

Virtual reality (VR) is a computer-based technology that allows users to engage with multimedia content that can closely emulate real-world experiences. By leveraging VR's distinctive features, users feel as though they are immersed in an alternative environment where they can interact with items and characters in a simulated space in real time. Most modern VR systems provide users with a panoramic, 360-degree perspective of the virtual surroundings and often incorporate user interfaces designed to facilitate interaction with objects and navigation within the virtual space.

Although VR technology has existed for decades, recent advances in computing paved the way for VR to fundamentally transform how humans of all ages interact with digital technology and revolutionize many aspects of our lives. It is estimated that the upcoming generation will spend up to 10 years immersed in VR throughout their lifetimes [1].

New technology often raises concerns about its potential impact on children [2], and VR is no exception. The immersive, multisensory, and embodied nature of VR sets it apart from previous technologies, leading to both increased potential and concern. Since childhood is a period

Jennifer M. Zosh contributed equally as co-first author.

J. Kaufman (✉)
Swinburne University of Technology, Melbourne, VIC, Australia
e-mail: jkaufman@swin.edu.au

J. M. Zosh
The Pennsylvania State University Brandywine, Media, PA, USA
e-mail: jzosh@psu.edu

J. O. Bailey
University of Oregon, Eugene, OR, USA

T. Keane
La Trobe University, Melbourne, VIC, Australia

P. Araiza-Alba
Swinburne University of Technology, Melbourne, VIC, Australia

Liminal VR, Melbourne, VIC, Australia

D. Cowie
Durham University, Durham, UK

E. Kim
Yonsei University College of Medicine, Seoul, South Korea

F. Mushtaq
University of Leeds, Leeds, UK

L. Tychsen
Washington University School of Medicine, St. Louis, MO, USA

St. Louis Children's Hospital, St. Louis, MO, USA

T. J. Smith
Creative Computing Institute, University of the Arts London, London, UK


D. A. Christakis, L. Hale (eds.), *Handbook of Children and Screens*,
https://doi.org/10.1007/978-3-031-69362-5_86

of high plasticity and growth [3], the potential impact of VR might be even more significant for children than for adults. Yet, many questions remain unanswered. This chapter summarizes the current state of knowledge and the remaining questions about VR's effects on children.

## 2 Current State

The current understanding of children using VR is still in its early stages. A limited number of empirical studies have explored the effects of VR on child development and education, but these studies face two significant constraints. First, they primarily examine short-term effects, as the technology remains under development, particularly for children. Second, until 2023, guidelines established by VR experience providers (e.g., Meta) and equipment manufacturers advised against the use of VR for children under 12 or 13 years of age. However, it is noteworthy that even during that time, children younger than 13 were engaging with VR [3].[1] Despite these limitations, some emerging themes have surfaced from this nascent research, and insights can be gleaned from studies examining children's use of other technologies.

### 2.1 Pain Distraction

Perhaps the only area of psychological VR research with clear, unambiguous outcomes is its use to distract from pain and anxiety in medical procedures. Research on VR as a distraction tool with children 4 years and older has revealed effectiveness in a range of procedures, such as venipuncture, chemotherapy, burn wound care, dental treatments, and immunizations [4, 5]. By creating engaging and immersive virtual environments, VR diverts the child's focus from the pain and anxiety associated with these procedures, reducing the need for sedatives and analgesics. The fact that VR is so effective at mitigating pain and anxiety in medical settings highlights its powerful ability to capture children's attention and fully immerse them. This observation raises important questions about the potential impact of VR on children's development, learning, and overall engagement with the real world outside of clinical settings.

### 2.2 Lessons from Pediatric Psychiatry

While child psychiatry applications of VR are largely outside the scope of this chapter, it is notable that VR is increasingly explored as a tool in child psychiatry, with applications in assessment, treatment, and research [4, 6]. One vibrant topic in childhood VR research is using VR to assess and treat neurodevelopmental disorders. For example, VR has shown promise in assessing children for attention disorders by examining attentional focus in a simulated classroom environment with built-in distractions [7]. These studies find that assessments implemented in a virtual classroom environment are at least as effective and sometimes more so than some traditional assessments at distinguishing between children with and without attention disorders. Like findings on pain distraction, these results further demonstrate the extent to which simulated environments in VR are processed as real by school-age children.

### 2.3 Education

VR is emerging as a promising tool in childhood education, promising several benefits for cognitive development and skill enhancement. VR has captured the attention of educators because of its ability to present abstract concepts concretely and in 3D. Indeed, the educational VR applications with the most promise are those that allow children to explore information from different perspectives or to explore novel environments [8]. Exploration from different perspectives facilitates mental rotation, memory, spatial represen-

[1] And, and as of September 2023, the minimum age for some Meta headsets has been lowered to 10+ years with a parent-managed account.

tation, effective problem-solving, and cognitive modifiability [9, 10]. Several recent reviews highlight the potential educational advantages of VR, particularly in STEM subjects, where tasks requiring visualization and interactivity greatly benefit from the VR medium [11–14]. However, there are significant limitations to the existing research on the effectiveness of VR in childhood education. These include a lack of studies focusing on arts education, limited quantitative measures of learning [15], and limited comparisons to other learning methods [4, 12].

Moreover, although VR technology has become more affordable and accessible, many obstacles remain to implement VR-enhanced learning programs in schools, including inadequate teacher training and IT services which inhibit the creation of VR content and its implementation in classrooms [16]. Additionally, although platforms and devices that afford social collaboration within VR immersive environments are increasing in number, they remain rare. In utilizing VR in isolation, the potential educational benefits may be offset by the sacrifice of social interaction and collaboration, which are well-established factors in promoting learning [17]. Finally, this technology is still prohibitively expensive for many, potentially creating another digital divide.

## 2.4 Safety Training

By simulating real-life situations in a safe and controlled environment, VR offers a secure environment for children to learn vital safety skills, such as recognizing potential risks at a beach or escaping a riptide [18], by simulating realistic conditions. This immersive experience enables children to practice decision-making and problem-solving without risk while boosting their motivation and interest in safety education, but notably, few studies have utilized modern VR technology in controlled experiments. Nevertheless, several effective implementations exist, and with advancing VR technology, its role in teaching safety skills to children will likely expand, opening new doors for engaging safety education.

## 2.5 VR and Visual Development

One area warranting further long-term investigation is the potential impact of VR on ophthalmological development and the immediate effects of this highly immersive and close-up technology. Initial studies suggested that children could be susceptible to issues like postural instability (difficulty maintaining balance) or decreased stereoacuity (depth perception from binocular cues) [19]. However, more recent research has not found an increased risk of VR-induced seizures in children with photosensitive epilepsy [20] or negative impacts on visuomotor function, postural stability, and motion sickness [14, 21]. Despite these findings, there are no data on whether such effects could emerge if children use VR for extended periods in a single sitting or consistently over months and years, or at younger ages. Thus, questions remain regarding long-term implications.

## 2.6 Insights from Screen Media Research

Finally, while VR is more immersive than typical screen media, some insights will likely prove relevant as we consider the impacts of VR on developing children. For example, research has shown that increased touchscreen device usage in infants and toddlers is associated with reduced sleep [22], a shift toward saliency-driven attention, and diminished cognitive control of attention [23], but also an earlier achievement of developmental milestones for fine-motor (e.g., finger) control compared to low touchscreen users [24]. Associations between cognitive development and the use of other screen mediums, including television [25] and video games [26], are well established. While causal evidence from randomized controlled trials is limited, the mechanisms by which screen time may influence developing cognition are apparent.

## 3 Future Research

The implications for VR for children and human society generally are vast and difficult to predict. The ways that VR is integrated into our lives will be influenced by technological advances, cultural acceptance, and scientific research on its psychological and physical effects. Its particular implications for children, whose brains are undergoing tremendous development and whose early experiences can have lifelong impacts, are even less predictable. Several areas deserve immediate investigation.

### 3.1 What Are the Potential Differential Impacts of VR on Children of Different Ages?

Children's experiences with digital interactions in VR differ from those with other technologies. Since VR enhances immersion and increases the intensity of children's interactions, it has the potential to affect their sense of embodiment. This can be positive, as learning is often supported by engaging, meaningful, iterative, socially interactive, and joyful experiences [27]. However, it may also amplify negative experiences, such as cyberbullying, losing track of time, isolation, and mental health concerns. Additionally, the intensity of the sensory experience and the complexity of the content should be considered. Fast-paced and fantastical content in videos can deplete children's executive functions, which are essential cognitive skills for regulating behavior [28]. The intensity of VR experiences, particularly those with minimal interaction [29], may have even more significant depletion effects.

As seen in the screen time debate, the impacts of technology on children are rarely entirely good or bad. Factors such as child age, quality of experience, time spent, individual differences/susceptibility, and the presence or absence of a caring adult to help navigate (and limit) the experience are all critical considerations. These effects may vary based on age, experience, and individual differences/susceptibility.

Therefore, more studies are needed to examine the longitudinal associations between VR use and child development in cognitive (especially attention control, vision, and executive functions), social, physical, creative, and motor development aspects. Concurrently, randomized controlled trials should be used to investigate the direct impact of VR use, with strong ethical controls to mitigate the risks of introducing VR.

As of 2024, most vendor guidelines recommend a minimum age of 10+ or 13 for VR usage. But as these headsets become more mainstream, younger children will use them, just as they use social media that shares similar age requirements [30]. To our knowledge, minimum ages for VR usage set by VR content and equipment vendors are not predicated on a robust evidence base concerning the specific developmental, cognitive, or physical impacts of VR technology on younger children. Instead, it appears to reflect a precautionary stance adopted by developers and manufacturers, driven by market acceptance, headset size, legal liability, and political pressure. As VR technology becomes more familiar to consumers, and its integration into daily life more seamless, we should expect that children younger than 10–13 years will increasingly encounter opportunities to use VR, particularly as they observe older family members engaging with the technology. The desire to include younger children in these experiences as well as children's own interest in engaging with VR may result in use that outpaces our scientific understanding of the implications, underscoring the need for research that transcends arbitrary age limits and examines VR's impact across ages.

### 3.2 How Will Increasing Familiarity with VR Technology Impact the Long-Term Effectiveness of VR Applications for Children?

As children become more accustomed to VR, researchers should assess how familiarity might influence the sustained benefits of VR applications in various domains, such as education, pain distraction, and safety training. Will the novelty and engagement of VR experiences decrease over time, leading to reduced effectiveness, or will continuous advancements in technology and the personalization of experiences counteract potential diminishing returns? Investigating the relationship between VR familiarity and its effectiveness in these areas will inform developers and educators how to adapt and evolve VR content to maintain its usefulness.

### 3.3 How Will Caregiver VR Usage Influence Parent–Child Interactions and Relationships, and What are the Implications for Children's Development?

If VR use becomes prevalent by adult caretakers, children might be regularly exposed to people using VR even if they are not using it themselves. This is important because caregiver use may affect the quality and quantity of caregiver–child interaction opportunities. It also normalizes and models VR usage from a very young age in the way parental usage of touchscreen devices does today. Based on existing data on screen use, there are warning signs about caregiver screen use impacting adult responsiveness and children's behavior [31]. Thus, not only will children's experiences with VR be more immersive, but so will their caregivers, which may impact caregiver–child relationships.

### 3.4 How Can We Leverage the Data Generated by VR Use for Good While Protecting Children's Data and Privacy from Targeted Advertising or Worse?

Major privacy concerns were highlighted by a recent Common Sense Media report highlighting the extensive personal data collected by headsets, including information such as body and eye position, facial expression, and skin color [32]. Given that individuals are personally identifiable with astonishingly limited use (e.g., less than 120 seconds), privacy remains paramount. Relatedly, research into memory formation in VR has not only shown that children can learn and generalize from VR materials but has also examined how false information and impossible events viewed in VR environments can impact children in real life [33, 34]. Specifically, VR experiences may make young children susceptible to forming false memories in VR that persist in real life; and to believe that impossible events are possible. This creates serious concern about children experiencing VR "realities" potentially as harmful as real life (e.g., abuse, bullying, and manipulation).

On the other hand, one can imagine the potential for individualized experiences based on an individual child's interests, knowledge, abilities, and goals. Today's curricula, texts, and even videos are somewhat one-size-fits-all—but VR and the use of AI and adaptive technologies have the potential to be individualized resources that can meet children exactly where they are and provide personalized experiences and information. But again, this also heightens the potential risk of targeted marketing and victimization as these devices generate more data than ever.

## 4 Recommendations

- *Policymakers*: Policymakers must recognize that our understanding of the potential impacts of VR on children is still in its infancy. As they are called upon to establish guidelines to protect children, consulting with scientists, researchers, pediatricians, and parents is essential, rather than relying solely on assurances of potential and safety from manufacturers. Several outstanding questions need to be addressed, such as who should regulate virtual environment platforms, and if regulation were to occur, how to balance the need to protect the public with the freedom of expression in such platforms. Additionally, as policymakers work toward providing greater access to VR technology, they should also consider issues related to diversity and equity, striving to bridge the digital divide and address potential disparities in access, content, and representation [34]. Ensuring that the benefits of VR technology are distributed fairly while mitigating potential negative impacts will require a comprehensive approach, including research, prospective data collection, and proper use of the collected data.

- *Educators and educational systems*: The prospect of VR enhancing education is undoubtedly enticing; however, we must remain cognizant of the limitations in our current understanding of children's learning experiences with VR. As of now, there is no evidence to suggest that VR-based programs outperform those developed by passionate, dedicated, and experienced educators. In light of our ongoing exploration of VR in education, it is advised that schools partner with researchers to study VR's potential to enhance learning in educational settings rather than relying on it as a replacement for high-quality teaching. Further, evidence-based professional development for educators and IT support will be necessary so that VR implementations add minimal disruption to the classroom.
- *Researchers, clinicians, and parents*: As virtual reality (VR) becomes more prevalent among children and adolescents, it is essential to consider how to protect them from potential harm and determine who will regulate its use. While current research has provided some insight into the possible long-term effects of VR, more is needed to provide clear guidance to parents and clinicians. As more research becomes available, it will be crucial to develop effective tools to help parents mitigate the risks for their children based on their age, developmental skills, and abilities. In summary, it is essential to exercise caution when using VR with young people and to take steps to ensure that they are adequately protected from any potential harm.
- *Developers*: A significant concern with VR is its tendency to be an individual activity, which can reduce opportunities for social interaction because it immerses the user in a virtual world isolated from those physically around them. This isolation limits shared experiences and direct interactions with family or peers during childhood, a time when social interaction is critical. To address this, we encourage developers to go beyond implementing typical parental controls such as screen time limits, content filtering, and activity monitoring and to focus on creating VR content and platforms that support group experiences, enabling children and their families or friends to enjoy VR together—in either the real or virtual world. Innovating VR games and educational activities for groups can transform VR from an isolating to a collaborative experience. Developing virtual spaces for interactive participation makes VR more engaging and promotes the developmental benefits of social interaction [35]. By prioritizing shared VR experiences and enhancing parental controls so that social interaction is not displaced by solo VR experiences, we aim to enhance the technology's role in supporting rather than detracting from children's social development.
- *All stakeholders*: Safe, effective, and age-appropriate experiences designed to support social, emotional, physical, and cognitive outcomes are the goal, but this will require a multi-sector approach. We recommend that teachers, designers, clinicians, and educators collaborate to provide a holistic approach to protecting children and using VR to enhance their lives. Equity and diversity must also be centered in designing and implementing VR technology to avoid bias, discrimination, and access issues. This will necessitate large-scale, multicenter, longitudinal research programs involving researchers, clinicians, families, hardware and software developers, and policymakers.

**Conflict of Interest and Funding Disclosures** DC's contribution to this chapter was supported by ESRC Grant number ES/W003120/1. FM is supported by the European Union's Horizon Research and Innovation programme under grant agreement no. 101070155 and the UKRI through the Horizon Europe Guarantee (#10039307).

## References


1. Allen C, McIntosh V. Safeguarding the metaverse: a guide to existing and future harms in virtual reality (VR) and the metaverse to support UK immersive technology policymaking. Institution of Engineering and Technology; 2023. https://www.theiet.org/digital. Accessed 24 Feb 2023.
2. Orben A. The Sisyphean cycle of technology panics. Perspect Psychol Sci. 2020;15(5):1143–57. https://doi.org/10.1177/1745691620919372.
3. Fox SE, Levitt F, Nelson CA. How the timing and quality of early experiences influence the development of brain architecture. Child Dev. 2010;81(1):28–40.
4. Araiza-Alba P, Keane T, Beaudry JL, Kaufman J. Immersive virtual reality implementations in developmental psychology. Dec 2020. https://doi.org/10.31234/osf.io/ga8sz.
5. Won AS, Bailey J, Bailenson J, Tataru C, Yoon IA, Golianu B. Immersive virtual reality for pediatric pain. Children. 2017;4(7):52. https://doi.org/10.3390/children4070052.
6. Kim S, Kim E. The use of virtual reality in psychiatry: a review. Soa Chongsonyon Chongsin Uihak. 2020;31(1):26–32. https://doi.org/10.5765/jkacap.190037. PMID: 32612410; PMCID: PMC7324842.
7. Rodríguez C, Areces D, García T, Cueli M, González-Castro P. Comparison between two continuous performance tests for identifying ADHD: traditional vs. virtual reality. Int J Clin Health Psychol. 2018;18(3):254–63. https://doi.org/10.1016/j.ijchp.2018.06.003.
8. Bailey JO, Bailenson JN. Immersive virtual reality and the developing child. Elsevier Inc.; 2017. https://doi.org/10.1016/B978-0-12-809481-5.00009-2.
9. Araiza-Alba P, et al. Immersive virtual reality as a tool to learn problem-solving skills. Comput Educ. 2021;164:104121.
10. Passig D, Tzuriel D, Eshel-Kedmi G. Improving children's cognitive modifiability by dynamic assessment in 3D Immersive Virtual Reality environments. Comput Educ. 2016;95:296–308. https://doi.org/10.1016/j.compedu.2016.01.009.
11. Maresky HS, Oikonomou A, Ali I, Ditkofsky N, Pakkal M, Ballyk B. Virtual reality and cardiac anatomy: exploring immersive three-dimensional cardiac imaging, a pilot study in undergraduate medical anatomy education. Clin Anat. 2019;32(2):238–43. https://doi.org/10.1002/ca.23292.
12. Hamilton D, McKechnie J, Edgerton E, Wilson C. Immersive virtual reality as a pedagogical tool in education: a systematic literature review of quantitative learning outcomes and experimental design. J Comput Educ. 2021;8(1):1–32. https://doi.org/10.1007/s40692-020-00169-2.
13. Kavanagh S, Luxton-Reilly A, Wuensche B, Plimmer B. A systematic review of virtual reality in education. Themes Sci Technol Educ. 2017;10(2):85–119.
14. Rauschenberger R, Barakat B. Health and safety of VR use by children in an educational use case. In: 2020 IEEE conference on virtual reality and 3D user interfaces (VR). IEEE; 2020. p. 878–84.
15. Southgate E, Smith SP, Cividino C, et al. Embedding immersive virtual reality in classrooms: ethical, organisational and educational lessons in bridging research and practice. Int J Child Comput Interact. 2019;19:19–29. https://doi.org/10.1016/j.ijcci.2018.10.002.
16. Araiza-Alba P, Keane T, Kaufman J. Are we ready for virtual reality in K–12 classrooms? Technol Pedagog Educ. 2022;31:1–21. https://doi.org/10.1080/1475939x.2022.2033307.
17. Hirsh-Pasek K, Zosh JM, Golinkoff RM, Gray JH, Robb MB, Kaufman J. Putting education in "educational" apps: lessons from the science of learning. Psychol Sci Public Interest. 2015;16(1):3–34. https://doi.org/10.1177/1529100615569721.
18. Araiza-Alba P, Keane T, Matthews B, et al. The potential of 360-degree virtual reality videos to teach water-safety skills to children. Comput Educ. 2021;163:104096. https://doi.org/10.1016/j.compedu.2020.104096.
19. Yamada-Rice D, Mushtaq F, Woodgate A, et al. Children and virtual reality: emerging possibilities and challenges. 12 Sept 2017. http://digilitey.eu/wp-content/uploads/2015/09/CVR-Final-PDF-reduced-size.pdf. Accessed 24 Feb 2023.
20. Tychsen L, Thio LL. Concern of photosensitive seizures evoked by 3D video displays or virtual reality headsets in children: current perspective. Eye Brain. 2020;12:45–8. https://doi.org/10.2147/EB.S233195.
21. Tychsen L, Foeller P. Effects of immersive virtual reality headset viewing on young children: visuomotor function, postural stability, and motion sickness. Am J Ophthalmol. 2020;209:151–9. https://doi.org/10.1016/j.ajo.2019.07.020.
22. Cheung C, Bedford R, Saez De Urabain IR, Karmiloff-Smith A, Smith TJ. Daily touchscreen use in infants and toddlers is associated with reduced sleep and delayed sleep onset. Sci Rep. 2017;7:46104.
23. Portugal AM, Bedford R, Cheung CHM, Gliga T, Smith TJ. Saliency-driven visual search performance in toddlers with low– vs high–touch screen use. JAMA Pediatr. 2021;175(1):96–7. https://doi.org/10.1001/jamapediatrics.2020.2344.
24. Bedford R, Saez de Urabain IR, Cheung CHM, Karmiloff-Smith A, Smith TJ. Toddlers' fine motor milestone achievement is associated with early touchscreen scrolling. Front Psychol. 2016;7:1108. https://doi.org/10.3389/fpsyg.2016.01108.
25. Nikkelen SWC, Valkenburg PM, Huizinga M, Bushman BJ. Media use and ADHD-related behaviors in children and adolescents: a meta-analysis. Dev Psychol. 2014;50(9):2228–41. https://doi.org/10.1037/a0037318.
26. Green CS, Bavelier D. Action video game modifies visual selective attention. Nature.

2003;423(6939):534–7. https://doi.org/10.1038/nature01647.
27. Zosh J, Hopkins E, Jensen H, et al. Learning through play: a review of the evidence. LEGO Fonden; 2017. https://www.legofoundation.com/en/research-and-learning/foundation-research/learning-through-play/. Accessed 24 Feb 2023.
28. Essex C, Gliga T, Singh M, Smith TJ. Understanding the differential impact of children's TV on executive functions: a narrative-processing analysis. Infant Behav Dev. 2022;66:101661.
29. Huber B, Yeates M, Meyer D, Fleckhammer L, Kaufman J. The effects of screen media content on young children's executive functioning. J Exp Child Psychol. 2018;170:72–85. https://doi.org/10.1016/j.jecp.2018.01.006.
30. Rideout V, Peebles A, Mann S, Robb M. Common sense census: media use by tweens and teens, 2021. San Francisco: Common Sense; 2022.
31. McDaniel BT, Radesky JS. Technoference: parent distraction with technology and associations with child behavior problems. Child Dev. 2018;89(1):100–9. https://doi.org/10.1111/cdev.12822.
32. Kelly G, Graham J, Bronfman J, Garton S. Privacy of virtual reality: our future in the metaverse and beyond. Common Sense Media; 2022. https://www.commonsensemedia.org/research/privacy-of-virtual-reality-our-future-in-the-metaverse-and-beyond. Accessed 20 Feb 2023.
33. Segovia KY, Bailenson JN. Virtually true: children's acquisition of false memories in virtual reality. Media Psychol. 2009;12(4):371–93. https://doi.org/10.1080/15213260903287267.
34. Schmitz A, Joiner R, Golds P. Is seeing believing? The effects of virtual reality on young children's understanding of possibility and impossibility. J Child Media. 2020;14(2):158–72. https://doi.org/10.1080/17482798.2019.1684964.
35. Hirsh-Pasek K, Zosh JM, Hadani HS, et al. A whole new world: education meets the metaverse. The Brookings Institution; 2022.

# Children's Understanding of Digital Tracking and Digital Privacy

Susan A. Gelman, Shaylene E. Nancekivell, Young-eun Lee, and Florian Schaub

## 1 Background

Digital technologies have proliferated into all aspects of life, for children and their families. With these technologies come not only benefits but also risks, including privacy risks with both interpersonal and institutional/commercial dimensions [1].

Regarding *interpersonal privacy*, children may expose private information about themselves and their families to peers and strangers, with implications for children's safety online and in the physical world [1, 2]. Sharing self-relevant information or problematic views online at a young age may affect one's opportunities years later when this information is found and taken out of context, for instance when applying for college or jobs [1, 3, 4].

*Institutional privacy* risks arise from the datafication of children's interactions with technology and uses of that data by institutions, companies, and governments. In addition to what children, parents, and caregivers explicitly share online, children's interactions with technologies are often tracked, analyzed, and commercialized in ways that are hidden from users. For instance, online behaviors are tracked on and across websites and apps, as well as across devices [4, 5], in order to infer individual characteristics and interests to which online advertisements are then targeted, which can be particularly manipulative for children [6]. This vast data collection of consumers, including children, is also monetized through selling and providing data access to third parties and data brokers [1, 5]. Further privacy risks arise from government and law enforcement access to companies' location and behavioral data about children and teenagers, with potential legal consequences, for instance in states and countries that outlaw gender affirming or abortion care.

While these privacy issues affect adults and children alike, children are particularly vulnerable—and recognized as such in privacy and data protection legislation—because of their limited understanding of digital privacy and tracking risks. Ubiquitous data collection from early childhood further contributes to the normalization of surveillance capitalism and datafication, as children are especially susceptible to descriptive regularities turning into prescriptive judgments [7]. In order to effectively meet and address digital privacy and tracking risks for children, it

Shaylene E. Nancekivell, Young-eun Lee and Florian Schaub contributed equally with all other contributors.

S. A. Gelman (✉) · F. Schaub
University of Michigan, Ann Arbor, MI, USA
e-mail: gelman@umich.edu

S. E. Nancekivell
University of Manitoba, Winnipeg, MB, Canada

Y.-e. Lee
Massachusetts Institute of Technology, Cambridge, MA, USA


D. A. Christakis, L. Hale (eds.), *Handbook of Children and Screens*,
https://doi.org/10.1007/978-3-031-69362-5_87

is necessary to understand how children conceptualize these risks, including what beliefs and misconceptions they may hold, what information they are lacking, what aspects are challenging to understand, and how children develop concepts of privacy.

## 2 Current State

In reviewing the current state of the literature on children's understanding and thinking about technology as it relates to privacy and tracking, we focus on children under 14 years of age and their parents, with occasional discussions of adolescents as relevant.

### 2.1 What Do Children Think Technology Can Know About Them?

An informed evaluation of digital tracking and digital privacy requires an understanding of what digital devices "know" about the user. This includes that data flows from the user outward to others; what kinds of data are gathered; how those data are used; where data are located, stored, and accessed; with whom data are shared; and what is required to remove data not only from one's device but also from the cloud. Children's understanding of these factors appears to be highly limited. Evidence suggests that children often do not recognize that information travels bi-directionally and may not understand more subtle forms of information flow (e.g., tracking of app use; collating information from multiple sources) [8]. They also may not understand the full range of devices that can track information about them, with even older children (11–15 years of age) primarily thinking of the internet in terms of traditional computing devices (computers, phones, and tablets) rather than connected toys, wearable devices, smart speakers, or household appliances [9]. Young children (below 10 years of age) may also underestimate the information that the device is tracking and storing (e.g., not realizing that a digital toy records their conversations, which later can be accessed by parents) [10].

Children tend to view the digital world in terms of interpersonal rather than institutional interactions [1]. Thus, younger children typically think that tracking them would require directly observing their behavior (e.g., viewing them through a camera), whereas older children or adults understand that data may be compiled broadly and automatically by recording a user's behavior [8]. Even when thinking about institutions, children 10–14 years of age often conceptualize companies in terms of people (e.g., characterizing Google as the employees who work there) [11]. This interpersonal stance is also seen in how children construe smartphones or smart speakers with which they can engage in conversations (such as Alexa or Google Home), often attributing both animate and inanimate qualities to these devices (e.g., being "a girl" and having wires and electricity) [12].

Although there are important developmental changes in children's understanding of technology, extensive research outside of this domain demonstrates that development is more nuanced than once thought. Cognitive development does not progress in qualitatively distinct "stages." Young children are capable of reasoning about subtle and nonobvious aspects of the world, children with expertise in a domain can outperform adults, and even complex ideas can be communicated to children as young as kindergarten age [12, 13]. Conversely, adults are not immune to the kinds of biases, reasoning errors, and egocentrism that can be seen in children [4, 12, 13]. It is therefore important to consider how knowledge, experience, and causal frameworks (such as ownership or trust in testimony) may scaffold children's understanding in the digital domain.

### 2.2 What Do Children Understand About Privacy in the Digital Domain?

Early in development, children's privacy concepts are grounded in physical space [14]. For example, when asked to describe what is "private," concerns about physical bathrooms and bedrooms dominate the responses of children under 10 years [14]. Young children also view privacy as an interpersonal issue and overlook institutional privacy concerns. For example, when asked about privacy threats, children rarely mention concerns about monetization of data or corporate malfeasance, but they do mention concerns around stalking or physical harm [2, 8, 15, 16]. Less is known about how young children think about parents' ability to track them, access, or share their information (e.g., uploading pictures or videos of them, also known as "sharenting," Ref. [1]) [17, 18]. However, by adolescence young people disapprove of "sharenting" and consider it embarrassing [18].

At the same time, children understand that the digital domain differs in important ways from the physical domain [19]. For example, they know that items can be transmitted wirelessly and believe that downloading a file has less serious moral consequences compared to taking a physical version of the same item [20]. By at least 8 years of age, children are sensitive to complex distinctions between personal information and other kinds of information [2, 21, 22]. For example, in one study, children judged that users own the personal information that is shared with apps (address, school name, and gender), but not analogous general facts (e.g., children go to school) [22].

Children will take some measures to keep their personal information private, such as using pseudonyms instead of real names [2, 21, 23]. However, they also will disclose their personal information, especially when incentivized to do so [23]. They rely heavily on visual cues to understand when apps are using or accessing their information [8]. After personal information has been knowingly shared, even teenagers have miscalibrated insights into how private it is [1, 24]. For example, on Facebook, teenagers overestimate the privacy of their school information, but underestimate the privacy of their email addresses [24].

## 2.3 How Do Children Conceptualize Digital Tracking?

A particular kind of privacy issue that has received recent attention is that of digital tracking, with the wide availability of phones, wearables, or apps that track children's location and activities (e.g., via Google Maps, Apple AirTag, or Life360), in addition to behavioral tracking by companies and other institutions. Although parents may view child-tracking apps as a tool to ensure their child's safety [25], this technology also has the potential for strangers as well as other family members to access information about a child. Younger children are especially positive in their attitudes regarding location and file tracking, with those aged 10 years and younger reporting it is okay or even a good thing to track others digitally, whereas older children and adults express negative views [26, 27]. A marked change with age can also be seen in children's qualitative responses to digital tracking. Whereas adults evoked moral principles (privacy, ownership, and permission) as well as potential negative material consequences (stalking, stealing), children focused on the functional benefits, such as being able to find lost items [27].

However, even young children do not approve of all sorts of digital tracking indiscriminately. Even 5-year-olds view the tracking of other people as less acceptable than that of oneself [27]. Further, children are sensitive to the trustworthiness of the tracker and the information being tracked. Specifically, 5- to 17-year-olds are more negative about digital tracking when the tracker seems less trustworthy (e.g., a person from a different social group, or a person who is characterized as "mean") and when a private photograph (e.g., messy bedroom) is shared [26]. These results show that even from age 5, children do not blindly trust digital tracking, and they are able to consider relevant information when evaluating its permissibility.

Several factors appear to contribute to younger children's relatively weaker understanding of the risks of digital tracking. These include focusing more on benefits than risks [4, 27], trusting technological devices such as voice assistants [28], and treating descriptive regularities as prescriptively correct [7], thereby potentially normalizing practices like tracking that erode digital privacy.

## 3 Future Research

Our chapter demonstrates that children's conceptualizations of privacy and tracking are complex. Even at a young age, children are sometimes reasoning in sophisticated ways about technology and privacy. At the same time, young children may be unaware of many potential digital privacy risks, in particular regarding institutional privacy and digital tracking. There is substantial development in children's thinking about privacy and tracking with age, and certain orientations, such as an interpersonal stance, dominate early thinking. We recommend three directions for future research, focused on: children's privacy risk understandings, improving children's digital privacy literacy and risk awareness, and designing child-appropriate privacy information and controls:

### 3.1 What Are the Risk Understandings of Children of Different Ages?

- How do younger children reason about digital tracking and privacy risks? Most studies are with children 12 years and older, and few are with children under 8 years [1, 15]. Given the widespread use of digital technologies with and by increasingly younger children, focusing on these younger ages is vital.
- How do children think about data that can be inferred from seemingly benign information or behaviors, such as location, search queries, browsing, video streaming, game play, ad-viewing, or purchases? In contrast to explicitly provided or shared data, such inferences are substantially harder to understand and require deeper awareness of risks around combining different data sources.
- How do children reason about data routinely gathered in trusted contexts such as healthcare or educational settings (including providers of learning software, class management systems, and health portals), as compared to data flows and privacy risks in commercial products and services?
- What can large-scale experimental and observational studies reveal? Much of the research in this area relies on qualitative interviews with small samples [15]; these are valuable for providing insights into children's reasoning but may underestimate children's sensitivity because they require verbalization and explicit reflection. We recommend research that assesses children's understanding using multiple methods and larger sample sizes, including experiments, observational data, implicit beliefs, and in situ behaviors—as well as explicit beliefs.
- What kinds of variation can be seen in children's privacy understanding, and what factors may contribute to such variation, beyond child age? Potentially relevant factors include technology experience, socioeconomic status, cultural context, marginalized identities, and individual differences. These are vastly understudied in psychological research as a whole. To date, little work has examined how and where children learn about digital privacy and tracking risks, including the degree to which internal processes (e.g., intuitive theories, hypothesis testing) and external processes (e.g., testimony, formal pedagogy) affect children's understanding of these concepts.

### 3.2 What Are Effective Ways to Educate Children About Digital Privacy Risks and to Counter Their Misconceptions?

- How can we help children better understand data flows, tracking, and both interpersonal and institutional privacy risks? Different conceptual frameworks should be considered to determine which may be most compelling to children at different ages (e.g., safety vs. ownership framework).

- How can we move from providing children with an understanding of privacy risks to helping them engage in appropriate protective behaviors? What might be effective settings and interventions for doing so?
- What are parents' beliefs, misconceptions, and concerns about digital tracking and privacy, and how are these communicated to children? Parents are potentially an important source of information, but research indicates they are ambivalent—wanting to educate their children, but also to shield them from learning about negative (frightening) elements [29, 30]. Parents may also be a source of privacy violations (e.g., sharenting; parental tracking). How can parents be better supported and educated in helping their children develop digital privacy literacy?

### 3.3 What Constitutes Child-Appropriate Design of Privacy Information and Controls?

- Recent regulation requiring child-appropriate design necessitates more research on what child-appropriate privacy information, controls, and protections should look like in different contexts. What are the effects of conveying privacy-related information and options through alternative means other than textual privacy notices and disclosures (e.g., with visuals to make hidden data flows more visible, or by leveraging comics, cartoons, and other child-oriented media to explain concepts and practices)?
- What are the effects of data collection/sharing defaults and dark patterns or deceptive designs that encourage children to reveal more information, on children's perceptions of norms around data sharing and collection?

## 4 Recommendations

- Education on digital privacy risks should begin at earlier ages. While more research is needed on effective ways to educate children about digital privacy risks, an apparent gap in the literature is that privacy risks are considered a topic that pertains to older children. Yet as our chapter indicates, this is an issue for younger children as well. An important goal is informing younger children and their parents of privacy risks they may be unaware of (such as behavioral tracking based on selections, behaviors, and ads) and means of protecting against them.
- Difficulties understanding privacy risks and protections might make it hard for children (and adults) to recognize risks of seemingly routine data collection, such as in health contexts, especially for vulnerable groups. Practitioners and educators should regularly talk to parents and children about the data they are storing/sharing and associated risks that children (and many adults) may overlook (e.g., reproductive information of LGBTQ+ youth).
- Regulatory requirements on child privacy protections should be based on research findings. Parental consent has proven difficult to implement and respective requirements are often circumvented by companies [5]. Age cutoffs for enhanced legal privacy protections are inconsistent (e.g., <14 in COPPA, <16 in GDPR). Emerging requirements of age-appropriate design in the United Kingdom and California are well intentioned but may compound privacy issues through age verification/profiling requirements and lack guidance on what actually constitutes appropriate design for children of different ages, how to account for developmental differences, and how to support development at different ages [31]. There is a need to develop research-informed guidance for age-appropriate design as part of respective public policy efforts.

- Besides educating children and parents about risks and improving regulation, services and apps with child users could take steps to reduce privacy risks for children, such as by practicing privacy by design and by centering respect for their (child) users rather than merely striving for legal compliance. This may include but is not limited to collecting only necessary data (data minimization), implementing privacy-friendly defaults, and exploring business models that do not rely on the extensive tracking of individual users within and across services.

**Conflict of Interest and Funding Disclosures** None.

## References

1. Livingstone S, Stoilova M, Nandagiri R. Children's data and privacy online: growing up in a digital age: an evidence review. 2019. https://eprints.lse.ac.uk/101283/1/Livingstone_childrens_data_and_privacy_online_evidence_review_published.pdf. Accessed 23 Mar 2023.
2. Zhao J, Wang G, Dally C, et al. I make up a silly name. In: Proceedings of the 2019 CHI conference on human factors in computing systems. New York: ACM; 2019. https://doi.org/10.1145/3290605.3300336.
3. O'Keeffe GS, Clarke-Pearson K. The impact of social media on children, adolescents, and families. Pediatrics. 2011;127(4):800–4. https://doi.org/10.1542/peds.2011-0054.
4. Acquisti A, Brandimarte L, Loewenstein G. Secrets and likes: the drive for privacy and the difficulty of achieving it in the digital age. J Consum Psychol. 2020;30(4):736–58. https://doi.org/10.1002/jcpy.1191.
5. Reyes I, Wijesekera P, Reardon J, Elazari Bar On A, Razaghpanah A, Vallina-Rodriguez N, Egelman S. "Won't somebody think of the children?": examining COPPA compliance at scale. Proc Priv Enhanc Technol. 2018;(3):63–83. https://doi.org/10.1515/popets-2018-0021.
6. Meyer M, Adkins V, Yuan N, Weeks HM, Chang Y-J, Radesky J. Advertising in young children's apps: a content analysis. J Dev Behav Pediatr. 2019;40(1):32–9. https://doi.org/10.1097/DBP.0000000000000622.
7. Roberts SO, Gelman SA, Ho AK. So it is, so it shall be: group regularities license children's prescriptive judgments. Cogn Sci. 2017;41(Suppl 3):576–600. https://doi.org/10.1111/cogs.12443.
8. Sun K, Sugatan C, Afnan T, Simon H, Gelman SA, Radesky J, Schaub F. "They see you're a girl if you pick a pink robot with a skirt": a qualitative study of how children conceptualize data processing and digital privacy risks. In: Proceedings of the 2021 CHI conference on human factors in computing systems. New York: ACM; 2021. p. 1–34.
9. Brodsky JE, Lodhi AK, Powers KL, Blumberg FC, Brooks PJ. "It's just everywhere now": middle-school and college students' mental models of the internet. Hum Behav Emerg Technol. 2021;3:495–511. https://doi.org/10.1002/hbe2.281.
10. McReynolds E, Hubbard S, Lau T, Saraf A, Cakmak M, Roesner F. Toys that listen: a study of parents, children, and internet-connected toys. In: Proceedings of the 2017 CHI conference on human factors in computing systems. New York: ACM; 2017. p. 5197–207.
11. Kodama C, St. Jean B, Subramaniam M, Taylor NG. There's a creepy guy on the other end at Google!: engaging middle school students in a drawing activity to elicit their mental models of Google. Inf Retr J. 2017;20:403–32.
12. Xu Y, Warschauer M. What are you talking to?: understanding children's perceptions of conversational agents. In: Proceedings of the 2020 CHI conference on human factors in computing systems. New York: ACM; 2020. p. 1–13.
13. Gelman SA, Frazier BN. Development of thinking in children. In: Holyoak KJ, Morrison RG, editors. The Oxford handbook of thinking and reasoning, Oxford library of psychology. Oxford University Press; 2012. p. 513–28. https://doi.org/10.1093/oxfordhb/9780199734689.013.0026.
14. Oates M, et al. Turtles, locks, and bathrooms: understanding mental models of privacy through illustration. Proc Priv Enhanc Technol. 2018;4:5–32. https://petsymposium.org/popets/2018/popets-2018-0029.php.
15. Stoilova M, Nandagiri R, Livingstone S. Children's understanding of personal data and privacy online – a systematic evidence mapping. Inf Commun Soc. 2021;24(4):557–75. https://doi.org/10.1080/1369118X.2019.1657164.
16. Dowthwaite L, Creswick H, Portillo V, Zhao J, Patel M, Perez Vallejos E, Koene A, Jirotka M. "It's your private information. It's your life." Young people's views of personal data use by online technologies. In: Proceedings of the interaction design and children conference. New York: ACM; 2020. p. 121–34.
17. Brosch A. When the child is born into the internet: sharenting as a growing trend among parents on Facebook. New Educ Rev. 2016;43(1):225–35.
18. Verswijvel K, Walrave M, Hardies K, Heirman W. Sharenting, is it a good or a bad thing? Understanding how adolescents think and feel about sharenting on social network sites. Child Youth Serv Rev. 2019;104:104401. https://doi.org/10.1016/j.childyouth.2019.104401.
19. Danovitch JH. Growing up with Google: how children's understanding and use of internet-based devices relates to cognitive development. Hum Behav Emerg

Technol. 2019;1(2):81–90. https://doi.org/10.1002/hbe2.142.
20. Lee Y, Gelman SA. The development of digital ownership in children. J Exp Child Psychol. 2022;224:1–11. https://doi.org/10.1016/j.jecp.2022.105519.
21. Kumar P, Naik SM, Devkar UR, Chetty M, Clegg TL, Vitak J. "No telling passcodes out because they're private": understanding children's mental models of privacy and security online. Proc ACM Hum Comput Interact. 2017;1:1–21. https://doi.org/10.1145/3134699.
22. Nancekivell SE, Fahey JB. Who owns your information? Young children's judgments of who owns the general and personal information users share with apps. Proc Annu Meet Cogn Sci Soc. 2022;44(44):2074–8.
23. Desimpelaere L, Hudders L, Van de Sompel D. Children's perceptions of fairness in a data disclosure context: the effect of a reward on the relationship between privacy literacy and disclosure behavior. Telematics Inform. 2021;61:101602.
24. Moll R, Pieschl S, Bromme R. Competent or clueless? Users' knowledge and misconceptions about their online privacy management. Comput Hum Behav. 2014;41:212–9. https://doi.org/10.1016/j.chb.2014.09.033.
25. Sukk M, Siibak A. Caring dataveillance and the construction of "good parenting": Estonian parents' and pre-teens' reflections on the use of tracking technologies. Communications. 2021;46(3):446–67.
26. Gelman SA, Cuneo N, Kulkarni S, Snay S, Roberts SO. The roles of privacy and trust in children's evaluations and explanations of digital tracking. Child Dev. 2021;92(5):1769–84. https://doi.org/10.1111/cdev.13572.
27. Gelman SA, Martinez M, Davidson NS, Noles NS. Developing digital privacy: children's moral judgments concerning mobile GPS devices. Child Dev. 2018;89(1):17–26. https://doi.org/10.1111/cdev.12826.
28. Girouard-Hallam LN, Danovitch JH. Children's trust in and learning from voice assistants. Dev Psychol. 2022;58(4):646–61. https://doi.org/10.1037/dev0001318.supp.
29. Mai A, Guelmino L, Pfeffer K, Weippl E, Krombholz K. Mental models of the internet and its online risks: children and their parent(s). In: International conference on human-computer interaction. Cham: Springer; 2022. p. 42–61.
30. Zhang-Kennedy L, Mekhail C, Abdelaziz Y, Chiasson S. From nosy little brothers to stranger-danger: children and parents' perception of mobile threats. In: Proceedings of the 15th international conference on interaction design and children. New York: ACM; 2016. p. 388–99.
31. Grace TD, Abel C, Salen K. Child-centered design in the digital world: investigating the implications of the age-appropriate design code for interactive digital media. In: Proceedings of the ACM interaction design and children conference. New York: ACM; 2023. p. 289–97. https://doi.org/10.1145/3585088.3589370.

# Correction to: Youth Participatory Politics: Understanding and Supporting Civic Engagement in the Social Media Era

Ellen Middaugh, Mariah Kornbluh, Ashley Lee, Neta Kligler-Vilenchik, Srividya Ramasubramanian, Lynn Schofield Clark, and Tanner Vea

**Correction to:**
**Chapter 35 in: D. A. Christakis, L. Hale (eds.), Handbook of Children and Screens, https://doi.org/10.1007/978-3-031-69362-5_35**

On Chapter 35, incorrect affiliations for a few authors need to be updated and to be updated in Contributors page in Front matter as well.

"The original version of this chapter has been revised."

The authors' affiliations in Chapter 35 need to be corrected.

The incorrect affiliations are as follows:

Srivi Ramasubramanian should be Syracuse University (she was noted as Penn State U, which was Tanner Vea's affiliation).

Ashley Lee and Neta Kligler-Vilenchik's affiliations were switched.

When corrected, the affiliations would appear as:

Srivi Ramasubramanian, Syracuse University, Syracuse, NY, USA

Ashley Lee, Harvard University, Cambridge, MA, USA

Neta Kligler-Vilenchik, Hebrew University of Jerusalem, Jerusalem, Israel

Tanner Vea, University of Washington, Seattle, WA, USA

Please note that as we crosschecked the front matter against the chapters, these errors are present and should be corrected in the List of Contributors as well.

---

The updated version of this chapter can be found at
https://doi.org/10.1007/978-3-031-69362-5_35


D. A. Christakis, L. Hale (eds.), *Handbook of Children and Screens*,
https://doi.org/10.1007/978-3-031-69362-5_88

# Index




D. A. Christakis, L. Hale (eds.), *Handbook of Children and Screens*,
https://doi.org/10.1007/978-3-031-69362-5

**D**

## S

## T



## V



## W



## Y

The manufacturer's authorised representative in the EU is Springer Nature Customer Service Centre GmbH, Europaplatz 3, 69115 Heidelberg, Germany. If you have any concerns regarding our products, please contact ProductSafety@springernature.com

Printed and bound by CPI Group (UK) Ltd, Croydon, CR0 4YY
30/09/2026
02225600-0020